REVIEW OF WIC FOOD PACKAGES

Improving Balance and Choice

Final Report

Committee to Review WIC Food Packages

Food and Nutrition Board

Health and Medicine Division

A Report of

The National Academies of

SCIENCES · ENGINEERING · MEDICINE

THE NATIONAL ACADEMIES PRESS

Washington, DC

www.nap.edu

THE NATIONAL ACADEMIES PRESS 500 Fifth Street, NW Washington, DC 20001

This activity was supported by Grant No. AG-3198-D-14-0050_0001-005 from the U.S. Department of Agriculture. Any opinions, findings, conclusions, or recommendations expressed in this publication do not necessarily reflect the views of any organization or agency that provided support for the project.

International Standard Book Number-13: 978-0-309-45016-4
International Standard Book Number-10: 0-309-45016-0
Digital Object Identifier: https://doi.org/10.17226/23655

Additional copies of this publication are available for sale from the National Academies Press, 500 Fifth Street, NW, Keck 360, Washington, DC 20001; (800) 624-6242 or (202) 334-3313; http://www.nap.edu.

Printed in the United States of America

Suggested citation: National Academies of Sciences, Engineering, and Medicine. 2017. *Review of WIC food packages: Improving balance and choice: Final report*. Washington, DC: The National Academies Press. doi: https://doi.org/10.17226/23655.

The National Academies of

SCIENCES • ENGINEERING • MEDICINE

The **National Academy of Sciences** was established in 1863 by an act of Congress, signed by President Lincoln, as a private, nongovernmental institution to advise the nation on issues related to science and technology. Members are elected by their peers for outstanding contributions to research. Dr. Marcia McNutt is president.

The **National Academy of Engineering** was established in 1964 under the charter of the National Academy of Sciences to bring the practices of engineering to advising the nation. Members are elected by their peers for extraordinary contributions to engineering. Dr. C. D. Mote, Jr., is president.

The **National Academy of Medicine** (formerly the Institute of Medicine) was established in 1970 under the charter of the National Academy of Sciences to advise the nation on medical and health issues. Members are elected by their peers for distinguished contributions to medicine and health. Dr. Victor J. Dzau is president.

The three Academies work together as the **National Academies of Sciences, Engineering, and Medicine** to provide independent, objective analysis and advice to the nation and conduct other activities to solve complex problems and inform public policy decisions. The National Academies also encourage education and research, recognize outstanding contributions to knowledge, and increase public understanding in matters of science, engineering, and medicine.

Learn more about the National Academies of Sciences, Engineering, and Medicine at **www.national-academies.org**.

The National Academies of
SCIENCES • ENGINEERING • MEDICINE

Reports document the evidence-based consensus of an authoring committee of experts. Reports typically include findings, conclusions, and recommendations based on information gathered by the committee and committee deliberations. Reports are peer reviewed and are approved by the National Academies of Sciences, Engineering, and Medicine.

Proceedings chronicle the presentations and discussions at a workshop, symposium, or other convening event. The statements and opinions contained in proceedings are those of the participants and have not been endorsed by other participants, the planning committee, or the National Academies of Sciences, Engineering, and Medicine.

For information about other products and activities of the National Academies, please visit nationalacademies.org/whatwedo.

COMMITTEE TO REVIEW WIC FOOD PACKAGES

KATHLEEN M. RASMUSSEN (*Chair*), Nancy Schlegel Meinig Professor of Maternal and Child Nutrition, Division of Nutritional Sciences, Cornell University

SHANNON E. WHALEY (*Vice Chair*), Director of Research and Evaluation, Public Health Foundation Enterprises WIC Program

SUSAN S. BAKER, Professor and Co-Chief, Digestive Diseases and Nutrition Center, Department of Pediatrics, Women and Children's Hospital of Buffalo

MARIANNE P. BITLER, Professor, Department of Economics, University of California, Davis

PATSY M. BRANNON, Professor, Division of Nutritional Sciences, Cornell University

ALICIA L. CARRIQUIRY, Distinguished Professor, Department of Statistics, Iowa State University

DAVID E. DAVIS, Professor, Department of Economics, South Dakota State University

MARY KAY FOX, Senior Fellow, Mathematica Policy Research, Inc.

TAMERA J. HATFIELD, Associate Professor, Obstetrics and Gynecology, Division of Maternal and Fetal Medicine, University of California, Irvine

HELEN H. JENSEN, Professor of Economics and Head, Food and Nutrition Policy Research of the Center for Agricultural and Rural Development, Iowa State University

RACHEL K. JOHNSON, Robert L. Bickford, Jr., Green and Gold Professor of Nutrition, Professor of Medicine, University of Vermont

ANGELA ODOMS-YOUNG, Associate Professor, Department of Kinesiology and Nutrition, University of Illinois at Chicago

RAFAEL PÉREZ-ESCAMILLA, Professor of Epidemiology and Public Health, Director, Office of Public Health Practice, Director, Global Health Concentration, Yale School of Public Health

A. CATHARINE ROSS, Professor of Nutrition, Dorothy Foehr Huck Chair, Department of Nutritional Sciences, Pennsylvania State University

CHARLENE RUSSELL-TUCKER, Chief Operating Officer, Connecticut Department of Education

Consultants

MEI CHUNG, Assistant Professor, Department of Public Health and Community Medicine, School of Medicine, Tufts University
ROSE GLADSTEIN, Consultant, R Gladstein Consulting LLC
HOECHEL JEON, Post-doctoral Research Associate, Center for Agricultural and Rural Development, Iowa State University
JOHN A. KIRLIN, Economist, U.S. Department of Agriculture, Economic Research Service
DAVID LEVIN, Economist, U.S. Department of Agriculture, Economic Research Service
SUZANNE P. MURPHY, Researcher (Professor) Emeritus, University of Hawaii Cancer Center
MIYOUNG OH, Post-doctoral Research Associate, Center for Agricultural and Rural Development, Iowa State University

Health and Medicine Division Staff

MARIE E. LATULIPPE, Study Director
MEGHAN E. QUIRK, Program Officer
BERNICE CHU, Research Associate
ALICE VOROSMARTI, Research Associate
AMBAR SAEED, Senior Program Assistant
ANN L. YAKTINE, Director, Food and Nutrition Board

Reviewers

This report has been reviewed in draft form by individuals chosen for their diverse perspectives and technical expertise. The purpose of this independent review is to provide candid and critical comments that will assist the institution in making its published report as sound as possible and to ensure that the report meets institutional standards for objectivity, evidence, and responsiveness to the study charge. The review comments and draft manuscript remain confidential to protect the integrity of the deliberative process. We wish to thank the following individuals for their review of this report:

LOREN BELL, Altarum Institute
RONETTE BRIEFEL, Mathematica Policy Research
JULIE A. CASWELL, University of Massachusetts at Amherst
SUSAN J. CROCKETT, University of Minnesota
STEPHEN R. DANIELS, University of Colorado School of Medicine
WILLIAM DIETZ, George Washington University
LUCIA KAISER, University of California, Davis
JACOB A. KLERMAN, Abt Associates, Inc.
BARBARA PETERSEN, Exponent
KAREN E. PETERSON, University of Michigan
LORRENE RITCHIE, University of California Division of Agriculture and Natural Resources
JUDITH S. STERN, University of California, Davis
JANET AUSTIN TOOZE, Wake Forest Baptist Medical Center

KENNETH W. WACHTER, University of California, Berkeley
JAMES P. ZILIAK, University of Kentucky

Although the reviewers listed above have provided many constructive comments and suggestions, they were not asked to endorse the conclusions or recommendations nor did they see the final draft of the report before its release. The review of this report was overseen by **Diane F. Birt,** Iowa State University, and **Elaine L. Larson,** Columbia University Mailman School of Public Health. They were responsible for making certain that an independent examination of this report was carried out in accordance with institutional procedures and that all review comments were carefully considered. Responsibility for the final content of this report rests entirely with the authoring committee and the institution.

Contents

Preface

The Special Supplemental Nutrition Program for Women, Infants, and Children (WIC) began 40 years ago as a pilot program and has since grown to serve more than 8 million pregnant women, and mothers and their infants and young children. Today the program serves more than a quarter of the pregnant women and half of the infants in the United States, at an annual cost of about \$6.2 billion. Through its contribution to the nutritional needs of pregnant, breastfeeding, and postpartum women; infants; and children under 5 years of age, this federally supported nutrition assistance program is integral to meeting national nutrition policy goals for a significant portion of the U.S. population.

To assure the continued success of WIC, Congress mandated that the Food and Nutrition Service of the U.S. Department of Agriculture (USDA) reevaluate the program's food packages every 10 years to assure they remain aligned with the goals of the *Dietary Guidelines for Americans* (DGA). In 2014, USDA asked the Institute of Medicine (IOM) to undertake this reevaluation. This complex task included consideration of whether or not WIC participants should be permitted to purchase white potatoes with the cash value voucher (CVV), a part of the benefit package that provides access to vegetables and fruits. In its first of three reports, published early in 2015, the committee recommended that white potatoes be allowed as a WIC-eligible vegetable for purchase with the CVV. The second report of this series, published in 2016, provided a summary of the work of phase I of the study as well as the analytical underpinnings for phase II. This is the third and final report in this series. It provides further data analyses, a regulatory impact analysis, and the committee's final recommendations.

The revised food packages were constrained to be cost neutral with the current food packages, which means that any increases in the costs of components of the packages or allowed substitutions had to be balanced by corresponding decreases in costs elsewhere. This required the committee to be creative in responding to its charge to align the packages with the DGA. When making these revisions, the committee considered the supplemental nature of the WIC program and used a systematic approach. The committee was able to make changes to the packages that improve their alignment with the DGA and, thus, the dietary balance of the packages. The committee was able to improve the number of substitution options included in the packages and, thus, the choices available to participants to meet their cultural and personal preferences. The revised packages increase the cash value voucher for all participants, although the amounts differ by food package, and include fish in nearly all food packages. In addition, the committee provided enhanced support for breastfeeding, both exclusive and partial breastfeeding, along with greater flexibility for breastfeeding in the first 30 days after delivery.

This report is the first review of the WIC food packages to contain a regulatory impact analysis. This may permit USDA to move more rapidly to implement the changes proposed. These changes build on administrative actions taken in response to the IOM's 2006 *Time for a Change* report for further ease of implementation. It is noteworthy that the regulatory impact analysis not only shows that the revisions to the food packages should be cost neutral when implemented but also that they are projected to provide substantial cost savings over time, savings that could be used to make further nutritional improvements to the food packages.

The work of the committee was greatly enhanced by the contributions of many individuals who participated in the study's public activities. The committee is grateful to the speakers in its data-gathering workshops who gave valuable insights as well as their time to assist the committee with its task. The committee also thanks the members of the public who provided comments in open sessions or through the committee's website. Lastly, the committee is indebted to the many WIC staff members who gave their time and expertise to help committee members better understand administration of and participation in the WIC program.

The size of this report is testimony to the magnitude of the committee's task. It exists thanks to the hard work of many individuals. Committee members volunteered many hours of their time to this work. Their collaborative spirit as well as careful thinking and writing are to be commended. The committee was supported in its work by several consultants. Suzanne Murphy provided critical insights based on her experience in leading the committee that produced the first major reevaluation of the WIC food packages, published in 2006. Her sage advice is much appreciated. Mei Chung led the development and execution of all of the committee's literature reviews. Rose Gladstein assisted with the regulatory impact analysis.

The committee would like to thank the staff of the Center for Agricultural and Rural Development (CARD) and the Department of Statistics at Iowa State University for their analysis of the data from the National Health and Nutrition Examination Survey (NHANES) and National Household Food Acquisition and Purchase Survey. Committee members Helen Jensen and Alicia Carriquiry guided the CARD's work, which was carried out by David Osthus, Miyoung Oh, and Hocheol Jeon. John A. Kirlin and David Levin of USDA's Economic Research Service reviewed the committee's application of the FoodAPS and IRI datasets to the study, and Kevin Dodd and Susan Krebs-Smith of the National Cancer Institute provided helpful guidance on analyses of NHANES.

To accomplish this task numerous staff members at the National Academies of Sciences, Engineering, and Medicine supported the work of the committee. Marie Latulippe served as the project's study director and provided leadership, creative ideas, and an optimistic and calm spirit against tight deadlines. She was assisted by Meghan Quirk after March 2015, who led the regulatory impact analysis. Bernice Chu assisted with literature reviews and data management, and Ambar Saeed dealt with administrative logistics. Leslie Pray assisted with report organization and editing, and Rebecca Morgan of the National Academies Library/Research Center with fact checking. Alice Vorosmarti assisted with literature reviews and other data-oriented tasks. Naisi Zhao assisted the committee from January to April 2016 as a Mirzayan Fellow. Ann Yaktine, director of the Food and Nutrition Board, supervised the work of the staff and provided useful insights at many points in the committee's deliberation. The committee owes them all a debt of gratitude for their hard work and professionalism.

Kathleen M. Rasmussen, *Chair*
Committee to Review WIC Food Packages

Summary

THE SPECIAL SUPPLEMENTAL NUTRITION PROGRAM FOR WOMEN, INFANTS, AND CHILDREN

Among the nutrition assistance programs available to low-income families, the Special Supplemental Nutrition Program for Women, Infants, and Children (WIC) is the only one that specifically targets the nutritional needs of pregnant, breastfeeding, and postpartum women; infants; and children less than 5 years of age. WIC also includes nutritional assessment, nutrition education, breastfeeding support and referrals to health and social services, in addition to a prescribed food package. WIC participation has grown from 88,000 individuals served in 1974 to approximately 8 million women, infants, and children served in 2015 with services provided through 1,900 local agencies operating in 10,000 clinic sites across the United States and its territories.

The program's goals have evolved to include promoting and supporting breastfeeding by providing the breastfeeding mother with benefits for up to 1 year; providing WIC participants with a wider variety of foods, including vegetables, fruits, and whole grains; and providing WIC state agencies greater flexibility in prescribing food packages to accommodate the food preferences of WIC participants. WIC, like some other nutrition assistance programs, has been aligned with the *Dietary Guidelines for Americans* (DGA). Additionally, the program goals align with two major *Healthy People 2020* goals and nearly 30 health objectives, specifically those related to birth weight, childhood and adult weight, and breastfeeding prevalence. Congress has now mandated that an evaluation of the WIC food packages occur every 10 years.

WIC Food Package Changes

The WIC food packages remained relatively unchanged until the U.S. Department of Agriculture's Food and Nutrition Service (USDA-FNS) asked the Institute of Medicine (IOM) to convene an expert committee to review and update the food packages in 2004. That committee's report recommended wide-ranging revisions to the WIC food packages. Following issuance of the "Interim Rule" in 2007, the majority of the IOM report's recommendations were implemented. These updates included providing whole wheat bread, several additional grain options, a cash value voucher (CVV) to purchase vegetables and fruits, a reduction in the amount of juice, eggs, milk, and formula, and the removal of whole milk for all participants except 1-year-old children.

Most local WIC agencies, vendors, and manufacturers adopted the food package revisions successfully. The variety of dairy and grain products in the marketplace and the availability of WIC-approved foods have improved since 2009. The increased flexibility offered to program participants was important for meeting their needs and preferences. For many participants, however, some foods (e.g., fluid milk, ready-to-eat cereals) may not align with personal or cultural preferences, leading to reduced redemption and consumption.

The Committee's Task

In response to the congressional mandate, in 2014, USDA-FNS asked the National Academies of Sciences, Engineering, and Medicine to convene an expert committee to review and assess the nutritional status and food and nutritional needs of the WIC-eligible population and provide specific scientifically-based recommendations based on its review and grounded in the most recently available science. In addition, the committee was charged to ensure that recommendations for revising the WIC food packages are consistent with the DGA and address the health and cultural needs of the WIC participant population. Finally, the committee's recommendations should operate efficiently and be effectively administered across the geographic scope of the program. The complete task is described in Chapter 1.

The committee has produced three reports. In *An Evaluation of White Potatoes in the Cash Value Voucher: Letter Report*, it recommended that white potatoes be allowed for purchase with the cash value voucher (CVV). In *Review of WIC Food Packages: Proposed Framework for Revisions*, the committee presented the evidence, analyses, and framework to be applied to develop the committee's recommendations. In this third report, the committee provides its final analyses, recommendations, and the supporting rationale.

The Committee's Process

To address its task, the committee formulated a strategy that included an ongoing comprehensive review of the published literature and other available evidence, consideration of information from public workshops and public comments, analyses of relevant data, and deliberation on topics related to its charge. This committee also benefitted from newly available data on redemption of WIC foods.

The committee designed a systematic and transparent process for identifying actions that could prompt consideration of a revision in the food packages, which included use of a decision tree to establish "priority nutrients" and "priority food groups" and to identify appropriate changes in the food packages (see Chapter 5, Figure 5-1). It also developed a set of criteria for inclusion of foods in the food packages (see Box S-1) and a framework to guide the decision-making process that included nutritional and cost trade-offs (see Figure S-1). Noteworthy among these criteria is the concept that the packages should provide a balanced supplement to participants' diets. Guided by information gathered, the committee used an iterative process to identify potential food package changes. The committee then compared the impact of potential changes against the criteria, within the constraints of the cost-neutral requirement, to develop its

BOX S-1

Criteria for Inclusion of Foods in the WIC Food Packages

1. The packages provide a balanced supplement to the diets of women and children.
2. The packages contribute to reduction of the prevalence of inadequate nutrient intakes and of excessive nutrient intakes.
3. The packages contribute to an overall dietary pattern that is consistent with the *Dietary Guidelines for Americans* for individuals 2 years of age and older.
4. The packages contribute to an overall diet that is consistent with established dietary recommendations for infants and children less than 2 years of age, including encouragement of and support for breastfeeding.
5. The foods in the packages are available in forms and amounts suitable for low-income persons who may have limited transportation options, storage, and cooking facilities.
6. The foods in the packages are readily acceptable, commonly consumed, are widely available, take into account cultural eating patterns and food preferences, and provide incentives for families to participate in the WIC program.
7. The foods in the packages do not create an undue burden on state agencies or vendors.

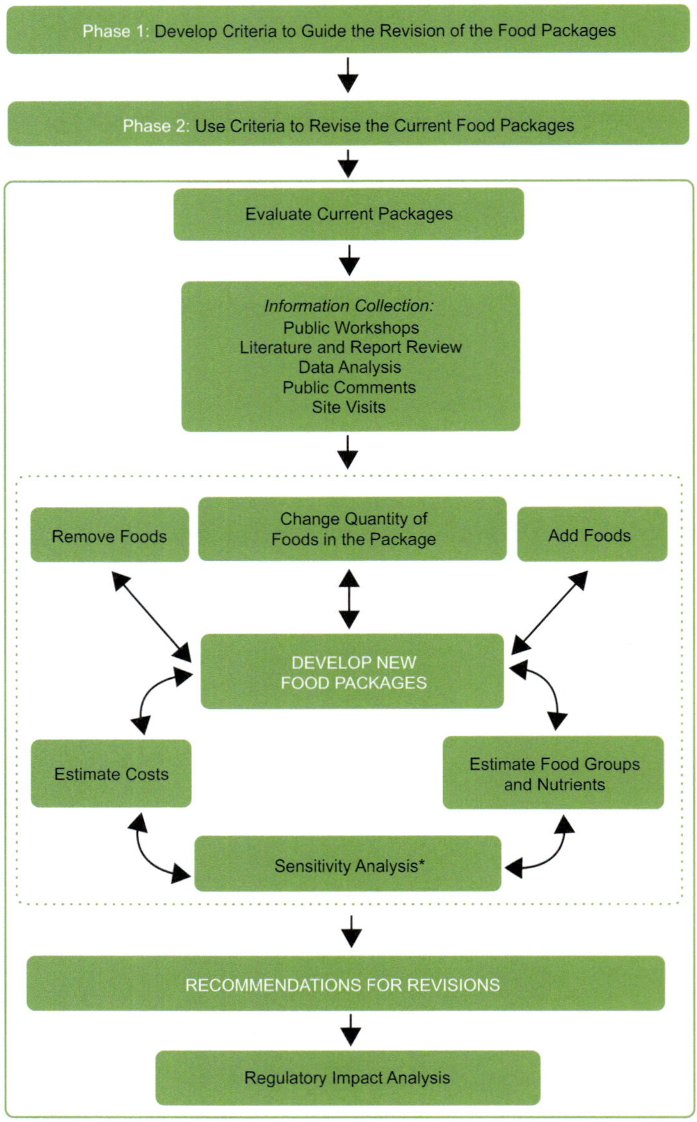

FIGURE S-1 Process for revising the WIC food packages.
NOTES: The dotted line indicates components of the process that iterate until the criteria for food package revisions are met (see criteria 1 through 6 presented above).

* The sensitivity analysis tests the assumptions applied to develop the cost-neutral revised food packages. A description of the sensitivity analysis is provided in Chapter 8.

recommendations. A sensitivity analysis (see Chapter 8) was conducted to test the committee's assumptions and a regulatory impact analysis (see Chapter 10) was conducted to assess the projected impact of the recommended food packages changes on program participation, the value of the food packages as selected, and program costs and administration.

The committee's analysis of data from the National Health and Nutrition Examination Survey (NHANES 2005–2012) was used to identify nutrients consumed in inadequate or excessive amounts and food groups consumed in less- or more-than-recommended amounts and to set nutrient and food group priorities.

The committee found that the current food packages provide 100 percent or more of the recommended intake of several nutrients and food groups. The committee considered these more-than-supplemental amounts (i.e., they provided more than a moderate proportion of an individual's requirement or recommended intake) and reduced them to be able to address other nutritional priorities. As a result of the diversity of nutrients that can be provided through the CVV, and participants' preference for this option, the committee considered it useful to increase the CVV to improve vegetable and fruit intakes. In other situations, the committee considered that an alternative form of food could be useful to promote intake of foods already included in the packages. The committee considered fish as a possible addition to the food packages because low-mercury seafood is recommended in the DGA and seafood intakes are below recommended amounts.

Available data also indicated that the current strategy of allowing breastfeeding women only two options in the first month (no formula or one can of formula) did not change breastfeeding initiation, but it did affect duration. While issuance of the partial breastfeeding package declined, there was an increased issuance of the fully formula-feeding package, along with an increased issuance of the fully breastfeeding package.

Challenges with the Process

The committee faced challenges that affected its ability to assess the data, meet the criteria, or revise the packages consistent with the potential actions identified from the decision tree. Briefly, these challenges included

- Some of the sample sizes in the NHANES dataset for population subgroups of interest were very small, so the committee combined survey years to obtain adequate numbers of participants for analysis. The need to combine survey years precluded fulfilling USDA's request for a pre-post 2009 food package change comparison.
- For women coded as "breastfeeding" in NHANES, the duration and intensity of breastfeeding were unknown, thus partially

breastfeeding women could not be distinguished from exclusively breastfeeding women.

- Women coded as "pregnant" in NHANES were treated as a single group to increase the sample size, although this precluded full adjustment for their varying needs by trimester.
- There is no available analytical method to resolve differences in estimates of nutrient inadequacy derived from Dietary Reference Intakes (DRIs) (Estimated Average Requirement [EAR] and Adequate Intake [AI]) with estimates of under-consumption relative to the DGA food groups. The committee used both to identify possible targets for supplementation.
- The cost-neutral constraint precluded inclusion of several of the identified potential actions for food package changes.

THE REVISED FOOD PACKAGES

The proposed revisions to the food packages in this report are designed to contribute positively to dietary quality of WIC-participating women, infants, and children. Most aspects of the current food packages are unchanged in the proposed new packages. However, a few foods have been added or amounts increased to enhance the quality of the packages. To maintain cost neutrality, amounts of some foods, primarily those that were provided in excess of the DGA recommended amounts or those that were poorly redeemed, were decreased. Overall, the proposed packages provide better adherence to the DGA and further increase flexibility and choice.

Among the factors that the committee considered in making decisions were: the value of the food packages to the mother–infant dyad; the practical importance of the CVV and its value to participants; and participant preferences (both cultural and personal). Constraints to changing foods in the package relative to foods in the marketplace, the capacity of the vendors who provide foods to participants, and state-level administrative concerns were also considered. Final adjustments were made in an iterative fashion, weighing cost with all priorities and factors. Table S-1 presents the food packages for fully breastfeeding, partially breastfeeding, and formula-feeding mother–infant dyads. Table S-2 presents the food packages for children and for pregnant women.

Summary of Recommendations to Revised WIC Food Packages

In response to its task, the committee recommended revisions to the WIC food packages that align with the DGA and are more consistent with the nutrition standards of other nutrition assistance programs that serve children. The committee targeted three primary areas: amounts of foods, specifications for foods, and additional substitution options for foods. To improve balance among food groups, most foods that are currently provided in more-than-supplemental amounts are reduced (i.e., juice, dairy [milk], peanut butter, legumes, and infant foods). Foods that are currently provided in lower amounts or were consumed in amounts below that recommended (i.e., whole grains, vegetables, fruits, and seafood) are increased. Food specifications are adjusted to increase the provision of whole grains (all breakfast cereals must meet the whole grain-rich criteria, all bread must be 100 percent whole wheat) and reduce the contribution of added sugars from foods that can substitute for milk (i.e., yogurt, soy beverage). The food choices allowed in the 2009 food package revisions were retained, and additional choices were added (i.e., a substitution of CVV for jarred infant fruits or vegetables or juice, some fish in place of some jarred infant food meats, an additional quart of yogurt for milk, additional grain choices, and options for vegan participants, including soy-based cheese and yogurt substitute products). The committee anticipates no increase in the administrative burden of these changes because the recommended revisions build upon the 2009 food package updates.

The overarching recommendations for revising the WIC food packages are presented below. Details about specific revisions to amounts of foods allowed and specifications are provided in Chapter 6.

6-1. **The U.S. Department of Agriculture's Food and Nutrition Service (USDA-FNS) should increase the dollar amount of the cash value voucher, add fish, and reduce the amounts of juice, milk, legumes, and peanut butter in all food packages for women and children (IV, V-A, V-B, and VII), to improve the balance of food groups in alignment with the 2015–2020 *Dietary Guidelines for Americans*. These changes also apply to food package VI, except that the amounts of milk are unchanged and the amounts of legumes are increased.**

6-2. **USDA-FNS should support the cultural food preferences and special dietary needs of WIC participants by requiring states to offer additional options for the WIC food categories, including substitution of a CVV in place of juice, additional forms and varieties of vegetables and fruits, both canned and dried legumes, and a range of options and sizes for grains and yogurt. A substitution of legumes for peanut butter or for eggs should be allowed for individuals who have a peanut allergy, or that are following a vegan diet, respectively.**

TABLE S-1 The Revised WIC Food Packages: Maximum Monthly Allowances Presented as the Benefits to the Mother–Infant Dyad in Food Packages I, II, III, V-B, VI, and VII

	Fully Breastfeeding Dyad		Partially (Mostly) Breastfeeding Dyad		Formula-Feeding Dyad	
WIC Food Categories	Infants 0 to 5 Months (FP I or III)	Infants 6 to 11 Months (FP II or III)	Infants 0 to 5 Months (FP I or III)	Infants 6 to 11 Months (FP II or III)	Infants 0 to 5 Months (FP I or III)	Infants 6 to 11 Months (FP II or III)
For Infants						
Formula	—	—	0 to 3 months: up to 364 fl oz 4 to 5 months: up to 442 fl oz	Up to 312 fl oz	0 to 3 months: up to 806 fl oz 4 to 5 months: up to 884 fl oz	Up to 624 fl oz
Infant cereal	—	16 oz	—	8 oz	—	8 oz
Infant food vegetables and fruits	—	128 oz or 64 oz and $10 CVV or 0 oz and $20 CVV	—	128 oz or 64 oz and $10 CVV or 0 oz and $20 CVV	—	128 oz or 64 oz and $10 CVV or 0 oz and $20 CVV
Infant food meats	—	40 oz	—	—	—	—

For Women	Fully Breastfeeding Women (FP VII)	Partially (Mostly) Breastfeeding Women (FP V-B)	Postpartum Women (FP VI)	
Vegetables and fruits	$35 CVV	$25 CVV	$15 CVV	No foods are provided to women after 6 months postpartum
Legumes	2 lb every 3 months	2 lb every 3 months	2 lb every 3 months	
Juice	64 fl oz	64 fl oz	—	
Dairy (milk)	16 qt	16 qt	16 qt	
Breakfast cereal	36 oz	36 oz	36 oz	
Whole grains	16 to 24 oz	16 to 24 oz	—	
Peanut butter	16 to 18 oz every 3 months	16 to 18 oz every 3 months	16 to 18 oz every 3 months	
Eggs	2 dozen	1 dozen	1 dozen	
Fish	60 oz every 3 months	30 oz every 3 months	10 oz every 3 months	

NOTES: — = the WIC food category is not authorized in the corresponding food package; CVV = cash value voucher; FP = food package. See Table 6-1 for additional details and all substitution options. See Table 6-4 for details related to WIC food specifications.

TABLE S-2 The Revised WIC Food Packages: Maximum Monthly Allowances Presented as the Benefits to Children and Pregnant Women in Food Packages IV, V-A, and III

WIC Food Category	Children 1 to Less Than 2 Years (FP IV-A)	Children 2 to Less Than 5 Years (FP IV-B)	Pregnant Women (FP V-A)	Special Dietary Needs (FP III)
WIC formula	—	—	—	Up to 455 fl oz of liquid concentrate, if appropriate
Vegetables and fruits	$12.00 CVV	$12.00 CVV	$15.00 CVV	Other foods in food packages IV and V-A are provided as appropriate
Legumes	1 lb every 3 months	1 lb every 3 months	2 lb every 3 months	
Juice	64 fl oz	64 fl oz	64 fl oz	
Dairy (milk)	12 qt	14 qt	16 qt	
Breakfast cereal	36 oz	36 oz	36 oz	
Whole grains	16–24 oz	16–24 oz	16–24 oz	
Peanut butter	16–18 oz every 3 months	16–18 oz every 3 months	16–18 oz every 3 months	
Eggs	1 dozen	1 dozen	1 dozen	
Fish	10 oz every 3 months	10 oz every 3 months	10 oz every 3 months	

NOTES: — = the food is not authorized in the corresponding food package; CVV = cash value voucher; FP = food package. See Table 6-2 for additional details and all substitution options. See Table 6-4 for details related to WIC food specifications.

6-3. USDA-FNS, as a means of supporting breastfeeding of any duration and intensity, should allow individual tailoring of the infant food packages to best meet the needs of the mother–infant dyad.

6-4. USDA-FNS should reduce the amounts of infant cereal across food package II for all infants, and reduce the amounts of jarred infant food vegetables and fruits and jarred infant food meats provided in food package II for fully breastfed infants. Caregivers should be permitted to substitute all or part of the jarred infant food vegetables and fruits with a cash value voucher, and a portion of jarred infant food meat with canned fish.

6-5. USDA-FNS should no longer require provision of a WIC formula to all participants that are issued food package III. Participants should be permitted access to the foods in the package appropriate for their age, physiological state, and medical condition. The health care provider may refer to the WIC registered dietitian and/or qualified nutritionist for identifying appropriate foods (excluding WIC formula) and their prescribed amounts as well as the length of time the participant requires the foods.

6-6. USDA-FNS should issue food package V-B to women who are pregnant with multiple fetuses and food package VII to women who are partially breastfeeding multiple infants.

6-7. USDA-FNS should modify required specifications for some WIC foods to improve their alignment with dietary guidance.

COST EVALUATION OF THE REVISED FOOD PACKAGES

The committee generated nutrient and cost profiles for the current and revised food packages using detailed assumptions about participation, food choices, food prices, and redemption rates. The weighted average, per-participant cost of the revised set of food packages is $37.32, 5 cents more than the cost of the current set of food packages (see Chapter 7, Table 7-2). The revised food packages therefore meet the task requirement for cost-neutrality (see Chapter 7).

The committee considered the financial value of the food packages to the mother–infant dyads (fully formula-feeding, partially breastfeeding, and fully breastfeeding) to evaluate how the packages support them and the perceived value of the packages to these dyads. As redeemed, the value of the revised food packages for breastfeeding dyads is higher than that of the current packages. The committee found it difficult, within cost-neutral constraints, to lower the value of the formula-feeding dyad packages without decreasing the amounts of infant formula required to provide close to 100 percent of infant needs in the first 6 months.

THE REVISED FOOD PACKAGES MEET SPECIFIED CRITERIA

The Revised Food Packages Provide Supplemental Amounts of Most Food Groups

To meet the criterion of providing a balanced supplement to participants' diets, the WIC packages were modified to reduce foods that provided more-than-supplemental amounts and increase foods needed to improve intakes of priority nutrients and food groups. The modifications accounted for participant preferences by evaluating available redemption data. For example, quantities of milk were reduced from providing 85 to 119 percent to 71 to 75 percent of recommended intakes. Juice was reduced and the CVV was increased correspondingly to shift the fruit consumption toward whole fruit, the preferred source of fruit in the DGA. In addition, the CVV was increased for all food packages to increase consumption of vegetables, which are poorly consumed, and fruit. Redemption of legumes and peanut butter is relatively low (approximately 50 percent), and the current food packages meet nearly 100 percent of the DGA recommended intake for several population subgroups, so amounts of legumes and peanut butter were reduced in several of the revised packages. Revisions to the whole grain requirement increase the ratio of whole-to-refined grains provided in the revised packages. Nearly all revised packages now provide some fish (although the amounts remain low).

The Revised Packages Provide at Least 50 Percent of the DRI of Most Priority Nutrients

Reductions in foods provided in more-than-supplemental amounts led to reductions in some nutrients in each food package. However, most nutrients prioritized by the committee are provided in amounts equivalent to at least 50 percent of the EAR or AI in the revised packages. However, potassium and fiber (higher priority across packages), choline (higher priority, pregnant women), vitamin D (lower priority, pregnant women), and copper (lower priority, postpartum women) are provided in amounts below 50 percent of the EAR or AI in the revised packages. The committee experienced the same limitations to meeting recommended amounts of all nutrients in a balanced diet as the DGAs did in developing their food patterns. The challenge was compounded by the committee's cost-neutrality constraint.

The Revised Packages Are More Consistent with Dietary Guidance

The revised food packages provide some of all DGA food groups, provide more whole than refined grains, and provide more whole fruit than fruit juice compared to the current packages. The amount of juice provided to children in the revised food packages is approximately 50 percent of the limit for juice that is recommended by the American Academy of Pediatrics. The amounts of "calories for other uses" (which include added sugars and saturated fat) were reduced across food packages. The specified limit for added sugars in yogurt was lowered but, nonetheless, the new yogurt option may increase added sugars. However, this is still in alignment with DGA guidance that some added sugars are appropriate in nutrient-dense foods to promote palatability. Sodium was reduced in all food packages.

The Revised Packages Enhance Options for Cultural Preferences and for Situations in Which Transportation, Storage, or Cooking Facilities Are Limited

The revised food packages include additional grain options suitable for various cultures (corn meal, corn masa flour, buckwheat, and teff), and allow additional yogurt, which may be more culturally suitable than fluid milk. The CVV offers the greatest degree of flexibility for meeting cultural needs and was increased in all food packages. The general increase in CVV as well as options to substitute additional amounts of CVV for juice or for jarred infant foods offers participants even more flexibility to meet their preferences. Volumes of foods difficult to transport have been reduced (e.g., milk, jarred infant foods) which lowers this burden. The requirement to provide canned legumes and a canned, frozen, or dried form of vegetable or fruit improves the suitability of the packages for various storage or cooking conditions.

The Revised Packages Consider WIC Agency and Vendor Burdens

Before changing the food specifications for yogurt and ready-to-eat cereal, the committee obtained information on market availability of these products to ensure vendors nationwide would be able to implement them. The revised food packages also consider that new food options are allowed in sizes commonly available to vendors and therefore accessible to participants.

RECOMMENDATIONS FOR IMPLEMENTATION AND RESEARCH

The committee was charged to outline recommendations for implementation of the revised food packages and research (including data collection) to support evaluation of the revised packages and the next 10-year review. These recommendations are outlined below, with the rationale supporting each provided in Chapter 11.

Recommendations for implementation are:

11-1. The U.S. Department of Agriculture's Food and Nutrition Service (USDA-FNS) should develop the tools and strategies needed to assist state agencies, local agencies, and vendors to inform participants about and support them to make the best use of the expanded options of the revised food packages.

11-2. USDA-FNS should maximize the extent to which the revised food packages motivate the choice to initiate and continue breastfeeding among all racial and ethnic groups by enhancing and stabilizing the funding available (independent of the food packages) for peer counseling and other lactation support staff in WIC sites.

To close the identified research gaps of highest priority, the committee recommends funding of research in the following areas:

11-3. USDA-FNS should fund research to evaluate the effects of the recommended revisions to the WIC food packages on participant satisfaction, participation in the program, redemption of WIC foods, and participants' diets and health.

11-3a. USDA-FNS should collect WIC state agency policies on an annual basis and establish a national database of electronic benefit transfer (EBT) expenditures by program participants.

11-3b. USDA-FNS and the Department of Health and Human Services should collaborate to achieve expansion of nationally representative collection of data on the dietary intakes for pregnant, breastfeeding, and postpartum women and breastfed infants in the National Health and Nutrition Examination Survey. USDA-FNS should request that the data on breastfeeding women include an indicator on the intensity of breastfeeding (i.e., exclusive or partial).

11-4. USDA-FNS should fund data collection and analysis of that data toward optimizing support for breastfeeding and increasing the proportion of WIC participants who choose to initiate and continue breastfeeding, and tailoring food package options to best meet the needs and goals of the breastfeeding dyad. USDA-FNS should examine how breastfeeding outcome data are captured in WIC Management Information Systems and work toward a set of universal breastfeeding indicators that can be captured across systems.

11-5. USDA-FNS should fund research to assess how inclusion of the cash value voucher as a component of WIC food packages affects: food package redemption rates, participant choice of vegetable and fruit varieties, overall diet quality, and vendor stocking practices.

11-6. USDA-FNS should fund research to evaluate the feasibility of adjusting the value of the cash value voucher in high-cost states and territories (Alaska, Guam, Hawaii, and the U.S. Virgin Islands).

USDA-FNS asked that the committee identify changes to the food packages that should be made if funding for the WIC food packages is 10 percent higher or is 10 percent lower than cost-neutrality. The following recommendations are offered in response:

11-7. The committee recommends that in the case that USDA-FNS has funding above cost-neutrality, the value of the CVV should be increased for all children on the program.

11-8. The committee recommends that in the case that USDA-FNS has funding below cost-neutrality, provision of juice should be further reduced or eliminated across food packages.

KEY MESSAGES FROM THE COMMITTEE FOR USDA AND FOR THE NEXT WIC REVIEW COMMITTEE

Although the committee completed its task, much work remains. Three major priorities emerged for future consideration: continued and improved support for breastfeeding, encouraging consumption of vegetables, and availability and use of WIC data.

Given the barriers to breastfeeding faced by low-income women, it is possible that WIC may be reaching nearly all those who are willing and able to breastfeed exclusively. To promote and encourage any breastfeeding, the committee maintained an enhanced food package for exclusively breastfeeding women. Moreover, it also enhanced the food package for partially breastfeeding women. This is essential for women who find exclusive breastfeeding incompatible with other constraints in their lives, but are nonetheless interested in and can be successful with partial breastfeeding. Reaching and supporting all breastfeeding women is a way for WIC to enhance its stated commitment to breastfeeding. This will require expansion and full coordination of the several WIC resources that promote and support breastfeeding, and the committee strongly encourages USDA-FNS to meet this challenge.

Although the committee was able to increase the amounts of the CVV, it remains a challenge to improve redemption of vegetables with it. This is because of WIC participants' preference for fruits. Those participants who received the largest increase in the CVV should be able to satisfy their preference for fruits and begin to purchase more vegetables. However, to increase vegetable redemption, the CVV may have to be substantially increased for all participants and accompanied by appropriate nutrition education and perhaps further incentives. In a cost-neutral environment, this may require reductions in the amount of other high-cost items, such as dairy products and infant formula, which are provided in amounts at the high end of supplemental in the revised packages.

The limited information available to this committee on redemption of WIC foods was crucial for understanding how participants use the program, but more such data (as well as many other kinds of data) were unavailable, so the committee provided recommendations to address these data needs for future decision making. It is essential that WIC identify ways to increase the availability of program data so that interested researchers can contribute their expertise to determine what aspects of the program work and how and also what aspects are cost-effective and scalable.

The committee's strategy for revisions includes several noteworthy innovations. These include the committee's development of the concept of supplemental as applied to the WIC food packages and its use as a criterion for the revision of the packages, use of data on redemption and the distribution of redemption to inform estimates of actual use of the food packages, and consideration of the dyadic nature of infant feeding related to the contents of the food packages. These innovations permitted the committee to make important revisions to the food packages within the constraint of cost neutrality. In particular, the committee was able to balance the food packages to increase the variety of foods included, increase participants' choices within food categories, and develop a comprehensive approach to the use of the packages to support breastfeeding of all intensities. To be fully effective, these revisions to the food package should be accompanied by the recommendations for implementation presented here. These revisions to the food packages are expected to improve both the attractiveness of the program to participants as well as its success in meeting the WIC program's goals to promote and support breastfeeding and to safeguard the health of low-income women, infants, and children through the provision of foods that provide key nutrients.

1

Introduction and the Process for Revising the WIC Food Packages

The Special Supplemental Nutrition Program for Women, Infants, and Children (WIC) was piloted by the U.S. Department of Agriculture's Food and Nutrition Service (USDA-FNS) in 1972 and enacted into legislation in 1975 (USDA/ERS, 2015). The WIC program is designed to provide specific foods with nutrients determined by nutritional research to be lacking in the diets of the WIC target population (7 C.F.R. § 246). The foods offered by WIC are referred to as the WIC food packages. The food package is comprised of a specific set of foods prescribed to each participant on a monthly basis. This and other terms referenced frequently in the report are defined in Box 1-1.

WIC program services are administered as a federal grant provided to the 50 states and the District of Columbia, Puerto Rico, Guam, American Samoa, the American Virgin Islands, the Northern Mariana Islands, and 34 Indian Tribal Organizations (ITOs) (USDA/FNS, 2015a). Services are administered through 90 state agencies which provide the food packages, breastfeeding support, nutrition education, and health and social service referrals to eligible individuals. Eligible individuals fulfill criteria related to age and physiological state, income, and nutritional risk, as summarized in Box 1-2.

In 2015, the WIC program served approximately 8 million women, infants, and children through 1,900 local agencies in 10,000 clinic sites (USDA/FNS, 2015a, 2016). Approximately 54 percent of infants and approximately 31 percent of children ages 1 to less than 5 years in the United States received WIC services in 2014 (USDA/FNS, 2016). WIC also served many mothers of the WIC-participating infants and children. WIC participants can receive benefits through vouchers to purchase the foods

BOX 1-1

Terms and Definitions

Cash value voucher (CVV): A monthly voucher in the WIC food packages (currently $11 for women and $8 for children) that allows for the purchase of a variety of vegetables and fruits.

Cost-neutral: Refers to condition that the weighted average per-participant cost of the revised set of food packages falls within 10 cents of the weighted average per-participant cost of the current set of food packages. Under this constraint, the effects of each food package on cost depend upon the number of participants represented by that package.

Electronic benefit transfer (EBT): An electronic system that allows a recipient to authorize transfer of their government benefits from a federal account to a retailer account to pay for products received.

Final rule: 7 C.F.R. § 246 in the *Federal Register* updated on March 4, 2014, to reflect revisions to the WIC food packages proposed in the 2006 IOM report, *WIC Food Packages, Time for a Change.*

Food package: A specific set of foods prescribed to each WIC participant on a monthly basis. There are currently seven food packages assigned by age and physiological state (pregnant; breastfeeding; or postpartum, non-breastfeeding). Participants are prescribed quantities of foods rather than dollar values with the exception of the cash value voucher.

Redemption (rate or data): Percentage of prescribed foods issued that are obtained by the participant at the WIC vendor.

WIC vendor: Authorized WIC retailer where participants may redeem WIC foods that are obtained using WIC benefits.

NOTE: See Appendix B for a comprehensive glossary.

specified in the package. Some states have migrated to an electronic benefit transfer (EBT) card to issue benefits, and all states are required to convert to EBT systems by 2020.

As with other federal nutrition assistance programs,[1] WIC is required to provide food and services in alignment with the *Dietary Guidelines*

[1] Other federal nutrition assistance programs include the Supplemental Nutrition Assistance Program, National School Lunch Program, National School Breakfast Program, Child and Adult Care Food Program, Summer Food Service Program, Fresh Fruit and Vegetable Program, and Special Milk Program, among others. WIC participants may also benefit from one or several of these programs. The committee was tasked with evaluation of the WIC food packages exclusively.

BOX 1-2

Life-Stage, Income, and Nutritional WIC Eligibility Criteria

Categorical eligibility: The individual is either a pregnant woman; a breastfeeding woman up to 1-year postpartum; a woman less than 6-months postpartum; an infant less than 12 months of age, or a child from 1 to less than 5 years of age.

Income eligibility: The individual is either living in a household with an income less than or equal to 185 percent of the federal poverty level or enrolled in the Temporary Assistance for Needy Families program, Supplemental Nutrition Assistance Program, or Medicaid program.

Nutritional risk: The individual has at least one of the nutritional risk factors approved by USDA-FNS as qualifying for WIC services.

for Americans (DGA) (U.S. Congress, P.L. 101-445, 1990;[2] USDA/HHS, 2016). Given that the DGA are revised every 5 years, review and update of nutrition assistance programs are needed at regular intervals. In 2006, the Institute of Medicine (IOM) proposed revisions to the program for the first time in its 35-year history (IOM, 2006). An evaluation of the food packages is now congressionally mandated to occur every 10 years (P.L. 101-147).[3] This report serves as the next required 10-year review (i.e., following the IOM report published in 2006). This introductory chapter provides an overview of the WIC services and food packages, as well as examining the committee's task and the process for determining what changes to the food packages might be appropriate.

OVERVIEW OF THE WIC PROGRAM

Program Goals

The mission of the WIC program has remained to safeguard the health of low-income women, infants, and children up to age 5 who are at nutritional risk by providing food, nutrition counseling, and access to health services (USDA/ERS, 2015). The program goals, however, have evolved since its introduction. Today they also include promoting and supporting breastfeeding by providing the breastfeeding mother with benefits for up to

[2] 101st Congress. 1990. Public law no. 101-445, National Nutrition Monitoring and Related Research Act of 1990.

[3] 101st Congress. 1989. Public law no. 101-147, Child Nutrition and WIC Reauthorization Act of 1989.

1 year; providing WIC participants with a wider variety of foods, including vegetables, fruits, and whole grains; and providing WIC state agencies greater flexibility in prescribing food packages to accommodate cultural eating patterns[4] of WIC participants (USDA/FNS, 2014). WIC supports the national health goals of *Healthy People 2020*, specifically those related to birth weight, childhood and adult weight, and breastfeeding prevalence (NWA, 2013; HHS, 2015).

The Role of Nutrition Education in WIC

Nutrition education is key in supporting WIC participants' choices to purchase healthy foods, prepare these foods in a healthful manner, and consume them as part of a diet aligned with the DGA. Indeed, WIC is the only federal supplemental nutrition assistance program to have a nutrition education component required by law (as specified in sections 17(b)(7), 17(f)(1)(C)(x), and 17(j) of the Child Nutrition Act of 1966, as amended, and the Federal WIC regulations in sections 246.2 and 246.11 [USDA/FNS, 2007]). Under these regulations, WIC nutrition education must be "available at no cost to participants; be easily understood by participants; bear a practical relationship to the participant's nutritional needs, household situation, and cultural preferences; and be designed to achieve the regulatory nutrition education goals" (USDA/FNS/NAL, 2006).

WIC state agencies have the responsibility to develop educational materials that fulfill these federal requirements (USDA/FNS/NAL, 2006). In addition, the food packages themselves provide foods that serve as a tool to meet the dietary goals of the DGA and around which education can be designed.

WIC Breastfeeding Promotion and Support Activities

WIC program activities intended to increase breastfeeding prevalence parallel the three categories of global strategies known to improve breastfeeding outcomes (protection, promotion, and support):

1. WIC breastfeeding *protection* activities include not providing infant formula during the first month after birth to mothers who have expressed their desire to breastfeed.[5]

[4] This is referenced in the Final Rule as "cultural food preferences."

[5] The Final Rule states: "The issuance of any formula to breastfed infants in the first month after birth is a State agency option. If a State agency chooses this option, it may issue one can of powder infant formula in the container size that provides closest to 104 reconstituted fluid ounces to partially breastfed infants on a case-by case basis. Breastfed infants who are provided this option are considered partially (mostly) breastfed" (USDA/FNS, 2014).

2. WIC breastfeeding *promotion* activities include providing enhanced WIC food packages for breastfeeding mothers compared to fully formula-feeding mothers; counseling on maternal–child health benefits of breastfeeding and of the food packages offered to breastfeeding mothers by WIC; and providing educational materials at WIC clinics.
3. WIC breastfeeding *support* activities include the WIC breastfeeding peer-counseling program, lactation management support offered by certified lactation consultants hired by the program (i.e., certified by the International Lactation Consultant Association), and the provision of breast pumps to women.[6]

WIC has been actively protecting, promoting, and supporting breastfeeding since 1989, when Congress enacted the first of a series of laws requiring WIC to develop standards to ensure adequate breastfeeding promotion and support at both state and local levels (USDA/FNS, 2013).[7] In 1992, Congress required that The U.S. Department of Agriculture (USDA) establish a national breastfeeding promotion program and provided various means by which this could be funded. Two years later, Congress passed the Healthy Meals for Healthy Americans Act, which requires that state WIC agencies spend $21 for each pregnant and breastfeeding woman in support of breastfeeding promotion.

Both WIC and non-WIC breastfeeding promotion and support activities appear to play a critical role in the improvement of breastfeeding initiation, duration, and exclusivity among WIC participants according to the committee's review of 15 interventional and 3 cross-sectional studies (see Anderson et al., 2005, 2007; Bonuck et al., 2005; Hayes et al., 2008; Meehan et al., 2008; Hopkinson and Konefal Gallagher, 2009; Petrova et al., 2009; Sandy et al., 2009; Bunik et al., 2010; Olson et al., 2010; Pugh et al., 2010; Kandiah, 2011; Whaley et al., 2012; Chapman et al., 2013; Haider et al., 2014; Hildebrand et al., 2014; Howell et al., 2014; Reeder et al., 2014; NASEM, 2016). This is in alignment with global

[6] Although these are common support activities, they are not available universally among WIC state agencies.

[7] Based on P.L. 101-147 (1989), states were required to conduct a yearly evaluation of their breastfeeding promotion and support activities, provide nutrition education and breastfeeding materials in languages other than English as appropriate; include in their state plan a plan to provide nutrition education and breastfeeding promotion and a plan to coordinate operations with local agency programs for breastfeeding promotion; and designate a breastfeeding coordinator to provide training on breastfeeding promotion and support to local agency staff responsible for breastfeeding. The annual evaluation of activities is no longer required.

strategies that have proven effective (Pérez-Escamilla and Chapman, 2012; Pérez-Escamilla et al., 2012).[8]

Additional details about the effects of breastfeeding promotion and support activities among WIC participants are provided in Chapter 2.

The Current WIC Food Packages

The WIC program provides seven types of food packages, as shown in Table 1-1. These packages (numbered I through VII) accommodate different physiological state categories of women, different ages of children, and different developmental stages of infants. In addition, food package III is issued to participants (women, infants, or children) with special medical needs as determined by a physician. The foods offered must meet minimum nutritional specifications, although additional nutritional standards are permitted at the state level. Participants are required to be issued a specific amount of foods in each category (the maximum monthly allowance [MMA]), with the exception of infant formula. Infants that are fully formula-fed may receive an amount of formula between the full nutrition benefit and the MMA. For all infants, the amount of formula should be tailored to meet the needs of the mother-infant dyad.

The revisions proposed by the IOM in 2006 resulted in dramatic changes to the nutrient density of foods in the food packages. For example, an upper limit was set for the amount of total sugars in yogurt, whole grains were required for bread and its substitution options, and the vegetable and fruit cash value voucher (CVV) was added as a new food instrument. These specifications and any modifications proposed by the committee are further reviewed in Chapter 6.

The changes were initially implemented in 2009 (USDA/FNS, 2007) and finalized in 2014 (USDA/FNS, 2014). Tables 1-2 and 1-3 present the composition (in maximum amounts) of the seven different WIC food packages, as defined in the March 2014 Final Rule (USDA/FNS, 2014). Most, but not all, of the IOM's (2006) recommendations were fully implemented; a few recommendations underwent modification before implementation or were not implemented (see Appendix C, Table C-1). Although most changes were implemented by fall of 2009 in accordance with the Interim Rule (USDA/FNS, 2007), implementation occurred over a period of 6 years (see

[8] Effective global strategies to improve breastfeeding outcomes include protection (e.g., enforcement of the WHO Code for the Marketing of Breastmilk Substitutes, labor legislation to support the needs of employed women), promotion (e.g., mass media campaigns, World Breastfeeding Week), and support activities (e.g., the Baby Friendly Hospital Initiative, breastfeeding peer counseling programs) (Pérez-Escamilla and Chapman, 2012; Pérez-Escamilla et al., 2012).

TABLE 1-1 Overview of the Current WIC Food Packages and Categorical Eligibility

Food Package Number	Individuals Eligible by Category*
I	Formula-fed, partially breastfed, or fully breastfed infants, ages 0 to less than 6 months
II	Formula-fed, partially breastfed, or fully breastfed infants, ages 6 to less than 12 months
III	Participants (women, infants, or children) with special medical needs as determined by a physician
IV	Children ages 1 to less than 5 years
V	Pregnant or partially breastfeeding women (up to 1 year)
VI	Postpartum, non-breastfeeding women (up to 6 months)
VII	Postpartum, fully breastfeeding women (up to 1 year)

* Individuals must also meet the income and nutritional risk requirements, as noted in Box 1-2.
SOURCE: USDA/FNS, 2014.

Appendix C, Table C-2). Additional details on the effects of these changes are provided in Chapter 2.

Substitutions Allowed Within the WIC Food Packages

An important change that has been implemented in the current WIC food packages is the ability to substitute foods within many of the food categories. These substitutions allow for more variety and more cultural sensitivity in foods provided by the packages. As noted in the Interim Rule, substitution for a food in the WIC food categories "must be nutritionally equivalent or superior to the food it is intended to replace" (USDA/FNS, 2007). The implication of this statement is that the nutrient content of substitutions for WIC foods should be similar, components (e.g., protein) should be of similar quality, and nutrients should be similarly bioavailable. Although allowed substitutions have been specified by USDA-FNS (2014), WIC state agencies are not required to implement all of them. Table 1-4 provides data on substitutions allowed by WIC state agencies, illustrating the variability in WIC-approved food lists among states.

TABLE 1-2 Full Nutrition Benefit and Maximum Monthly Allowances of Supplemental Foods for Infants in Food Packages I, II, and III

	Fully Formula Fed (FF)		Partially (Mostly) Breastfed (BF/FF)		Fully Breastfed (BF)	
Foods	FP I–FF & III–FF A: 0 through 3 months B: 4 through 5 months	FP II–FF & III–FF 6 through 11 months	FP I–BF/FF & III BF/FF A: 0 to 1 month[a,b] B: 1 through 3 months C: 4 through 5 months	FP II–BF/FF & III BF/FF 6 through 11 months	FP I–BF 0 through 5 months	FP II–BF 6 through 11 months
WIC formula[c,d,e,f]	A: FNB = 806 fl oz, MMA = 823 fl oz, reconstituted liquid concentrate or 832 fl oz RTF or 870 fl oz reconstituted powder B: FNB = 884 fl oz, MMA = 896 fl oz, reconstituted liquid concentrate or 913 fl oz RTF or 960 fl oz reconstituted powder	FNB = 624 fl oz, MMA = 630 fl oz, reconstituted liquid concentrate or 643 fl oz RTF or 696 fl oz reconstituted powder	A: 104 fl oz reconstituted powder B: FNB = 364 fl oz, MMA = 388 fl oz, reconstituted liquid concentrate or 384 fl oz RTF or 435 fl oz reconstituted powder C: FNB = 442 fl oz, MMA = 460 fl oz, reconstituted liquid concentrate or 474 fl oz RTF or 522 fl oz reconstituted powder	FNB = 312 fl oz, MMA = 315 fl oz, reconstituted liquid concentrate or 338 fl oz RTF or 384 fl oz reconstituted powder	—	—

Infant cereal	—	24 oz	—	24 oz	—	24 oz
Infant food vegetables and fruits	—	128 oz	—	128 oz	—	256 oz
Infant food meat	—	—	—	—	—	77.5 oz

NOTES: — = the food is not authorized in the corresponding food package; BF = fully breastfed; BF/FF = partially (mostly) breastfed; FF = fully formula fed; FNB = full nutrition benefit; FP = food package; MMA = maximum monthly allowance; RTF = ready-to-feed.

[a] State agencies have the option to issue not more than one can of powder infant formula in the container size that provides closest to 104 reconstituted fluid ounces to breastfed infants on a case-by-case basis.

[b] Liquid concentrate and ready-to-feed (RTF) may be substituted at rates that provide comparable nutritive value.

[c] *WIC formula* means infant formula, exempt infant formula, or WIC-eligible nutritionals. Infant formula may be issued for infants in food packages I, II and III. Medical documentation is required for issuance of infant formula, exempt infant formula, WIC-eligible nutritionals, and other supplemental foods in food package III. Only infant formula may be issued for infants in food packages I and II.

[d] The full nutrition benefit is defined as the minimum amount of reconstituted fluid ounces of liquid concentrate infant formula as specified for each infant food package category and feeding variation (e.g., food package IA—fully formula fed).

[e] The maximum monthly allowance is specified in reconstituted fluid ounces for liquid concentrate, RTF liquid, and powder forms of infant formula and exempt infant formula. Reconstituted fluid ounce is the form prepared for consumption as directed on the container.

[f] State agencies must provide at least the full nutritional benefit authorized to non-breastfed infants up to the maximum monthly allowance for the physical form of the product specified for each food package category. State agencies must issue whole containers that are all the same size of the same physical form. Infant formula amounts for breastfed infants, even those in the fully-formula fed category should be individually tailored to the amounts that meet their nutritional needs.

SOURCE: Modified from 7 C.F.R. § 246 (USDA/FNS, 2014).

TABLE 1-3 Maximum Monthly Allowances of Supplemental Foods for Children and Women in Food Packages IV, V, VI, and VII

	Children	Women		
Foods	FP IV: 1 through 4 years	FP V: Pregnant and Partially (Mostly) BF (up to 1 year PP)[a]	FP VI: Postpartum (up to 6 months PP)[b]	FP VII: Fully Breastfeeding (up to 1 year PP)[c,d]
Juice, single strength[e]	128 fl oz	144 fl oz	96 fl oz	144 fl oz
Milk, fluid	16 qt[f,g,h,i,j]	22 qt[f,g,h,i,k]	16 qt[f,g,h,i,k]	24 qt[f,g,h,i,k]
Breakfast cereal[l]	36 oz	36 oz	36 oz	36 oz
Cheese	—	—	—	1 lb
Eggs	1 dozen	1 dozen	1 dozen	2 dozen
Fresh vegetables and fruits[m,n]	$8.00 in CVV	$11.00 in CVV	$11.00 in CVV	$11.00 in CVV
Whole wheat or whole grain bread[o]	2 lb	1 lb	—	1 lb
Fish (canned)	—	—	—	30 oz
Legumes[p] and/or peanut butter	1 lb or 18 oz	1 lb and 18 oz	1 lb or 18 oz	1 lb and 18 oz

NOTES: — = the food is not authorized in the corresponding food package; BF = breastfeeding; CVV = cash value voucher; FP = food package; PP = postpartum.

[a] Food package V is issued to two categories of WIC participants: Women participants with singleton pregnancies; breastfeeding women whose partially (mostly) breastfed infants receive formula from the WIC program in amounts that do not exceed the maximum formula allowances, as appropriate for the age of the infant.

[b] Food package VI is issued to two categories of WIC participants: Nonbreastfeeding postpartum women and breastfeeding postpartum women whose infants receive more than the maximum infant formula allowances, as appropriate for the age of the infant.

[c] Food package VII is issued to four categories of WIC participants: Fully breastfeeding women whose infants do not receive formula from the WIC Program; women pregnant with two or more fetuses; women partially (mostly) breastfeeding multiple infants from the same pregnancy; and pregnant women who are also fully or partially (mostly) breastfeeding singleton infants.

[d] Women fully breastfeeding multiple infants from the same pregnancy are prescribed 1.5 times the maximum allowances.

[e] Combinations of single-strength and concentrated juices may be issued provided that the total volume does not exceed the maximum monthly allowance for single-strength juice.

[f] Whole milk is the standard milk for issuance to 1-year-old children (12 through 23 months). At state agency option, fat-reduced milks may be issued to 1-year-old children for whom overweight or obesity is a concern. The need for fat-reduced milks for 1-year-old children must be based on an individual nutritional assessment and consultation with the child's health care provider if necessary, as established by state agency policy. Low-fat (1%) or nonfat milks are the standard milk for issuance to children ≥24 months of age and women. Reduced fat (2%) milk is authorized only for participants with certain conditions, including but not limited to, underweight and maternal weight loss during pregnancy. The need for reduced fat (2%) milk for children ≥24 months of age (food package IV) and women (food packages V–VII) must be based on an individual nutritional assessment as established by state agency policy.

[g] Evaporated milk may be substituted at the rate of 16 fl oz of evaporated milk per 32 fl oz of fluid milk or a 1:2 fluid ounce substitution ratio. Dry milk may be substituted at an equal reconstituted rate to fluid milk.

[h] For children and women, cheese may be substituted for milk at the rate of 1 lb of cheese per 3 qt of milk. For children and women in food packages IV–VI, no more than 1 lb of cheese may be substituted. For fully breastfeeding women in food package VII, no more than 2 lb of cheese may be substituted for milk. State agencies do not have the option to issue additional amounts of cheese beyond these maximums even with medical documentation. (No more than a total of 4 qt of milk may be substituted for a combination of cheese, yogurt or tofu for children and women in food packages IV–VI. No more than a total of 6 qt of milk may be substituted for a combination of cheese, yogurt, or tofu for women in food package VII.)

[i] For children and women, yogurt may be substituted for fluid milk at the rate of 1 qt of yogurt per 1 quart of milk; a maximum of 1 qt of milk can be substituted. Additional amounts of yogurt are not authorized. Whole yogurt is the standard yogurt for issuance to 1-year-old children (12 through 23 months). At state agency option, low-fat or nonfat yogurt may be issued to 1-year-old children for whom overweight and obesity is a concern. The need for lowfat or nonfat yogurt for 1-year-old children must be based on an individual nutritional assessment and consultation with the child's health care provider if necessary, as established by state agency policy. Low-fat or nonfat yogurts are the only types of yogurt authorized for children ≥ 24 months of age and women. (No more than a total of 4 qt of milk may be substituted for a combination of cheese, yogurt, or tofu for children and women in food packages IV–VI. No more than a total of 6 qt of milk may be substituted for a combination of cheese, yogurt, or tofu for women in Food Package VII.)

[j] For children, issuance of tofu and soy-based beverage as substitutes for milk must be based on an individual nutritional assessment and consultation with the participant's health care provider if necessary, as established by state agency policy. Such determination can be made for situations that include, but are not limited to, milk allergy, lactose intolerance, and vegan diets. Soy-based beverage may be substituted for milk for children on a quart-for-quart basis up to the total maximum allowance of milk. Tofu may be substituted for milk for children at the rate of 1 lb of tofu per 1 quart of milk. (No more than a total of 4 qt of milk may be substituted for a combination of cheese, yogurt, or tofu for children in Food Package IV.) Additional amounts of tofu may be substituted, up to the maximum allowance for fluid milk for lactose intolerance or other reasons, as established by state agency policy.

continued

TABLE 1-3 Continued

[k] For women, soy-based beverage may be substituted for milk on a quart-for-quart basis up to the total maximum allowance of milk. Tofu may be substituted for milk at the rate of 1 lb of tofu per 1 qt of milk. (No more than a total of 4 qt of milk may be substituted for a combination of cheese, yogurt, or tofu for women in food packages V and VI. No more than a total of 6 quarts of milk may be substituted for a combination of cheese, yogurt, or tofu for women in food package VII.). Additional amounts of tofu may be substituted, up to the maximum allowances for fluid milk, for lactose intolerance or other reasons, as established by state agency policy.

[l] At least one-half of the total number of breakfast cereals on the state agency's authorized food list must have whole grain as the primary ingredient and meet labeling requirements for making a health claim as a "whole grain food with moderate fat content" as defined in the Final Rule.

[m] Both fresh fruits and fresh vegetables must be authorized by state agencies. Processed vegetables and fruits, meaning canned (shelf-stable), frozen, and/or dried vegetables and fruits may also be authorized to offer a wider variety and choice for participants. State agencies may choose to authorize one or more of the following processed vegetables and fruits: canned fruit, canned vegetables, frozen fruit, frozen vegetables, dried fruit, and/or dried vegetables. The cash-value voucher may be redeemed for any eligible vegetables and fruits. State agencies may not selectively choose which vegetables and fruits are available to participants. For example, if a state agency chooses to offer dried fruits, it must authorize all WIC-eligible dried fruits.

[n] The monthly value of the fruit/vegetable cash-value vouchers will be adjusted annually for inflation as described in § 246.16(j).

[o] Whole wheat and/or whole grain bread must be authorized. State agencies have the option to also authorize brown rice, bulgur, oatmeal, whole-grain barley, whole wheat macaroni products, or soft corn or whole wheat tortillas on an equal weight basis.

[p] Canned beans may be substituted for dry beans at the rate of 64 oz (e.g., four 16-oz cans) of canned beans for 1 lb dry beans. In food packages V and VII, both beans and peanut butter must be provided. However, when individually tailoring food packages V or VII for nutritional reasons (e.g., food allergy, underweight, participant preference), state agencies have the option to authorize the following substitutions: 1 lb dry and 64 oz canned beans/peas (and no peanut butter); or 2 lb dry or 128 oz canned beans/peas (and no peanut butter); or 36 oz peanut butter (and no beans).

SOURCE: Modified from 7 C.F.R. § 246 (USDA/FNS, 2014), updated with WIC Policy Memorandum #2015-3 and WIC Policy Memorandum #2015-4.

Introduction of the Cash Value Voucher

Implementation of the food packages in 2009 introduced not only new foods, but also the CVV,[9] a new type of benefit with a specific dollar value for purchasing vegetables and fruits. States are now required to allow "split tender," meaning participants may pay the difference out of pocket (or with benefits from the Supplemental Nutrition Assistance Program) if their vegetable and fruit purchase exceeds the amount on the CVV (USDA/FNS, 2014).

Overview of the WIC Shopping Process

At the time of this writing, 18 states had implemented the EBT system, and the remainder of states continue to use paper vouchers. With a paper voucher, a participant is required to purchase all WIC foods listed on a voucher in a single shopping trip.[10] In contrast, the EBT card allows participants to redeem any portion of the foods issued (for any participating family member) at any time during the month. In either case, the foods must be redeemed in the issued month. In the store, participants must find and choose the state-specific WIC authorized foods. Foods may be identified in a number of ways, for example, by use of a state-prepared food buying guide or by labels posted on the shelf. When using the CVV, participants must calculate the amount of vegetables and fruits that can be covered with $8 or $11 (any overage may be paid out-of-pocket).

When paper vouchers are used, the participant may be required to separate WIC foods from other foods at checkout (see CDPH, 2016). With the EBT system, separation is not typically necessary. For the WIC benefits to be accepted by the vendor, the vendor must have the Universal Product Code (UPC) properly entered into their check-out system.

THE COMMITTEE'S TASK

In response to a request from Congress, USDA-FNS charged the Health and Medicine Division (HMD) of the National Academies of Sciences, Engineering, and Medicine's[11] current Committee to Review the WIC Food Packages to conduct a two-phase evaluation of the WIC food packages and

---

[9] In states issuing electronic benefit transfer (EBT) cards, the cash value voucher (CVV) is referred to as a cash value benefit (CVB).

[10] In some states, specific food categories are issued on a separate check, such as infant formula and the CVV. Other foods are grouped together on one check. Foods like milk are typically issued across multiple vouchers so not all milk has to be purchased at one time.

[11] As of March 15, 2016, the Health and Medicine Division continues the consensus studies and convening activities previously undertaken by the Institute of Medicine.

TABLE 1-4 Substitutions Allowed by WIC State Agencies, Fiscal Year 2015

Authorized Forms	All WIC State Agencies: Number of Agencies	All WIC State Agencies: Percent of Agencies	Percent of WIC Participants Covered by This Option[a]
	Milk and milk substitutes		
Soy beverages	82	95	99.9
Tofu	54	63	72.7
Nonfat, 1%, and 2% milk[b]	61	71	69.1
Nonfat and 1% milk[b]	22	26	28.8
	Cheese		
Low sodium	22	26	48.3
Fat free	16	19	37.1
Low cholesterol	11	13	18.3
	Peanut butter		
Low sodium	25	29	45.3
Low sugar	17	20	34.4
Reduced fat	17	20	15.6
	Beans and peas[c]		
Canned beans	73	85	84.9
	Whole grains[d]		
Brown rice	83	97	99.8
Tortillas	77	90	99.6
Oats	66	77	85.9
Bulgur and/or barley	22	26	22.8
Whole wheat pasta	25	29	29.7
	Canned fish[e]		
Any tuna	86	100	100
Any salmon	80	93	97.7
Sardines	54	63	45.7
Any mackerel	20	23	6.9
	Forms of vegetables and fruits		
Frozen	70	81	85.5
Canned	51	59	63.4
Dried	5	6	16.5

TABLE 1-4 Continued

NOTES: Data are from the WIC Food Package Policy Options II study (USDA/FNS, 2015b); responses for the study were received from 86 of 90 state agencies, covering 99.98 percent of WIC participants.

[a] Percentages represent the number of WIC participants linked to the state agencies offering the option.

[b] The Final Rule established 1% and nonfat milk as standard issuance for women and children ages 2 and older (a change from the Interim Rule, which also included 2 percent milk as standard issuance). The final rule authorizes 2% milk, soy-based beverages, and tofu as substitutions for 1% and nonfat milk based on nutrition assessment and consultation with a healthc are provider if necessary. The Final Rule also permitted yogurt as a milk alternative for women and children. However, since this option was not implemented until after data collection for the study from which this table was derived was completed, data on number of state agencies authorizing yogurt are not documented here.

[c] The Final Rule permits any type of mature dry beans, peas, or lentils in dry or canned forms. All WIC state agencies authorize some form of dry beans and peas; 81 percent of state agencies authorize all varieties of dry beans and peas.

[d] WIC state agencies are required to offer whole wheat or whole-grain bread. They also have the option to offer whole-grain alternatives.

[e] WIC state agencies are required to offer at least two types of canned fish.

SOURCES: USDA/FNS, 2014a, 2015b.

develop recommendations for revising the packages to be consistent with the *Dietary Guidelines for Americans* (DGA) (USDA/HHS, 2016). The committee was also charged to consider the health and cultural needs of a diverse WIC-participating population while ensuring the program remains cost-neutral, efficient for nationwide distribution, and straightforward to administer in national, state, and local agencies. The statement of task for this study is presented in Box 1-3. In addition to this, the committee was asked to develop a prioritized set of recommendations for implementation research focusing on data collection, analyses, and other methodological approaches to documenting the impact of the recommended changes to the WIC food packages on anticipated outcomes.

This report is the final of three reports fulfilling the USDA-FNS request. The first report in the series, *An Evaluation of White Potatoes in the Cash Value Voucher: Letter Report* (IOM, 2015), assessed the impact on food and nutrient intakes of the WIC-participating population of the 2009 regulation to allow the purchase of vegetables and fruits, excluding white potatoes, with a CVV and recommended that white potatoes be allowed as a WIC-eligible vegetable. The second (interim) report, *Proposed Framework for Revisions: Interim Report* (NASEM, 2016), included a comprehensive review of evidence to support the development of recommendations. This, the final report, includes any relevant updates to the interim report as well as the final recommendations for changes to the WIC food packages. The

BOX 1-3

Statement of Task

An ad hoc committee will undertake a two-phase comprehensive examination of the U.S. Department of Agriculture's Special Supplemental Nutrition Program for Women, Infants, and Children (WIC) food packages (i.e., the foods provided to supplement the diet of participants, tailored to their age and health status). The committee will first review and assess the nutritional status and food and nutritional needs of the WIC-eligible population and the impact of the 2009 regulation, finalized in 2014, to exclude white potatoes from WIC food packages against key recommendations of the 2010 *Dietary Guidelines for Americans*, on nutrient intake and indicators of diet quality; and changes in nutrient and food intake values and indices of diet quality if fresh white potatoes are included in the WIC benefit.

The committee will then review and assess the WIC food packages and make specific evidence-based recommendations, based on its evidence review and grounded in the most recently available science. Recommendations for changes to the WIC food packages will build on the revisions recommended in the 2006 IOM report *WIC Food Packages: Time for a Change* and implemented in 2009. Recommended revisions to WIC food packages will be consistent with the 2015 *Dietary Guidelines for Americans*, the Dietary Reference Intakes, and advice from the American Academy of Pediatrics. The recommendations will take into account the health and cultural needs of the WIC participant population, support efficient program operations, and allow effective administration across the geographic scope (national plus some U.S. territories) of the program. The goal is to recommend changes in the food packages, as appropriate, while ensuring that

remainder of this chapter describes the committee's task and approach to determining what changes to the food packages might be appropriate.

Special Tasks Requested by the Food and Nutrition Service

In the context of the overall task (see Box 1-3), USDA-FNS requested that the committee evaluate certain foods and food specifications as part of this review. The committee was asked to (1) consider the inclusion of additional fish species in food packages, and consider inclusion of fish across food packages; (2) consider the current science on functional ingredients[12]

[12] At the time this report was written, the U.S. Food and Drug Administration (FDA) had not established a definition for functional foods or ingredients. Functional ingredients are permitted in foods if evidence indicates the ingredients are safe at estimated national levels of consumption, but efficacy of these ingredients is not evaluated or regulated by the FDA.

the recommendations are practical, economical, reflect current nutritional science, and allow the program to effectively meet the nutritional and cultural needs of the WIC-participating population.

The study will be carried out in two phases and produce three reports. An initial phase I letter report will include dietary and energy intake analyses, food intake analyses relative to the *Dietary Guidelines for Americans*, diet quality indices, and a sensitivity analysis to determine the impact of exclusion of white potatoes in WIC food packages on consumption of other foods and the ability of WIC participants to meet key recommendations of the *Dietary Guidelines for Americans*. The letter report will contain findings and recommendations for white potatoes that: are consistent with the current *Dietary Guidelines for Americans*, consider the health and cultural needs of the WIC-participating population, and can be administered effectively and efficiently nationwide and in a cost-effective manner. A phase I (interim) report will contain a description of the evidence-based review strategy, dietary and energy intake analyses, data on breastfeeding trends and variability, and food expenditure analysis, and it will recommend general food groups that could be used to address specific nutritional deficits. The phase II (final) report will be based on the findings in phase I, evidence gathered from the literature review, evaluation of costs, and assessment of sensitivity and regulatory impact analyses, and it will recommend revisions for WIC packages that are culturally suitable,* cost neutral, efficient for nationwide distribution, and nonburdensome to administration.

---

* The term *culturally suitable* was not clearly defined. The committee's interpretation is that foods in the package should align with food preferences and feeding practices based on a participant's ethnic identity and religion.

added to foods for infants, children, and adults to determine how USDA-FNS might approach the inclusion of foods containing these ingredients in the WIC food packages; and (3) evaluate the evidence related to the current requirement that infant formula be issued based on a reconstituted energy density of 20 kcal/ounce. The related recommendations (as appropriate) are presented in Chapters 6 and 11.

Definition of Supplemental Foods

WIC was designed to be a supplemental food program. The definition of supplemental in this context has evolved since the program's inception (see Appendix C, "Chronology of Statutes Pertaining to the Definition of

---

Broadly, functional foods and ingredients are thought to provide a "health benefit beyond basic nutrition," and may be beneficial to long-term health (Crowe and Francis, 2013).

WIC Supplemental Foods" for a summary of the definition over time). Most recently, the 2007 Interim Rule defined supplemental foods as

> those foods containing nutrients determined by nutritional research to be lacking in the diets of pregnant, breastfeeding, and postpartum women, infants, and children, and foods that promote the health of the population served by the WIC program as indicated by relevant nutrition science, public health concerns, and cultural eating patterns, as prescribed by the Secretary in § 246.10. (P.L. 95-627, § 17)[13]

The USDA-FNS task to the committee (see Box 1-3) covers all components of this definition (i.e., nutrition, health, breastfeeding practices, and cultural eating patterns of the WIC-participating population), and the recommendations in this report were developed with an awareness of the supplemental nature of the food packages. The committee's application of this term is further detailed in Chapter 6.

Limitations to the Task

The recommendations in this report were limited by the statement of task, presented in Box 1-3, and are not permitted to go beyond the task. Although the committee acknowledges that WIC participants prepare WIC foods in various ways (e.g., some WIC participants add saturated fats, added sugars, and sodium to foods included in their WIC packages), the committee was not asked to consider how WIC participants modify WIC foods before consumption. In addition, foods considered for the packages were to be readily available or soon to be available in the marketplace by the time the newly revised food packages could be reasonably in place. Finally, changes to USDA-FNS programs that are linked to the WIC food packages but are fiscally independent (e.g., farmers' markets) were considered for context, but no changes to the functions of such programs are suggested.

THE PROCESS FOR REVISING THE WIC FOOD PACKAGES

In the interim report for this study (NASEM, 2016), the committee outlined an approach to the evaluation and revision of the food packages. The committee's first step was to design strategies to ensure collection of the required information and to analyze this information as described previously. Next, the committee developed and subsequently modified (see below, "Criteria for Food Package Revisions") the criteria that it would use to evaluate potential changes to the food packages. The committee also

[13] 95th Congress. 1978. P.L. 95-627, § 17: Child care food program.

developed an iterative framework for testing possible changes against the criteria. The three general components of this overall approach (information collection, criteria for revisions, and the iterative framework), plus additional decision tools required to support these activities, are further described in this section.

Approach to Information Collection

The committee developed an approach to the collection of information needed to support the task. The strategies applied are summarized here, with details of the methodologies and findings available in the indicated chapters or appendixes.

Convening Workshops

Over the course of this study, four information-gathering public workshops were held, three in Washington, DC, and one in Irvine, California. Each workshop was followed by a public comment session. The agendas for these workshops are available in Appendix D. Comments provided are available in the public access file for this study.[14]

Conducting a Comprehensive Literature and Report Review

The committee was tasked with conducting a comprehensive literature review to gather evidence to support its final recommendations.[15] In collaboration with HMD staff and committee consultants, draft key research questions were developed based on the statement of task, literature review questions developed for the letter report (IOM, 2015), and other topics outlined by USDA-FNS for committee consideration. The key questions, literature search strategy, and study eligibility criteria were refined using an iterative process. Key findings from the literature review are presented throughout the report where applicable. Details of the literature review methodology are available in Appendix D.

---

[14] Files may be accessed by emailing paro@nas.edu.

[15] Time and resources were inadequate to carry out a full systematic review. Specifically, the last two steps of a systematic review process were not completed: (1) risk of bias evaluation, and (2) evidence synthesis (which includes evaluation of the strength of the evidence).

Analyzing Food and Nutrient Intakes and Diet Quality of WIC and WIC-Eligible Populations[16]

HMD was tasked with carrying out two comparisons: (1) nutrient intake of WIC participants compared to WIC-eligible nonparticipants, and (2) nutrient intake of WIC participants before the 2009 food package changes compared to after the 2009 food package changes. For this task, the committee analyzed data from survey years 2005 to 2012 of the National Health and Nutrition Examination Survey (NHANES). Details of the analysis and results are available in Chapter 4 and Appendix J.

Determining WIC Food Package Food, Nutrient, and Cost Profiles

The food group and nutrient contributions and costs of the current food packages served as the baseline from which to evaluate food package changes. Details of the food group and nutrient contributions of the current food packages, along with a comparison to dietary intake recommendations, are presented in Chapter 3. Details of the food group and nutrient contributions of the revised food packages are included in Chapter 9 and Appendix T. A cost analysis is presented in Chapter 7. Appendix R details the assumptions applied to develop the nutrient and cost profiles.

Conducting Sensitivity and Regulatory Impact Analyses

A sensitivity analysis was applied to the revised food package profiles to assess the effects of alternative potential food package changes on (1) the nutrient and food group composition of the packages relative to the DGA recommended food groups and subgroups, and (2) cost. This analysis considered different potential changes to food amounts, redemption, and/or participation to develop the cost-neutral revised food packages. In addition to the sensitivity analysis, a regulatory impact analysis (RIA) was conducted to evaluate the effect of the committee's recommended changes in WIC food packages on program participation, the value of selected food packages, and program cost and administration. Details of the sensitivity and RIA approaches and results are presented in Chapters 8 and 10, respectively.

Conducting a Food Expenditure Analysis

The committee was required to conduct an evaluation of the food costs of WIC-participating households, including individual expenditures on

[16] In accordance with the task, data were also generated for low-income women that were ineligible because they were not pregnant, breastfeeding, or postpartum.

separate food groups, to assess the relative contribution of the WIC food packages to household total food expenditures. The methods for and results of this analysis are presented in Chapter 2. Additional details are provided in the phase I report (NASEM, 2016).

Visiting WIC Sites and Shopping for WIC Foods

USDA-FNS asked that the majority of committee members visit a WIC site and experience shopping as a WIC participant prior to development of the phase I (interim) report. Between March and June 2015, committee members visited a total of 14 WIC sites and vendors either in their home state, another state, or both. The visits were organized to ensure geographic and cultural diversity, a balance of sites issuing paper vouchers versus using EBT, and activity at the site (e.g., participant flow and provision of nutrition education). A list of sites visited by city and state, as well as a summary of the committee's impressions from this experience, is presented in Appendix D.

Reviewing Public Comments

As required by USDA-FNS, comments were solicited through the HMD study website and in-person at five public comment sessions over the course of the study. A summary of common themes is presented in Appendix D.

Criteria for Food Package Revisions

Criteria for food package revisions were presented in the committee's phase I report (NASEM, 2016). To develop the criteria, the committee examined the criteria outlined by the 2006 IOM committee. The committee used these criteria for this review, with only slightly modified language. This was because, after a thorough review of the evidence, the committee concluded that the 2006 criteria were comprehensive and remained appropriate to include. After phase I, an additional criterion (criterion 1) was added because the committee determined that it was required to guide its work and permit it to meet its task. The final criteria, presented in Box 1-4, reflect the committee's priorities, first, to meet the goals of the WIC program; second, to respond to the requirement that the WIC food packages be aligned with the DGA; and third, to provide a package that is acceptable to participants and feasible to implement at every level. In this section, the rationale supporting each criterion is described. The degree to which the revised food packages meet these criteria is evaluated in Chapter 9.

BOX 1-4

Criteria for Inclusion of Foods in the WIC Food Packages

1. The packages provide a balanced supplement to the diets of women and children.
2. The packages contribute to the reduction of the prevalence of inadequate nutrient intakes and of excessive nutrient intakes.
3. The packages contribute to an overall dietary pattern that is consistent with the *Dietary Guidelines for Americans* for individuals 2 years of age and older.
4. The packages contribute to an overall diet that is consistent with established dietary recommendations for infants and children less than 2 years of age, including encouragement of and support for breastfeeding.
5. The foods in the packages are available in forms and amounts suitable for low-income persons who may have limited transportation options, storage, and cooking facilities.
6. The foods in the packages are readily acceptable, commonly consumed, widely available, take into account cultural eating patterns and food preferences, and provide incentives for families to participate in the WIC program.
7. The foods in the packages do not create an undue burden on state agencies or vendors.

Criterion 1: Providing a Supplement to the Diet

The packages provide a balanced supplement to the diets of women and children.

Rationale The concept of the WIC program providing a supplemental amount of food to participants is part of the full name of the WIC program, namely the Special Supplemental Nutrition Program for Women, Infants, and Children. The current food packages provide widely varying proportions of required nutrients and recommended food groups (see Chapter 3) and a better balance in these proportions would permit the committee to align the food packages more adequately with the DGA. The committee decided that, because WIC participants (other than formula-fed infants in the first 6 months of life), consume foods and beverages not supplied by the WIC food packages that meet some portion of their nutrient needs, the supplementation target (i.e., proportion of requirement) should be to meet a moderate proportion of an individual's requirement for a particular nutrient or recommended amount of a food group. Furthermore, the committee decided that the supplementation target may differ depending on the nutrient requirement and the degree to which foods appropriate for the food package and available in the marketplace could meet this requirement.

Criterion 2: Optimizing Nutrient Intakes

The packages contribute to reduction of the prevalence of inadequate nutrient intakes and of excessive nutrient intakes.

Rationale WIC is a supplemental food program designed to provide specific nutrients determined by nutritional research to be lacking in the diets of the WIC-participating population. As described in Chapter 4, the committee's evaluation of nutrient intakes among WIC-eligible populations led to the identification not only of nutrients for which intakes were inadequate, but also nutrients for which intakes were excessive. Restrictions on food types, as well as on added salt, sugars, and saturated fats, are all intended to reduce excessive intake of these nutrients. Nutrition education through WIC that is linked to the food packages also helps to ensure that participants' overall diets align with their energy and nutrient needs as well as with the DGA. However, inasmuch as WIC is a "supplemental nutrition program," it cannot be expected to alleviate all nutritional deficits or excesses in participants' diets. Nutrient intake is evaluated in Chapter 4, and nutrients are prioritized based on the prevalence of inadequate or excessive intakes in Chapter 5. The committee's interpretation of the term *supplemental* is described above and discussed further in Chapter 6.

Criterion 3: Aligning with the Most Recent Dietary Guidelines for Americans

The packages contribute to an overall dietary pattern that is consistent with the DGA for individuals 2 years of age and older.

Rationale A goal of the final recommendations is to ensure that WIC food packages are consistent with the DGA. The food package composition was compared to the DGA food patterns appropriate for the age and physiological state of package recipients. Food packages were also evaluated for provision of nutrients of public health concern and nutrients to limit (added sugars, saturated fat, and sodium).

Criterion 4: Aligning with the Most Recent Dietary Guidance for Individuals Younger Than 2 Years of Age

The packages contribute to an overall diet that is consistent with established dietary recommendations for infants and children less than 2 years of age, including encouragement of and support for breastfeeding.

Rationale Because the DGA do not apply to infants and children less than 2 years of age, WIC food packages should be consistent with guidance from other authorities for subgroups within this age range, including the American Academy of Pediatrics, the Academy of Nutrition and Dietetics, and the World Health Organization. Promotion of breastfeeding is an overarching goal of the WIC program, however, the proportion of WIC women who breastfeed falls below the proportion of overall low-income women and well below the *Healthy People 2020* objectives (Ryan et al., 2002; CDC, 2015; HHS, 2015). Therefore, attention was paid to how the revised food packages can motivate breastfeeding. Chapter 3 contains additional detail on the dietary guidance identified by the committee and its application to infants and children less than 2 years of age.

Criterion 5: Suitability and Safety for Individuals with Limited Transportation, Storage Options, and Cooking Facilities

The foods in the packages are available in forms and amounts suitable for low-income persons who may have limited transportation options, storage, and cooking facilities.

Rationale Access to WIC vendors is limited in many areas where WIC participants live, as are cooking and food-storage facilities in their homes. As a result, the WIC food packages must be designed to consider these barriers to acquisition, transportation, and safe consumption of WIC foods.

Criterion 6: Acceptability, Availability, and Perceived Value

The foods in the packages are readily acceptable, commonly consumed, widely available, take into account cultural eating patterns and food preferences, and provide incentives for families to participate in the WIC program.

Rationale Consumption of WIC foods may be influenced by the acceptability, preferences for, or availability of foods that are issued in the food packages. Definitions of acceptability, availability, and related terms are provided below; acceptability, accessibility, and cultural considerations are reviewed in Chapters 2 and 3.

Acceptability Food acceptability means that foods provided are easily incorporated into the diet, considering many different factors. Employment is one factor that may affect dietary patterns and the extent to which acquired or purchased WIC foods are actually consumed. Time constraints and a need for convenience are important when considering possible modifications to the WIC food packages. Additionally, some individuals have food-triggered, immune-mediated sensitivities that require specific foods or diets. These include food allergies, celiac disease, non-celiac gluten sensitivity, and lactose intolerance. The committee considered how the current food packages could be improved to meet the needs of the diverse WIC-participating population.

Commonly consumed USDA's strategy for generating the DGA recommended food intake patterns starts with understanding the actual eating patterns of Americans to ensure that recommendations are compatible with these patterns. Similarly, it was important for the committee to consider the current food packages and possible changes in the context of what WIC participants actually eat. Redemption data and national food intake data were key sources of this information.

Food availability and accessibility Measures of food accessibility include the distance of WIC participants to WIC vendors, how participants access stores (by car or other transportation), and where (at large or small stores) participants primarily shop for foods. Using one's own vehicle allows more flexibility in store choice; lack of a vehicle limits the ability to transport large or heavy items or a large number of items. The committee also considered the availability of food types and sizes in the marketplace.

Cultural considerations Culture can be defined as shared beliefs, values, and behaviors of groups of people that influence their specific needs and preferences (NWA, 2003). The committee interpreted *culturally suitable foods* as foods that align with food preferences and feeding practices based on a participant's ethnic identity and religion. Such foods could complement cultural eating practices or behaviors while still providing nutrients for which intake is found to be lacking. Several changes to the food packages in 2009 were made to allow flexibility with consideration to cultural needs (IOM, 2006). The current committee also considered how WIC food packages accommodate preferences for vegetarian and vegan diets, food-related religious practices (e.g., Kosher and Halal diets), and other preferences.

Perceived value Participation in WIC and redemption and consumption of WIC foods may be somewhat dependent upon the perceived value of the food packages (as an incentive) and other services provided. Food packages that draw participation can encourage continued enrollment and use of the nutrition education, breastfeeding support, and health services accessible through WIC. The converse may also be true, meaning that providing these services and support may help WIC participants attach more value to their WIC foods. The committee examined additional possibilities for promoting the choice to breastfeed, which are reflected in the revised food packages presented in Chapter 6.

Criterion 7: Moderating Administrative Burden

The foods in the packages do not create an undue burden on state agencies or vendors.

Rationale The WIC program is administered by USDA-FNS and numerous state and local agencies. As specified in the task, the proposed changes should not unduly add to the administrative burden of these agencies.[17] Likewise, changes should not unduly add to WIC vendor burden, given that the ease of WIC program administration is closely linked to the ability of WIC-authorized vendors to provide WIC foods. Additional detail on the committee's evaluation of the effect of the 2009 food packages changes on state agency and vendor burden is presented in Chapter 2.

Framework for Revisions

The committee's overall process for revising the WIC food packages is illustrated in Figure 1-1. The objective was to ensure that the revisions fell within the criteria outlined in the previous section. First, the current food packages were evaluated for the nutrients and food groups provided as well as the challenges faced during implementation. After reviewing this information, the committee identified priority changes in the food packages and tested possible changes in an iterative fashion to align with the criteria. The sensitivity analysis was used to determine the extent to which particular changes affected nutrients, food groups, and costs. As a final step, the revised packages were further changed to ensure cost-neutrality, considering the committee's priority changes. This process involved nutritional and cost trade-offs, with final recommendations guided by the criteria and cost constraints. Once the iterations resulted in changes meeting the criteria, recommendations were finalized. A regulatory impact analysis was then conducted to assess the projected effect of changes in WIC food packages on program participation, the value of the food packages as selected, and program costs and administration.

[17] Administrative burden includes adding unreasonably to staff time and effort, requiring additional systems that are not already in place, or requiring any program modifications that would be disproportionate to the benefit of the change.

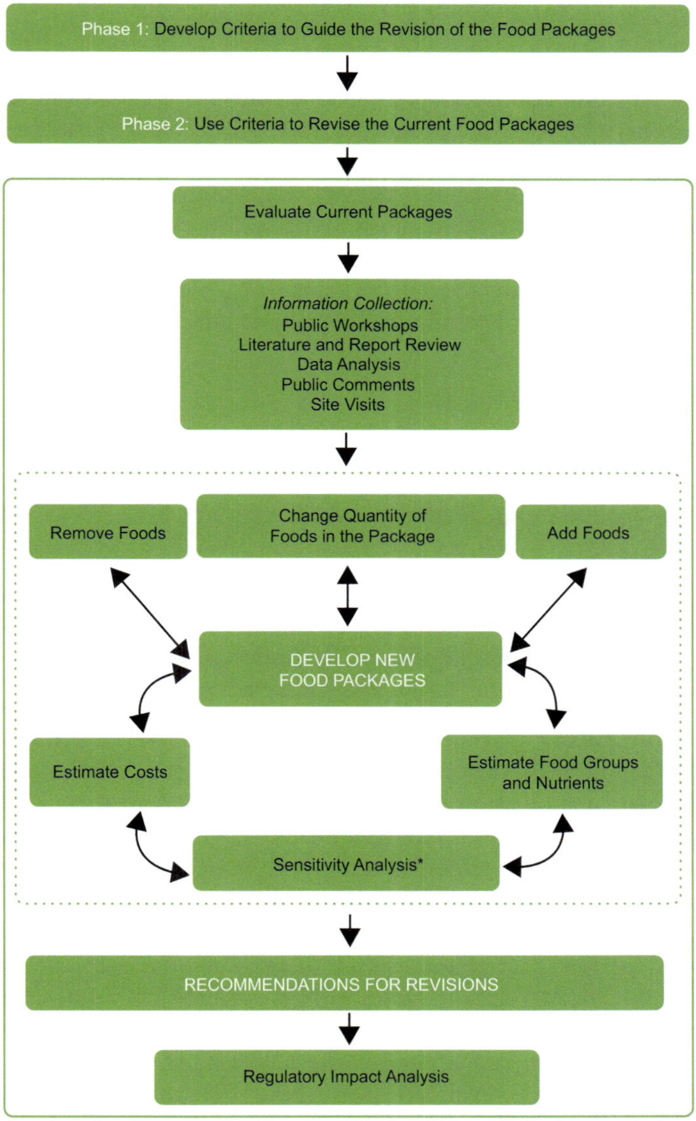

FIGURE 1-1 Process for revising the WIC food packages.

NOTES: The dotted line indicates components of the process that iterate until the criteria for food package revisions are met (see criteria 1 through 7 presented above).

* The sensitivity analysis tests the assumptions applied to develop the cost-neutral revised food packages. For example, if redemption of a food in the final revised package was assumed to be 80 percent, the sensitivity analysis could test effects on cost, nutrients, and food groups should redemption rise to 90 percent. A description of the sensitivity analysis is provided in Chapter 8.

Qualitative Assessment of Food Package Changes

The committee considered additional dimensions that could be affected by changes to the food packages. These included the effects of changes on participation (uptake) in the program and/or effects on the redemption rates of foods within each package, over the 5 years following implementation. These changes were particularly relevant for conducting the RIA, and several major changes were included as an option in the RIA (see Chapter 10 and Appendix U for details on the execution and results of the RIA). Examples include an increase in the rates of CVV redemption or shifts of participants from fully formula feeding to partially breastfeeding.

Variations from Cost-Neutral

Although the committee was tasked with ensuring overall cost-neutrality for recommended changes to the WIC food packages, it was also asked to offer prioritized recommendations in the event that USDA-FNS's WIC funding is either above or below the cost-neutral level. These priorities appear in Chapter 11.

Determining Foods to Be Added, Deleted, or Changed in the Food Packages

The committee's consideration of possible changes to the food packages was based on the concept of the food packages as supplemental. (See Chapter 6 for a discussion of the committee's interpretation of "supplemental.") As such, the food packages should supplement participants' diets with foods containing nutrients that are both underconsumed and linked to health outcomes relevant to the WIC-participating population. The committee considered whether to add foods or to allow for additional or more costly food options that could address these inadequacies as well as alignment with the DGA. To make these changes possible, the committee identified foods currently in the food packages that could be reduced or removed. To do this, the committee evaluated the packages for foods that (1) were provided in more than a supplemental amount in comparison to the DGA; (2) were not associated with nutrient inadequacies and food groups for which intake was below recommended amounts or were of lower priority related to these inadequacies; (3) contributed to either excess energy intake or excess intake of saturated fat, added sugars, sodium, and refined grains, and (4) were poorly redeemed or were not redeemed because of food preference, availability, or other reasons. These concepts were considered in balance with cost. The committee also sought opportunities to improve the value of the breastfeeding packages.

Aligning Guidance for Nutrients and Foods

The committee faced a fundamental challenge when evaluating dietary adequacy for nutrients, which are based on nutrient requirements described in the Dietary Reference Intakes (DRI), compared to food groups, which are based on recommendations in the DGA. This challenge stems from differences in the methods used to establish dietary adequacy and differences in how the two sets of guidelines are used to plan diets for groups of individuals.

To evaluate dietary adequacy for nutrients based on the DRI, the Estimated Average Requirement (EAR) is used. The EAR is the daily intake estimated to meet the nutrient requirement of half the healthy individuals in a particular life stage, sex, and age group. Thus, it is the median of the distribution of requirements in that group. In planning diets for groups, the objective is to minimize the proportion of individuals with usual daily intakes below the EAR (IOM, 2003). In the committee's deliberations, nutrients were considered underconsumed if the prevalence of inadequacy was 5 percent or greater, meaning that at least 5 percent of individuals in the subgroup consumed less than the EAR. Using this approach, the committee identified 15 nutrients as being consumed in inadequate amounts in at least one subgroup of WIC women. A proportion of the reported dietary inadequacies could have resulted from underreporting of energy intake, which is a common problem in dietary surveys, including NHANES (Briefel et al., 1997; Macdiarmid and Blundell, 1998; McKenzie et al., 2002; CDC, 2010; Archer et al., 2013; Murakami and Livingstone, 2015; Subar et al., 2015). As a result of this problem, the committee gave priority to those nutrients for which the prevalence of inadequacy was greater than 50 percent, followed by those for which the prevalence was between 10 and 50 percent and, finally, by those for which the prevalence was between 5 and 10 percent (see Chapter 5).

In contrast to nutrients, food group intakes are assessed using the DGA food patterns, which are designed to ensure that the nutrient requirements of nearly all (97.5 percent) individuals in a particular life stage, sex, and age group are met. The DGA food patterns are based on providing the Recommended Dietary Allowances (RDAs) for all (or most) nutrients; the RDA for each nutrient is the DRI value for that nutrient that is two standard deviations above its EAR. Inasmuch as the food patterns are designed to meet all (or most) of the RDAs, recommended intakes for some of the more easily obtained nutrients can be well above their RDAs (Britten et al., 2012). For example, because protein-containing foods are also good sources of iron and zinc, food patterns designed to meet the RDAs for iron and zinc (less easily obtained nutrients) can result in a recommended intake of protein (a more easily obtained nutrient) being well above its RDA. Inasmuch as the

DGA recommendation may be higher than even the RDA, the prevalence of intakes that are below recommended food patterns may be higher than the prevalence of intakes that are below the nutrient EARs. This discrepancy was evident among children 2 to less than 5 years old, among whom inadequate nutrient intakes were rare, but food-group intakes below the food pattern recommendations were common.

As a result of these considerations, the committee first used the prevalence of nutrient inadequacy, in conjunction with evidence of a health consequence relevant to the WIC-participating population, to identify the priority nutrients among groups of WIC participants. Alignment of the food packages with the DGA food groups took place at a later step and involved a similarly structured process. The committee chose a less-restrictive approach for selecting the foods group intakes that should be improved than the one (described above) that was used for selecting which nutrient intakes should be improved. For food groups, if 50 percent or more of the population group fell below the recommended intake, then the committee thought that improving intake of this food group should be a priority; if 75 percent or more of the population group fell below the recommended intake, then the committee thought that improving intake of this food group should be a higher priority.

SUMMARY AND ORGANIZATION OF THIS REPORT

In summary, the committee applied the iterative process of the framework (see Figure 1-1) to ensure that the revised food packages met the seven overarching criteria (see Box 1-4). The remainder of this report provides details on the methodologies applied, as well as the findings, conclusions and recommendations resulting from the process. The chapter contents are as detailed below:

Chapter 2—Changes Since the Last Review and Continuing Challenges
Chapter 3—Alignment of the Current Food Packages with Dietary Guidance, Special Dietary Needs, and Cultural Eating Practices or Food Preferences
Chapter 4—Nutrient and Food Group Intakes of WIC Participants
Chapter 5—Nutrient and Food Group Priorities for the Food Packages
Chapter 6—The Revised Food Packages
Chapter 7—Evaluation of Cost
Chapter 8—Sensitivity Analysis
Chapter 9—How the Revised Food Packages Meet the Criteria Specified
Chapter 10—The Regulatory Impact Analysis (Abridged)
Chapter 11—Recommendations for Implementation and Research

Overall, this report presents findings and other information intended to guide the USDA's Food and Nutrition Service to improve the supplemental food portion of the WIC program, improve the nutritional status of WIC participants, promote breastfeeding, and, indirectly, facilitate making the nutrition education component of the WIC program more consistent with the DGA (USDA/HHS, 2016).

REFERENCES

Anderson, A. K., G. Damio, S. Young, D. J. Chapman, and R. Peréz-Escamilla. 2005. A randomized trial assessing the efficacy of peer counseling on exclusive breastfeeding in a predominantly Latina low-income community. *Archives of Pediatrics & Adolescent Medicine* 159(9):836–841.

Anderson, A. K., G. Damio, D. J. Chapman, and R. Peréz-Escamilla. 2007. Differential response to an exclusive breastfeeding peer counseling intervention: The role of ethnicity. *Journal of Human Lactation* 23(1):16–23.

Archer, E., G. A. Hand, and S. N. Blair. 2013. Validity of U.S. nutritional surveillance: National Health and Nutrition Examination Survey caloric energy intake data, 1971–2010. *PLoS One* 8(10):e76632.

Bonuck, K. A., K. Freeman, and M. Trombley. 2005. Country of origin and race/ethnicity: Impact on breastfeeding intentions. *Journal of Human Lactation* 21(3):320–326.

Briefel, R. R., C. T. Sempos, M. A. McDowell, S. Chien, and K. Alaimo. 1997. Dietary methods research in NHANES III: Under-reporting of energy intake. *American Journal of Clinical Nutrition* 65(S):1203S–1209S.

Britten, P., L. E. Cleveland, K. L. Koegel, K. J. Kuczynski, and S. M. Nickols-Richardson. 2012. Updated US Department of Agriculture food patterns meet goals of the 2010 dietary guidelines. *Journal of the Academy of Nutrition and Dietetics* 112(10): 1648–1655.

Bunik, M., P. Shobe, M. E. O'Connor, B. Beaty, S. Langendoerfer, L. Crane, and A. Kempe. 2010. Are 2 weeks of daily breastfeeding support insufficient to overcome the influences of formula? *Academic Pediatrics* 10(1):21–28.

CDC (Centers for Disease Control and Prevention). 2010. *Obesity and socioeconomic status in adults: United States, 2005–2008.* http://www.cdc.gov/nchs/data/databriefs/db50.pdf (accessed December 20, 2016).

CDC. 2015. *Bridged-race population estimates 1990–2014 request.* http://wonder.cdc.gov/bridged-race-v2014.html (accessed August 29, 2016).

CDPH (California Department of Public Health). 2016. *WIC authorized food list shopping guide.* http://www.cdph.ca.gov/programs/wicworks/WIC%20Foods/WICAuthorizedFoodListShoppingGuide-3-28-2016.pdf (accessed October 27, 2016).

Chapman, D. J., K. Morel, A. Bermudez-Millan, S. Young, G. Damio, and R. Peréz-Escamilla. 2013. Breastfeeding education and support trial for overweight and obese women: A randomized trial. *Pediatrics* 131(1):e162–e170.

Crowe, K. M., and C. Francis. 2013. Position of the Academy of Nutrition and Dietetics: Functional foods. *Journal of the Academy of Nutrition Dietetics* 113(8):1096–1103.

Haider, S. J., L. V. Chang, T. A. Bolton, J. G. Gold, and B. H. Olson. 2014. An evaluation of the effects of a breastfeeding support program on health outcomes. *Health Services Research* 49(6):2017–2034.

Hayes, D. K., C. B. Prince, V. Espinueva, L. J. Fuddy, R. Li, and L. M. Grummer-Strawn. 2008. Comparison of manual and electric breast pumps among WIC women returning to work or school in Hawaii. *Breastfeeding Medicine* 3(1):3–10.

HHS (U.S. Department of Health and Human Services). 2015. *Healthy People 2020: Maternal, infant, and child health objectives.* https://www.healthypeople.gov/2020/topics-objectives/topic/maternal-infant-and-child-health/objectives (accessed December 20, 2016).

Hildebrand, D. A., P. McCarthy, D. Tipton, C. Merriman, M. Schrank, and M. Newport. 2014. Innovative use of influential prenatal counseling may improve breastfeeding initiation rates among WIC participants. *Journal of Nutrition Education and Behavior* 46(6):458–466.

Hopkinson, J., and M. Konefal Gallagher. 2009. Assignment to a hospital-based breastfeeding clinic and exclusive breastfeeding among immigrant Hispanic mothers: A randomized, controlled trial. *Journal of Human Lactation* 25(3):287–296.

Howell, E. A., S. Bodnar-Deren, A. Balbierz, M. Parides, and N. Bickell. 2014. An intervention to extend breastfeeding among black and Latina mothers after delivery. *American Journal of Obstetrics and Gynecology* 210(3):239.e231–e235.

IOM (Institute of Medicine). 2003. *Dietary Reference Intakes: Applications in dietary planning.* Washington, DC: The National Academies Press.

IOM. 2006. *WIC food packages: Time for a change.* Washington, DC: The National Academies Press.

IOM. 2015. *Review of WIC food packages: An evaluation of white potatoes in the cash value voucher: Letter report.* Washington, DC: The National Academies Press.

Kandiah, J. 2011. Teaching new mothers about infant feeding cues may increase breastfeeding duration. *Food and Nutrition Sciences* 2(4):259–264.

Macdiarmid, J., and J. Blundell. 1998. Assessing dietary intake: Who, what and why of under-reporting. *Nutrition Research Reviews* 11(2):231–253.

McKenzie, D. C., R. K. Johnson, J. Harvey-Berino, and B. C. Gold. 2002. Impact of interviewer's body mass index on underreporting energy intake in overweight and obese women. *Obesity Research and Clinical Practice* 10(6):471–477.

Meehan, K., G. G. Harrison, A. A. Afifi, N. Nickel, E. Jenks, and A. Ramirez. 2008. The association between an electric pump loan program and the timing of requests for formula by working mothers in WIC. *Journal of Human Lactation* 24(2):150–158.

Murakami, K. and M. B. Livingstone. 2015. Prevalence and characteristics of misreporting of energy intake in US adults: NHANES 2003–2012. *British Journal of Nutrition* 114(8):1294–1303.

NASEM (National Academies of Sciences, Engineering, and Medicine). 2016. *Review of WIC food packages: Proposed framework for revisions: Interim report.* Washington, DC: The National Academies Press. doi: 10.17226/21832.

NWA (National WIC Association). 2003.WIC culturally sensitive food prescription recommendations. Washington, DC: National WIC Association. https://s3.amazonaws.com/aws.upl/nwica.org/WIC_Culturally_Sensitive_Food_Prescription.pdf (accessed August 24, 2016).

NWA. 2013. *The role of WIC in public health.* Washington, DC: National WIC Association. https://s3.amazonaws.com/aws.upl/nwica.org/WIC_Public_Health_Role.pdf (accessed December 20, 2016).

Olson, B. H., S. J. Haider, L. Vangjel, T. A. Bolton, and J. G. Gold. 2010. A quasi-experimental evaluation of a breastfeeding support program for low income women in Michigan. *Maternal and Child Health Journal* 14(1):86–93.

Pérez-Escamilla, R., and D. J. Chapman. 2012. Breastfeeding protection, promotion, and support in the United States: A time to nudge, a time to measure. *Journal of Human Lactation* 28(2):118–121.

Pérez-Escamilla, R., L. Curry, D. Minhas, L. Taylor, and E. Bradley. 2012. Scaling up of breastfeeding promotion programs in low- and middle-income countries: The "breastfeeding gear" model. *Advances in Nutrition* 3(6):790–800.

Petrova, A., C. Ayers, S. Stechna, J. A. Gerling, and R. Mehta. 2009. Effectiveness of exclusive breastfeeding promotion in low-income mothers: A randomized controlled study. *Breastfeeding Medicine* 4(2):63–69.

Pugh, L. C., J. R. Serwint, K. D. Frick, J. P. Nanda, P. W. Sharps, D. L. Spatz, and R. A. Milligan. 2010. A randomized controlled community-based trial to improve breastfeeding rates among urban low-income mothers. *Academic Pediatrics* 10(1):14–20.

Reeder, J. A., T. Joyce, K. Sibley, D. Arnold, and O. Altindag. 2014. Telephone peer counseling of breastfeeding among WIC participants: A randomized controlled trial. *Pediatrics* 134(3):e700–e709.

Ryan, A., Z. Wenjun, and A. Acosta. 2002. Breastfeeding continues to increase into the new millennium. *Pediatrics* 11(6):1103–1109.

Sandy, J. M., E. Anisfeld, and E. Ramirez. 2009. Effects of a prenatal intervention on breastfeeding initiation rates in a Latina immigrant sample. *Journal of Human Lactation* 25(4):404–411; quiz 458–459.

Subar, A. F., L. S. Freedman, J. A. Tooze, S. I. Kirkpatrick, C. Boushey, M. L. Neuhouser, F. E. Thompson, N. Potischman, P. M. Guenther, V. Tarasuk, J. Reedy, and S. M. Krebs-Smith. 2015. Addressing current criticism regarding the value of self-report dietary data. *Journal of Nutrition* 145(12):2639–2645.

USDA/ERS (U.S. Department of Agriculture/Economic Research Service). 2015. *The WIC program: Background, trends, and economic issues, 2015 edition*. Washington, DC: USDA/ERS. http://www.ers.usda.gov/media/159295/err73.pdf (accessed December 20, 2016).

USDA/FNS (U.S. Department of Agriculture/Food and Nutrition Service). 2007. *Special Supplemental Nutrition Program for Women, Infants and Children (WIC): Revisions in the WIC food packages; Interim Rule*. 7 C.F.R. § 246.

USDA/FNS. 2013. *WIC participant and program characteristics 2012 final report*. Alexandria, VA: USDA/FNS. http://www.fns.usda.gov/sites/default/files/WICPC2012.pdf (accessed December 20, 2016).

USDA/FNS. 2014. *Special Supplemental Nutrition Program for Women, Infants, and Children (WIC): Revisions in the WIC food packages; final rule*. 7 C.F.R. § 246.

USDA/FNS. 2015a. *About WIC—WIC at a glance*. http://www.fns.usda.gov/wic/about-wic-wic-glance (accessed December 20, 2016).

USDA/FNS. 2015b. *WIC food packages policy options II, final report*. Alexandria, VA: USDA/FNS. http://www.fns.usda.gov/wic-food-package-policy-options-ii (accessed November 11, 2015).

USDA/FNS. 2016. *Frequently asked questions about WIC*. http://www.fns.usda.gov/wic/frequently-asked-questions-about-wic (accessed May 22, 2016).

USDA/FNS/NAL (U.S. Department of Agriculture/Food and Nutrition Service/National Agricultural Library). 2006. *WIC program nutrition education guidance*. http://www.nal.usda.gov/wicworks/Learning_Center/ntredguidance.pdf (accessed September 4, 2015).

USDA/HHS (U.S. Department of Agriculture/U.S. Department of Health and Human Services). 2016. *2015–2016 Dietary Guidelines for Americans*. Washington, DC: U.S. Government Printing Office. https://health.gov/dietaryguidelines/2015 (accessed August 29, 2016).

Whaley, S. E., M. Koleilat, M. Whaley, J. Gomez, K. Meehan, and K. Saluja. 2012. Impact of policy changes on infant feeding decisions among low-income women participating in the Special Supplemental Nutrition Program for Women, Infants, and Children. *American Journal of Public Health* 102(12):2269–2273.

2

The WIC Program: Changes Since the Last Review and Continuing Challenges

The first major changes to the Special Supplemental Nutrition Program for Women, Infants, and Children (WIC) food packages in 35 years were recommended by the Institute of Medicine (IOM) in 2006 and implemented by state agencies in 2009 as a result of the U. S. Department of Agriculture's Food and Nutrition Service (USDA-FNS) 2007 interim regulation. Since then, there have also been numerous changes in the WIC environment. This chapter presents a review of changes in the food packages themselves as well as the numerous other changes that have occurred since 2006 and that could potentially affect any updates to the WIC food packages. These include changes in the number and types of WIC participants, economic factors such as participants' food expenditures and the costs of the program, and dietary guidance. Also included here is a description of the experience of WIC participants today. The chapter concludes with a summary of key findings and conclusions reached by the committee upon examination of the evidence described throughout the chapter.

ADAPTATION TO THE WIC FOOD PACKAGE CHANGES PROPOSED IN 2006

A description of the WIC food package changes implemented in response to the 2006 IOM recommendations is provided in Chapter 1 and in Appendix C, Table C-1. Although the 2006 recommendations were based on the best science available, a number of research activities have been undertaken since then to continue to evaluate the impact of WIC generally and the food package changes specifically. As described in Appendix E,

Table E-1, USDA-sponsored investigators have studied changes in the behavior of vendors, the availability of vegetables and fruits for purchase with the cash value voucher (CVV), the availability of foods in new sizes, and the pattern of household-level food purchases. The information presented below and throughout this chapter is based on key findings from these and other studies.

Challenges to Implementation of the 2009 Food Package Changes

Implementation of the 2009 food packages involved challenges at the federal, state, and local agency levels, as well as for vendors and manufacturers. A summary of the key challenges and actions taken to resolve these challenges is presented in Table 2-1 and described in detail in the phase I report (NASEM, 2016). For the most part, these challenges have since been overcome, but they remain relevant to consider in future rounds of food package revisions.

At the state agency level, notable challenges included production and distribution of the 1-pound loaf of bread, dealing with the "dangling quart" of milk, changes to container sizes available in the marketplace (e.g., juice and peanut butter), and implementation of the CVV (a description of the CVV is provided in Chapter 1). But along with these challenges, as noted in Chapter 1, a key benefit of the 2009 food package changes, finalized in 2014, was the ability for states to tailor packages (USDA/FNS, 2007a). Although the additional options led to some inconsistencies in specific foods available from state to state, it enabled state administrators to make decisions that maximize the suitability of the foods for their own population and that also contain costs. For example, the Final Rule allows children ages 12 to 24 months to receive fat-reduced milks if overweight or obesity is a concern (USDA/FNS, 2014a). As of 2015, 72 percent of WIC state agencies had adopted this option, covering 60 percent of WIC participants (USDA/FNS, 2015A).

At the vendor level, despite challenges to ensuring WIC foods were available, most evidence suggests that the food package revisions were beneficial for vendors, increasing both sales and profitability for the items offered in the revised food package (Andreyeva et al., 2011) and increasing sales of newly eligible food items to non-WIC customers (Gittelsohn et al., 2012). However, the revised food packages were designed to be cost-neutral to WIC. Thus, while sales apparently increased from WIC foods for some items (reduced-fat milk, whole grains, fruits, and vegetables), sales likely decreased for others (whole milk, juice) (Andreyeva et al., 2013a; Andreyeva and Luedicke, 2013b, 2014). Although some vendors reported difficulty finding and maintaining suppliers for some foods, available evidence finds that prices for these items did not increase, suggesting that

TABLE 2-1 Challenges to Implementation of the 2009 Food Package Revisions

Stakeholder	Challenge	Resolution
Federal	Dangling quart: after substitution options, a quart of milk remained, creating a stocking challenge for vendors	Yogurt substitution option in place of the "dangling quart"; states are permitted to authorize purchase of quart sizes of milk (USDA/FNS, 2014a)
	Container size: change in sizes of peanut butter from 18 to 16 ounces, and in some juices from 64 to 59 ounces	Permission for state authorization of different sizes as approved by USDA-FNS[a] (USDA/FNS, 2016a)
	CVV: A new food instrument based on a fixed cash value	Permission for "split tender" so that participants can cover any overage with cash (USDA/FNS, 2014a)
Federal/State	CVV: A new food instrument based on a cash value; difficult for participants to select an amount of produce that exactly matched the value	Education to staff, participants, and vendors
State agency	CVV in lieu of jarred infant food vegetables and fruits (currently fresh only) for infants 9 to 11 months of age; difficult if states offer canned, frozen, or dried vegetables and fruits for other participants	No resolution; some states have not implemented the option because of Management Information System limitations
	EBT: requires development of a database for WIC-approved foods	Established strategies by early EBT adopters, a model for later adopters; development of a national UPC database is required for state use (P.L. 111-296, Healthy, Hunger-Free Kids Act of 2010)
	Cost containment: balancing with diversity and availability of foods	Not fully resolved: rebates contain costs, but limit program ability to support breastfeeding; cost-containment may limit vendors, brands, sizes, forms, or prices (e.g. "least expensive brand"[b] requirements)

continued

TABLE 2-1 Continued

Stakeholder	Challenge	Resolution
	Container size: change in sizes of peanut butter from 18 to 16 ounces, and in some juices from 64 to 59 ounces and in some juices from 64 to 59 ounces	Permission for state authorization of different sizes as approved by USDA-FNS
Local agency	Introduction of new foods or changes to foods	Staff and participant education
Vendor	Requirement in the Final Rule to stock at least two different fruits and two different vegetables	Vendors' choice of less perishable options or canned/frozen varieties if the state authorizes canned, frozen, or dried options (USDA/FNS, 2015a)
	Stocking the specific size; maintaining freshness (Gleason et al., 2011)	Higher prices for WIC foods (Tisone et al., 2014; USDA/ERS, 2014a)
	Difficulty finding distributors and suppliers for specific food items (Andreyeva et al., 2011; Gittelsohn et al., 2012)	ND
Manufacturer	Specific size or product with the WIC food specification not available	At higher cost, modified production streams to manufacture the required product; or prohibitive cost so the product is not manufactured[c]

NOTES: CVV = cash value voucher; EBT = electronic benefit transfer; ND = No data are available as to whether this continues to be a challenge; UPC = Universal Product Code; USDA-FNS = U.S. Department of Agriculture's Food and Nutrition Service.

[a] States are permitted to authorize different sizes only if there is limited availability of the prescribed specified size and nutritional integrity is not compromised (see USDA/FNS, 2016a).

[b] The "least expensive brand" requirement is a strategy selected by some states by which participants are directed to the products that are the least expensive among all products offered by that store that meet WIC specifications.

[c] Personal communication, National Pasta Association, July 16, 2015. Report is available in the public access file for this study (Email: paro@nas.edu).

SOURCES: As cited in the table.

vendors adjusted their supply quantities without incurring increased costs (Zenk et al., 2014).

At the local level, results from multiple studies have documented the effect of WIC nutrition education on participant knowledge, attitudes, and behavior change (USDA/ERS, 2007; Kavanagh et al., 2008; Ritchie et al., 2010; USDA/FNS, 2010; Sullivan et al., 2011; Whaley et al., 2012a,b;

Hildebrand et al., 2014; Isbell et al., 2014; USDA/FNS, 2016c). A few of these studies have examined the effects of nutrition education on participant adaptation to the 2009 food package changes in particular. In California, Ritchie et al. (2010) demonstrated that nutrition education alone led to increased consumption of low-fat milk and whole grains even before the 2009 changes to the WIC food packages. Following the change, consumption of these foods increased further (Whaley et al., 2012b). A study of the effect of the 2009 breastfeeding food package change on rates of breastfeeding demonstrated significant increases in exclusive breastfeeding in the 6 months prior to the policy change when staff training and participant education focused on the upcoming policy changes (Whaley et al., 2012a). Similar changes were not evident in other states where staff training and participant education specific to the breastfeeding food package changes were not a focus prior to the food package change. Together, these studies suggest that achieving the intended health impact of the WIC food packages and 2009 revisions is facilitated by staff training and participant education.

Finally, the electronic benefit transfer (EBT) system is designed to enhance efficiency across the program by limiting purchases to only those foods authorized by the program. However, the linked databases that code "WIC-approved" foods must be updated continually in response to changes in the marketplace, which poses an administrative burden. USDA-FNS is in the process of developing a nationally representative Universal Product Code (UPC) database in collaboration with states, which should help to alleviate some of this burden. Because WIC benefits are grouped by EBT systems at the household rather than individual level, an additional benefit of the EBT system is the flexibility it allows in food acquisition when more than one family member is a WIC participant. Another vendor-level benefit of the EBT system was demonstrated by Phillips et al. (2014), who reported that EBT implementation both improved the ability of vendors to track inventory and stabilized inventory because participants were able to make purchases throughout the month instead of during a single visit. In addition, vendor reimbursement occurred more quickly.

CHANGES IN THE WIC-PARTICIPATING POPULATION

This section provides an overview of key characteristics of the WIC-participating population and changes since 2006. Specifically, the committee examined participation rates, demographics (including income and employment status), expenditures of the WIC-participating population on food, and breastfeeding trends of the WIC-participating population compared to the U.S. population generally.

WIC Participation Rates

Although the national WIC caseload increased between 2006 and 2010 (see Figure 2-1), reaching a peak of approximately 9 million in 2010, participation declined thereafter to approximately 8 million by 2014 and continued to decline into 2015 (USDA/ERS, 2015a). The year 2014 marked the fourth consecutive year—and only the fourth year in the program's history—that participation for women, infants, and children all fell (see Figure 2-2). In parallel, between fiscal years (FYs) 2013 and 2014, overall expenditures across USDA nutrition assistance programs decreased 5 percent and participation in the Supplemental Nutrition Assistance Program (SNAP) and the National School Lunch Program decreased by 2 and 1 percent, respectively. However, during the same period, participation in the School Breakfast Program and the number of meals served in the Child and Adult Care Food Program both increased by 2 percent (USDA/ERS, 2015b).

The reasons for the overall decline in WIC participation since 2010 are unclear, but the decline may be at least partially attributable to decreasing U.S. birthrates, as well as to the nation's improving economic health. From 2007 to 2009, the United States experienced an economic downturn that may have caused more individuals to have incomes low enough to ensure eligibility for WIC. During the recession, Medicaid, SNAP, and Temporary Assistance for Needy Families (TANF), experienced increases in participation and received increased funding through the American Recovery and Reinvestment Act of 2009 (KFF, 2009, 2015; CBO, 2012; EOPUS, 2014). Participants in these programs who meet WIC age and physiological state criteria are automatically eligible for WIC. Not only has the country been experiencing a still-incomplete recovery from the recession that began in 2008, but other recent changes in Medicaid, SNAP, and TANF may have affected WIC eligibility and participation as well. Additionally, between October 1 and 16, 2013, the federal government experienced a shutdown, which resulted in a gap in funding for the WIC program at the beginning of the fiscal year. Although most states maintained WIC services, some offered modified services; program recovery was slow in some states, lasting up to a year.

In addition to these demographic and economic changes that may have influenced WIC participation between 2010 and 2015, the committee considered whether the food package changes initially implemented in 2009 may have contributed as well. To do this, the committee used state-level data on participation and the number eligible for WIC from 2006–2012 (USDA/FNS, 2011a, 2013, 2014b, 2015b; Bitler and Hoynes, 2013). The analysis considered the effects of national trends, time invariant state factors, the date of implementation of the new food package, unemployment rate, births per capita, and participation in TANF/SNAP/Unemployment Insurance (UI). Details of the estimation method are discussed in Appendix F.

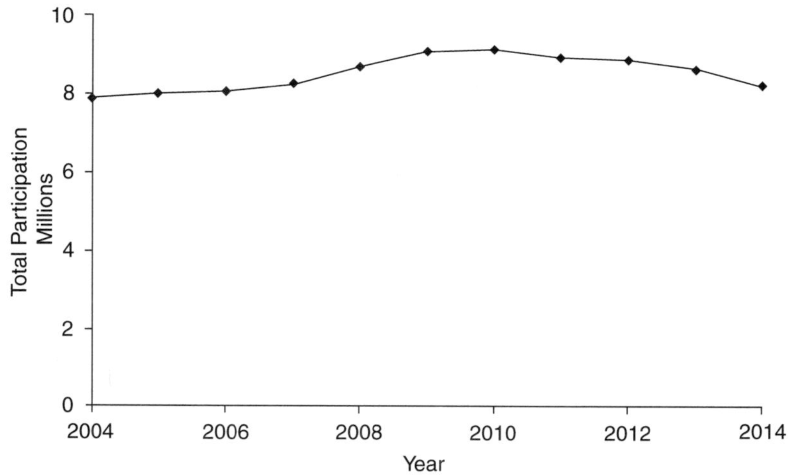

FIGURE 2-1 Annual number of participants in the WIC program constructed from monthly averages of participants, FY2004–2015.
NOTES: FY2014 is the latest complete data. Data for FY2015 may be incomplete.
SOURCE: USDA/FNS, 2016b.

The results suggest no significant difference between participation before versus after implementation of the new food packages. The estimated effect was not statistically significant, and it was small in magnitude.

Demographics of the WIC-Participating Population

WIC Participation by Age and Physiological State

The proportion of WIC participants varies among women by physiologic state and among children by age, but this proportion has remained relatively stable since 2006 (see Table 2-2). Data from 2012 indicate that 63 percent of individuals eligible for WIC nationwide participated in the program (USDA/FNS, 2015b). This includes 85 percent of eligible infants, 53 percent of eligible children, 71 percent of eligible pregnant women, and 77 percent of eligible postpartum women (USDA/FNS, 2015b). The majority of women who participate in WIC are pregnant. Of the remaining women, approximately half are breastfeeding and half are postpartum but not breastfeeding. More than half of infants are fully formula-fed. Of the remaining infants, approximately half are fully and half are partially breastfed. The majority of WIC participants are children (53 percent in 2014) (USDA/FNS, 2015c). Many eligible children discontinue participation after

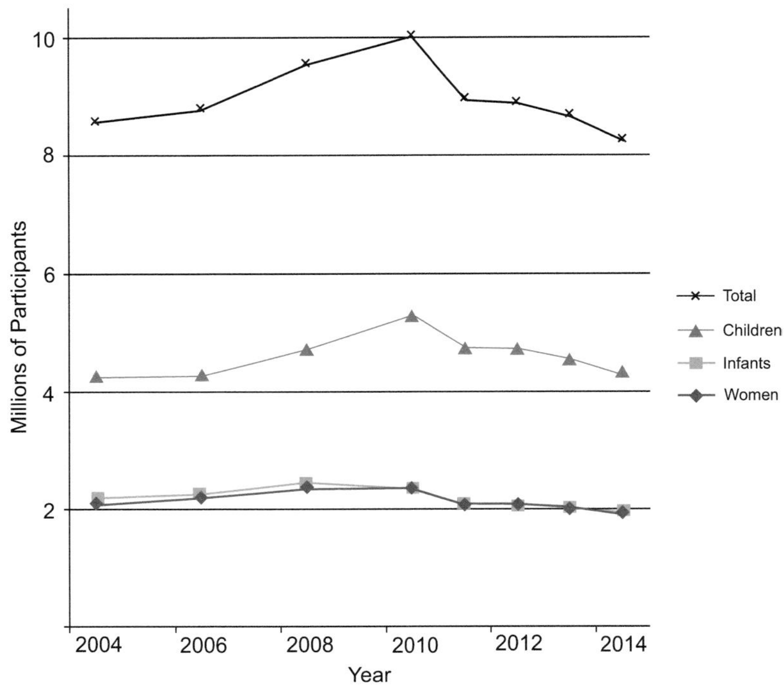

FIGURE 2-2 Average annual WIC participation by participant category, 2004–2014
NOTE: No participation data were available for 2005, 2007, or 2009.
SOURCES: USDA/FNS, 2007b, 2010, 2015b.

1 year of age (USDA/FNS, 2011a), although the specific reasons for this behavior are unknown.

Racial and Ethnic Composition of the WIC-Participating Population

WIC serves a population with a diverse racial and ethnic composition, and this composition, based on major race and ethnicity categories, has not changed more than 3 percent between 2006 and 2014 (USDA/FNS, 2007a, 2015c) (see Figures 2-3a and 2-3b). Of note in the figures below, the percentage of WIC participants who reported being white increased between 2006 and 2014 by a few percentage points (see Figure 2-3a), yet the percentage of Hispanic/Latino participants remained the same despite an increase in proportions of Hispanic people in the U.S. population (see Figure 2-3b) (USCB, 2011). There was also a decrease in the percentage of WIC participants who reported being American Indian and Alaskan Native

TABLE 2-2 Participation of Women and Children in WIC by Physiological State or Feeding Mode, FY2005–2006 and 2015–2016

	April 2006			2015–2016		
		Proportion of the WIC-Participating Population (%)			Proportion of the WIC-Participating Population (%)	
Group or Subgroup	Number of Participants Nationwide	Of Women	Of All WIC Participants	Number of Participants Nationwide	Of Women	Of All WIC Participants
Nationwide	8,772,217			8,023,742		
Total women	**2,205,594**	—	**25**	**1,923,171**	—	**24**
Pregnant women	986,433	45	11	772,151	40	10
Postpartum women	634,372	29	7	557,464	29	7
Partially BF women	NR	—	—	345,371	18	4
Fully BF women	NR	—	—	248,186	13	3
BF women	584,789	27	7	593,557	31	7
		Of Infants	Of All WIC Participants		Of Infants	Of All WIC Participants
Total infants	**2,272,626**	—	26	**1,939,740**	—	**24**
FF infants	NR	—	—	1,340,943	69	17
Partially BF infants	NR	—	—	349,113	18	4
Fully BF infants	NR	—	—	249,684	13	3
Total children	**4,293,997**	—	49	**4,160,832**	—	**52**

NOTES: BF = breastfeeding/breastfed; FF = formula-fed; NR = not reported.
SOURCES: USDA/FNS, 2007b, 2016b.

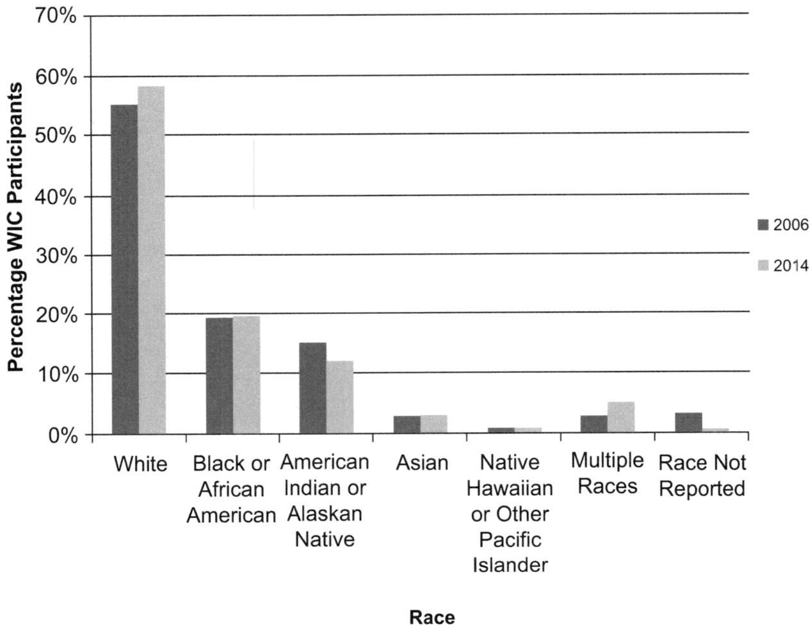

FIGURE 2-3a Distribution of race of WIC participants, 2006 and 2014.
SOURCES: USDA/FNS, 2007b, 2015c.

between 2006 and 2014. The U.S. population has increased 9 percent since 2005, with the greatest contributions to population growth from immigration, temporary and permanent residency, and other population shifts (DHS, 2014). According to the U.S. Census Bureau, the majority of growth in the U.S. population from 2000 to 2010 resulted from an increase in Hispanic and Asian populations (USCB, 2011). The 2010 American Community Survey found that 92 percent of the U.S. Hispanic population comprises 10 subgroups, with the top three being Mexican, Puerto Rican, and Cuban (Motel and Patten, 2012). Although there are no available national data on racial and ethnic subgroups in the WIC-participating population, these subgroup proportions likely reflect a national trend.

Income Distribution

The WIC-participating population is exceptionally poor compared to the general U.S. population. WIC household income is generally much lower than the qualifying income requirement of not more than 185 percent of the federal poverty-to-income ratio. In 2014, 74 percent of all WIC participants

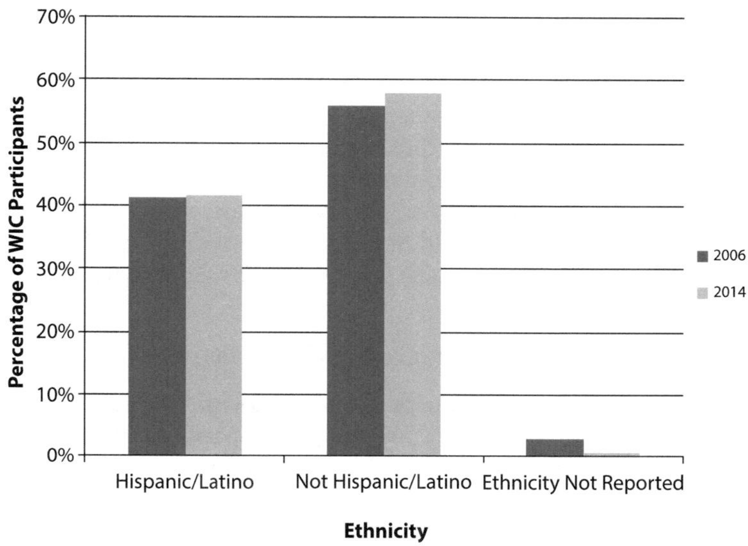

FIGURE 2-3b Distribution of ethnicity of WIC participants, 2006 and 2014.
SOURCES: USDA/FNS, 2007b, 2015c.

reported incomes at or below federal poverty guideline, with 38 percent reporting incomes equal to or less than 50 percent of the Federal poverty guideline (USDA/FNS, 2015c). This 74 percent figure represents an increase from 2006, when 67 percent of WIC participants had household incomes that fell at or below the federal poverty guideline (USDA/FNS, 2007b).

Employment Status of WIC Participants

Although data on the employment status of WIC participants were not available to the committee, U.S. Census Bureau data for 2014 indicate that 20 percent of working women (15.2 million women) were below 185 percent of poverty. Forty-one percent of these women were working full-time (6.2 million), and 59 percent were working part-time (9.0 million) (USCB, 2015). The number of low-income working families in the United States rose from 10.2 million in 2010 to 10.4 million in 2011 (Roberts et al., 2013). In 2012, 39 percent of these families were headed by working mothers (Povich et al., 2014). Among all families, the share of low-income, female-headed working families increased from 54 percent in 2007 to 58 percent in 2012 (Povich et al., 2014).

Data from the American Time Use Survey (2003–2011) indicate that full-time employment appears to be associated with significantly reduced time spent preparing food (Sliwa et al., 2015). Data from the same survey (2006–2008) show that lower income and the presence of young children are both associated with significantly more time spent in food preparation (Senia et al., 2014). A smaller study of more than 2,000 mothers in Minnesota supports this finding, and indicates that those with full-time employment spent less time on food preparation and consumed fewer vegetables and fruits compared to mothers with part-time or no employment (Bauer et al., 2012). Working mothers may also experience additional time stress that can affect preparation of healthy meals at home (Jabs and Devine, 2006; Beshara et al., 2010).

Food Expenditures of WIC Participants

The committee was tasked with planning and implementing an analysis of food expenditures for the WIC-participating population using national data. Data from the Food Acquisition and Purchase Survey (FoodAPS) (USDA/ERS, 2015c) were used in phase I to compare household expenditures on total food, food at home, and food away from home among three groups: (1) WIC-participating households, (2) WIC-eligible, nonparticipating households (i.e., households with incomes less than or equal to 185 percent of the poverty-to-income ratio and with a pregnant woman or child less than 5 years old), and (3) WIC-ineligible, nonparticipating households (i.e., households with incomes greater than 185 percent of the poverty-to-income ratio) with a pregnant woman or children less than 5 years of age (NASEM, 2016).[1]

These data also allow for examination of detailed expenditures by WIC-participating households for specific WIC food categories. As described in further detail in Chapter 10 of the phase I report (NASEM, 2016), FoodAPS is a nationally representative, stratified sampling of 4,826 households from April 2012 through January 2013. Data on food expenditures were collected over a 7-day period, with all household members asked to track and report their food purchases or acquisitions during the survey week. Information on each "event" (i.e., purchase or acquisition) included whether the food was purchased or acquired at home or away from home, total expenditure, and source of payment (i.e., specifically whether the event included use of payment with a WIC voucher and, if so, the amount of payment allotted to WIC items). Although in most cases it was not possible to know exactly which foods were obtained with the WIC food voucher (because more than one type of tender may have been reported), by examining individual food codes, purchased items could be categorized as WIC food items. Data were weighted using the household

[1] Significant differences detected in these comparisons cannot necessarily be attributed to WIC participation.

weights provided in the FoodAPS documentation.[2] Mean food expenditures were compared between WIC-participating households and both types of non-WIC-participating households using *t*-tests and the Pearson chi-square statistic (Rao and Scott, 1984).[3]

The analysis of the FoodAPS data provides evidence on the total food expenditures and expenditures on food groups for WIC-participating households to assess the relative contribution of the WIC food packages to their food expenditures. Overall, as shown in Table 2-3 (i.e., updated from Table 10-2 in the phase I report [NASEM, 2016]), the average weekly expenditures for food at home (FAH) for WIC-participating households was $124.20/week, similar to weekly expenditures of WIC-eligible, non-participating households ($113.20/week). WIC-participating households had marginally greater (p = 0.10) expenditures on food away from home (FAFH) expenditures ($60.59/week) than those of WIC-eligible, non-participating households ($47.06/week). The average value of WIC expenditures for these WIC-participating households was $10.75/week. Among all WIC-participating households (i.e., both those that made WIC purchases during the week and those that did not), this represents 8.8 percent of total FAH expenditures. Among the nearly one-third of WIC-participating households (32.3 percent) that made a purchase with a WIC benefit during the week, WIC expenditures represented 24.3 percent of reported FAH expenditures for that week.

The data also allowed comparison of expenditures for specific WIC food items among the three groups of households. As shown in Table 2-4, the overall average level of expenditures on identified WIC food items ($21.55/week) was significantly larger for WIC-participating households than for eligible non-WIC-participating households ($14.82/week, p = 0.01), and was similar to the average expenditures of the non-WIC-participating households with income greater than 185 percent of the poverty income ratio ($21.31/week). The share of WIC food items in FAH expenditures was higher for WIC-participating households than for the other households (18 percent overall for WIC-participating households, and 13 percent and 13.5 percent of total FAH expenditures for the low-income and higher-income non-WIC-participating households, respectively; p = 0.01). Among households with WIC expenditures during the week (WIC paid >0),

---

[2] All standard errors account for oversampling and the complex survey design of FoodAPS Sampling weights were constructed based on the FoodAPS survey stratification of households with the survey target groups determined by SNAP receipt and poverty status, and used to produce estimates that are nationally representative of U.S. households. To apply sampling weights, the committee used the *svyset* command in STATA (a data analysis and statistical software package) and followed guidance in FoodAPS Users Guide (USDA/ERS, 2016b).

[3] These data were generated under contract with the Center for Agricultural and Rural Development at Iowa State University, then checked by committee members.

TABLE 2-3 Summary Statistics for Weekly Food Expenditures for WIC-Participating and Other Households

	Mean Weekly Expenditures in Dollars (SE)		
Expenditure Variable	WIC-Participating Households (N = 461)	Non-WIC, Income ≤185% PIR (Pregnant, or Child <5 years) (N = 306)	Non-WIC, Income >185% PIR (Pregnant, or Child <5 years) (N = 241)
Food Expenditures (1 week)			
Total food expenditures ($)	184.78 (10.33)	160.21 (10.66)[b]	242.46 (15.45)[a]
Food at home (FAH) ($)	124.20 (6.12)	113.20 (8.10)	164.14 (13.09)[a]
Food away from home (FAFH) ($)	60.59 (6.6)	47.06 (4.92)[b]	7 8.33 (6.35)[b]
WIC Expenditure Patterns (1 week)			
% of households using WIC in week (% of total)	32.3 (3.8)		
Average value of WIC expenditures in week ($)	10.75 (1.82)		
WIC expenditures as share of total food expenditures (all WIC-participating households) (%)	5.8 (0.9)		
WIC expenditures as share of total FAH expenditures (for all WIC-participating households) (%)	8.8 (1.3)		
WIC expenditures as share of total FAH expenditures (for households with WIC event in week) (%)	24.3 (2.5)		

NOTES: FAFH = food away from home; FAH = food at home; PIR = federal poverty-to-income ratio; SE = standard error; SNAP = Supplemental Nutrition Assistance Program. Population weights were applied. This table is reproduced from Table 10-2 from the WIC committee phase I report.

[a] Significantly different from the WIC-participating households at a 1 percent level of statistical significance.

[b] Significantly different from the WIC-participating households at a 10 percent level of statistical significance.

SOURCE: USDA/ERS, 2015c.

expenditures on WIC food items averaged 29 percent of total FAH expenditures. Because WIC-participating households also used other resources to acquire WIC food items, the average value of WIC food items acquired was greater than the value of reported WIC expenditures in the week.[4]

Also shown in Table 2-4, for most of the identified food items, WIC-participating households spent more than other households. For example, WIC-participating households spent a weekly average of $1.42 on eggs, compared to $0.72 for WIC-eligible, nonparticipating households and $1.00 for non-WIC-participating higher-income households; and WIC-participating households spent $3.98 per week on milk, compared to $3.05 per week for eligible, non-WIC-participating households and $3.88 per week for non-WIC-participating higher- income households. Weekly expenditures on breakfast cereals were close in value across the three groups. WIC-participating households spent less on vegetables and fruits ($1.79/week) than did the other higher-income households ($2.60/week).[5]

The FoodAPS data show how expenditures on WIC food items were made in the "shopping trip" (event) among the household groups. At the level of purchase and acquisition events, as shown in Table 2-5, the average value of WIC expenditures as a purchase event was $21.74. Expenditures for most WIC food items were larger when WIC vouchers were used at the shopping event (WIC Paid >0) than otherwise (WIC Paid = 0). Compared to when WIC vouchers were used during an event (WIC paid >0) ($15.68/event),[6] average spending on identified WIC food items was less when WIC vouchers were not used (WIC paid = 0) ($3.58/event). The same pattern holds for most individual food items. For example, when WIC vouchers were used (WIC paid >0), WIC-participating households spent an average $3.43 on milk during a single shopping trip, compared to, on average, $0.59 when vouchers were not used (WIC paid = 0).[7] Among the low

---

[4] This could also be due to misclassification of some items as WIC-qualifying when in fact they are not. The misclassification errors would be similar across the household categories.

[5] The amount reported here as "vegetables and fruits" includes processed vegetables and fruits (with "food codes").

[6] For purchase events when WIC was used (WIC Paid >0), the analysis captured only 81 percent of the reported total WIC value spent. Possible reasons to explain why the sum of item expenses differs from the reported total WIC expenditures include the fact that not all items have a reported expenditure or imputed expenditure. This would include some of the WIC items in our calculations, including vegetables and fruits purchased with a CVV.

[7] Of note is the relatively low value of expenditures on vegetables and fruits during WIC shopping events ($0.10), compared to what participants redeemed when vouchers were not used ($0.45). The very small value recorded for expenditures on vegetables and fruits when WIC benefits were used in the event (WIC Paid >0) may reflect misreporting of the vegetables and fruits expenditures when using the CVV. Underreporting and misclassification of food expenditures acquired with WIC benefits would mean that the total amount of WIC expenditures is underestimated.

TABLE 2-4 Weekly Household Expenditures: Total Expenditures, Expenditures When WIC Is Used (WIC Paid >0) and When WIC Is Not Used (WIC Paid = 0)

	WIC Participating Households			Non-WIC, Income ≤185% (Pregnant or Child <5)	Non-WIC, Income >185% (Pregnant or Child <5)
		WIC Paid >0	WIC Paid = 0		
	N = 461	N = 150	N = 311	N = 306	N = 241
Total food at home expenditure (FAH) ($)	124.18 (7.62)	160.92 (9.30)	106.77 (9.66)	113.15 (8.07)	164.14 (13.09)
Total WIC expenditure ($)	10.75 (1.82)	33.42 (4.09)			
WIC food item expenditure ($)	21.55 (2.03)	41.44 (3.58)	12.13 (1.60)	14.82 (1.24)[a]	21.31 (2.01)
WIC items/Total FAH Expenditure (%)	17.90 (1.37)	29.21 (2.51)	11.55 (1.01)	13.14 (1.10)[a]	13.46 (0.82)[a]
	($)	($)	($)	($)	($)
Breakfast cereal	2.40 (0.38)	5.08 (0.80)	1.13 (0.30)	2.49 (0.29)	2.31 (0.35)
Infant cereal	0.03 (0.03)	0.01 (0.01)	0.04 (0.04)	0.02 (0.02)	0.02 (0.02)
Infant vegetable and fruit	0.56 (0.21)	1.08 (0.55)	0.31 (0.16)	0.34 (0.15)	0.45 (0.20)

Infant meat	0.02 (0.01)	0.02 (0.02)	0.02 (0.02)	0.09 (0.07)	0.01 (0.01)
Infant formula	3.21 (1.23)	9.62 (3.72)	0.17 (0.12)	0.48 (0.21)[b]	0.96 (0.59)[c]
Milk	3.98 (0.40)	7.19 (0.68)	2.46 (0.40)	3.05 (0.31)[c]	3.88 (0.39)
Cheese	3.20 (0.37)	4.90 (0.55)	2.44 (0.46)	2.54 (0.32)	5.07 (1.04)[c]
Soy milk	0.27 (0.11)	0.55 (0.32)	0.15 (0.08)	0.22 (0.09)	0.23 (0.08)
Eggs	1.42 (0.21)	2.04 (0.30)	1.13 (0.26)	0.72 (0.09)[a]	1.00 (0.17)
Legumes	0.64 (0.14)	0.77 (0.27)	0.57 (0.16)	0.61 (0.16)	0.43 (0.11)
Peanut butter	0.35 (0.10)	0.78 (0.23)	0.14 (0.09)	0.26 (0.08)	0.09 (0.03)[b]
Vegetable and fruit	1.79 (0.31)	2.53 (0.53)	1.45 (0.37)	1.44 (0.27)	2.60 (0.37)[c]
Fish	0.21 (0.07)	0.21 (0.08)	0.21 (0.10)	0.25 (0.08)	0.05 (0.02)[b]
Bread	0.49 (0.14)	1.33 (0.36)	0.09 (0.04)	0.19 (0.07)[b]	0.34 (0.11)[b]
Juice	1.76 (0.27)	3.32 (0.63)	1.03 (0.17)	1.13 (0.18)[c]	1.49 (0.29)
Yogurt	1.21 (0.24)	2.12 (0.48)	0.78 (0.25)	0.96 (0.20)	2.18 (0.43)[b]
Tofu	– (–)	– (–)	– (–)	0.02 (0.01)	0.19 (0.13)

NOTES: FAH = food at home. Population weights were applied.
[a] Significantly different from the WIC-participating households at a 1 percent level of statistical significance.
[b] Significantly different from the WIC-participating households at a 5 percent level of statistical significance.
[c] Significantly different from the WIC-participating households at a 10 percent level of statistical significance.
SOURCE: USDA/ERS, 2015c.

TABLE 2-5 Food Expenditures Events During Week: Total for Event, Amount WIC Paid (WIC Paid >0) and Other Paid (WIC Paid = 0)

	WIC Participating Households			Non-WIC, Income ≤185% (Pregnant or Child <5)	Non-WIC, Income >185% (Pregnant or Child <5)
		WIC Paid >0	WIC Paid = 0		
	N = 1,967	N = 252	N = 1,715	N = 1,055	N = 826
Total food at home (FAH) expenditure in event ($)	29.54 (1.37)	25.42 (3.03)	30.09 (1.5)	33.6 (2.03)	47.82 (3.16)[a]
Total WIC expenditure in event ($)		21.74 (2.26)			
WIC food item expenditure in event ($)	4.96 (0.33)	15.68 (1.54)	3.58 (0.28)	4.31 (0.32)	6.15 (0.54)
WIC items/total FAH expenditure in events (%)	21.73 (1.60)	68.02 (4.42)	15.13 (1.54)	14.88 (1.90)	13.73 (1.06)[c]
WIC items/WIC expenditure in events (%)		81.47 (8.18)			
	$	$	$	$	$
Breakfast cereal	0.55 (0.08)	1.39 (0.25)	0.45 (0.09)	0.72 (0.09)	0.67 (0.10)
Infant cereal	0.01 (0.01)	-	0.01 (0.01)	0.00 (0.00)	0.01 (0.00)
Infant vegetable and fruit	0.13 (0.05)	0.55 (0.36)	0.07 (0.03)	0.1 (0.03)	0.13 (0.05)

Infant meat	0.01 (0.00)	– (–)	0.01 (0.00)	0.03 (0.02)	0.00 (0.00)
Infant formula	0.74 (0.20)	5.61 (1.62)	0.11 (0.05)	0.14 (0.06)[a]	0.28 (0.13)[c]
Milk	0.91 (0.09)	3.43 (0.38)	0.59 (0.08)	0.89 (0.08)	1.12 (0.12)
Cheese	0.74 (0.09)	1.24 (0.27)	0.67 (0.09)	0.74 (0.09)	1.46 (0.25)
Soy milk	0.06 (0.03)	0.15 (0.08)	0.05 (0.03)	0.06 (0.02)	0.07 (0.02)
Eggs	0.33 (0.05)	0.64 (0.12)	0.29 (0.05)	0.21 (0.03)[b]	0.29 (0.05)
Legumes	0.15 (0.03)	0.23 (0.05)	0.14 (0.03)	0.18 (0.05)	0.13 (0.03)
Peanut butter	0.08 (0.02)	0.33 (0.09)	0.05 (0.02)	0.07 (0.02)	0.03 (0.01)[b]
Vegetable and fruit	0.41 (0.05)	0.10 (0.03)	0.45 (0.06)	0.42 (0.08)	0.75 (0.10)[a]
Fish	0.05 (0.02)	0.01 (0.01)	0.05 (0.02)	0.42 (0.08)[a]	0.02 (0.01)[c]
Bread	0.11 (0.03)	0.63 (0.15)	0.05 (0.02)	0.07 (0.02)	0.10 (0.03)
Juice	0.41 (0.05)	1.36 (0.27)	0.28 (0.04)	0.06 (0.02)[a]	0.43 (0.08)
Yogurt	0.28 (0.05)	0.03 (0.02)	0.31 (0.06)	0.28 (0.06)	0.63 (0.13)[b]
Tofu	– (–)	– (–)	– (–)	0.01 (0.00)	0.05 (0.04)

NOTES: Population weights were applied.

[a] Significantly different from the WIC-participating households at a 1 percent level of statistical significance.

[b] Significantly different from the WIC-participating households at a 5 percent level of statistical significance.

[c] Significantly different from the WIC-participating households at a 10 percent level of statistical significance.

SOURCE: USDA/ERS, 2015c.

income households, WIC-participating households had higher expenditures for infant formula, eggs, and juice in shopping trips (shopping events) compared with other low income households.

The analysis of expenditure patterns among the three groups of households shows that the expenditures of WIC-participating households differ from other households in several ways. In comparison to other eligible households with income less than 185 percent of the poverty-to-income threshold, WIC-participating households spent more on total food expenditures and more on FAFH. Comparable households with higher-income spent more than WIC-participating households both in total and for FAH and FAFH. WIC-participating households spent more on identified WIC food items in a week than did comparable households with income less than 185 percent of the poverty-to-income ratio. The amount spent on identified WIC food items was comparable to the spending level of the higher-income, non-WIC-participating households.

Breastfeeding Trends in the WIC-Participating Population Compared to the U.S. Population

Healthy People 2020's goals for breastfeeding are presented in Table 2-6 (HHS, 2015). In 2011, the U.S. Surgeon General called for action to support these goals, recommending that families, communities, health care centers, and employment sites provide the support necessary for women to initiate and continue breastfeeding (HHS, 2011). To assess progress toward reaching these goals, the U.S. Centers for Disease Control and Prevention (CDC) estimates breastfeeding prevalence across the United States every 2 years, using data from the U.S. National Immunization Survey. The most recent estimates reflect statistics for children born in 2013 and represent survey data from 2014 and 2015 (see Table 2-6). As shown in the table,

TABLE 2-6 *Healthy People 2020* Breastfeeding Objectives Compared to 2014–2015 Proportion (%) of Children Who Were Breastfed at Various Ages

Breastfeeding Behavior and Infant Age	*Healthy People 2020*: Objectives	2014–2015 U.S. Breastfeeding Prevalence
Proportion who ever breastfed	81.9	81.1
Proportion breastfed at 6 months	60.6	51.8
Proportion breastfed at 1 year	34.1	30.7
Proportion exclusively breastfed at 3 months	46.2	44.4
Proportion exclusively breastfed at 6 months	25.5	22.3

SOURCES: HHS, 2015; CDC, 2016a.

although the national goal for initiation of breastfeeding has nearly been achieved, goals for duration of breastfeeding have been more challenging to meet (CDC, 2016a). This may result, in part, from differences in breastfeeding behavior related to racial and ethnic groups, maternal education and age, and WIC participation (CDC, 2010).

In addition to varying by income, the proportion of women that breastfeed varies among racial and ethnic groups. In 2009 and 2013, for example, the prevalence of breastfeeding at 6 months was consistently lowest for non-Hispanic African Americans (33 and 39 percent of infants, respectively) and non-Hispanic American Indian/Alaska Native (39 and 41 percent, respectively) and highest for non-Hispanic Asian (86 and 84 percent, respectively) (see Table 2-7). Studies of breastfeeding prevalence in the WIC-participating population show similar variation, with fewer African-American women initiating and sustaining breastfeeding compared to other racial and ethnic groups (Hurley et al., 2008; Marshall et al., 2013; McKinney et al., 2016). The underlying reasons for racial and ethnic differences in breastfeeding prevalence are not well understood at this time, but differences among racial/ethnic groups in ever breastfeeding are now relatively small (from 79 to 99 percent of the proportion of non-Hispanic whites who ever breastfed) (see Figure 2-4). There are much larger differences among racial/ethnic groups in continued breastfeeding at 6 months (from 36 to 111 percent of the proportion of non-Hispanic whites who continued to breastfeed at 6 months) (see Figure 2-4).

In the WIC-participating population, the most recent WIC Participant and Program Characteristics (PC2014) report indicated that, in 2014,

TABLE 2-7 Prevalence of Ever Breastfeeding and Breastfeeding at 6-Months Postpartum by Race: 2009 and 2013

	Breastfeeding Prevalence (%)			
	Ever Breastfed		Still Breastfeeding at 6 Months	
Race/Ethnicity	2009	2013	2009	2013
Hispanic	80.1	83.0	47.4	45.6
Non-Hispanic white	77.7	84.3	48.6	57.9
Non-Hispanic African American	60.7	66.3	33.4	39.1
Non-Hispanic Asian	86.3	83.8	65.2	64.4
Non-Hispanic American Indian/Alaska Native	69.1	68.3	39.4	41.3
Two or more races	72.9	79.0	44.4	51.0

NOTES: Data are not adjusted for income.
SOURCE: CDC, 2016b.

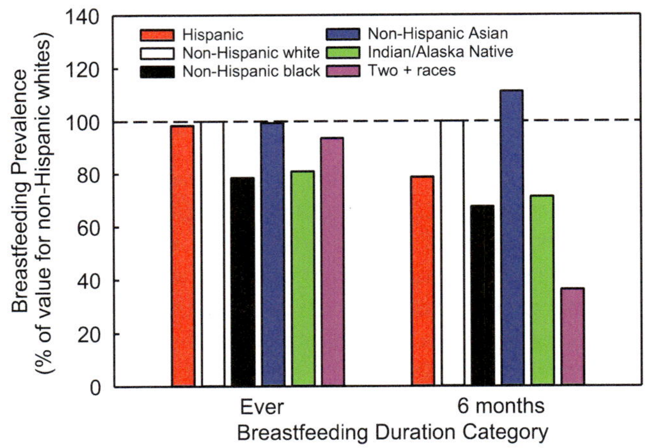

FIGURE 2-4 Breastfeeding prevalence by racial/ethnic group expressed as a percentage of values for non-Hispanic whites: United States, 2013.
SOURCE: HHS, 2015.

70 percent of infants (served by agencies that provided data) were ever breastfed (USDA/FNS, 2015c). Although other measures of breastfeeding prevalence were available to the committee, the longest time-series for which all-infant and WIC-infant prevalence of breastfeeding could be compared was at 6 months of age (see Figure 2-5) (1971 through 2013 for U.S. infants; 1978–2013 for WIC infants) (Ryan et al., 2002; CDC, 2015). In 2013, all-infant 6-month breastfeeding prevalence was 49 percent, while the WIC-infant estimate was 39 percent. Although a lower proportion of WIC infants were breastfed than those in the general population, the prevalence of breastfeeding in both groups has been increasing since the late 1970s.

Six-month breastfeeding prevalence in the U.S. population has consistently tracked with income. As shown in Table 2-8, from 2008 to 2013, 6-month breastfeeding prevalence ranged from as low as 33 to 38 percent for women under 100 percent of the poverty level to as high as 60 to 70 percent in women at 600 percent or more of the poverty level (CDC, 2016b). Although breastfeeding increased during this time period for women in all income levels, increases between 2008 and 2013 were highest among women with income above 200 percent of the poverty level. Other available data indicate that between 2004 and 2008, breastfeeding prevalence was lower for WIC-participating women compared to WIC-eligible, nonparticipating women, with substantial differences across racial/ethnic groups (CDC, 2010).

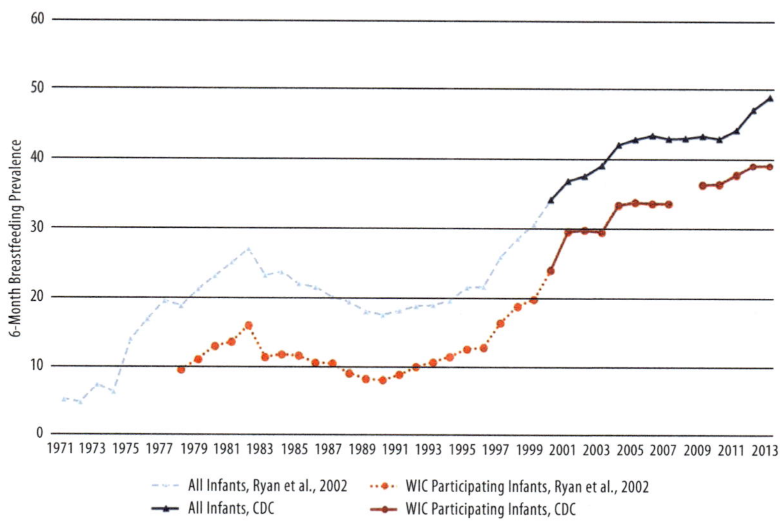

FIGURE 2-5 Six-month breastfeeding prevalence: 1971–2013.
NOTES: Data exclusively for WIC eligible, nonparticipants were not available. Therefore, the comparison of all infants to WIC infants is an underestimate of the difference of interest, namely WIC nonparticipants vs. WIC-participating infants. Two data sources were used to construct this time series: the Ross Laboratories Mothers' Survey (Ryan et al., 2002) and the Centers for Disease Control and Prevention (CDC, 2015). The Ross Laboratories Mothers' Survey is a large national survey conducted by Ross Laboratories, a manufacturer of infant formula. Ross sent questionnaires each month to a sample of mothers. Nearly 1 million surveys were sent annually in the 1990s (Ryan, 2005). For example, in 1996, 744,000 questionnaires were mailed (Ryan et al., 2002). Data for 1971 to 1999 are from the Ross Mothers' Survey. Line breaks indicate missing data.
SOURCES: Ryan et al., 2002; CDC, 2015.

TABLE 2-8 6-Month Breastfeeding Prevalence (%) in the United States by Income from 2008 to 2013

Income Relative to Poverty Level	2008	2009	2010	2011	2012	2013
Less than 100%	33.5	35.7	38.1	37.8	37.7	38.2
100–199%	41.3	44.7	42.5	45.5	49.1	47.0
200–399%	50.0	53.4	55.1	57.7	59.5	60.4
400–599%	55.1	61.1	59.3	61.9	66.3	65.9
600% or greater	60.2	61.7	65.4	67.9	70.4	70.1

SOURCE: National Immunization Survey Data, as analyzed by the Centers for Disease Control and Prevention (CDC, 2016b).

Promotion of Breastfeeding in the WIC Program

A number of breastfeeding promotion and support strategies have been in place as part of *Healthy People 2020* that may have helped to increase the prevalence of breastfeeding in both WIC-participating and non-WIC-participating populations. These include strategies to increase the proportion of employers that have worksite lactation support programs, reduce the proportion of breastfed newborns that receive formula supplementation within the first 2 days of life, and increase the proportion of live births that occur in facilities that provide recommended care for lactating mothers and their infants (HHS, 2015). The Baby-Friendly Hospital Initiative has been assisting hospitals with meeting these goals (IOM, 2011b; WHO, 2012).

Additionally, since the food package revisions implemented in 2009, there has been a concerted effort within WIC to increase the proportion of women who breastfeed. The committee's phase I review of breastfeeding (see Chapter 7 in NASEM, 2016) found that the 2009 changes to the food package were associated with small improvements in breastfeeding initiation (USDA/FNS, 2011a; Whaley et al., 2012a; Chiasson et al., 2013; Langellier et al., 2014; Joyce and Reeder, 2015). However, it was not possible to determine whether these improvements resulted from the food package changes themselves, the enhanced breastfeeding promotion and support activities begun at about the same time, or both.

As of 1996, states were no longer required to conduct an annual evaluation of breastfeeding promotion and support activities (P.L. 104-193, Personal Responsibility and Work Opportunity Reconciliation Act of 1996). As a result, other than in Whaley et al. (2012a), little information exists as to which specific breastfeeding promotion and support activities within WIC have been the most successful. Implementation of the USDA's Loving Support© program is one way that WIC breastfeeding activities are supported, but implementation varies depending upon available state-level resources.

USDA-FNS Guidance Related to Provision of Infant Formula

Provision of Infant Formula in the First Month

The choice to breastfeed is complex; protection, promotion, and support activities must be in place to ensure success (Pérez-Escamilla and Chapman, 2012; Pérez-Escamilla et al., 2012).[8] The introduction of formula during the first weeks after birth is a risk factor for both shorter duration of exclusive and also any breastfeeding (Walker, 2015). In accordance,

[8] The committee recognizes that some women are unable to breastfeed fully.

the most recent WIC breastfeeding guidance issued by USDA-FNS states that the WIC program's intent is that all women be supported to breastfeed exclusively. For women who want to breastfeed, it states: "Infant formula in the first month may only be issued after careful assessment of the mother and infant by staff with breastfeeding training. If it is determined some formula is appropriate for the infant in the first month, the mother should be advised on the appropriate amount of formula to feed the infant" (USDA/FNS, 2016a). The current WIC food packages reflect this guidance. The food packages for breastfed infants from 0–1 month of age have no formula, or (at the state's option) up to one can of powder infant formula in the container size that provides closest to 104 reconstituted fluid ounces on a case-by-case basis. Infants who need more than 104 ounces of formula in the first month (or need any formula in states that do not allow one can) must be issued the fully formula-fed package.

Tailoring the Amounts of Formula Issued

The USDA-FNS guidance document referenced above also advises tailoring of infant formula issuance: "The goal is to provide as *minimal* an amount of supplemental formula as is needed, while offering counseling and support, in order to help the mother establish and maintain successful milk production" (USDA/FNS, 2016a). The full nutrition benefit is designed to provide close to 100 percent of the nutritional needs of the nonbreastfed infant from birth to 6 months. There are currently limited data available that describe the feeding patterns of women who receive the full nutrition benefit. One study conducted in California (Whaley et al., 2012a) documented that food packages are generally well aligned with actual feeding practices, but there is still some misalignment: 12 percent of mothers who receive the full formula package from 0–6 months reported doing some breastfeeding. This suggests the potential for overfeeding and supports the need for careful assessment of the mother and infant by staff with breastfeeding training to adequately assess the formula needs of all dyads. A larger study of food package alignment with feeding behavior was recently included in the *USDA FNS 2016 Research and Evaluation Plan* (USDA/FNS, 2016c).

Evidence for the Benefits of Breastfeeding Promotion and Support in WIC

At present, the availability and implementation of breastfeeding support and promotion activities at the state level are highly variable. Some variation is linked to available resources, and some may reflect differing needs of state-specific WIC-participating populations. The best example of these activities in the WIC program is in California, where Whaley et al.

(2012a) found that when breastfeeding support and promotion efforts were paired with the new food packages, the proportion of WIC participants who chose to fully breastfeed increased by 86 percent. The specific activities implemented included two statewide campaigns. First, the Healthy Habits for Life campaign was the staff wellness component of the campaign that started 9 months prior to the food package changes and included training materials to help WIC staff make healthy lifestyle changes in preparation for helping WIC participants to make those same changes.[9] Second, the Healthy Habits Begin at Birth campaign, started 6 months before the food package changes, focused on pregnant women, postpartum and breastfeeding women, and infants. This helped prepare WIC families for the upcoming food package changes that related to infant feeding, especially breastfeeding and introducing baby foods. The finding that the proportion of women choosing the fully breastfeeding packages started to increase before the actual food package changes, and then increased even more substantially after the changes and have been maintained, suggests that pairing support and educational activities with policy changes has maximal effect on participant behavior change. However, as a result of budget constraints, breastfeeding support resources are not universally available to all women participating in WIC who choose to breastfeed.

Effects of the 2009 Food Package Changes on the Choice to Breastfeed

The food packages implemented in 2009 were designed to encourage exclusive breastfeeding by allowing very limited issuance of infant formula to breastfeeding women in the first 30 days postpartum. States may allow the issuance of one can of formula in the infant's first month of life, but they are not permitted to create food packages that routinely issue formula to breastfeeding women during this period (USDA/FNS, 2014a). Although the intention of this policy was to support breastfeeding in the immediate postpartum period, evidence indicates the policy had an unintended consequence because women had to choose between two options: (1) receive no formula from WIC, or (2) receive the maximum formula allowance provided to nonbreastfeeding mothers. In some states, a third option to receive 1 can of formula is available in the first month. The results of the largest study of the impact of the food package changes on breastfeeding rates showed that there were no changes in breastfeeding initiation that could be attributed to the revised food packages (USDA/FNS, 2011b). Although

[9] A full description of the Healthy Habits campaigns can be found at https://www.cdph.ca.gov/programs/wicworks/Pages/WICHealthyHabits2009.aspx (accessed December 19, 2016).

issuance of the full breastfeeding package (the first option noted above) increased in the first month, there was also an increase in issuance of the full-formula package (the second option noted above) (USDA/FNS, 2011b). The results of this study also indicated that although issuance of the full breastfeeding package was higher in the first month after implementation of the 2009 food packages, the transition of infants out of this package and into a partially breastfeeding or fully formula-feeding package occurred at a significantly faster rate compared to before implementation of the 2009 food packages. Although there is some evidence that the allowance of one can of formula in the first month helps support breastfeeding, data are not available on either the impact of a one-can policy or its breadth of implementation.

Barriers and Incentives to Breastfeeding in the WIC-Participating Population

The committee's phase I report (NASEM, 2016, Chapter 7) covered barriers, motivators and incentives for breastfeeding as well as the effect of the WIC breastfeeding food package on breastfeeding promotion, initiation, and duration among both WIC and low-income populations. Identified barriers to breastfeeding were numerous and included social norms, cultural factors, social structures, employment,[10] and biomedical factors (see Table 7-4 in NASEM, 2016), although the influence of each specific barrier on breastfeeding in the WIC-participating population could not be determined.

There is some evidence that breastfeeding promotion and support provided through the WIC program improves breastfeeding initiation (Olson et al., 2010; Whaley et al, 2012a; Haider et al., 2014; Hildebrand et al., 2014) and duration (Bonuck et al., 2005; Olson et al., 2010; Pugh et al., 2010; Chapman et al., 2013; Haider et al., 2014; Reeder et al., 2014). Data are less convincing for the effects of promotion and support on exclusivity of breastfeeding (Anderson et al., 2005, 2007; Bonuck et al., 2005; Hayes et al., 2008; Meehan et al., 2008; Hopkinson and Konefal Gallagher, 2009; Petrova et al., 2009; Sandy et al., 2009; Bunik et al., 2010; Olson et al., 2010; Pugh et al., 2010; Kandiah, 2011; Chapman et al., 2013; Haider et al., 2014; Hildebrand et al., 2014; Howell et al., 2014; Reeder et al., 2014). WIC participants may perceive that the program delivers conflicting messages by supporting breastfeeding while also distributing infant formula at no cost to participants (Holmes et al., 2009).

[10] Following the release of the phase I report, the literature search update identified additional references. In Dunn et al. (2015), employment status was significantly associated with breastfeeding duration. Over half of women breastfeeding for 6 months or longer were not employed full time or part time.

WIC participation has been associated with a lower proportion of women who initiate breastfeeding and shorter durations of exclusive and any breastfeeding compared to women not participating in WIC (Li et al., 2005; Hendricks et al., 2006; Ryan and Zhou, 2006; Jacknowitz and Tiehen, 2007; Flower et al., 2008; Bunik et al., 2009; Ziol-Guest and Hernandez, 2010; Jensen, 2012; Mao et al., 2012; Marshall et al., 2013; Ma et al., 2014; Bullinger and Gurley-Calvez, 2016; Gregory et al., 2016). However, these findings are dependent upon methodology applied and treatment of selection bias.[11] Using variation in food prices as an instrumental variable (as a means of controlling for selection bias), it was reported that WIC participation decreases the proportion of women that exclusively breastfeed by nearly 50 percent (Bullinger and Gurley-Calvez, 2016). Yet, Gregory et al. (2016), using a propensity-matching method, reported that WIC participation was not associated with a lower likelihood of breastfeeding at 3 months and that WIC participants and nonparticipants differed with respect to baseline factors that predict breastfeeding. Both studies used the Infant Feeding Practices II dataset to develop their samples. Evidence on the effect of timing of entry into WIC on these outcomes is not conclusive (Joyce et al., 2008; Ziol-Guest and Hernandez, 2010; Tenfelde et al., 2011; Langellier et al., 2012; Ma and Magnus, 2012; Jacobson et al., 2015; Metallinos-Katsaras et al., 2015).

WIC PROGRAM COSTS OVER TIME

Any changes to the food packages to be recommended by the committee are required to be cost-neutral so the current average food package cost (with adjustments for inflation) can be maintained. Total WIC costs, including Food and Nutrition Services administration, were $6.2 billion in 2015, representing a decrease of almost $1 billion from 2011, when total costs were $7.2 billion. Average per participant monthly food costs have also declined, to $43.37 in 2015, from $46.69 in 2011 (USDA/FNS, 2016b) (see Table 2-9).

Major cost savings are made available to the WIC program through the infant formula rebate system. The total dollar value of rebates received from infant formula manufacturers by WIC state agencies in FY2015 was $1.8 billion, an increase of about $124 million since 2012, when $1.69 billion in rebates were received (USDA/FNS, 2016b) (see Table 2-10).

[11] See Chapter 4 for a discussion of selection bias.

TABLE 2-9 WIC Program Costs, 2005–2015

Year	Participation (millions)	Program Costs for Food (millions of dollars)	Average Monthly Food Cost Per Person (dollars)
2005	8,023	3,602.80	37.42
2006	8,088	3,597.50	37.07
2007	8,285	3,881.10	39.04
2008	8,705	4,534.00	43.40
2009	9,122	4,640.90	42.40
2010	9,175	4,561.80	41.43
2011	8,961	5,020.20	46.69
2012	8,908	4,810.50	45.00
2013	8,663	4,497.10	43.26
2014	8,258	4,324.40	43.64
2015	8,024	4,176.20	43.37

NOTES: Participation data are annual averages in millions. In addition to food and nutrition services and administrative costs, total expenditures include funds for program evaluation, Farmers' Market Nutrition Program (FY1989 onward), special projects and infrastructure. Nutrition services includes nutrition education, preventative and coordination services (such as health care), and promotion of breastfeeding and immunization. FY2015 data are preliminary; all data are subject to revision.
SOURCE: USDA/FNS, 2016b.

TABLE 2-10 WIC Infant Formula and Food Rebates, 2005–2015

Fiscal Year	Rebates (millions of dollars)
2005	1,709.77
2006	1,774.95
2007	1,902.74
2008	2,006.80
2009	1,937.42
2010	1,692.04
2011	1,314.10
2012	1,688.17
2013	1,876.85
2014	1,812.34
2015	1,799.20

NOTES: Data for 2008–2011 are rebates billed during the fiscal year. Data for 2012–2015 are rebates received during a fiscal year. Values reflect rebates on infant formula and, to a lesser extent, infant food.
SOURCES: USDA/FNS, 2016b (years 2008–2015); Personal communication, V. Oliveira, USDA-ERS, July 23, 2014 (years 2005–2007).

RELEVANT CHANGES IN THE ENVIRONMENT SINCE 2006: DIETARY PATTERNS, THE FOOD SUPPLY, AND DIETARY GUIDANCE

In this section, changes in the environment since the previous food package review that have implications for the revised food packages are summarized. These include changes in dietary patterns in the U.S. population, an expansion of the variety of foods available in the marketplace, and changes in dietary guidance.

Dietary Patterns of Americans Have Changed

There have been several changes in consumption of food groups by the U.S. population since the 2006 report. Most notably, after decades of increases, mean energy intake decreased significantly between 2003–2004 and 2009–2010 for the U.S. population overall (Ford and Dietz, 2013). Additionally, between 2007–2008 and 2011–2012 (periods immediately before and after the 2009 food package changes), in women 20 years and older, consumption of whole grains increased 34 percent, consumption of seafood low in omega-3 fatty acids increased by 26 percent, and consumption of nuts and seeds increased by 28 percent (see Table 2-11). In contrast, consumption of soy products decreased by 30 percent. Between 2007–2008 and 2011–2012, in children ages 2–5 years, consumption of seafood high in omega-3 doubled, yogurt consumption increased by 83 percent, and consumption of whole grains increased by 46 percent (see Table 2-12). The committee's analysis (see Chapter 4) indicated that, despite these increases, intakes of whole grains and seafood are nonetheless below recommended amounts for both WIC-eligible women and children. Economic Research Service (ERS) data indicate that per capita wheat product consumption (whole grain and refined) has declined since 2000 (USDA/ERS, 2016a), a trend which could be related to consumer interests in lowering carbohydrate intake or in gluten-free products. Although comparison of 2007–2008 and 2011–2012 is provided for discussion, the direction and magnitude of change varies depending upon the survey years compared.

Expansion of the Variety of Foods Available in the Marketplace Since 2006

According to an ERS report on trends in new food products in the United States (USDA/ERS, 2014a), from 2006 to 2010, the share of new products in the categories of fruit and vegetables, dairy products, pasta and rice, and infant food increased while the share of new snack product

TABLE 2-11 Trends in Food Consumption from Selected Food Groups: Mean Intakes for U.S Women, 20 Years and Older, NHANES 2005–2012

Food Group	Mean Intake Per Day				Percent Change from Before to After the 2009 FP Changes (2007–2008 to 2011–2012)[b]
	2005–2006[a]	2007–2008	2009–2010	2011–2012	
Total fruit (c-eq)	0.88	0.92	1.06	0.96	4
Total vegetables (c-eq)	1.48	1.42	1.46	1.51	6
Whole grains (oz-eq)	0.67	0.68	0.81	0.91	34
Refined grains (oz-eq)	4.87	4.71	4.75	4.92	4
Seafood low omega-3 (oz-eq)	0.43	0.31	0.46	0.39	26
Seafood high omega-3 (oz-eq)	0.16	0.12	0.15	0.12	0
Eggs (oz-eq)	0.42	0.41	0.43	0.43	5
Soy products (oz-eq)	0.06	0.10	0.08	0.07	-30
Nuts and seeds (oz-eq)	0.54	0.54	0.58	0.69	28
Total protein foods (oz-eq)	4.89	4.72	4.87	4.82	2
Milk (c-eq)	0.85	0.75	0.78	0.70	-7
Cheese (c-eq)	0.59	0.57	0.63	0.63	11
Yogurt (c-eq)	0.06	0.06	0.08	0.07	17
Total dairy (c-eq)	1.51	1.41	1.50	1.43	1
Oils (g-eq)	19.20	19.06	19.92	22.83	20
Solid fat (g-eq)	33.94	33.02	30.84	30.64	-7
Added sugars (tsp-eq)	14.83	15.80	15.24	15.37	-3

NOTES: c-eq = cup-equivalents; FP = food package; g-eq = gram-equivalents; oz-eq = ounce-equivalents; tsp-eq = teaspoon-equivalents.

[a] During this time period, the revised food packages were conceived by the Institute of Medicine committee (see IOM, 2006).

[b] The direction of these changes varies if different sets of survey years are compared. The changes are not associated with the WIC food packages.

SOURCES: USDA/ARS, 2005–2012; USDA/ARS, 2014.

and beverage introductions decreased. The variety of available fresh fruit has been robust over the past decade, possibly spurred by a greater ethnic diversity of consumers (Bentley and Pérez, 2015). On the other hand, the availability of 100% fruit juice has fallen steadily since its peak in 1977. Availability per capita of 100% orange juice, which accounts for half of the availability all fruit juice in the United States, decreased 54 percent between 1977 and 2012 (Bentley and Pérez, 2015).

TABLE 2-12 Trends in Food Consumption from Selected Food Groups: Mean Intakes for U.S. Children, 2 to 5 Years of Age, NHANES 2005–2012

Food Group	Mean Intake Per Day				Percent Change from Before to After the 2009 FP Changes (2007–2008 to 2011–2012)[b]
	2005–2006[a]	2007–2008	2009–2010	2011–2012	
Total fruit (c-eq)	1.38	1.49	1.46	1.41	-5
Total vegetables (c-eq)	0.74	0.70	0.67	0.66	-6
Whole grains (oz-eq)	0.49	0.46	0.70	0.67	46
Refined grains (oz-eq)	4.20	4.05	4.03	4.41	9
Seafood low omega-3 (oz-eq)	0.17	0.11	0.12	0.13	18
Seafood high omega-3 (oz-eq)	0.04	0.01	0.03	0.02	100
Eggs (oz-eq)	0.28	0.34	0.31	0.32	-6
Soy products (oz-eq)	0.03	0.03	0.04	0.03	0
Nuts and seeds (oz-eq)	0.27	0.24	0.32	0.29	21
Total protein foods (oz-eq)	2.86	2.90	3.00	2.90	0
Milk (c-eq)	1.63	1.67	1.70	1.62	-3
Cheese (c-eq)	0.47	0.49	0.59	0.56	14
Yogurt (c-eq)	0.07	0.06	0.08	0.11	83
Total dairy (c-eq)	2.18	2.23	2.38	2.30	3
Oils (g-eq)	13.83	13.23	13.03	15.00	13
Solid fat (g-eq)	29.21	29.88	28.96	29.77	0
Added sugars (tsp-eq)	13.72	12.96	12.45	12.92	0

NOTES: c-eq = cup-equivalents; FP = food package; g-eq = gram-equivalents; oz-eq = ounce-equivalents; tsp-eq = teaspoon-equivalents.

[a] During this time period, the revised food packages were conceived by the Institute of Medicine committee (see IOM, 2006).

[b] The direction of these changes varies if different sets of survey years are compared. The changes are not associated with the WIC food packages.

SOURCES: USDA/ARS, 2005–2012; USDA/ARS, 2014.

The introduction of new-product claims gives some indication of changes in the food supply that result from changes in consumer preferences. In 2010, "no gluten" ranked among the top 10 claims for the first time, with nearly triple the number of products making this claim compared to 2006 (USDA/ERS, 2014a). "Low or no fat" product claims also moved to the top 10 claims for the first time since 2006. From 2006 to 2010, launches of new products with "whole grain" claims doubled worldwide (Oldways Whole Grains Council, 2016).

The Food Supply and the WIC Program

Several recent changes in the U.S. food supply with implications for the revised food packages can be attributed to the influence of WIC itself. For example, since the Child Nutrition and WIC Reauthorization Act of 2004, which included provisions for infant formula manufacturers to bid for state WIC contracts, manufacturers have been bidding for formulas supplemented with the fatty acids docosahexaenoic acid (DHA) and arachidonic acid (ARA).[12] When bidding began, these products were relatively new additions to formula options in the marketplace (USDA/ERS, 2011a). At present, nearly all infant formulas sold in the United States are supplemented with DHA and ARA, an indication of WIC's significant influence on the infant formula market (USDA/ERS, 2011a). Another example of WIC's influence on the U.S. food supply is anecdotal evidence suggesting that increased availability of 1-pound loaves of whole wheat bread can be attributed to the addition of this item to the WIC food packages in 2009 (Oliveira and Frazao, 2015).

Changes in Dietary Guidance

The 2006 IOM review of WIC food packages drew on the 2005 *Dietary Guidelines for Americans* (DGA) (USDA/HHS, 2005). The DGA are updated every 5 years, and since the 2006 review, the 2010 and the 2015–2020 DGA have been issued. As described in the statement of task, the committee was charged with aligning WIC food packages for individuals ages 2 years and older with the most current DGA. Recommendations for infants and children less than 2 years of age draw on the recommendations of the American Academy of Pediatrics (AAP) and other authoritative groups. Changes in dietary guidance since 2005 relevant to the WIC food packages are summarized below.

In addition to these changes, the Dietary Guidelines Advisory Committee reported strong evidence that the seafood industry has rapidly expanded to meet demand and that fisheries are increasingly employing sustainable management strategies to avoid long-term collapse (USDA/HHS, 2015). This is important given WIC's broad reach and recommendations included herein related to fish in the food packages.

---

[12] There were some state/alliance bids that specified DHA/ARA formula products as early as 2002 (see https://ideas.repec.org/p/sda/workpa/12008.html, accessed December 19, 2016).

Changes to Recommended Food Group Intakes

This review presents an opportunity to improve the alignment of the food packages after two changes in the DGA and after introduction of the 2009 food package changes. Compared to the 2005 DGA (see Table 2-13), the 2010 DGA reorganized the vegetable food group into five

TABLE 2-13 USDA Food Intake Patterns for Kcal Levels of Interest: Comparison of 2005 and 2015–2020 DGA

		Kcal Pattern					
		1,300[a]		2,300[b]		2,600	
Food Group	Units	2005	2015–2020	2005	2015–2020	2005	2015–2020
Fruits	c-eq/d	1¼	1¼	2	2	2	2
Vegetables	c-eq/d	1½	1½	3	3	3½	3½
Dark green	c-eq/wk	1½	1	3	2	3	2½
Red/orange	c-eq/wk	1	3	2	6	2½	7
Dry beans and peas[c]	c-eq/wk	1	½	3	2	3½	2½
Starchy	c-eq/wk	2½	3½	6	6	7	7
Other	c-eq/wk	4½	2½	7	5	8½	5½
Grains	oz-eq/d	4½	4½	7½	7½	9	9
Whole grains	oz-eq/d	2¼	2¼	3¾	3¾	4½	4½
Other grains	oz-eq/d	2¼	2¼	3¾	3¾	4½	4½
Protein Foods [d]		3½	3½	6¼	6¼	6½	6½
Meat, poultry, eggs	oz-eq/wk		16½		29½		31
Seafood	oz-eq/wk		5		9½ ↓[e]		10
Nuts, seeds, soy (oz-eq/wk)	oz-eq/wk		2½ ↑ [e]		5		5
Dairy	c-eq/d	2	2½	3	3	3	3
Oils	g/d	17	17	30	30	34	34
Limits for:							
Calories for Other Uses [f]	kcal	171	105	326	315	410	380
(% of calories) [f]	%	13	8	14	14	16	15

NOTES: c-eq = cup-equivalents; DGA = *Dietary Guidelines for Americans*; oz-eq = ounce-equivalents.

[a] Serving equivalents for the 1,300-kcal food pattern are the average of the 1,200- and 1,400-kcal patterns.

[b] Serving equivalents for the 2,300-kcal food pattern are the average of the 2,200- and 2,400-kcal patterns.

TABLE 2-13 Continued

[c] In the USDA food patterns, dry beans and peas are first counted toward the protein foods group until recommendations for that group are met, then are counted toward the dry beans and peas vegetable subgroup (USDA, 2015).

[d] In 2005, key protein sources were categorized as "lean meats and beans," without protein subgroups.

[e] An arrow indicates that the recommended food group amount changed from 2010 to 2015–2020 by 1 unit in the specified direction. Other 2015–2020 food pattern amounts are unchanged from 2010.

[f] In 2005, solid fats and added sugars were built into a "discretionary calorie allowance" instead of specific gram levels of intake. These values are shown as a comparator to "calories for other uses" from the 2015–2020 DGA, which include added sugars, alcohol, added refined starches, saturated (solid) fats, or more than the recommended amount of nutrient-dense foods.

SOURCES: USDA/HHS, 2005, 2010, 2016.

subgroups. The recommended food intakes increased for "red-orange vegetables," "starchy vegetables," and "beans and peas." The recommended quantities of "dark-green vegetables" and "other vegetables" decreased. There were no changes in recommended intakes of total fruit, grains, protein foods, or oils. Recommended intakes of dairy foods were slightly increased for two levels of caloric intake. Compared to the 2010 DGA, the 2015–2020 DGA included no changes to the recommended amounts from each of the major food groups or food subgroups, except for small changes to the subgroups of protein foods. In summary, the major change in the DGA since the 2005 edition relevant to this review is the reformulation of the vegetable subgroups. This reformulation has already resulted in the committee's recommendation that WIC participants should be allowed to acquire white potatoes with their CVV (IOM, 2015).

Changes to Food Patterns

The food patterns in the 2010 DGA included templates for several variations in the USDA Food Patterns, including the Dietary Approaches to Stop Hypertension (DASH) Eating Plan, and Mediterranean, vegetarian, and vegan patterns. The 2015–2020 DGA included a healthy U.S.-style, healthy Mediterranean, and healthy vegetarian patterns (USDA/HHS, 2016).

Shortfall Nutrients and Nutrients of Public Health Concern

The 2015–2020 DGA identified nine nutrients (vitamin A, vitamin D, vitamin E, vitamin C, folate, calcium, magnesium, fiber, and potassium) as "shortfall" nutrients, that is, nutrients that are underconsumed relative to Dietary Reference Intake recommendations (see Table 2-14 for

TABLE 2-14 Shortfall Nutrients and Nutrients of Public Health Concern Noted in the *Dietary Guidelines for Americans*: 2005, 2010, and 2015–2020

	2005	2010	2015–2020
		Adults	
Calcium	✓*	✓*	✓*
Potassium	✓*	✓*	✓*
Choline		✓	
Fiber	✓*	✓*	✓*
Magnesium	✓		✓
Vitamin A	✓	✓	✓
Vitamin C	✓	✓	✓
Vitamin E	✓*	✓	✓
Vitamin D		✓*	✓*
Vitamin K		✓	
Folate	✓		✓
		Children and Adolescents	
Calcium	✓*	✓*	✓*
Potassium	✓*	✓*	✓*
Fiber	✓*	✓*	✓*
Magnesium		✓	✓
Phosphorus		✓	
Vitamin A		✓	✓
Vitamin C		✓	✓
Vitamin E	✓*	✓	✓
Vitamin D		✓*	✓*
		Women of Reproductive Age	
Iron	✓*	✓*	✓*
Folate	✓*	✓*	✓

NOTES: ✓ = shortfall nutrient; ✓* = nutrient of public health concern; nutrients of public health concern are those shortfall nutrients that are linked to adverse health outcomes.
SOURCES: USDA/HHS, 2005, 2010, 2015.

a comparison across the 2005, 2010, and 2015–2020 DGA). Calcium, vitamin D, fiber, and potassium were further classified as nutrients of public health concern because their underconsumption has been linked to adverse health outcomes. For adolescent and premenopausal females, iron was also identified as a shortfall nutrient because of risk of iron-deficiency.

Compared to the 2010 DGA, the 2015–2020 DGA no longer identified choline and vitamin K in adults, phosphorus in children, and vitamin B12 in adults over 50 as shortfall nutrients. In the 2010 DGA, folate was not identified as a shortfall nutrient, rather a nutrient of concern for women capable of becoming pregnant; the newer guidelines continue to recommend that women of reproductive age supplement a diet rich in vegetables, fruits, and grains with foods enriched with folic acid or that include folic acid supplements. The 2015–2020 DGA still consider iron a nutrient of public health concern.

Limiting Added Sugars, Saturated Fats, and Other Food Components

Both the 2010 DGA (USDA/HHS, 2010) and 2015–2020 DGA (USDA/HHS, 2016) focused on limiting added sugars in the diet, with the 2015–2020 DGA specifically recommending limiting added sugars to no more than 10 percent of total calories. The 2015–2020 DGA also retained the 2010 DGA recommendation to limit saturated fat to no more than 10 percent of total calories. (In the 2010 DGA, a maximum percentage of total energy intake from both saturated fats and added sugars was also provided.) Depending on energy needs, the 2015-2020 DGA specify that recommended limits for energy intakes for added sugars and saturated fats (plus energy from other "calories for other uses" [COU][13]) could actually be lower (or greater) than 10 percent. For example, most calories in a 1,200- to 1,800-kcal food pattern are needed to meet nutrient intake needs, leaving less than 10 percent of total calories for other uses (i.e., intake from all COU combined must be less than 10 percent of total calories).

The 2010 DGA recommended that adults up to 50 years of age limit their sodium intake to 2,300 mg per day and that adults 51 years and older, African Americans, and adults with hypertension, diabetes, or chronic kidney disease limit sodium intake to 1,500 mg daily. In contrast, the 2015–2020 DGA recommend a sodium limit of 2,300 mg per day for all adults.

The 2010 DGA recommendation to limit cholesterol was not retained, although the 2015–2020 DGA recommend limiting intake to as little dietary cholesterol as possible while maintaining a healthy eating pattern (USDA/HHS, 2016). This position is consistent with recommendations made by the American College of Cardiology/American Heart Association (ACC/AHA, 2013). Eggs, a primary source of cholesterol in the American diet, are currently included in the WIC food packages for children and women.

---

[13] In the 2015–2020 DGA, calories from added sugars and saturated fat, along with calories from added refined starch, as well as additional calories from the recommended food groups, and alcohol, are termed "calories for other uses" (COU). In the 2010 DGA, calories from added sugars, saturated fats, and alcohol were termed "discretionary calories."

Amounts were reduced in 2009 primarily to allow room for additional foods and, secondarily, to reduce the total amount of cholesterol in the package (IOM, 2006). Contributions of the WIC foods to COU are further reviewed in Chapter 3.

Changes in Dietary Guidance for Infants and Children Up to 2 Years of Age

Since the 2006 IOM report, minor updates have been made to dietary guidance for individuals less than 2 years of age. In 2008, the AAP issued guidance recommending reduced-fat milks for children over the age of 1 year for whom overweight or obesity are concerns (AAP, 2008). As denoted in the Final Rule, USDA-FNS permits the issuance of reduced-fat milks for children 1 year of age and over who fall into this category (USDA/FNS, 2014a). Also in 2008, the AAP published a statement reporting insufficient data to document a protective effect of any dietary intervention on allergy development beyond 4 to 6 months of age (Greer et al., 2008). Results of the committee's review of current dietary guidance for infants and children up to 2 years of age and alignment of the food packages are presented in Chapter 3.

Updates to Nutrient Intake Recommendations and Evidence for Importance in Growth and Development

The DGA apply the Dietary Reference Intakes (DRI) as the basis for identifying nutrient inadequacies. The DRI are also part of the process used to generate food patterns for specific kcal levels. Since the 2006 review of WIC food packages, the IOM has issued one report updating the DRI for calcium and vitamin D (IOM, 2011a). Also since 2006, the importance of choline, omega-3 fatty acids, and vitamin D in fetal growth and development has become clearer. The evidence for the role of these nutrients was reviewed in more detail in the phase I report (NASEM, 2016, Chapter 6).

THE WIC PARTICIPANT EXPERIENCE TODAY

The WIC participant experience today, illustrated in Figure 2-6, is influenced by a number of factors related both to the food packages themselves and to the WIC environment. These factors include racial and ethnic subgroup differences in food preferences and infant and child feeding practices; behavioral barriers and motivators; environmental and economic factors affecting the availability and access to food; and administrative and vendor challenges associated with the WIC food packages. The committee considered the interplay of these factors to ensure that WIC food packages are culturally suitable, efficient for nationwide distribution, and not burdensome to administer. Details of the committee's review of these components are available in Chapter 2 of the phase I report (NASEM, 2016). Key points from that review are summarized here.

Cultural Variation in Satisfaction with the 2009 Food Package Changes

Multiple studies have documented moderate to high satisfaction with the 2009 changes in the WIC food packages (Gleason and Pooler, 2011; Whaley et al., 2012b; Ishdorj and Capps, 2013; Bertmann et al., 2014; Ritchie et al., 2014). However, evidence also indicates cultural variation in participants' satisfaction with certain types or amounts of food items. Black et al. (2009) conducted interviews and focus groups with WIC participants and caregivers throughout Maryland to assess perceptions of the proposed food package changes and examine differences in food preferences by race and ethnicity. Although food preferences appeared to be similar between non-Hispanic black and non-Hispanic white participants, Hispanic respondents were more likely than non-Hispanic respondents to prefer beans compared to peanut butter and to express dislike for frozen and canned vegetables. In a statewide survey of nearly 3,000 mostly (79 percent) Hispanic WIC participants and caregivers in California, Ritchie et al. (2014) reported that nearly all (91 percent) respondents were satisfied with the new food items introduced (vegetables and fruits, whole grains, and lower-fat milk). Additionally, a higher proportion of primarily Spanish speakers (compared to primarily English speakers) were satisfied with vouchers for whole grains, vouchers for lower-fat milk, and the amount of juice; and a higher proportion of primarily English speakers (compared to primarily Spanish speakers) were satisfied only with the amount of milk and not with the amounts of other foods. Actual consumption of foods was difficult to ascertain. In a quasi-experimental study in northern Illinois, Zenk et al. (2012) found that the availability of fresh fruit and vegetables at authorized WIC retailers increased significantly after the 2009 package changes for African-American culturally specific vegetables and fruits, but not for Latino culturally specific vegetables and fruits.[14]

Redemption of WIC Foods

In addition to published studies of the acceptability of the 2009 food packages, the committee also examined state data on foods actually purchased (i.e., from states that have implemented the EBT system). A summary of redemption data gathered from a sample of states at various time points between 2012 and 2016 is presented in Table 2-15 (see the table

[14] See Appendix G, Table G-2, for detail from Zenk et al. (2012).

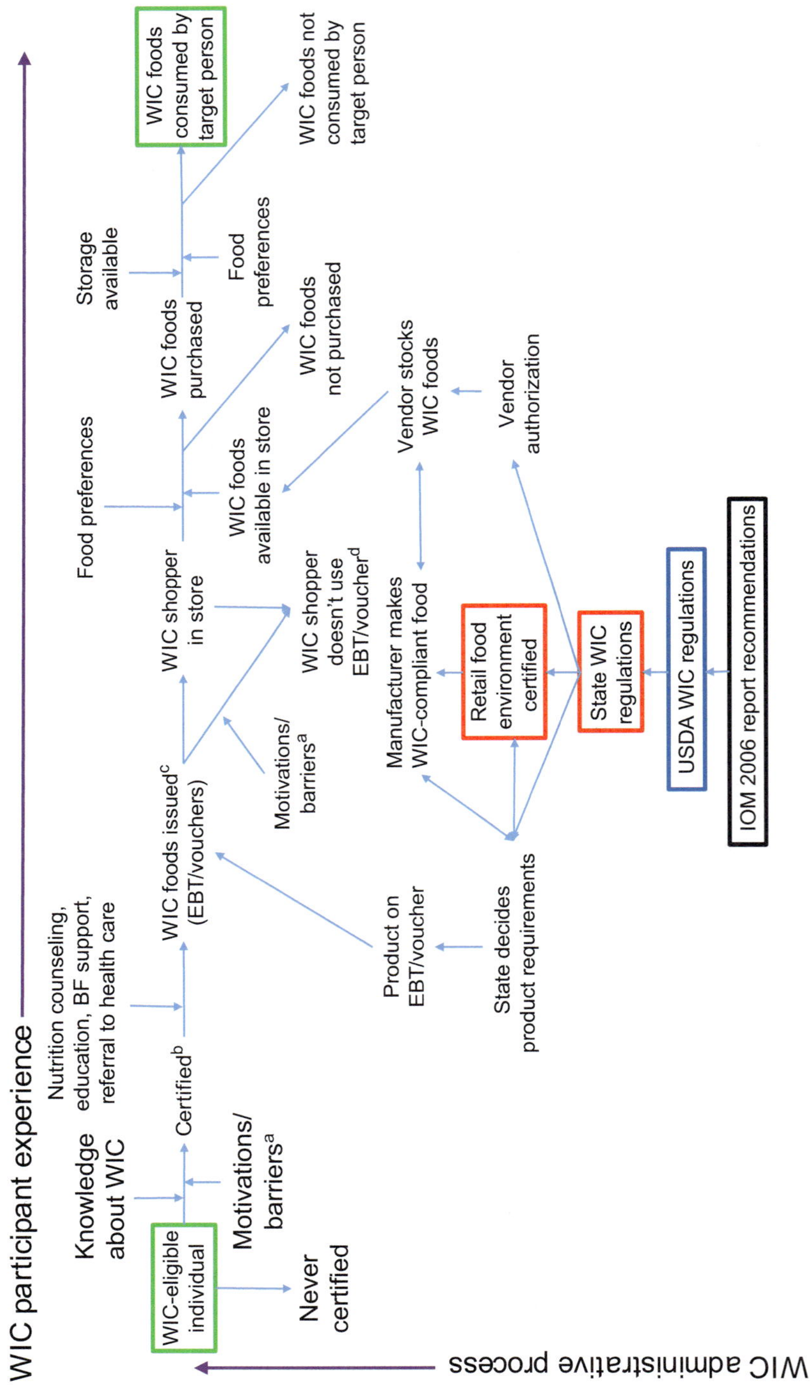
WIC participant experience
WIC administrative process
WIC-eligible individual
Never certified
Knowledge about WIC
Motivations/ barriers[a]
Certified[b]
Nutrition counseling, education, BF support, referral to health care
WIC foods issued[c] (EBT/vouchers)
Product on EBT/voucher
State decides product requirements
Motivations/ barriers[a]
WIC shopper in store
WIC shopper doesn't use EBT/voucher[d]
Manufacturer makes WIC-compliant food
Retail food environment certified
State WIC regulations
USDA WIC regulations
IOM 2006 report recommendations
Food preferences
WIC foods available in store
Vendor stocks WIC foods
Vendor authorization
WIC foods purchased
WIC foods not purchased
Storage available
Food preferences
WIC foods consumed by target person
WIC foods not consumed by target person

FIGURE 2-6 Overview of the WIC program administrative and participant processes. Legislative mandates may also affect WIC regulations.

NOTES: This figure is a theoretical representation; it does not consider effects of other individual or household resources.

[a] Potential participant barriers may include lack of access to transportation to the WIC site and/or the vendor, time required to visit a WIC site, inconvenient WIC clinic hours, lack of knowledge about the program, or lack of preference for WIC foods, among other barriers.

[b] Certification for WIC requires the individual to be categorically eligible (pregnant, postpartum woman, infant, child up to age 5), meet income eligibility guidelines (<185 percent of the federal poverty level), provide proof of residence in the state where benefits are issued and have a nutritional risk. Women certified during pregnancy are certified for the duration of pregnancy plus up to 6 weeks postpartum. Postpartum recertification following the birth of the infant is for either 6 months (if not breastfeeding) or 12 months (if breastfeeding), after which time the mother is no longer eligible for WIC. In the case of a fetal or pregnancy loss, women remain eligible and can be recertified for the program for 6 months after the end of the pregnancy. Beginning in 2013, the Federal Rule gave states the discretion to certify infants and children for either a 6- or 12-month period (USDA/FNS, 2015b). As of this writing, certification periods for infants and children are 6 or 12 months depending on state-level decisions. The need for the participant to visit the program site for recertification is not illustrated in this diagram.

[c] EBT benefits/food vouchers are valid for a 1-month period. States have the discretion to decide whether the 1-month benefit period is a calendar month (e.g., June 1–30) or a rolling month based on the date of benefit issuance (e.g., June 20–July 19). For an individual who is certified, up-to-date on all required documentation, and has no high-risk conditions, benefits can be issued for up to a 3-month period. This means that, although WIC foods are issued for a 1-month period, a participant may be issued up to 3 months of benefits at one visit. Only the current month of benefits can be used immediately. The remaining benefits issued for use in future month(s) must be retained and used only in the future month(s). Valid dates for future month benefits are printed on the voucher or included on the EBT receipt. The need for the participant to visit the program site to obtain EBT benefits/food vouchers is not illustrated in this diagram.

[d] Significant lack of redemption or under-redemption of a WIC food is information used by WIC state agencies to make decisions about available products. This feedback loop is not represented in this diagram.

TABLE 2-15 Redemption of WIC Foods, 2013–2016

WIC Food Category	Average Percent Redemption (Range)	Relevant Food Package(s)
Infant formula	94 (88–98)[a,b,c]	I, II
Eggs	80 (71–85)[e]	IV through VII
Cash value voucher	77 (69–89)[e]	IV through VII
Whole milk	75 (63–84)[a,b,d]	IV-A[h]
Juice	70 (53–80)[e]	IV through VII
Cheese	70 (54–80)[a,b,d,f]	IV through VII
Fish	69 (54–65)[e]	VII
WIC-eligible medical foods	66 (57–75)[a,g]	All packages
Low-fat milk	65 (49–75)[e]	IV-B[i] through VII
Breakfast cereal	60 (46–69)[e]	IV through VII
Whole grain bread	53 (39–65)[e]	IV through V and VII
Infant food fruits/vegetables	51 (34–65)[a,b,d,g]	II
Peanut butter/legumes	51 (44–66)[e]	IV through VII
Infant cereal	47 (38–59)[a,b,d,g]	II
Infant food meats	31 (24–43)[a,b,d,f,g]	II

NOTES: The following prioritization was applied to select redemption rates for the current food package nutrient and cost profiles: First priority = the average of redemption data from 5 unidentified states, provided to the committee by FNS; if not available, second priority = the average of redemption data provided to the committee by individual states. Data span several months or an entire year, but provide a general picture of the typical food category redemption. The "average percent redemption" indicates the value applied in the nutrient and cost profiles, with the source indicated by superscript. The range indicates the range considering all values made available to the committee.

[a] Average and range include data from Massachusetts for 2015.

[b] Average and range include data from Kentucky for 2015.

[c] Average and range include data from California for 2015.

[d] Average and range include data from Chickasaw Nation for 2015.

[e] Average represents the average of redemption from 5 unidentified states, fiscal year 2013–2014, data provided by USDA-FNS. A description of this data source is available in Chapter 7 and Appendix R. Range includes data from all sources made available to the committee.

[f] Average and range include data from Texas for 2015.

[g] Average and range include data from Wyoming, late 2015 to early 2016.

[h] Food package IV-A is for children ages 1 to less than 2 years.

[i] Food package IV-B is for children ages 2 to less than 5 years.

SOURCES: USDA/ERS, 2014b; other data referenced are available in the public access file for this study (Email: paro@nas.edu).

footnotes for time ranges). Available data indicate that redemption was variable for most food categories, but consistently high for infant formula and consistently low for jarred infant meats. For foods provided in more than one food package, it was not possible to determine if redemption was different among food packages. There were not enough data to determine whether states with high concentrations of particular racial and ethnic groups have higher redemption for specific items (e.g., tortillas or beans are common Hispanic staples). Nonetheless, the committee considered possible regional differences in food and substitution preferences in its deliberations.

Barriers to WIC Participation and Redemption

Key barriers to WIC participation and redemption of WIC foods are summarized in Box 2-1, and details of the committee's review are available in Appendix G, Table G-1. Although the quantitative evidence identified by the committee was sufficient to support only an association, not a causal relationship, between these barriers and either participation or redemption, possibilities for maximizing both participation and redemption include: streamlining the registration process (Gilbert et al., 2014), enhancing customer service and reducing wait times for participants (Christie et al.,

BOX 2-1

Summary of Literature Findings on Barriers to WIC Participation and Redemption

Barriers to Participation

- Long wait times; crowded physical environment
- Lack of transportation
- Belief that family is ineligible; changing eligibility restrictions
- Program requires too much effort, difficult paperwork
- Language barriers

Barriers to Redemption

- Embarrassment, negative interactions in stores
- Gaps in knowledge (e.g., determining amount of F/V with CVV)
- Limited selection of WIC foods at local vendors; products not available in allowable forms
- Vendor challenges anticipating demand and maintaining adequate supply of some WIC foods
- Maintaining food freshness at the vendor (particularly small vendors)

SOURCE: See Appendix G, Table G-1.

2006), informing participants of local vendors (Gleason et al., 2014), ensuring culturally-appropriate nutrition messaging (Phillips et al., 2014), enhancing the perceived value of packages (Gleason and Pooler, 2011), and examining the impact of minimum stocking requirements on food availability (Gleason et al., 2011). As the EBT system is implemented nationwide (by 2020), it may remove several of the identified barriers (Phillips et al., 2014).

The WIC Participant Shopping Experience

Although studies are limited, qualitative work among WIC programs nationwide suggests that the participant shopping experience can be another key barrier to participation and redemption of WIC foods. Prior to the food package revisions, a survey administered to parents and caretakers of WIC participants in New York State found that issues with food procurement (store policies, food availability) and the WIC food packages (adequacy, satisfaction with the items) were barriers to participation (Woelfel et al., 2004).[15] Several small studies were carried out after implementation of the 2009 food package changes to evaluate the perception and use of the CVV by WIC participants (Christie et al., 2006; Gleason and Pooler, 2011; Najjar, 2013; Bertmann et al., 2014; Gleason et al., 2014). Bertmann et al. (2014) reported that CVVs were inconsistently redeemed in Arizona. They identified the following barriers to redemption: participants' perception of annoyance or anger expressed by cashier or other shoppers; cashiers' lack of training; fluctuation in enforcement of WIC redemption rules from store to store and week to week; and feelings of embarrassment or judgment when using the CVV. The authors cautioned, however, that their findings might not be generalizable to other WIC-participating populations. In a Wisconsin study of WIC participant CVV redemption patterns, Gleason and Pooler (2011) reported positive responses overall to the package changes, but with differences in non-use and maximum use of the CVV among some WIC subpopulations. Some participants described a level of discomfort with having to do math in the store, which the researchers hypothesized may be enough to deter use of the benefits. Additionally, the authors identified several vendor-level challenges, including difficulties in maintaining fresh foods (particularly in smaller stores), anticipating client demand, and having the correct sizes available. Najjar (2013) reported that helpful vendors and both vendor and participant understanding about the use of the CVV can positively affect the WIC shopping experience.

The effect of allowing split tender for CVV purchases (using a different payment method for the amount over the CVV benefit) on redemption has

[15] Although this study fell outside the committee's search parameters for publication year, the committee considered its findings to be particularly applicable.

yet to be comprehensively evaluated. Inasmuch as WIC provides vouchers for all other foods based on quantity, not value, WIC participants may pay less attention to food prices when redeeming their vouchers (Hoynes and Schanzenbach, 2015). The CVV, however, is a cash benefit, and purchasing power may vary regionally. In a study of 26 metropolitan market areas, Leibtag and Kumcu (USDA/ERS, 2011b) found that the 20 most commonly purchased vegetables and fruits cost 30 to 70 percent more in the highest-priced compared to the lowest-priced market areas.

WIC Participant Shopping Venues

The types of stores from which WIC benefits are typically redeemed is relevant when considering the availability of WIC foods in specific store types and food package changes that may affect small and large vendors differently. Based on the most recent ERS evaluation (USDA/ERS, 2016c), WIC participants redeem their benefits mostly (77 percent) at large stores (super stores, supermarkets, and large grocery stores). Approximately 63 percent of WIC vendors can be classified as large stores. However, data indicate that the proportion of WIC redemptions at large stores varies by state, ranging from 50 to 99 percent. In some states, smaller stores play a significant role, accounting for as many as 70 percent of WIC retail vendors (Rhode Island) and capturing as much as 50 percent of WIC retail redemptions (California) (USDA/ERS, 2016c). An earlier study (conducted in 2009) which showed a similar focus on large stores indicated that most WIC participants used their vouchers and did most other food shopping at the same store (84 percent); reasons provided for shopping at a different store for WIC foods included convenience (44 percent) and cost (32 percent) (USDA/FNS, 2012).

Although Ford and Dzewaltowski (2010) found that WIC mothers had access to many food stores within a 3-mile radius of their home, whether residing in a micropolitan or metropolitan area, and a recent study of SNAP and WIC-participating households using nationally representative data from USDA's National Household Food Acquisition and Purchase Survey (FoodAPS) indicated that the nearest store was an average of 2.0 miles from the household, the same FoodAPS data also indicated that the store primarily used for grocery shopping was, on average, 3.4 miles from the household (USDA/ERS, 2015). FoodAPS also indicated that the vast majority (88 percent) of WIC-participating households accessed grocery stores using their own vehicle, and 7 percent of WIC-participating households reported walking, biking, using public transport, shuttle, delivery, or some other form of transportation (USDA/ERS, 2015d).

Availability of WIC Foods

Several research groups have examined the effects of the 2009 changes to the WIC food packages on food availability and, therefore, access to WIC foods. Studies comparing vendor inventory before versus after the 2009 changes in Illinois (Zenk et al., 2012), Connecticut (Andreyeva et al., 2011), Baltimore, Maryland (Cobb et al., 2015), Hartford, Connecticut (Havens et al., 2012), and New Orleans, Louisiana (O'Malley et al., 2014; Rose et al., 2014) have indicated improved availability of fruits, vegetables, lower-fat milks, juices, jarred infant vegetables and fruits, and/or whole grains among WIC vendors. Cobb et al. (2015) found that both becoming WIC-authorized and the WIC policy change itself were associated with significant increases in WIC-relevant "healthy food availability"[16] scores. Havens et al. (2012) likewise reported improvements in "healthy food supply"[17] scores among WIC convenience and grocery stores, although the improvements varied from 16 percent in higher-income neighborhoods to 39 percent in lower-income areas. A systematic review of four studies confirmed overall improved availability of WIC foods at WIC-authorized vendors (Schultz et al., 2015). Andreyeva et al. (2011) and Zenk et al. (2014) noted some carryover in improved availability to stores that did not participate in WIC, possibly attributable to changes in the food supply chain.

Nationwide Distribution and Costs of Food

As part of its consideration of changes to the food packages, the committee evaluated information on the cost and national distribution of foods (including to low-income neighborhoods). The purpose of this evaluation was to ensure that foods in the revised packages are accessible to WIC participants living in different geographic areas of the United States, including both rural and urban areas. The committee factored into its considerations seasonal variability in food availability, pricing (including regional price differences and price variability of product substitutions), the impact of shelf stability on nationwide distribution, vendor requirements for inventory turnover limits of perishable food products, and types of vendors in different locales (e.g.,

---

[16] The "healthy food availability" scores, ranging from 0 to 27 points, that were allotted based on the presence and number of varieties available of the following items: fruit (4 points), vegetables (4 points), low-fat milk (1 point), lean beef and chicken (4 points), healthy frozen meals (1 point), whole-wheat bread (4 points), low-sodium alternatives (2 points), and low-sugar cereal (2 points) as well as the relative shelf space of healthy versus unhealthy alternatives of milk and frozen food (Cobb et al., 2015).

[17] The "healthy food supply" score was a composite of data on availability, variety, quality, and prices of foods including cow's milk; soy milk; tofu; fresh, canned, and frozen fruit and vegetables; canned sardines and salmon; whole-grain bread and tortillas; brown rice; and whole-grain cereals (Andreyeva et al., 2012).

TABLE 2-16 Changes and Challenges Since the IOM 2006 Review: Key Findings and Conclusions

Challenge or Environmental Change Evaluated	Finding(s) and Conclusion(s)
Adaptation to the 2009 Food Package Implementation	State and local agencies, vendors, and manufacturers were largely able to adapt; some continuing challenges are related to sizes available in the marketplace. Consideration to the feasibility of potential food package changes from the perspective of states, local agencies, vendors, and manufacturers is critical for implementation success.
	Evidence indicates that targeted nutrition education in advance of food package changes can result in positive behavior change. This strategy could be applied at the state level to future food package changes.
Changes in WIC Participation	WIC participation has been declining since 2010, although the proportions of participants according to food package categories have remained consistent. The underlying cause of the decline is not clear but is not related to the 2009 food package changes (see Appendix F). Attention to retention of the program's value and reduction of participation barriers is warranted. Inasmuch as children ages 1 to less than 5 years comprise the majority of the WIC-participating population, changes to this food package (IV) will have the greatest effect on overall program costs for food.
Food Expenditures of WIC Participants	WIC benefits cover an important share of food expenditures for participating households. Despite some limitations to the data, the new evidence shows WIC-participating households spend more on WIC food items than do other households with low income.
Changes in Breastfeeding Prevalence	Breastfeeding prevalence among WIC participants is lower than that of other low-income women. Evidence is inconclusive about whether the 2009 food package changes affected the choice to breastfeed.
Associations Between WIC Participation and Breastfeeding	WIC participation was associated with a lower likelihood of breastfeeding initiation, duration, and exclusivity. Available data indicate that breastfeeding promotion and support among WIC participants is associated with the choice to breastfeed. These activities may improve breastfeeding prevalence in WIC when linked closely to food package changes.
	Evidence suggests that the 2009 food package policy that limited formula in the first month resulted in more women being issued the full formula-feeding package. Allowing a greater degree of flexibility in formula issuance in the first month may better support any degree of breastfeeding for women who choose a mixed-feeding option.

continued

TABLE 2-16 Continued

Challenge or Environmental Change Evaluated	Finding(s) and Conclusion(s)
Ability of the Current Food Packages to Meet Participants' Needs	The current food packages offer a degree of flexibility both at the state and participant level. Available information suggests that the current food packages are satisfactory and meet needs, but redemption data suggest that improvements can be made.
Changes in Dietary Guidance	Key changes to the *Dietary Guidelines for Americans*, guidance for individuals less than 2 years of age, and to Dietary Reference Intakes have been made since the IOM 2006 review. These changes may have implications for both amounts of and specifications for foods in the WIC food packages.
Nationwide Availability of WIC Foods	The marketplace has expanded substantially since 2006 and now includes a wider variety of dairy and grain products, which may have improved the nationwide availability of foods that meet WIC specifications. Although most WIC participants shop at larger stores, smaller stores may be the only option for some WIC participants. Availability of WIC foods at both types of stores remains important.

supermarket versus trading post). Although most WIC redemptions occur at large stores, some participants may have access primarily to smaller vendors, so all store sizes were important to consider (USDA/ERS, 2016c).

KEY FINDINGS AND CONCLUSIONS

This chapter includes a review of the many WIC programmatic and other environmental changes of relevance to the review of food packages. Table 2-16 summarizes the key findings and conclusions reached by the committee upon examination of the evidence described in this chapter.

REFERENCES

AAP (American Academy of Pediatrics) Committee on Nutrition. 2008. Lipid screening and cardiovascular health in childhood. *Pediatrics* 122(1):198–208.

ACC/AHA (American College of Cardiology/American Heart Association). 2013. *Guideline on the treatment of blood cholesterol to reduce atherosclerotic cardiovascular risk in adults: A report of the American College of Cardiology/American Heart Association Task Force on Practice Guidelines.* http://circ.ahajournals.org/content/circulationaha/early/2013/11/11/01.cir.0000437738.63853.7a.full.pdf (accessed November 6, 2016).

Andreyeva, T., J. Luedicke, A. E. Middleton, M. W. Long, and M. B. Schwartz. 2011. *Changes in access to healthy foods after implementation of the WIC food package revisions.* Washington, DC: USDA/ERS.

Andreyeva, T., J. Luedicke, A. E. Middleton, M. W. Long, and M. B. Schwartz. 2012. Positive influence of the revised Special Supplemental Nutrition Program for Women, Infants, and Children food packages on access to healthy foods. *Journal of the Academy of Nutrition Dietetics* 112(6):850–858.

Andreyeva, T., J. Luedicke, A. S. Tripp, and K. E. Henderson. 2013a. Effects of reduced juice allowances in food packages for the Women, Infants, and Children program. *Pediatrics* 131(5):919–927.

Andreyeva, T., and J. Luedicke. 2013b. Federal food package revisions: Effects on purchases of whole-grain products. *American Journal of Preventive Medicine* 45(4):422–429.

Andreyeva, T., J. Luedicke, K. E. Henderson, and M. B. Schwartz. 2014. The positive effects of the revised milk and cheese allowances in the Special Supplemental Nutrition Program for Women, Infants, and Children. *Journal of the Academy of Nutrition and Dietetics* 114(4):622–630.

Bauer, K. W., M. O. Hearst, K. Escoto, J. M. Berge, and D. Neumark-Sztainer. 2012. Parental employment and work-family stress: Associations with family food environments. *Social Science and Medicine* 75(3):496–504.

Bentley, J., and A. Pérez. 2015. *Fresh fruit makes up a growing share of U.S. fruit availability*. USDA/ERS. https://www.ers.usda.gov/amber-waves/2015/may/fresh-fruit-makes-up-a-growing-share-of-us-fruit-availability (accessed December 21, 2016).

Bertmann, F. M., C. Barroso, P. Ohri-Vachaspati, J. S. Hampl, K. Sell, and C. M. Wharton. 2014. Women, infants, and children cash value voucher (CVV) use in Arizona: A qualitative exploration of barriers and strategies related to fruit and vegetable purchases. *Journal of Nutrition Education and Behavior* 46(3 Suppl):S53–S58.

Beshara, M., A. Hutchinson, and C. Wilson. 2010. Preparing meals under time stress. The experience of working mothers. *Appetite* 55(3):695–700.

Bitler, M., and H. Hoynes. 2013. The more things change, the more they stay the same? The safety net and poverty in the great recession. *Journal of Labor Economics* (working paper). doi: 10.3386/w19449.

Black, M. M., K. M. Hurley, S. E. Oberlander, E. R. Hager, A. E. McGill, N. T. White, and A. M. Quigg. 2009. Participants' comments on changes in the revised Special Supplemental Nutrition Program for Women, Infants, and Children food packages: The Maryland Food Preference Study. *Journal of the American Dietetic Association* 109(1): 116–123.

Bonuck, K. A., K. Freeman, and M. Trombley. 2005. Country of origin and race/ethnicity: Impact on breastfeeding intentions. *Journal of Human Lactation* 21(3):320–326.

Bullinger, L. R., and T. Gurley-Calvez. 2016. WIC participation and maternal behavior: Breastfeeding and work leave. *Contemporary Economic Policy* 34(1):158–172.

Bunik, M., N. F. Krebs, B. Beaty, M. McClatchey, and D. L. Olds. 2009. Breastfeeding and WIC enrollment in the Nurse Family Partnership program. *Breastfeeding Medicine* 4(3):145–149.

Bunik, M., P. Shobe, M. E. O'Connor, B. Beaty, S. Langendoerfer, L. Crane, and A. Kempe. 2010. Are 2 weeks of daily breastfeeding support insufficient to overcome the influences of formula? *Academic Pediatrics* 10(1):21–28.

CBO (Congressional Budget Office). 2012. *The Supplemental Nutrition Assistance Program*. Washington, DC: Congressional Budget Office. https://www.cbo.gov/sites/default/files/cbofiles/attachments/04-19-SNAP.pdf (accessed December 21, 2016).

CDC (Centers for Disease Control and Prevention). 2010. Racial and ethnic differences in breastfeeding initiation and duration, by state—National Immunization Survey, United States, 2004-2008. *Morbidity and Mortality Weekly Report* 59(11):327–334.

CDC. 2015. *Nutrition, physical activity and obesity data, trends and maps web site*. https://nccd.cdc.gov/NPAO_DTM (accessed December 21, 2016).

CDC. 2016a. *Breastfeeding report card*. https://www.cdc.gov/breastfeeding/pdf/2016breastfeedingreportcard.pdf (accessed December 21, 2016).

CDC. 2016b. *National Immunization Survey (NIS)*. https://www.cdc.gov/breastfeeding/data/nis_data/index.htm (accessed October 14, 2016).

Chapman, D. J., K. Morel, A. Bermudez-Millan, S. Young, G. Damio, and R. Pérez-Escamilla. 2013. Breastfeeding education and support trial for overweight and obese women: A randomized trial. *Pediatrics* 131(1):e162–e170.

Chiasson, M. A., S. E. Findley, J. P. Sekhobo, R. Scheinmann, L. S. Edmunds, A. S. Faly, and N. J. McLeod. 2013. Changing WIC changes what children eat. *Obesity (Silver Spring)* 21(7):1423–1429.

Christie, C., J. A. Watkins, A. Martin, H. Jackson, J. E. Perkin, and J. Fraser. 2006. Assessment of client satisfaction in six urban WIC clinics. *Florida Public Health Review* 3:35–42.

Cobb, L. K., C. A. M. Anderson, L. Appel, J. Jones-Smith, U. Bilal, J. Gittelsohn, and M. Franco. 2015. Baltimore city stores increased the availability of healthy food after WIC policy change. *Health Affairs* 34(11):1849–1857.

DHS (U.S. Department of Homeland Security). 2014. *2013 yearbook of immigration statistics*. Washington, DC: U.S. Department of Homeland Security, Office of Immigration Statistics.

Dunn, R. L, K. A. Kalich, R. Fedrizzi, and S. Phillips. 2015. Barriers and contributors to breastfeeding in WIC mothers: A social ecological perspective. *Breastfeeding Medicine* 10(10):493–501.

EOPUS (Executive Office of the President of the United States). 2014. The economic impact of the American Recovery and Reinvestment Act five years later: Final report to Congress. https://www.whitehouse.gov/sites/default/files/docs/cea_arra_report.pdf (accessed December 21, 2016).

Flower, K. B., M. Willoughby, R. J. Cadigan, E. M. Perrin, and G. Randolph. 2008. Understanding breastfeeding initiation and continuation in rural communities: A combined qualitative/quantitative approach. *Maternal and Child Health Journal* 12(3):402–414.

Ford, P. B., and D. A. Dzewaltowski. 2010. Limited supermarket availability is not associated with obesity risk among participants in the Kansas WIC program. *Obesity (Silver Spring)* 18(10):1944-1951.

Ford, E. S., and W. H. Dietz. 2013. Trends in energy intake among adults in the United States: Findings from NHANES. *American Journal of Clinical Nutrition* 97(4):848–853.

Gilbert, D., J. Nanda, and D. Paige. 2014. Securing the safety net: Concurrent participation in income eligible assistance programs. *Maternal and Child Health Journal* 18(3):604–612.

Gittelsohn, J., M. N. Laska, T. Andreyeva, G. Foster, D. Rose, J. Tester, S. H. Lee, S. N. Zenk, A. Odoms-Young, T. McCoy, and G. X. Ayala. 2012. Small retailer perspectives of the 2009 women, infants and children program food package changes. *American Journal of Health Behavior* 36(5):655–665.

Gleason, S., and J. Pooler. 2011. The effects of changes in WIC food packages on redemptions: Final report. Altarum Institute. http://naldc.nal.usda.gov/download/50613/PDF (accessed December 21, 2016).

Gleason, S., R. Morgan, L. Bell, and J. Pooler. 2011. Impact of the revised WIC food package on small WIC vendors: Insight from a four-state evaluation. Altarum Institute. http://www.calwic.org/storage/FourStateWICFoodPackageEvaluation-Full_Report-20May11.pdf (accessed December 21, 2016).

Gleason, S., D. McGuire, and R. Morgan. 2014. Opportunities to enhance American Indian access to the WIC food package: Evidence from three case studies. Altarum Institute. http://altarum.org/sites/default/files/uploaded-publication-files/Opportunities%20to%20Enhance%20Am%20Indian%20Access%20to%20the%20WIC%20FP_fmt_04.pdf (accessed December 21, 2016).

Greer, F. R., S. H. Sicherer, A. W. Burks, and American Academy of Pediatrics Committee on Nutrition. 2008. Effects of early nutritional interventions on the development of atopic disease in infants and children: The role of maternal dietary restriction, breastfeeding, timing of introduction of complementary foods, and hydrolyzed formulas. *Pediatrics* 121(1):183–191.

Gregory, E. F., S. M. Gross, T. Q. Nguyen, A. M. Butz, and S. B. Johnson. 2016. WIC participation and breastfeeding at 3 months postpartum. *Maternal and Child Health Journal* 20(8):1735–1744.

Haider, S. J., L. V. Chang, T. A. Bolton, J. G. Gold, and B. H. Olson. 2014. An evaluation of the effects of a breastfeeding support program on health outcomes. *Health Services Research* 49(6):2017–2034.

Havens, E. K., K. S. Martin, J. Yan, D. Dauser-Forrest, and A. M. Ferris. 2012. Federal nutrition program changes and healthy food availability. *American Journal of Preventive Medicine* 43(4):419–422.

Hayes, D. K., C. B. Prince, V. Espinueva, L. J. Fuddy, R. Li, and L. M. Grummer-Strawn. 2008. Comparison of manual and electric breast pumps among WIC women returning to work or school in Hawaii. *Breastfeeding Medicine* 3(1):3–10.

Hendricks, K., R. Briefel, T. Novak, and P. Ziegler. 2006. Maternal and child characteristics associated with infant and toddler feeding practices. *Journal of the American Dietetic Association* 106(1 Suppl 1):S135–S148.

HHS (U.S. Department of Health and Human Services). 2011. The Surgeon General's call to action to support breastfeeding. http://www.surgeongeneral.gov/library/calls/breastfeeding/calltoactiontosupportbreastfeeding.pdf (accessed December 21, 2016).

HHS. 2015. *Healthy People 2020: Maternal, infant, and child health objectives*. https://www.healthypeople.gov/2020/topics-objectives/topic/maternal-infant-and-child-health/objectives (accessed December 21, 2016).

Hildebrand, D. A., P. McCarthy, D. Tipton, C. Merriman, M. Schrank, and M. Newport. 2014. Innovative use of influential prenatal counseling may improve breastfeeding initiation rates among WIC participants. *Journal of Nutrition Education and Behavior* 46(6):458–466.

Holmes, A. V., N. P. Chin, J. Kaczorowski, and C. R. Howard. 2009. A barrier to exclusive breastfeeding for WIC enrollees: Limited use of exclusive breastfeeding food package for mothers. *Breastfeeding Medicine* 4(1):25–30.

Hopkinson, J., and M. Konefal Gallagher. 2009. Assignment to a hospital-based breastfeeding clinic and exclusive breastfeeding among immigrant Hispanic mothers: A randomized, controlled trial. *Journal of Human Lactation* 25(3):287–296.

Howell, E. A., S. Bodnar-Deren, A. Balbierz, M. Parides, and N. Bickell. 2014. An intervention to extend breastfeeding among black and Latina mothers after delivery. *American Journal of Obstetrics and Gynecology* 210(3):239.e1–239.e5.

Hoynes, H., and D. W. Schanzenbach. 2015. U.S. food and nutrition programs. http://www.nber.org/chapters/c13488.pdf (accessed October 26, 2016).

Hurley, K. M., M. M. Black, M. A. Papas, and A. M. Quigg. 2008. Variation in breastfeeding behaviours, perceptions, and experiences by race/ethnicity among a low-income statewide sample of Special Supplemental Nutrition Program for Women, Infants, and Children (WIC) participants in the United States. *Maternal and Child Nutrition* 4(2):95–105.

IOM (Institute of Medicine). 2006. *WIC food packages: Time for a change*. Washington, DC: The National Academies Press.

IOM. 2011a. *Dietary Reference Intakes for calcium and vitamin D*. Washington, DC: The National Academies Press.

IOM. 2011b. *Early childhood obesity prevention policies*. Washington, DC: The National Academies Press.

IOM. 2015. *Review of WIC food packages: An evaluation of white potatoes in the cash value voucher: Letter report*. Washington, DC: The National Academies Press.

Isbell, M. G., J. G. Seth, R. D. Atwood, and T. C. Ray. 2014. A client-centered nutrition education model: Lessons learned from Texas WIC. *Journal of Nutrition Education and Behavior* 46(1):54–61.

Ishdorj, A., and O. Capps. 2013. The effect of revised WIC food packages on native American children. *American Journal of Agricultural Economics* 95(5):1266–1272.

Jabs, J., and C. M. Devine. 2006. Time scarcity and food choices: An overview. *Appetite* 47(2):196–204.

Jacknowitz, A., and L. Tiehen. 2007. Transitions into and out of the WIC program: A cause for concern? *Social Service Review* 83(2):151–183.

Jacobson, L. T., P. Twumasi-Ankrah, M. L. Redmond, E. Ablah, R. B. Hines, J. Johnston, and T. C. Collins. 2015. Characteristics associated with breastfeeding behaviors among urban versus rural women enrolled in the Kansas WIC program. *Maternal and Child Health Journal* 19(4):828–839.

Jensen, E. 2012. Participation in the Supplemental Nutrition Program for Women, Infants and Children (WIC) and breastfeeding: National, regional, and state level analyses. *Maternal and Child Health Journal* 16(3):624–631.

Joyce, T., and J. Reeder. 2015. Changes in breastfeeding among WIC participants following implementation of the new food package. *Maternal and Child Health Journal* 19(4):868–876.

Joyce, T., A. Racine, and C. Yunzal-Butler. 2008. Reassessing the WIC effect: Evidence from the Pregnancy Nutrition Surveillance System. *Journal of Policy Analysis and Management* 27(2):277–303.

Kandiah, J. 2011. Teaching new mothers about infant feeding cues may increase breastfeeding duration. *Food and Nutrition Sciences* 2(4):259–264.

Kavanagh, K. F., R. J. Cohen, M. J. Heinig, and K. G. Dewey. 2008. Educational intervention to modify bottle-feeding behaviors among formula-feeding mothers in the WIC program: Impact on infant formula intake and weight gain. *Journal of Nutrition Education and Behavior* 40(4):244–250.

KFF (Henry J. Kaiser Family Foundation). 2009. *A foundation for health reform: Findings of a 50 state survey of eligibility rules, enrollment and renewal procedures, and cost-sharing practices in Medicaid and CHIP for children and parents during 2009*. Washington, DC: Henry J. Kaiser Family Foundation. https://kaiserfamilyfoundation.files.wordpress.com/2013/01/8028.pdf (accessed December 21, 2016).

KFF. 2015. *Medicaid financing: How does it work and what are the implications?* Menlo Park, CA: The Henry J. Kaiser Family Foundation. http://files.kff.org/attachment/issue-brief-medicaid-financing-how-does-it-work-and-what-are-the-implications (accessed December 21, 2016).

Langellier, B. A., M. Pia Chaparro, and S. E. Whaley. 2012. Social and institutional factors that affect breastfeeding duration among WIC participants in Los Angeles County, California. *Maternal and Child Health Journal* 16(9):1887–1895.

Langellier, B. A., M. P. Chaparro, M. C. Wang, M. Koleilat, and S. E. Whaley. 2014. The new food package and breastfeeding outcomes among women, infants, and children participants in Los Angeles County. *American Journal of Public Health* 104(Suppl 1):S112–S118.

Li, R., N. Darling, E. Maurice, L. Barker, and L. M. Grummer-Strawn. 2005. Breastfeeding rates in the United States by characteristics of the child, mother, or family: The 2002 National Immunization Survey. *Pediatrics* 115(1):e31–e37.

Ma, P., and J. H. Magnus. 2012. Exploring the concept of positive deviance related to breastfeeding initiation in black and white WIC enrolled first time mothers. *Maternal and Child Health Journal* 16(8):1583–1593.

Ma, X., J. Liu, and M. Smith. 2014. WIC participation and breastfeeding in South Carolina: Updates from prams 2009–2010. *Maternal and Child Health Journal* 18(5):1271–1279.

Mao, C. Y., S. Narang, and J. Lopreiato. 2012. Breastfeeding practices in military families: A 12-month prospective population-based study in the national capital region. *Military Medicine* 177(2):229–234.

Marshall, C., L. Gavin, C. Bish, A. Winter, L. Williams, M. Wesley, and L. Zhang. 2013. WIC participation and breastfeeding among white and black mothers: Data from Mississippi. *Maternal and Child Health Journal* 17(10):1784–1792.

McKinney, C. O., J. Hahn-Holbrook, P. L. Chase-Lansdale, S. L. Ramey, J. Krohn, M. Reed-Vance, T. N. Raju, M. U. Shalowitz, and Community Child Health Research Network. 2016. Racial and ethnic differences in breastfeeding. *Pediatrics* 138(2).

Meehan, K., G. G. Harrison, A. A. Afifi, N. Nickel, E. Jenks, and A. Ramirez. 2008. The association between an electric pump loan program and the timing of requests for formula by working mothers in WIC. *Journal of Human Lactation* 24(2):150–158.

Metallinos-Katsaras, E., L. Brown, and R. Colchamiro. 2015. Maternal WIC participation improves breastfeeding rates: A statewide analysis of WIC participants. *Maternal and Child Health Journal* 19(1):136–143.

Motel, S., and E. Patten. 2012. The 10 largest Hispanic origin groups: Characteristics, rankings, top counties. Washington, DC: Pew Research Center.

Najjar, S. 2013. Barriers to WIC benefits redemption among participants in Washington State. Master's thesis, Seattle: University of Washington, School of Public Health.

NASEM (National Academies of Sciences, Engineering, and Medicine). 2016. *Review of WIC food packages: Proposed framework for revisions: Interim report.* Washington, DC: The National Academies Press. doi: 10.17226/21832.

Oldways Whole Grain Council. 2016. *Whole grain statistics.* http://wholegrainscouncil.org/newsroom/whole-grain-statistics (accessed December 21, 2016).

Oliveira, V., and E. Frazao. 2015. Painting a more complete picture of WIC: How WIC impacts nonparticipants. USDA/ERS. https://www.ers.usda.gov/amber-waves/2015/april/painting-a-more-complete-picture-of-wic-how-wic-impacts-nonparticipants (accessed December 21, 2016).

Olson, B. H., S. J. Haider, L. Vangjel, T. A. Bolton, and J. G. Gold. 2010. A quasi-experimental evaluation of a breastfeeding support program for low income women in Michigan. *Maternal and Child Health Journal* 14(1):86–93.

O'Malley, K., B. G. Luckett, L. F. Dunaway, J. N. Bodor, and D. Rose. 2015. Use of a new availability index to evaluate the effect of policy changes to the Special Supplemental Nutrition Program for Women, Infants, and Children (WIC) on the food environment in New Orleans. *Public Health Nutrition* 18(1):25-32.

Pérez-Escamilla, R., and D. J. Chapman. 2012. Breastfeeding protection, promotion, and support in the United States: A time to nudge, a time to measure. *Journal of Human Lactation* 28(2):118–121.

Pérez-Escamilla, R., L. Curry, D. Minhas, L. Taylor, and E. Bradley. 2012. Scaling up of breastfeeding promotion programs in low- and middle-income countries: The "breastfeeding gear" model. *Advances in Nutrition* 3(6):790–800.

Petrova, A., C. Ayers, S. Stechna, J. A. Gerling, and R. Mehta. 2009. Effectiveness of exclusive breastfeeding promotion in low-income mothers: A randomized controlled study. *Breastfeeding Medicine* 4(2):63–69.

Phillips, D., L. Bell, R. Morgan, and J. Pooler. 2014. Transition to EBT in WIC: Review of impact and examination of participant redemption patterns: Final report. Altarum Institute. http://altarum.org/sites/default/files/uploaded-publication-files/Altarum_Transition%20to%20WIC%20EBT_Final%20Report_071614.pdf (accessed December 21, 2016).

Povich, D., B. Roberts, and M. Mather. 2014. *Low-income working mothers and state policy: Investing for a better economic future.* Chevy Chase, MD: The Working Poor Families Project.

Pugh, L. C., J. R. Serwint, K. D. Frick, J. P. Nanda, P. W. Sharps, D. L. Spatz, and R. A. Milligan. 2010. A randomized controlled community-based trial to improve breastfeeding rates among urban low-income mothers. *Academic Pediatrics* 10(1):14–20.

Rao, J. N. K., and A. J. Scott. 1984. On Chi-squared tests for multiway contingency tables with cell proportions estimated from survey data. *Annals of Statistics* 12(1): 46–60.

Reeder, J. A., T. Joyce, K. Sibley, D. Arnold, and O. Altindag. 2014. Telephone peer counseling of breastfeeding among WIC participants: A randomized controlled trial. *Pediatrics* 134(3):e700–e709.

Ritchie, L. D., S. E. Whaley, P. Spector, J. Gomez, and P. B. Crawford. 2010. Favorable impact of nutrition education on California WIC families. *Journal of Nutrition Education and Behavior* 42(3 Suppl):S2–S10.

Ritchie, L. D., S. E. Whaley, and N. J. Crocker. 2014. Satisfaction of California WIC participants with food package changes. *Journal of Nutrition Education and Behavior* 46(3 Suppl):S71–S78.

Roberts, B., D. Povich, and M. Mather. 2013. *Low-income working families: The growing economic gap.* Chevy Chase, MD: The Working Poor Families Project.

Rose, D., K. O'Malley, L. F. Dunaway, and J. N. Bodor. 2014. The influence of the WIC food package changes on the retail food environment in New Orleans. *Journal of Nutrition Education and Behavior* 46(3 Suppl):S38-S44.

Ryan, A. S. 2005. More about the Ross Mothers Survey. *Pediatrics* 115(5):1450–1451.

Ryan, A. S., and W. Zhou. 2006. Lower breastfeeding rates persist among the Special Supplemental Nutrition Program for Women, Infants, and Children participants, 1978–2003. *Pediatrics* 117(4):1136–1146.

Ryan, A., Z. Wenjun, and A. Acosta. 2002. Breastfeeding continues to increase into the new millennium. *Pediatrics* 11(6):1103–1109.

Sandy, J. M., E. Anisfeld, and E. Ramirez. 2009. Effects of a prenatal intervention on breastfeeding initiation rates in a Latina immigrant sample. *Journal of Human Lactation* 25(4):404–411; quiz 458–459.

Schultz, D. J., C. Byker Shanks, and B. Houghtaling. 2015. The impact of the 2009 Special Supplemental Nutrition Program for Women, Infants, and Children food package revisions on participants: A systematic review. *Journal of the Academy of Nutrition and Dietetics* 115(11):1832–1846.

Senia, M. C., H. H. Jensen, and O. Zhylyevskyy. 2014. Time in eating and food preparation among single adults. *Review of Economics of the Household*: 1–34. doi: 10.1007/s11150-014-9258-5

Sliwa, S. A., A. Must, F. Perea, and C. D. Economos. 2015. Maternal employment, acculturation, and time spent in food-related behaviors among Hispanic mothers in the United States. Evidence from the American Time Use Survey. *Appetite* 87:10–19.

Sullivan, E. M., W. E. Bignell, A. Andrianos, and A. K. Anderson. 2011. Impact of education and training on type of care provided by community-based breastfeeding counselors: A cross-sectional study. *International Breastfeeding Journal* 6:12.

Tenfelde, S., L. Finnegan, and P. D. Hill. 2011. Predictors of breastfeeding exclusivity in a WIC sample. *Journal of Obstetric, Gynecologic, and Neonatal Nursing* 40(2):179–189.

Tisone, C. A., S. A. Guerra, W. Lu, E. L. McKyer, M. Ory, D. Dowdy, S. Wang, J. Miao, A. Evans, and D. M. Hoelscher. 2014. Food-shopping environment disparities in Texas WIC vendors: A pilot study. *American Journal of Health Behavior* 38(5):726–736.

USCB (U.S. Census Bureau). 2011. Overview of race and Hispanic origin: 2010. http://www.census.gov/content/dam/Census/library/publications/2011/dec/c2010br-02.pdf (accessed December 21, 2016).

USCB. 2015. *Population clock*. http://www.census.gov (accessed December 21, 2016).

USDA (U.S. Department of Agriculture). 2015. *Beans and peas are unique foods*. https://www.choosemyplate.gov/vegetables-beans-and-peas (accessed August 29, 2016).

USDA/ARS (U.S. Department of Agriculture/Agricultural Research Service). 2005–2012. *What we eat in America, NHANES 2005–2012*. Beltsville, MD: USDA/ARS. http://www.cdc.gov/nchs/nhanes/wweia.htm (accessed December 21, 2016).

USDA/ARS. 2014. *Food patterns equivalents database 2011–2012: Methodology and user guide*. Beltsville, MD: USDA/ARS. http://www.ars.usda.gov/SP2UserFiles/Place/80400530/pdf/fped/FPED_1112.pdf (accessed December 21, 2016).

USDA/ERS (U.S. Department of Agriculture/Economic Research Service). 2007. *Could behavioral economics help improve diet quality for nutrition assistance program participants?* Washington, DC: USDA/ERS. http://ben.cornell.edu/pdfs/USDA-BeEcon.pdf (accessed December 21, 2016).

USDA/ERS. 2011a. *The infant formula market. Consequences of a change in contract brand*. Washington, DC: USDA/ERS. https://www.ers.usda.gov/webdocs/publications/err124/6918_err124.pdf?v=41056 (accessed January 30, 2017).

USDA/ERS. 2011b. *The WIC fruit and vegetable cash voucher: Does regional price variation affect buying power?* Washington, DC: USDA/ERS. http://www.ers.usda.gov/media/127579/eib75.pdf (accessed March 2, 2015).

USDA/ERS. 2014a. *Cost containment in the WIC program: Vendor peer groups and reimbursement rates*. Washington, DC: USDA/ERS. https://www.ers.usda.gov/webdocs/publications/err171/48701_err171_summary.pdf (accessed December 21, 2016).

USDA/ERS. 2014b. Transition to EBT in WIC: Review of impact and examination of participant redemption patterns: Final report. Altarum Institute. http://altarum.org/sites/default/files/uploaded-publication-files/Altarum_Transition%20to%20WIC%20EBT_Final%20Report_071614.pdf (accessed December 21, 2016).

USDA/ERS. 2015a. *The WIC program: Background, trends, and economic issues*. 2015 edition. Washington, DC: USDA/ERS. https://www.aap.org/en-us/advocacy-and-policy/federal-advocacy/Documents/USDAWIC2015Report.pdf (accessed December 21, 2016).

USDA/ERS. 2015b. *The food assistance landscape FY 2014 annual report*. Washington, DC: USDA/ERS. http://www.ers.usda.gov/webdocs/publications/eib137/52406_eib137_summary.pdf (accessed November 7, 2016).

USDA/ERS. 2015c. *FoodAPS national household Food Acquisition and Purchase Survey*. Washington, DC: USDA/ERS. http://www.ers.usda.gov/data-products/foodaps-national-household-food-acquisition-and-purchase-survey.aspx (accessed December 21, 2016).

USDA/ERS. 2015d. *Where do Americans shop for food and how do they travel to get there?* Washington, DC: USDA/ERS. https://www.ers.usda.gov/webdocs/publications/eib138/eib138_errata.pdf?v=42636 (accessed January 30, 2017).

USDA/ERS. 2016a. *Wheat's role in the U.S. diet has changed over the decades*. Washington, DC: USDA/ERS. http://www.ers.usda.gov/topics/crops/wheat/wheats-role-in-the-us-diet.aspx (accessed December 21, 2016).

USDA/ERS. 2016b. *National household food acquisition and purchase survey (FoodAPS). User's guide to survey design, data collection, and overview of datasets.* http://www.ers.usda.gov/webdocs/DataFiles/FoodAPS_National_Household_Food_Acquisition_and_Purchase_Survey_17984//53285_UserGuideFoodAPS.pdf (accessed December 21, 2016).

USDA/ERS. 2016c. *Where do WIC participants redeem their food benefits? An analysis of WIC food dollar redemption patterns by store type.* Washington, DC: USDA/ERS. http://www.ers.usda.gov/webdocs/publications/eib152/57246_eib152.pdf (accessed November 7, 2016).

USDA/FNS (U.S. Department of Agriculture/Food and Nutrition Research Service). 2007a. *Special Supplemental Nutrition Program for Women, Infants and Children (WIC): Revisions in the WIC food packages; Interim Rule*, 7 C.F.R. § 246. Alexandria, VA: USDA/FNS.

USDA/FNS. 2007b. *WIC participant and program characteristics 2006.* Alexandria, VA: USDA/FNS. http://www.fns.usda.gov/sites/default/files/pc2006.pdf (accessed December 21, 2016).

USDA/FNS. 2010. *WIC participant and program characteristics 2008.* Alexandria, VA: USDA/FNS. http://www.fns.usda.gov/sites/default/files/pc2008_0.pdf (accessed December 21, 2016).

USDA/FNS. 2011a. *National and state-level estimates of Special Supplemental Nutrition Program for Women, Infants, and Children (WIC) eligibles and program reach, 2000–2009.* Alexandria, VA: USDA/FNS.

USDA/FNS. 2011b. *Evaluation of the birth month breastfeeding changes to the WIC food packages.* Alexandria, VA: USDA/FNS. http://www.fns.usda.gov/sites/default/files/BirthMonth.pdf (accessed December 21, 2016).

USDA/FNS. 2012. *National survey of WIC participants II.* Alexandria, VA: USDA/FNS. http://www.fns.usda.gov/national-survey-wic-participants-ii (accessed December 21, 2016).

USDA/FNS. 2013. *National and state-level estimates of Special Supplemental Nutrition Program for Women, Infants, and Children (WIC) eligibles and program reach, 2010.* Alexandria, VA: USDA/FNS. http://www.fns.usda.gov/sites/default/files/WICEligibles2010Vol1.pdf (accessed December 21, 2016).

USDA/FNS. 2014a. *Special Supplemental Nutrition Program for Women, Infants and Children (WIC): Revisions in the WIC food packages; Final Rule*, 7 C.F.R. § 246.

USDA/FNS. 2014b. *National and state-level estimates of the Special Supplemental Nutrition Program for Women, Infants, and Children (WIC) eligibles and program reach, 2011, Vol I.* Alexandria, VA: USDA/FNS. http://www.fns.usda.gov/sites/default/files/WICEligibles2011Volume1.pdf (accessed December 21, 2016).

USDA/FNS. 2015a. *WIC food packages policy options II, final report.* Alexandria, VA: USDA/FNS. http://www.fns.usda.gov/wic-food-package-policy-options-ii (accessed December 21, 2016).

USDA/FNS. 2015b. *National and state-level estimates of the Special Supplemental Nutrition Program for Women, Infants, and Children (WIC) eligibles and program reach, 2012, Vol I.* Alexandria, VA: USDA/FNS. http://www.fns.usda.gov/sites/default/files/ops/WICEligibles2012-Volume1.pdf (accessed December 21, 2016).

USDA/FNS. 2015c. *WIC participant and program characteristics 2014: Final report.* Alexandria, VA: USDA/FNS. http://www.fns.usda.gov/sites/default/files/ops/WICPC2014.pdf (accessed December 21, 2016).

USDA/FNS. 2016a. *Special Supplemental Nutrition Program for Women, Infants and Children (WIC): Food package policy and guidance.* Alexandria, VA: USDA/FNS. http://www.fns.usda.gov/sites/default/files/wic/WIC-Food-Package-Policy-Guidance.pdf (accessed August 26, 2016).

USDA/FNS. 2016b. *WIC program*. Alexandria, VA: USDA/FNS. http://www.fns.usda.gov/pd/wic-program (accessed July 13, 2016).

USDA/FNS. 2016c. *Food and Nutrition Service Research and Evaluation Plan—Fiscal Year 2016*. Alexandria, VA: USDA/FNS. http://www.fns.usda.gov/sites/default/files/ops/study-and-evaluation-plan-2016.pdf (accessed September 16, 2016).

USDA/HHS (U.S. Department of Agriculture/U.S. Department of Health and Human Services). 2005. *Dietary Guidelines for Americans 2005*. U.S. Government Printing Office. http://www.health.gov/dietaryguidelines/dga2005/document/pdf/DGA2005.pdf (accessed December 21, 2016).

USDA/HHS. 2010. *Dietary Guidelines for Americans 2010*. U.S. Government Printing Office. http://www.health.gov/dietaryguidelines/dga2010/dietaryguidelines2010.pdf (accessed December 21, 2016).

USDA/HHS. 2015. *The report of the Dietary Guidelines Advisory Committee on the Dietary Guidelines for Americans, 2015, to the Secretary of Agriculture and the Secretary of Health and Human Services*. USDA/HHS. http://www.health.gov/dietaryguidelines/2015-scientific-report/PDFs/Scientific-Report-of-the-2015-Dietary-Guidelines-Advisory-Committee.pdf (accessed December 21, 2016).

USDA/HHS. 2016. *Dietary Guidelines for Americans 2015*. U.S. Government Printing Office. https://health.gov/dietaryguidelines/2015 (accessed August 29, 2016).

Walker, M. 2015. Formula supplementation of breastfed infants: Helpful or hazardous? *ICAN: Infant, Child, & Adolescent Nutrition* 7(4):198–207.

Whaley, S. E., M. Koleilat., M. Whaley, J. Gomez, K. Meehan, K. Saluja. 2012a. Impact of policy changes on infant feeding decisions among low-income women participating in the Special Supplemental Nutrition Program for Women, Infants, and Children. *American Journal of Public Health* 102(12):2269–2273.

Whaley, S. E., L. D. Ritchie, P. Spector, and J. Gomez. 2012b. Revised WIC food package improves diets of WIC families. *Journal of Nutrition Education and Behavior* 44(3):204–209.

WHO (World Health Organization). 2012. Baby-friendly hospital initiative. World Health Organization. http://www.who.int/nutrition/topics/bfhi/en (accessed December 21, 2016).

Woelfel, M. L., R. Abusabha, R. Pruzek, H. Stratton, S. G. Chen, and L. S. Edmunds. 2004. Barriers to the use of WIC services. *Journal of the American Dietetic Association* 104(5):736–743.

Zenk, S. N., A. Odoms-Young, L. M. Powell, R. T. Campbell, D. Block, N. Chavez, R. C. Krauss, S. Strode, and J. Armbruster. 2012. Fruit and vegetable availability and selection: Federal food package revisions, 2009. *American Journal of Preventive Medicine* 43(4):423–428.

Zenk, S. N., L. M. Powell, A. M. Odoms-Young, R. Krauss, M. L. Fitzgibbon, D. Block, and R. T. Campbell. 2014. Impact of the revised Special Supplemental Nutrition Program for Women, Infants, and Children (WIC) food package policy on fruit and vegetable prices. *Journal of the Academy of Nutrition and Dietetics* 114(2):288–296.

Ziol-Guest, K. M., and D. C. Hernandez. 2010. First- and second-trimester WIC participation is associated with lower rates of breastfeeding and early introduction of cow's milk during infancy. *Journal of the American Dietetic Association* 110(5):702–709.

3

Alignment of the Current Food Packages with Dietary Guidance, Special Dietary Needs, and Cultural Eating Practices or Food Preferences

As described in the Statement of Task, recommended revisions to WIC food packages are required to be consistent with the 2015–2020 *Dietary Guidelines for Americans* (DGA)[1] (for individuals ages 2 years and older), advice from the American Academy of Pediatrics (AAP) or other authoritative groups (for individuals less than 2 years of age), and the Dietary Reference Intakes (DRIs). This chapter provides an evaluation of the alignment of the current food packages with these updated sets of guidance and with special dietary needs, preferences, or practices (e.g., medical conditions, vegetarian or vegan diets, cultural eating practices).

ALIGNMENT OF THE FOOD PACKAGES WITH DIETARY GUIDANCE FOR INDIVIDUALS AGES 2 YEARS AND OLDER

As noted in Chapter 1, the Special Supplemental Nutrition Program for Women, Infants, and Children (WIC) is required to provide foods and services in alignment with the DGA (U.S. Congress, P.L. 101-445, 1990), which are applicable to individuals ages 2 years and older. In this section, the contributions of the food packages to the DGA food patterns are evaluated, including the contribution of WIC-approved foods to intakes of sodium, added sugars, saturated fat, and "calories for other uses" (COU) (see Chapter 2 for a description of COU).

[1] References to the DGA in this chapter are specific to 2015–2020 unless otherwise noted.

Amounts of Foods in the Current Food Packages Compared to the USDA Food Patterns

Understanding the contribution of the WIC food packages to the U.S. Department of Agriculture (USDA)-recommended food patterns as outlined in the DGA (USDA/HHS, 2016) was required before the committee could consider how the food packages might be adjusted. As shown in Tables 3-1 through 3-4, the proportion of the DGA recommended amounts of food groups provided to women and children in the food packages varies across food groups and across food packages. The packages provide nearly 100 percent of recommendations for dairy in most cases and over 100 percent of recommended amounts of several other food groups and subgroups (i.e., dairy for fully breastfeeding women, juice for children,[2] peanut butter in most food packages, and legumes in food packages for children). In contrast, amounts of total grains, total protein foods, and total vegetables provided is generally less than 50 percent of recommended amounts. This variation suggested to the committee that there were opportunities for improvement in the alignment of the food packages with the DGA recommendations as well as with providing a more balanced supplement to participants' diets.

Of note, the WIC food packages serve individuals with a wide range of energy needs.[3] The data presented in tables 1 through 4 are therefore only approximations of the contribution of a WIC food package to a specific individual's energy needs. Additionally, the data in these tables are based on an assumption that all foods in the packages are consumed by the intended beneficiaries.

Alignment of the WIC Food Packages with Dietary Guidance for Intake of Fish

The USDA's Food and Nutrition Service (USDA-FNS) specifically tasked the committee to evaluate the inclusion of fish across food packages. As is evident in Tables 3-1 through 3-4, fish is provided only in food package VII for breastfeeding women. The DGA encourage consumption of high omega-3, low-mercury fish species (USDA/HHS, 2016), agreeing with the U.S. Food and Drug Administration/Environmental Protection Agency (FDA/EPA) joint federal fish advisory (2014). Intake of fish high in omega-3 fatty acids is recommended not only in the DGA, but also by the American Heart Association (AHA, 2015), AAP (AAP, 2014), and the

[2] Based on the lower end of the AAP range of 4 to 6 ounces per day.

[3] The food patterns applied in this report were selected based on the Estimated Energy Requirements calculated or assumed for each age and physiological-state subgroup, as outlined in Appendix J.

World Health Organization (PAHO/WHO, 2003). Table 3-5 presents the guidance from each of these groups. Generally, the recommended intake is between approximately 1 ounce and 2 ounces per day, depending on the target population.

These recommendations take into account the risks and benefits of fish intake, given that some fish species contain mercury, specifically methylated (organic) mercury, which can be detrimental to human health. Pregnant women are at the greatest risk. The 2015 Dietary Guidelines Advisory Committee (DGAC) report (USDA/HHS, 2015) reviewed and concurred with the Food and Agriculture Organization/World Health Organization (FAO/WHO) Expert Consultation on the Risks and Benefits of Fish Consumption (FAO/WHO, 2010), which stated that the health benefits of low-mercury fish consumption (whether farm raised or wild) outweigh risks with respect to both offspring development and mortality from cancers and cardiovascular diseases. The fish species for which the FDA advises limiting consumption are not included in the food packages.

Alignment of the WIC Food Packages with Dietary Guidance for Nutrients to Limit

The DGA recommend an upper sodium limit of 2,300 mg per day and upper limits of 10 percent of total calories from saturated fat and 10 percent of total calories from added sugars (USDA/HHS, 2016). Alignment of the WIC food packages with each of these recommendations is discussed below.

Sodium in the WIC Food Packages

The DGA recommendation to limit sodium to 2,300 mg per day aligns with the Tolerable Upper Intake Level (UL, a DRI value) for sodium for adults, ages 19 and older (IOM, 2005). In the WIC food packages, sodium is found primarily in cheese, canned vegetables, and canned fish. Sodium is otherwise limited in most other food categories. Although USDA/FNS (2014) encourages states to offer lower-sodium options, the low-sodium versions of some products cost more than their higher-sodium counterparts which may affect their inclusion on state WIC food lists.[4] The sodium content of representative allowable WIC foods is presented in Table 3-6.

[4] States may implement cost-containment practices in order to reduce the average food cost per WIC participant. This may include limiting food selection by size, form, or price, as well as mandating the use of particular brands.

TABLE 3-1 WIC Maximum Allowance Compared to the 2015–2020 DGA Food Pattern: Food Package V, Pregnant and Partially Breastfeeding Women, Up to 1 Year Postpartum

WIC Food Category	DGA Food Group	Units/d	WIC Maximum Allowance	DGA 2,600-kcal Food Pattern	% of 2,600-kcal DGA Recommendation[a]
Total fruit	*Total fruit*	c-eq	1.0	2.0	52
Juice, 100%[b]	Fruit, as juice	c-eq	0.6	1.0	60
Fruit, 67% of CVV[c]	Fruit, whole	c-eq	0.4	1.0	45
Total vegetables	*Total vegetables*	c-eq	0.5	3.5	13
Vegetable, 33% of CVV[d]		c-eq	0.2	3.5	6
Legumes (as a vegetable)[e]	Beans and peas	c-eq	0.3	0.4	71
Total dairy	*Total dairy*	c-eq	2.9	3.0	98
Milk		c-eq	2.9	3.0	98
Total grains	*Total grains*	oz-eq	1.7	9.0	19
Breakfast cereal[f]	Refined grains	oz-eq	1.0	4.5	22
Breakfast cereal	Whole grains	oz-eq	0.2	4.5	17[g]
Whole wheat bread	Whole grains	oz-eq	0.5		

Total protein foods	*Total protein foods*	oz-eq	1.6	6.5	28
Peanut butter	Nuts, seeds, and soy	oz-eq	1.2	0.7	168
Eggs	Meat, poultry, and eggs	oz-eq	0.4	4.4	9
Fish	Seafood	oz-eq	0.0	1.4	0

NOTES: c-eq = cup-equivalents; CVV = cash value voucher; DGA = *Dietary Guidelines for Americans*; oz-eq = ounce-equivalents.

[a] This kcal level most closely matched the calculated Estimated Energy Requirement for pregnant or breastfeeding WIC-participating women in NHANES 2005–2012. In the current WIC food packages, pregnant women and partially breastfeeding women receive the same benefits. Percentages represent the proportion of the recommended food pattern amount in the corresponding row of the DGA food pattern column.

[b] The DGA recommend that not more than 50 percent of total fruit intakes come from 100 percent fruit juice (USDA/HHS, 2016).

[c] Assumes that 67 percent of the CVV is used to purchase fruits, based on redemption data from Texas and Wyoming. A weighted composite cost of fruit ($0.55/c-eq) was developed, based on a composite of the most commonly consumed fruits (bananas, apples, oranges, berries, grapes, melon [watermelon was used in this case]) from an average of Massachusetts, Texas, and Wyoming redemption data. Only fresh fruit was included as all states allow fresh forms; ERS 2013 price data were updated with a consumer price index to 2015 values.

[d] Assumes that 33 percent of the CVV is used to purchase vegetables, based on redemption data from Texas and Wyoming. A weighted composite cost of vegetables ($0.55/c-eq) was developed, based on a composite of the most commonly consumed vegetables (tomatoes, avocados, potatoes, peppers, lettuce) from an average of Massachusetts, Texas, and Wyoming redemption data. Only fresh vegetables were included as all states allow fresh forms; ERS 2013 price data were updated with a consumer price index to 2015 values. Because potatoes were not yet available in Wyoming, the same proportion of potatoes was assumed for this state as for Texas.

[e] Legumes can also be assessed as a protein, but were placed in the vegetable group because a higher proportion of individuals had low intakes of vegetables across WIC participating subgroups compared to protein.

[f] In the current food packages, a ratio of 81 percent refined grains and 19 percent whole grains was applied, based on redemption data.

[g] To compare the food package contribution to the DGA recommended amounts of whole grains, the whole grain portion of breakfast cereal was added to the whole grain contribution of bread.

SOURCES: USDA/ARS, 2014; USDA/FNS, 2014; USDA/HHS, 2016. State-specific data are available in the public access file for this study (Email: paro@nas.edu).

TABLE 3-2 WIC Maximum Allowance Compared to the 2015–2020 DGA Food Pattern: Food Package VI, Women Up to 6 Months Postpartum

WIC Food Category	DGA Food Group	Units/d	WIC Maximum Allowance	DGA 2,300-kcal Food Pattern	% of 2,300-kcal DGA Recommendation[a]
Total fruit	*Total fruit*	c-eq	0.8	2.0	42
Juice, 100%[b]	Fruit, juice	c-eq	0.4	1.0	40
Fruit, 67% of CVV[c]	Fruit, whole	c-eq	0.4	1.0	45
Total vegetables	*Total vegetables*	c-eq	0.3	3.0	12
Vegetable, 33% of CVV[d]		c-eq	0.2	3.0	7
Legumes (as a vegetable)[e,f]	Beans and peas	c-eq	0.1	0.3	44
Total dairy	*Total dairy*	c-eq	2.1	3.0	71
Milk		c-eq	2.1	3.0	71
Total grains	*Total grains*	oz-eq	1.2	7.5	16
Breakfast cereal[g]	Refined grains	oz-eq	1.0	3.8	26
Breakfast cereal	Whole grains	oz-eq	0.2	3.8	6
Total protein foods	*Total protein foods*	oz-eq	1.3	6.3	20
Peanut butter[f]	Nuts, seeds, and soy	oz-eq	0.6	0.7	84
Eggs	Meat, poultry, and eggs	oz-eq	0.4	4.2	10
Fish	Seafood	oz-eq	0.0	1.4	0

NOTES: c-eq = cup-equivalents; CVV = cash value voucher; DGA = *Dietary Guidelines for Americans*; oz-eq = ounce-equivalents; PP = postpartum.

[a] The 2,300-kcal food pattern level most closely matched the calculated Estimated Energy Requirement for postpartum WIC-participating women in NHANES 2005–2012. Percentages represent the proportion of the recommended food pattern amount in the corresponding row of the DGA food pattern column.

[b] The DGA recommend that not more than 50 percent of total fruit intake come from 100 percent fruit juice (USDA/HHS, 2016).

[c] Assumes that 67 percent of the CVV is used to purchase fruits, based on redemption data from Texas and Wyoming. A weighted composite cost of fruit ($0.55/c-eq) was developed, based on a composite of the most commonly consumed fruits (bananas, apples, oranges, berries, grapes, melon [watermelon was used in this case]) from an average of Massachusetts, Texas, and Wyoming redemption data. Only fresh fruit was included as all states allow fresh forms; ERS 2013 price data were updated with a consumer price index to 2015 values.

[d] Assumes that 33 percent of the CVV is used to purchase vegetables, based on redemption data from Texas and Wyoming. A weighted composite cost of vegetables ($0.55/c-eq) was developed, based on a composite of the most commonly consumed vegetables (tomatoes, avocados, potatoes, peppers, lettuce) from an average of Massachusetts, Texas, and Wyoming redemption data. Only fresh vegetables were included as all states allow fresh forms; ERS 2013 price data were updated with a consumer price index to 2015 values. Because potatoes were not yet available in Wyoming, the same proportion of potatoes was assumed for this state as for Texas.

[e] Legumes can also be assessed as a protein, but were placed in the vegetable group because a higher proportion of individuals had low intakes of vegetables across WIC participating subgroups compared to protein.

[f] Assumes 50 percent legumes and 50 percent peanut butter. Because these values account for the proportion of the maximum allowance of legumes and peanut butter provided per month, they are lower than those presented in the phase I report (NASEM, 2016).

[g] In the current food packages, a ratio of 81 percent refined grains and 19 percent whole grains was applied, based on redemption data.

SOURCES: USDA/ARS, 2014; USDA/FNS, 2014; USDA/HHS, 2016. State-specific data are available in the public access file for this study (Email: paro@nas.edu).

TABLE 3-3 WIC Maximum Allowance Compared to the 2015–2020 DGA Food Pattern: Food Package VII, Fully Breastfeeding Women Up to 1 Year Postpartum

WIC Food Category	DGA Food Group	Units/d	WIC Maximum Allowance	DGA 2,600-kcal Food Pattern	% of 2,600-kcal DGA Recommendation[a]
Total fruit	*Total fruit*	c-eq	1.0	2.0	52
Juice, 100%[b]	Fruit, juice	c-eq	0.6	1.0	60
Fruit, 67% of CVV[c]	Fruit, whole	c-eq	0.4	1.0	45
Total vegetables	*Total vegetables*	c-eq	0.5	3.5	13
Vegetable, 33% of CVV[d]		c-eq	0.2	3.5	6
Legumes (as a vegetable)[e]	Beans and peas	c-eq	0.3	0.4	71
Total dairy	*Total dairy*	c-eq	3.6	3.0	119
Milk		c-eq	3.2	3.0	107
Cheese		c-eq	0.4	3.0	12
Total grains	*Total grains*	oz-eq	1.7	9.0	19
Breakfast cereal[f]	Refined grains	oz-eq	1.0	4.5	22
Breakfast cereal	Whole grains	oz-eq	0.2	4.5	17[g]
Whole wheat bread	Whole grains	oz-eq	0.5		
Total protein foods	*Total protein foods*	oz-eq	3.3	6.5	50
Peanut butter	Nuts, seeds, and soy	oz-eq	1.2	0.7	168
Eggs	Meat, poultry, and eggs	oz-eq	0.8	4.4	18
Fish	Seafood	oz-eq	1.0	1.4	70

NOTES: c-eq = cup-equivalents; CVV = cash value voucher; DGA = *Dietary Guidelines for Americans*; oz-eq = ounce-equivalents.

[a] The 2,600-kcal food pattern level most closely matched the calculated Estimated Energy Requirement for breastfeeding WIC-participating women in NHANES 2005–2012. Percentages represent the proportion of the recommended food pattern amount in the corresponding row of the DGA food pattern column.

[b] The DGA recommend that not more than 50 percent of fruit intakes come from 100 percent fruit juice (USDA/HHS, 2016)

[c] Assumes that 67 percent of the CVV is used to purchase fruits, based on redemption data from Texas and Wyoming. A weighted composite cost of fruit ($0.55/c-eq) was developed, based on a composite of the most commonly consumed fruits (bananas, apples, oranges, berries, grapes, melon [watermelon was used in this case]) from an average of Massachusetts, Texas, and Wyoming redemption data. Only fresh fruit was included as all states allow fresh forms; ERS 2013 price data were updated with a consumer price index to 2015 values.

[d] Assumes that 33 percent of the CVV is used to purchase vegetables, based on redemption data from Texas and Wyoming. A weighted composite cost of vegetables ($0.55/c-eq) was developed, based on a composite of the most commonly consumed vegetables (tomatoes, avocados, potatoes, peppers, lettuce) from an average of Massachusetts, Texas, and Wyoming redemption data. Only fresh vegetables were included as all states allow fresh forms; ERS 2013 price data were updated with a consumer price index to 2015 values. Because potatoes were not yet available in Wyoming, the same proportion of potatoes was assumed for this state as for Texas.

[e] Legumes can also be assessed as a protein, but were placed in the vegetable group because a higher proportion of individuals had low intakes of vegetables across WIC participating subgroups compared to protein.

[f] In the current food packages, a ratio of 81 percent refined grains and 19 percent whole grains was applied, based on redemption data.

[g] To compare the food package contribution to the DGA recommended amounts of whole grains, the whole grain portion of breakfast cereal was added to the whole grain contribution of bread.

SOURCES: USDA/ARS, 2014; USDA/FNS, 2014; USDA/HHS, 2016. State-specific data are available in the public access file for this study (Email: paro@nas.edu).

TABLE 3-4 WIC Maximum Allowance Compared to the 2015–2020 DGA Food Pattern: Food Package IV, Children 2 to Less Than 5 Years of Age*

WIC Food Category	DGA Food Group	Units/d	WIC Maximum Allowance	DGA 1,300-kcal Food Pattern	% of 1,300-kcal DGA Recommendation[b]
Total fruit	*Total fruit*	c-eq	0.9	1.25	69
Juice, 100%	Fruit, juice	c-eq	0.5	0.5[h]	107
Fruit, 67% of CVV[c]	Fruit, whole	c-eq	0.3	0.7	43
Total vegetables	*Total vegetables*	c-eq	0.3	1.5	19
Vegetable, 33% of CVV[d]		c-eq	0.2	1.5	11
Legumes (as a vegetable)[e,f]	Beans and peas	c-eq	0.13	0.07	177
Total dairy	*Total dairy*	c-eq	*2.1*	2.5	85
Milk		c-eq	2.1	2.5	85
Total grains	*Total grains*	oz-eq	*2.3*	4.5	50
Breakfast cereal[g]	Refined grains	oz-eq	1.0	2.3	43
Breakfast cereal	Whole grains	oz-eq	0.2	2.3	58[i]
Whole wheat bread	Whole grains	oz-eq	1.1		
Total protein foods	*Total protein foods*	oz-eq	1.0	3.5	29
Peanut butter[f]	Nuts, seeds, and soy	oz-eq	0.6	0.4	167
Eggs	Meat, poultry, and eggs	oz-eq	0.4	2.4	17
Fish	Seafood	oz-eq	0.0	0.6	0

NOTES: c-eq = cup-equivalents; CVV = cash value voucher; DGA = *Dietary Guidelines for Americans*; NR = no recommendation; oz-eq = ounce-equivalents.

*Some values in this table are corrected from the original prepublication version.

[a] The DGA apply to individuals ages 2 years and older; therefore, although food package IV is issued to younger children, the table is applicable only to those ages 2 to less than 5 years.

[b] For children ages 2 to less than 5 years, the median calculated Estimated Energy Requirement was 1,517 kcals. A food pattern of 1,300 kcal was selected for this age group because (1) 1,500 kcal/d may reflect recent increases in body weights for young children and was considered too high for normal weight children in this age group, particularly in light of efforts to reduce and/or contain the prevalence of childhood obesity, and (2) the 1,300-kcal pattern was applied in both the previous WIC food package review (IOM, 2006) and the Child and Adult Care Food Program (CACFP) report (IOM, 2011a) and should similarly be appropriate for current WIC participating children of the same ages. Percentages represent the proportion of the recommended food pattern amount in the corresponding row of the DGA food pattern column.

[c] Assumes that 67 percent of the CVV is used to purchase fruits, based on redemption data from Texas and Wyoming. A weighted composite cost of fruit ($0.55/c-eq) was developed, based on a composite of the most commonly consumed fruits (bananas, apples, oranges, berries, grapes, melon [watermelon was used in this case]) from an average of Massachusetts, Texas, and Wyoming redemption data. Only fresh fruit was included as all states allow fresh forms; ERS 2013 price data were updated with a consumer price index to 2015 values.

[d] Assumes that 33 percent of the CVV is used to purchase vegetables, based on redemption data from Texas and Wyoming. A weighted composite cost of vegetables ($0.55/c-eq) was developed, based on a composite of the most commonly consumed vegetables (tomatoes, avocados, potatoes, peppers, lettuce) from an average of Texas, Wyoming, and Massachusetts redemption data. Only fresh vegetables were included as all states allow fresh forms; ERS 2013 price data were updated with a consumer price index to 2015 values. Because potatoes were not yet available in Wyoming, the same proportion of potatoes was assumed for this state as for Texas.

[e] Legumes can also be assessed as a protein, but were placed in the vegetable group because a higher proportion of individuals had low intakes of vegetables across WIC participating subgroups compared to protein.

[f] Assumes 50 percent legumes and 50 percent peanut butter. Because these values account for the proportion of the maximum allowance of legumes and peanut butter provided per month, they are lower than those presented in the phase I report (NASEM, 2016).

[g] In the current food packages, a ratio of 81 percent refined grains and 19 percent whole grains was applied, based on redemption data.

[h] Equivalent to 4 oz per day, the lower end of AAP guideline of not more than 4–6 ounces per day.

[i] To compare the food package contribution to the DGA recommended amounts of whole grains, the whole grain portion of breakfast cereal was added to the whole grain contribution of bread.

SOURCES: USDA/ARS, 2014; USDA/FNS, 2014; USDA/HHS, 2016. State-specific data are available in the public access file for this study (Email: paro@nas.edu)

TABLE 3-5 Authoritative Recommendations for Intake of Fish High in Omega-3 Fatty Acids and Low in Mercury

Recommending Authority	Recommendation: Quantity of Seafood Recommended (oz per day)	Target Population
2015–2020 DGA	1.3	Adults, 2,200 kcal diet
2015–2020 DGA	1.0	Children, 1,300 kcal diet
2015–2020 DGA	1.1–1.7	Pregnant or breastfeeding women
FDA-EPA	1.1–1.7	Pregnant or breastfeeding women
AHA	1.0	Children and adults
AAP	0.6–1.1	Breastfeeding women
AAP	1–5 of flesh foods, including fish	Children ages 2 to 4
WHO	Flesh foods, including fish, as often as possible	Infants beginning complementary feeding

NOTES: AAP = American Academy of Pediatrics; AHA = American Heart Association; DGA = Dietary Guidelines for Americans; FDA-EPA = Food and Drug Administration-Environmental Protection Agency; WHO = World Health Organization.
SOURCES: PAHO/WHO, 2003; AAP, 2014; FDA-EPA, 2014; AHA, 2015; USDA/HHS, 2016.

Saturated Fat in the Food Packages

Although the DGA do not include an upper limit for total fat intake, as mentioned above and in Chapter 2, they do include an upper limit of 10 percent of total energy from saturated fat. They also include replacing saturated fats with polyunsaturated alternatives and replacing solid animal fats with nontropical vegetable oils and nuts. Additionally, the DGA describe a healthy food pattern as one that includes "fat-free or low-fat dairy, including milk, yogurt, cheese" (USDA/HHS, 2016, p. 15). Aligning with these recommendations, since 2012, the National School Lunch Program has required that all milk served in schools be low-fat or nonfat and, if flavored, nonfat. Although flavored milks are permitted in the National School Lunch Program, the overall food pattern energy levels limit the levels of added sugars in allowable milks (USDA/FNS, 2012). Another federal nutrition assistance program, the Child and Adult Care Food Program, also requires that all milk provided to individuals 2 years of age or older be low-fat or nonfat (USDA/FNS, 2016a). Similarly, the current WIC food packages allow only 1 percent or nonfat milk for individuals ages 2 years and older. Additionally, depending on the food package, quantities of cheese are limited to 1 or 2 pounds per month. The saturated fat content of various WIC-allowable foods is presented in Table 3-7.

TABLE 3-6 Sodium Content of Representative Currently Allowable WIC Foods

Daily Limit or Food and Serving-Equivalent	Sodium (mg)
DGA daily limits	
1,300 kcal pattern	1,500
2,300 and 2,600 kcal patterns	2,300
Food option and serving-equivalent[a]	
Canned green beans, 1 c-eq	424
Canned sweet corn, 1 c-eq	422
Canned whole tomatoes, 1 c-eq	218
Cheese, 1 oz-eq	185
Yogurt, plain, low fat, 1 c-eq	172
Chocolate milk, 1%, reduced sugar, 1 c-eq	162
Chocolate milk, 1%, 1 c-eq	159
Yogurt, vanilla, low fat, 1 c-eq[b]	140
Cereal, toasted oats, 1 oz-eq	139
Cereal, oat flakes with almonds, 1 oz-eq	118
Canned light tuna, packed in oil, 1 oz-eq	118
Soymilk, generic, 1 c-eq	115
Milk, 1%, 1 c-eq	108
Milk, nonfat, 1 c-eq	103
Soymilk, original, 1 c-eq[c]	95
Soymilk, vanilla, 1 c-eq[c]	85
Whole wheat bread, 1 oz-eq	73
Egg, 1 oz-eq	71
Canned light tuna, packed in water, 1 oz-eq	70
Peanut butter, salted, 1 oz-eq	68
Instant oats, 1 oz-eq	62
Canned pinto beans, 1 c-eq	41
Tofu, 1 oz-eq	9

NOTES: c-eq = cup-equivalents; DGA = *Dietary Guidelines for Americans*; oz-eq = ounce-equivalents. Nutrient amounts are from the National Nutrient Database for Standard Reference, release 28 (USDA/ARS, 2016) except where noted. For comparison, limits noted at the top of the table indicate 10 percent of kcal.

[a] Cup- and ounce-equivalent servings are per the Food Patterns Equivalents Database 2011–2012: Methodology and User Guide (USDA/ARS, 2014).

[b] Values based on the food label of a WIC-approved low-fat vanilla yogurt.

[c] Values based on the food label of a WIC-approved soymilk.

SOURCES: USDA/ARS, 2014, 2016; USDA/FNS, 2014; USDA/HHS, 2016; other sources where noted.

TABLE 3-7 Saturated Fat Content of Representative Currently Allowable WIC Foods

Daily Limit or Food and Serving-Equivalent	Saturated Fat (g)
DGA daily limits	
1,300 kcal pattern	14.4
2,300 kcal pattern	25.6
2,600 kcal pattern	28.9
Food option and serving-equivalent[a]	
Cheese, 1 oz-eq	5.3
Yogurt, plain, low fat, 1 c-eq	2.5
Peanut butter, salted, 1 oz-eq	1.7
Milk, 1%, 1 c-eq	1.6
Egg, 1 oz-eq	1.6
Chocolate milk, 1%, reduced sugar, 1 c-eq	1.5
Chocolate milk, 1%, 1 c-eq	1.4
Yogurt, vanilla, low fat, 1 c-eq[b]	1.0
Tofu, 1 oz-eq	0.9
Soymilk, generic, 1 c-eq	0.5
Soymilk, original, 1 c-eq[c]	0.5
Cereal, toasted oats, 1 oz-eq	0.4
Instant oats, 1 oz-eq	0.4
Canned light tuna, packed in oil, 1 oz-eq	0.4
Canned pinto beans, 1 c-eq	0.3
Cereal, oat flakes with almonds, 1 oz-eq	0.2
Milk, nonfat, 1 c-eq	0.1
Whole wheat bread, 1 oz-eq	0.1
Canned light tuna, packed in water, 1 oz-eq	0.1
Soymilk, vanilla, 1 c-eq[c]	0

NOTES: c-eq = cup-equivalents; DGA = *Dietary Guidelines for Americans*; oz-eq = ounce-equivalents. Nutrient amounts are from the National Nutrient Database for Standard Reference, release 28 (USDA/ARS, 2016) except where noted. For comparison, limits noted at the top of the table indicate 10 percent of kcal.

[a] Cup- and ounce-equivalent servings are per the Food Patterns Equivalents Database 2011–2012: Methodology and User Guide (USDA/ARS, 2014).

[b] Values based on the food label of a WIC-approved low fat vanilla yogurt.

[c] Values based on the food label of a WIC-approved soymilk.

SOURCES: USDA/ARS, 2014, 2016; USDA/FNS, 2014; USDA/HHS, 2016; other sources where noted.

TABLE 3-8 Added Sugars Content of Representative Currently Allowable WIC Foods

Daily Limit or Food and Serving-Equivalent	Added Sugars (g)[b]
DGA daily limits	
1,300 kcal pattern	32.5
2,300 kcal pattern	57.5
2,600 kcal pattern	65.0
Food option and serving-equivalent[a]	
Yogurt, vanilla, low fat, 1 c-eq[c]	16.6
Chocolate milk, 1%, 1 c-eq	11.6
Soymilk, vanilla, 1 c-eq[d]	11.0
Soymilk, generic, 1 c-eq	8.9
Soymilk, original, 1 c-eq[d]	6.0
Cereal, oat flakes with almonds, 1 oz-eq	5.4
Chocolate milk, 1%, reduced sugar, 1 c-eq[e]	5.1
Whole wheat bread, 1 oz-eq	1.4
Peanut butter, salted, 1 oz-eq	1.0
Cereal, toasted oats, 1 oz-eq	0.9
Milk, nonfat, 1 c-eq	0
Milk, 1%, 1 c-eq	0
Cheese, 1 oz-eq	0
Yogurt, plain, low fat, 1 c-eq	0
Tofu, 1 oz-eq	0
Egg, 1 oz-eq	0
Instant oats, 1 oz-eq	0
Canned light tuna, packed in water, 1 oz-eq	0
Canned light tuna, packed in oil, 1 oz-eq	0
Canned pinto beans, 1 c-eq	0

NOTES: c-eq = cup-equivalents; DGA = *Dietary Guidelines for Americans*; oz-eq = ounce-equivalents. Nutrient amounts are from the National Nutrient Database for Standard Reference, release 28 (USDA/ARS, 2016) except where noted. For comparison, limits noted at the top of the table indicate 10 percent of kcal.

[a] Cup- and ounce-equivalent servings are per the Food Patterns Equivalents Database 2011–2012: Methodology and User Guide (USDA/ARS, 2014).

[b] Added sugars were calculated by subtracting naturally occurring sugar from total sugar in the food option. The USDA Final Rule permits ≤40 grams of total sugar per cup of yogurt and ≤6 grams per ounce of breakfast cereal.

continued

TABLE 3-8 Continued

[c] Values based on the food label of a WIC-approved low fat vanilla yogurt containing 31.6 grams of total sugars. The plain low fat version of this yogurt contains 15 grams of sugar.

[d] Values based on the food label of a WIC-approved soymilk.

[e] Based on flavored milks approved for the School Meals Program that are not commercially available.

SOURCES: USDA/ARS, 2014, 2016; USDA/FNS, 2014; USDA/HHS, 2016; other sources where noted.

Added Sugars in the Food Packages

As noted above and in Chapter 2, as with saturated fats, the DGA recommend limiting added sugars to no more than 10 percent of total calories. Added sugars are sweeteners of various types added to foods (e.g., corn syrup, fruit juice concentrate, fructose, maltose) and do not include naturally occurring sugars such as those in 100% fruit juice or lactose in dairy products (USDA/HHS, 2016). The DGA further state that added sugars may have a role in increasing the palatability of nutrient-dense foods and specifically cited whole grain breakfast cereals and nonfat yogurts as examples (USDA/HHS, 2016).

Added sugars are limited in the WIC food packages. Although the FDA has issued a proposed rule on labeling of added sugars, at present, manufacturers are required to include only total sugars on the food label. Thus, specifications for some WIC foods, including ready-to-eat breakfast cereals and yogurt are for total sugars (not added sugars) (USDA/FNS, 2014). At present, USDA does not provide specifications for total sugars for soy beverages or flavored milk in the WIC food packages. The added sugars content of various WIC-allowable foods is presented in Table 3-8.

Alignment of the Current WIC Food Packages with Dietary Guidance for "Calories for Other Uses"

The concept of COU was introduced in the 2015–2020 DGA (replacing the 2010 DGA concept of "discretionary calories"). COU include calories from saturated fats (solid fats), added sugars, added refined starches, and alcohol, as well as additional calories from the food groups beyond amounts recommended. As described in Chapter 2, the limits for COU vary among food patterns, depending on how many "leftover" calories are available after the food group intake recommendations are met. For example, only 100 calories are available to be used as COU in a 1,200-kcal pattern, compared to 390 COU in a 2,600-kcal pattern.

As shown in Table 3-9, based on the committee's calculations of estimated contributions of the food packages to COU,[5] assuming full redemp-

[5] These estimates are based on several assumptions, as described in detail in Appendix R.

TABLE 3-9 Contributions of the Food Packages to the DGA Daily Limit for "Calories for Other Uses*

Percent of Total Daily kcals Available for COU[a]	Total kcal in FP[b]	FP COU Daily Limit[c]	Amount Provided by the Food Package Per Day: Saturated Fat[b] g	Saturated Fat[b] kcal	Added Sugar[b] g	Added Sugar[b] kcal	Total COU kcal in the FP[d]	Proportion of the Total Daily COU Limit (%)[e]	Proportion of Food Package COU Daily Limit (%)[f]
FP V: Women, Pregnant and Partially Breastfeeding (based on a 2,600-kcal pattern)									
15	787	118	9	77	7	30	107	27	90
FP VI: Women, Postpartum (based on a 2,300-kcal pattern)									
14	572	80	6	58	7	27	85	26	106
FP VII: Women, Fully Breastfeeding (based on a 2,600-kcal pattern)									
15	918	138	13	115	7	27	142	36	103
FP IV: Children ages 2 to less than 5 years (based on a 1,300-kcal pattern)									
8	648	52	7	59	7	27	87	83	167

NOTES: COU = calories for other uses, defined in the DGA as the combined calories from saturated fats (solid fats), added sugars, refined carbohydrates, and alcohol; DGA = 2015–2020 *Dietary Guidelines for Americans*; FP = food package. Kcal patterns were selected based on the calculated Estimated Energy Requirement for WIC participants, using NHANES 2011–2012 (children) or 2005–2012 (women). Calculations assume full redemption of the food packages.

*Some values in this table are corrected from the original prepublication version.

[a] Based on the DGA food pattern indicated.

[b] Based on the nutrient profiles of the food packages as developed using the methodology described in Appendix R, and presented in Appendix T.

[c] (percent of total daily kcals available for COU) × (total kcal in the food package). To calculate this value, it was considered that the COU provided by the package should be in the same proportion as the COU in the USDA daily food pattern. For example, the USDA food pattern for a 2,600-kcal diet allows 15 percent of calories from COU. Thus, if food package V provides approximately 787 kcal, 15 percent, or 118 kcal, can be proportionally allotted to COU.

[d] (saturated fat kcal) + (added sugars kcal).

[e] (total COU kcal in the package × 100)/(number of COU kcal for the food pattern [data not shown]).

[f] (proportion of the total daily COU limit × 100)/(FP COU daily limit). For example, food package V provides 107 kcal from COU, an amount that is 90 percent of 118 kcal.

SOURCES: USDA/ARS, 2016; USDA/HHS, 2016.

tion, all food packages provide less than the recommended total limit for COU for the diet as a whole. Considering the kcal provided by the package, the COU provided in each package are generally proportional to or slightly exceed the proportional limit for COU. Food packages for children exceed the proportional recommended limit for COU. The primary contributors to COU are dairy foods. Given that the current food packages are relatively limited in added sugars and saturated fat, these results indicate there is little room for additional COU in foods and beverages outside the WIC food packages. These results also suggest that it is a challenge for many WIC participants, especially children, to ensure that their overall diets fall within the recommended limits for COU.

ALIGNMENT OF THE FOOD PACKAGES WITH DIETARY GUIDANCE FOR INDIVIDUALS LESS THAN 2 YEARS OF AGE

The DGA do not currently include dietary guidance for individuals from birth to 24 months of age, although the Agricultural Act of 2014, also known as the Farm Bill, has officially called for future (i.e., 2020) DGA to include infants and toddlers (U.S. Congress, P.L. 113-79, 2014). Meanwhile, without this guidance, it is significantly more difficult to assess the appropriateness of the WIC food packages for children less than 2 years of age. To carry out its task, the committee compiled recommendations from the AAP, the Academy of Nutrition and Dietetics (AND), the World Health Organization (WHO), and other authoritative groups (see Table 3-10) and compared this guidance with the components of the food packages.

The committee found that the food packages are generally aligned with dietary guidance for infants and children ages 0 to less than 2 years, with the exception of juice, infant cereal, and jarred infant meat. Specifically, although the amount of juice provided in food package IV (which is provided to children 1 to 2 years of age) falls within the AAP recommended range of 4 to 6 ounces per day, this range is an upper limit. Moreover, the AAP guidelines emphasize whole fruit over 100% juice. Additionally, the AAP recommends a maximum of 4 tablespoons of infant cereal per day and a maximum of 1 to 2 ounces of jarred infant meat per day. The current infant food packages (food package II) provide 6 tablespoons of infant cereal per day (150 percent of the recommended amount) to all infants ages 6 to less than 12 months of age and 2.6 ounces of jarred infant meat (130 percent of the recommended amount) to fully breastfed infants of the same ages.

ALIGNMENT WITH THE DIETARY REFERENCE INTAKES

The committee also evaluated the alignment of the food packages with the DRI values appropriate for each age and physiological-state subgroup (see Appendix J, Tables J-1a to J-1c for a compilation of DRIs). For women and children, most nutrients have an associated Estimated Average Requirement (EAR), which is the intake level at which 50 percent of individuals in a population will meet their needs. Nutrient contributions of the food packages as percentages of EARs are presented in Tables 3-11 through 3-13 (EARs are specific to each target population). For nutrients with only an Adequate Intake (AI), the proportion of the AI offered in the packages is also presented, but interpretation should take into account that, in contrast to the EAR, mean intakes should fall at or above the AI. For infants, most of the DRIs are expressed as AIs. A detailed description of the methodology applied to create the food package nutrient profiles is provided in Appendix R.[6]

Highlights of the nutrient profiles presented in Tables 3-11 through 3-13 are summarized here, with a focus on the provision of shortfall nutrients. As discussed in Chapter 2, the DGA identified 10 shortfall nutrients: vitamin A, vitamin D, vitamin E, vitamin C, folate, calcium, magnesium, fiber, iron, and potassium. Of these, four were identified further as nutrients of public health concern: calcium, vitamin D, fiber, and potassium, as well as iron for adolescent and premenopausal females. All of the food packages provide relatively small amounts of vitamin E, choline, and potassium. Similarly, the majority of the USDA food patterns do not assure adequacy of these nutrients, or of vitamin D (USDA/HHS, 2016), a factor that was considered when determining options for improving nutrient composition of the food packages. None of the food packages exceeded the UL for any nutrient.

Food Packages for Women

Food Package V for Pregnant and Partially Breastfeeding Women

For pregnant women, food package V contributes more than 100 percent of the EAR for calcium, vitamin C, vitamin A, phosphorus, riboflavin, and vitamin B12; close to 100 percent of the EAR for folate; and between approximately 60 and 80 percent of the EAR for iron, magnesium, zinc, selenium, vitamin B6, thiamin, niacin, and vitamin D. Food package V provides approximately 8 g per day of fiber and 1,800 mg per day of potassium, or about one-third of the AI for these nutrients (see Table 3-11).

The DRI for breastfeeding women assumes exclusive breastfeeding. Therefore, it was not possible to estimate the contribution of the food packages to the needs of partially breastfeeding women in reference to a DRI value as no appropriate DRI is available.

---

[6] To develop the food package nutrient profiles, the nutrient contribution of each WIC food category (i.e., "milk" or "bread") was determined. The category may include the nutrient contributions of substitution options (i.e., cheese for milk) as described in Appendix R.

TABLE 3-10 Dietary Guidance for Breastfeeding Mothers and Infants and Children Less Than 2 Years of Age

Feeding Mode	Reference
Breastfeeding—Guidance for Infant Nutrition	
All infants should be exclusively breastfed for about 6 months, followed by continued breastfeeding as complementary foods are introduced, with continuation of breastfeeding for 1 year or longer as mutually desired by mother and infant.[a]	WHO, 2009; IOM, 2011b; AAP, 2014; AND, 2015
To improve the intake of long-chain omega-3 fatty acids by breastfed infants, it is recommended that their mothers consume 1–2 servings of "ocean-going" fish per week to achieve a maternal intake of 200–300 mg of omega-3 long-chain fatty acids.[b]	AAP, 2014
All breastfed infants should receive an oral supplement of vitamin D, 400 IU per day, beginning at hospital discharge.	AAP, 2012
Starting at 4 months of age exclusively breastfed infants should be supplemented with iron.	AAP Committee on Nutrition, 2010
Formula Feeding	
For infants who are not breastfed, iron-fortified formula is the recommended alternative for feeding the baby during the first year of life.	AAP, 2014
Supplementary fluoride should not be provided to formula-fed infants during the first 6 months of life. After 6 months of age, the need for fluoride supplementation depends on the fluoride concentration of water used to prepare formula.	AAP, 2014
There are a limited number of medical conditions in which breastfeeding is contraindicated.	AAP, 2012, 2014
Therapeutic (noncontract) formula should be made available through physician prescription for specific medical conditions.	AAP, 2014
Complementary Feeding	
Complementary foods should be gradually introduced to infants at approximately 6 months of life.	AAP, 2014
Complementary food rich in iron and zinc (fortified cereals and meats) should be introduced to exclusively breastfed infants at about 6 months of age depending on developmental readiness. Recommended amounts are 2 servings per day of cereal (2 tablespoons per serving) or 1 to 2 oz of meat per day.	AAP Committee on Nutrition, 2010; AAP, 2012, 2014
Introduce single-ingredient new foods, one at a time, observing for adverse reactions or intolerance.	AAP, 2014

TABLE 3-10 Continued

Feeding Mode	Reference
Avoid cow's milk until 1 year of age. Whole milk may be provided at 1 year of age. During the second year of life, low-fat milk may be considered if weight gain is appropriate, if weight gain is excessive, or family history is positive for obesity, dyslipidemia, or cardiovascular disease. Recommended total daily milk intake is 16 to 24 ounces. Intakes above 25 ounces/day may contribute to iron deficiency.	AAP Committee on Nutrition, 2008; NHLBI, 2011; AAP, 2014
Introduce a variety of foods. By 7 to 8 months, infants should be consuming foods from all food groups. Provide foods of varying textures (e.g., pureed, blended, mashed, finely chopped, and soft lumps). Gradually increase table foods. Avoid mixed textures, such as broth with vegetables.	AAP, 2014
Avoid foods that could cause choking or aspiration (e.g., hot dogs, nuts, grapes, raisins, raw carrots, popcorn, hard candies); avoid eating peanut butter from a spoon.	AAP Committee on Injury, Violence, and Poison Prevention, 2010; AAP, 2014
Developing Healthy Eating Patterns	
Allow lower-fat milks for children 1 year of age and older for whom obesity or overweight is a concern.	AAP Committee on Nutrition, 2008
Total daily juice intake should be limited to 4 to 6 ounces per day from 1 to 6 years of age. Encourage whole fruit over juice.	AAP, 2014
Avoid added sugar and added salt.	AAP, 2014
Repeat exposure to new foods and flavors may be required to optimize acceptance. Early exposure may promote the selection of a varied diet later in life.	AAP, 2014

[a] There is some controversy regarding whether exclusive breastfeeding meets energy requirements of infants at 6 months of age in developed countries. Fewtrell et al. (2007, p. 637S) states, "A reasonable interpretation of the available scientific data is that there are currently insufficient grounds to confidently recommend an optimal duration of exclusive breastfeeding of 6 as opposed to 4–6 months for infants in developed countries."

[b] This level of maternal fish intake has been associated with improved neurobehavioral development in infants. Concern regarding the possible risk from intake of excessive mercury or other contaminants is offset by the neurobehavioral benefits of an adequate DHA intake and can be minimized by avoiding the intake of predatory fish (e.g., pike, marlin, mackerel, tilefish, swordfish) (AAP, 2014).

SOURCES: As noted in the Reference column.

TABLE 3-11 Nutrients Provided per Day in the Current Food Packages Compared to Dietary Reference Intakes: Pregnant, Breastfeeding, and Postpartum Women

				FP V, Pregnant		FP VII, Breastfeeding		FP VI, Postpartum*	
Nutrient	EAR/AI Pregnant	EAR/AI Breastfeeding	EAR/AI Postpartum	Amount	% DRI	Amount	% DRI	Amount	% DRI
Energy (kcal)	2,625[a]	2,492[a]	2,350[a]	787	30	918	37	572	24
Protein (g)	71[b]	71[b]	46[b]	39	55	52	74	27	60
Fiber (g)	28[c]	29[c]	25[c]	8.0	29	8.0	28	5.7	23
Calcium (mg)	800	800	800	1,029	129	1,232	154	739	92
Copper (mg)	0.8	1	0.7	0.4	55	0.5	48	0.3	42
Iron (mg)	22	6.5	8.1	13.5	62	14	221	12.3	152
Magnesium (mg)	290/300[d]	255/265[d]	255/265[d]	198	68/68	214	84/81	132	52/50
Phosphorus (mg)	580	580	580	976	168	1,178	203	690	119
Selenium (μg)	49	59	45	31.6	65	64	108	25	56
Zinc (mg)	9.5	10.4	6.8	6.6	69	7.7	74	5.2	76
Potassium (mg)	4,700[c]	5,100[c]	4,700[c]	1,837	39	1,958	38	1,302	28
Vitamin A (μg RAE)	550	900	500	646	117	754	84	522	104
Vitamin E (mg)	12	16	12	3.6	30	4.0	25	2.5	20
Vitamin D (IU)	400	400	400	291	73	371	93	213	53
Vitamin C (mg)	70	100	60	72	103	72	72	57	95
Thiamin (mg)	1.2	1.2	0.9	0.9	76	0.9	78	0.7	81

Riboflavin (mg)	1.2	1.3	0.9	1.8	148	2.0	153	1.4	153
Niacin (mg)	14	13	11	9.9	71	13	98	8.0	72
Vitamin B6 (mg)	1.6	1.7	1.1	1.3	79	1.4	83	1.1	97
Folate (µg DFE)	520	450	320	473	91	487	108	425	133
Vitamin B12 (µg)	2.2	2.4	2	4.4	198	5.6	234	3.6	180
Choline (mg)	450[c]	550[c]	425[c]	75	17	147	27	71	17
Nutrients to Limit									
Added sugars (g)	65[e]	65[e]	57.5[e]	7.4	12	6.6	10	6.9	12
Saturated fat (g)	29[e]	29[e]	26[e]	8.5	29	13	44	6.4	25
Sodium (mg)	1,500[c]	1,500[c]	1,500[c]	727	48	1,007	67	527	35

NOTES: AI = adequate intake; DGA = *Dietary Guidelines for Americans*; EAR = Estimated Average Requirement; FP = food package; RAE = retinol activity equivalents; RDA = Recommended Dietary Allowance; Nutrient profiles were developed by applying the assumptions outlined in Appendix R.

*Some values in these columns are corrected from the original prepublication version.

[a] Value is the median estimated energy requirement (EER) calculated by the committee. Values differ slightly from those in Chapter 4 because EER values for that chapter were re-calculated in a different statistical program to generate percentiles. The means are equivalent for the two analyses.

[b] Values represent an RDA. The RDA is used for evaluation of the food package protein content because the EAR for protein is in units of g per kg body weight and therefore must be calculated for an individual.

[c] Indicates an AI. Other values are an EAR unless otherwise noted.

[d] Magnesium has two values: 19-30y/31-50y;

[e] Based the DGA recommended limit of 10 percent of kcal.

SOURCES: IOM, 1997, 1998, 2000, 2001, 2002/2005, 2005, 2011a; USDA/ARS, 2016; USDA/HHS, 2016.

TABLE 3-12 Nutrients Provided per Day in the Current Food Packages for Infants Less Than 12 Months of Age*

Nutrient	AI, Infants Less Than 6 Months	EAR/AI, Infants 6 to Less Than 12 Months	FF 0–3 mo	FF 4–5 mo	0–1 mo	BF/FF 1–3 mo	BF/FF 4–5 mo	FF 6–11 mo	BF/FF 6–11 mo	BF 6–11 mo
Energy (kcal)	617[a]	727[a]	588	645	71	289	347	621	409	300
Protein (g)	9.1[b]	11[b]	13	14	1.6	6.4	7.7	14	8.8	13
Fiber (g)	ND	ND	0	0	0	0	0	3.7	3.7	5.9
Calcium (mg)	200	260	560	607	68	276	327	604	404	208
Copper (mg)	0.2	0.22	0.48	0.52	0.06	0.24	0.28	0.52	0.35	0.28
Iron (mg)	0.27	6.9[c]	11	12	1.3	5.3	6.3	21	17	14
Magnesium (mg)	30	75	46	50	5.5	23	27	68	52	58
Phosphorus (mg)	100	275	342	369	41	168	199	388	266	220
Selenium (μg)	15	20	15	16	1.8	7.2	8.6	18	13	14
Zinc (mg)	2	2.5[c]	5.1	5.6	0.6	2.5	3.0	5.9	4.1	3.3
Potassium (mg)	400	700	641	702	77	316	377	830	599	669
Vitamin A (μg RAE)	400	500	531	582	64	262	313	550	358	262
Vitamin E (mg)	4	5	7.2	7.8	0.9	3.5	4.2	7.0	4.4	2.2
Vitamin D (IU)	400	400	348	370	42	171	199	313	192	58
Vitamin C (mg)	40	50	62	68	7.4	30	37	71	49	46
Thiamin (mg)	0.2	0.30	0.5	0.6	0.1	0.3	0.3	0.70	0.52	0.35

Riboflavin (mg)	0.3	0.40	0.78	0.87	0.09	0.39	0.47	0.92	0.63	0.47
Niacin (mg)	2	4	6.3	6.9	0.8	3.1	3.7	9.7	7.4	7.5
Vitamin B6 (mg)	0.10	0.30	0.36	0.40	0.04	0.18	0.21	0.29	0.16	0.09
Folate (µg DFE)	65	80	152	159	18	75	86	158	105	62
Vitamin B12 (µg)	0.4	0.5	1.8	1.9	0.2	0.9	1.0	2.1	1.4	1.2
Choline (mg)	125	150	100	113	12	49	61	100	63	60
Nutrients to Limit										
Added sugars (g)	NA	NA	0	0.7	0	0	0.4	0.5	0.3	0
Saturated fat (g)	NA	NA	13.4	14.6	1.6	6.6	7.8	10.7	5.9	1.4
Sodium (mg)	120	370	178	194	21	88	104	156	93	64

NOTES: AI unless otherwise noted; AI = adequate intake; BF = breastfed; BF/FF = partially breastfed; DFE = dietary folate equivalents; DGA = *Dietary Guidelines for Americans*; EAR = Estimated Average Requirement; FF = formula fed; RAE = retinol activity equivalents; RDA = Recommended Dietary Allowance. Nutrient profiles were developed by applying the assumptions outlined in Appendix R. *Some values in this table are corrected from the original prepublication version.

[a] Value is the median estimated energy requirement (EER) calculated by the committee.

[b] Value represents an RDA. The RDA is used for evaluation of the food package protein content because the EAR for protein is in units of g per kg body weight and therefore must be calculated for an individual.

[c] Value represents an EAR.

SOURCES: IOM, 1997, 1998, 2000, 2001, 2002/2005, 2005, 2011a; USDA/ARS, 2016; USDA/FNS, 2016b.

TABLE 3-13 Nutrients Provided per Day in the Current Food Packages Compared to Dietary Reference Intakes: Children Ages 1 to Less Than 5 Years of Age*

			Children 1 to Less Than 2 Years		Children 2 to Less Than 5 Years		
Nutrient	EAR/AI, 1–3 y	EAR/AI, 4–8 y	Amount	% DRI	Amount	% DRI, 1–3 y	% DRI, 4–5 y
Energy (kcal)	917[a]	1,517[a]	725	79	648	71	43
Protein (g)	13[b]	19[b]	29	224	31	236	162
Fiber (g)	19[c]	25[c]	7.1	38	7.1	38	29
Calcium (mg)	500	800	717	143	787	157	98
Copper (mg)	0.26	0.34	0.42	161	0.35	134	102
Iron (mg)	3	4.1	13.4	445	13.5	449	328
Magnesium (mg)	65	110	138	212	154	237	140
Phosphorus (mg)	380	405	690	182	762	201	188
Selenium (µg)	17	23	35.2	207	32	187	138
Zinc (mg)	2.5	4	5.5	221	5.7	227	142
Potassium (mg)	3,000[c]	3,800[c]	1,267	42	1,357	45	36
Vitamin A (µg RAE)	210	275	417	199	532	253	194
Vitamin E (mg)	5	6	1.1	22	3.0	60	50
Vitamin D (IU)	400	400	254	63	213	53	53
Vitamin C (mg)	13	22	56	429	60	458	271
Thiamin (mg)	0.4	0.5	0.8	211	0.8	206	165
Riboflavin (mg)	0.4	0.5	1.4	345	1.4	353	282

Niacin (mg)	5	6	8.9	179	9.0	179	150
Vitamin B6 (mg)	0.4	0.5	1.1	268	1.1	277	222
Folate (μg DFE)	120	160	430	358	431	359	269
Vitamin B12 (μg)	0.7	1	3.8	546	3.6	514	360
Choline (mg)	200[c]	250[c]	71	36	77	38	31
Nutrients to Limit							
Added sugars (g)	NA	32.5[d]	8.4	NA	6.9	21	21
Saturated fat (g)	NA	14.4[d]	11.9	NA	6.6	47	46
Sodium (mg)	1,000[c]	1,200[c]	587	59	639	64	53

NOTES: AI = adequate intake; DFE = dietary folate equivalents; DGA = *Dietary Guidelines for Americans*; EAR = Estimated Average Requirement; NA = not applicable; RAE = retinol activity equivalents. Nutrient profiles were developed by applying the assumptions outlined in Appendix R.*Some values in this table are corrected from the original prepublication version.

[a] Value is the median estimated energy requirement (EER) calculated by the committee.

[b] Values represent a Recommended Dietary Allowance (RDA). The RDA is used for evaluation of the food package protein content because the EAR for protein is in units of g per kg body weight and therefore must be calculated for an individual.

[c] Indicates an AI. Other values are an EAR unless otherwise noted.

[d] For added sugars and saturated fat, value is the percent of the *Dietary Guidelines for Americans* (DGA) limit.

SOURCES: IOM, 1997, 1998, 2000, 2001, 2002/2005, 2005, 2011a; USDA/ARS, 2016; USDA/HHS, 2016.

Food Package VI for Postpartum Women

Food package VI for women who are postpartum (up to 6 months) provides more than 100 percent of the EAR for iron, folate, phosphorus, riboflavin, vitamin B12, and vitamin A, and nearly 100 percent of calcium, vitamin B6, and vitamin C EARs are provided in the food package. The package also provides between 70 and 80 percent of the EAR for zinc and niacin and approximately 50 percent of the EAR for vitamin D. This food package provides 6 g per day of fiber and approximately 1,300 mg per day of potassium, well below the AIs for these nutrients (see Table 3-11).

Food Package VII for Fully Breastfeeding Women

Food package VII for women who are fully breastfeeding (up to 12 months) provides more than 100 percent of the EAR for calcium, phosphorus, selenium, vitamin C, riboflavin, vitamin B12, and iron. Between 70 and 100 percent of the EAR for protein, zinc, thiamin, niacin, vitamin B6, folate, and vitamin D is provided. This food package provides 8 g of fiber per day and approximately 1,900 mg per day of potassium. As for other food packages, these amounts are below the AI for these nutrients (see Table 3-11).

Food Packages for Infants

Assessment of the contributions of the infant food packages to nutrient requirements was made more challenging by the lack of EAR values for these age groups. Although a full analysis of the food package nutrients was conducted, the committee focused on iron and zinc, which are commonly considered nutrients of concern for infants, particularly if breastfed (AAP, 2014), and for which EAR values have been determined. The results of this analysis are presented in Table 3-12.

For infants ages 6 to less than 12 months, food package II provides between 14 and 21 mg per day of iron depending on the feeding mode (formula fed, partially breastfed, or fully breastfed), compared to an EAR of 6.9 mg per day. The same food package provides between approximately 3 and 6 mg per day of zinc, compared to an EAR of 2.5 mg, again depending on feeding mode.

Food Package IV for Children Ages 1 to Less Than 5 Years

The nutrient contributions of the food package are different between children ages 1 to less than 2 years compared to children ages 2 to less than 5 years because the former are required to be issued whole milk products (see

Table 3-13). Overall, provision of most nutrients is well over 100 percent of the EAR, with some as high as approximately 400 percent (iron and vitamin C). For children ages 2 to less than 5 years, the food package provides over 100 percent of the EAR for calcium, iron, vitamins C and A, and folate among other nutrients. The package provides approximately 50 percent of the average vitamin D requirements for children of all qualifying ages.

FORMS AND COMPOSITION OF FOODS PROVIDED IN THE FOOD PACKAGES AND ALIGNMENT WITH DIETARY GUIDANCE

In addition to evaluating the quantities of nutrients and food groups provided by the food packages, the committee evaluated the appropriateness of the types of food for the intended recipients. Table 3-14 lists the current WIC foods that are authorized across food packages and the dietary guidance related to food types and food composition. In nearly all cases, the foods provided are consistent with this guidance. For example, only whole milk is provided to children 1 to less than 2 years of age, and milk provided to individuals ages 2 years and older is low-fat or nonfat. In only two cases are the foods provided not well aligned with dietary guidance. First, juice provided to children meets 100 percent of the lower end of the AAP limit. Yet whole fruit is the preferred form of fruit (see Table 3-10). Second, although intake of fish, particularly varieties high in omega-3 and low in mercury, is recommended for children and women (see Table 3-5), fish is currently provided only to fully breastfeeding women in food package VII.

ALIGNMENT OF THE FOOD PACKAGES WITH SPECIAL DIETARY NEEDS AND PREFERENCES

In Chapters 8 and 9 of the phase I report for this study, the ability of the food packages to meet the needs of WIC participants with particular medical conditions, cultural eating patterns, or food preferences was reviewed (NASEM, 2016). In this section, key components of that review that affected the committee's decisions on food package changes are summarized along with additional relevant information collected in phase II.

Foods to Address Medical Conditions

The current WIC food packages can accommodate a wide range of medical conditions. This section summarizes, first, the circumstances under which food package III can be issued and, second, the extent to which the WIC food packages accommodate the dietary needs of individuals with food allergies and other food-triggered sensitivities.

TABLE 3-14 Dietary Guidance Related to Types or Composition of Foods in Current WIC Food Packages

Foods in Current WIC Food Packages	Dietary Guidance for Infants and Children Less Than 2 Years*	Dietary Guidance for Children and Women*
100% juice with vitamin C, starting at 1 year of age	Infants less than 1 year of age should not consume juice; total daily juice intake should be limited to 4 to 6 ounces per day for children 1 to 6 years of age; encourage whole fruit over juice (AAP, 2014)	Young children (up to 6 years of age) should limit their juice intake to 4 to 6 ounces per day (AAP, 2014) Individuals more than 2 years of age should not consume more than 50% of their total fruit intake as juice (USDA/HHS, 2016)
Milk, whole for those 1 to 2 years of age, nonfat or 1% for older participants; fat-reduced milks to be issued to 1-year-old children (12 months to 2 years of age) for whom overweight or obesity is a concern	Avoid cow's milk until 1 year of age. Whole milk may be provided at 1 year of age. Lower fat milk may be allowed for children 1 year of age if obesity or overweight is a concern (AAP Committee on Nutrition, 2008; AAP, 2014; NHLBI, 2011) Intakes above 32 ounces/day may contribute to iron deficiency in children 1 to 2 years of age (AAP, 2014)	Most dairy consumed by individuals ages 2 and older should be low-fat (USDA/HHS, 2016)
Breakfast cereal, iron-fortified: may be hot or ready-to-eat, refined or whole grain	Infant cereal should be fortified with iron and zinc; two servings per day are recommended (1–2 T per serving) (AAP Committee on Nutrition, 2010a; AAP, 2012, 2014)	At least 50% of total grain intake should be from whole grains
Cheese, starting at 1 year of age	NR	Appropriate intake depends upon the total dairy intake recommendations as well as the amount of saturated fat and sodium in the overall diet; one strategy to reduce saturated fat intake is to replace regular cheese with low-fat cheese (USDA/HHS, 2016)
Eggs, starting at 1 year of age	Eggs may be introduced along with other complementary foods (PAHO/WHO, 2003; WHO, 2005; AAP, 2014)	No specific recommendations related to eggs

TABLE 3-14 Continued

Foods in Current WIC Food Packages	Dietary Guidance for Infants and Children Less Than 2 Years*	Dietary Guidance for Children and Women*
Vegetables and fruits, CVV option for breastfeeding infants, ages 9 to 11 months	Provide foods of varying textures (e.g., pureed, blended, mashed, finely chopped, and soft lumps); gradually increase table foods. Avoid mixed textures, such as broth with vegetables (AAP, 2014)	Whole fruit should be encouraged over juice (AAP, 2014)
Whole wheat or whole grain bread, starting at 1 year of age	NR	At least 50% of total grains intake should be from whole grains (USDA/HHS, 2016)
Fish (canned), fully breastfeeding women only	Infants should consume flesh foods, including fish, as soon as possible (PAHO/WHO, 2003)	Children should consume 1 oz of low-mercury seafood per day (USDA/HHS, 2016) Pregnant or breastfeeding women should consume between 1.1 and 1.3 ounces of low-mercury seafood per day (AAP, 2014; FDA-EPA, 2014; USDA/HHS, 2016)
Legumes and/or peanut butter, starting at 1 year of age	NR	No specific recommendations on types or composition of legumes or peanut butter
Iron-fortified infant formula	For infants that are not breastfeeding, iron-fortified formula is the recommended alternative for feeding the baby during the first year of life (AAP, 2014)	NA
Infant food meat, single-ingredient	Complementary foods should be introduced gradually to infants after 6 months of life; 1–2 ounces of meat or 1–2 small jars of commercially prepared meat per day (AAP Committee on Nutrition, 2010b; AAP, 2012, 2014)	NA

NOTES: DGA = *Dietary Guidelines for Americans*; NA = not applicable; NR = no recommendation; T = tablespoon.

* Sources of guidance as cited in parentheses.

The Special Case of Food Package III

At the discretion of a health care provider, participants may be considered "medically fragile" and can receive food package III for either themselves or their children. There exists no generally accepted definition of medical fragility. Examples include an infant with failure to thrive and an adult with a wired jaw. Individual states have policies regarding who may qualify under WIC. Approximately 3 percent of WIC participants are recipients of this package, 75 percent of whom are infants, 25 percent children, and less than 1 percent adults (USDA/FNS, 2016b).

Depending on a participant's specific medical needs, food package III is tailored to include either infant formula, noncontract[7] infant formulas with unique nutritional composition, or WIC-eligible nutritionals (a "WIC formula"[8]). Most WIC participants who are issued food package III receive non-contract formulas (USDA/FNS, 2016b). The WIC definition for WIC-eligible nutritionals (see Box 3-1) is similar to the FDA definition of a medical food (Section 5(b)(3) of the Orphan Drug Act (21 U.S.C. 360ee(b)(3)), except that the WIC definition does not include "administered under the supervision of a physician" and does not acknowledge "distinctive nutritional requirements, based on recognized scientific principles ... established by medical evaluation." However, a medical professional prescription or recommendation is still needed for a participant to receive food package III, therefore in practice, the definitions are essentially the same and the WIC definition was considered by the committee to be appropriate.

The types and quantities of WIC formula and supplemental foods must be determined by the medical professional with appropriate documentation provided to the state agency. State agencies may allow the health care provider to refer to the WIC registered dietitian and/or qualified nutritionist for identifying appropriate supplemental foods (excluding WIC formula) and their prescribed amounts, as well as the length of time the participant requires the supplemental foods. Participants receiving food package III may be issued 455 ounces of WIC formula per month in addition to the maximum allowance of all other foods in the package appropriate for their life stage. Exceptions to these food package

[7] Any formula that is noncontract is not subject to rebates. Exempt infant formula is always noncontract. By federal regulation, for WIC participants who are also on Medicaid, the Medicaid program is the primary payer for exempt infant formulas, as well as for WIC-eligible nutritionals. WIC is not the primary payer for Medicaid beneficiaries but may be the payer for those not on Medicaid. Some private insurance may also cover exempt formula.

[8] WIC formula refers to infant formula, exempt infant formula, or a WIC-eligible nutritional.

BOX 3-1

Definition of WIC-Eligible Nutritionals*

(7 C.F.R. § 246.3)

WIC-eligible nutritionals means certain enteral products that are specifically formulated to provide nutritional support for individuals with a qualifying condition, when the use of conventional foods is precluded, restricted, or inadequate. Such WIC-eligible nutritionals must serve the purpose of a food, meal, or diet (may be nutritionally complete or incomplete) and provide a source of calories and one or more nutrients; be designed for enteral digestion via an oral or tube feeding; and may not be a conventional food, drug, flavoring, or enzyme. WIC-eligible nutritionals include many, but not all, products that meet the definition of medical food in Section 5(b)(3) of the Orphan Drug Act (21 U.S.C. 360ee(b)(3)).

* The term *WIC-eligible medical foods* was changed to *WIC-eligible nutritionals* in the Final Rule (USDA/FNS, 2014).

regulations may be made as necessary and as dictated by the Final Rule (USDA/FNS, 2014).[9]

In some cases, participants under the care of a health care provider may be prescribed foods atypical for the participant's age category, such as when jarred infant foods are issued to individuals over 1 year of age. Under current regulations, participants must be prescribed a WIC formula to be issued food package III, whether or not it is included in the health care provider prescription and whether or not this required issuance suits the participant's condition (i.e., a participant 2 years of age or older who is prescribed whole milk is unlikely to also be in need of a WIC formula).[10]

Food-Triggered Immune-Mediated Sensitivities

All of the food packages can support the nutritional needs of several different types of food-triggered immune-mediated sensitivities, including food allergies, celiac disease, non-celiac gluten sensitivity (NCGS), and lactose intolerance. Chapter 8 of the phase I report included a summary

[9] As specified in the Final Rule, exceptions to the maximum monthly allowance of all other foods may be made for recipients of food package III, including (1) whole milk may be provided to children over 2 years of age and to women with a qualifying condition; (2) state agencies have the flexibility to provide children and women the option of receiving commercial jarred infant food fruits and vegetables in lieu of the cash value voucher; and (3) WIC formula may be provided in lieu of foods at 6 months of age.

[10] Text in this paragraph is updated from the original prepublication version.

of evidence from the literature on the nutritional needs of individuals with these medical conditions (NASEM, 2016). Here, the ways that the current food packages accommodate individuals with these conditions and potential gaps are highlighted.

Food allergies Allergy has been defined as a hypersensitivity disorder of the immune system where the immune system reacts to substances in the environment normally considered harmless (CDC, 2013). The most common food allergies are allergies to peanut, tree nuts, seafood, milk, hen's eggs, wheat, fish, and soy (Chafen et al., 2010), all of which were considered relevant to this review.

The committee's review of the literature indicated that, for infants at risk of developing allergy, most experts recommend breastfeeding for approximately 6 months and the provision of hydrolyzed[11] protein formula for nonbreastfed infants (Greer et al., 2008; Chafen et al., 2010; Fleischer et al., 2013). Historically, the AAP Committee on Nutrition (2000) recommended avoidance of some foods by breastfeeding mothers. However, authors of a recent systematic review of maternal intake during pregnancy or lactation did not find any conclusive evidence of an effect of maternal diet on the development of allergy in infants (Netting et al., 2014). In accordance with these recommendations, hydrolyzed protein infant formulas for allergy at-risk infants are available to formula-fed WIC infants with a physician's prescription.

There is no currently defined role for WIC-provided infant foods in allergy prevention because it is not fully understood how introduction of solid foods in the first year of life might influence the development of allergy. However, there is some evidence that early introduction of peanut protein reduces the likelihood of peanut allergy (Du Toit et al., 2008, 2015; Gruchalla and Sampson, 2015). Based on this evidence, the AAP issued interim guidance in September 2015 for the early (between 4 and 11 months of age) introduction of peanut protein to high-risk infants under care of a health care provider (Fleischer et al., 2015). In the fall of 2016, the National Institute of Allergy and Infectious Disease is set to release a policy to formally recommend the introduction of peanut to high-risk children at between 4 to 6 months of age (Greenhawt, 2016).

For children and adults, the current WIC packages include substitutions for allergenic foods so individuals with most major food allergies can be accommodated (see Table 3-15). However, as noted in the table, there is no current substitution for individuals with egg or fish allergies or those allergic to both cow's milk and soy. The committee considered the latter

[11] Hydrolyzed refers to formulas containing cow's milk proteins that have been extensively broken down so they are unlikely to cause an allergic reaction.

TABLE 3-15 Options in WIC Food Package Categories Potentially Unsuitable for Special Diets and Major Allergies

	Special Diet				Major Allergen					
WIC Food Category	Vegetarian	Vegan	Gluten Free	Lactose Free	Milk	Eggs	Fish	Peanuts	Wheat	Substitutions Allowed (% of state agencies allowing substitution)
Ready to eat cereal			✓						✓	Gluten-free corn cereal (88); gluten-free rice cereal (86)
Whole wheat bread			✓						✓	Brown rice (97); certified gluten-free corn tortillas (86); certified gluten-free oats (77)
Milk		✓		✓	✓					Soy beverage (95); tofu (63); lactose-free milk (>44)
Cheese		✓		✓	✓					No substitution
Eggs		✓				✓				No substitution
Peanut butter								✓		Canned legumes (85); dry legumes (100)
Canned fish	✓	✓					✓			No substitution

NOTES: ✓ Indicates that the primary food in the category is not likely to be suitable for the particular diet or allergy unless a suitable substitution is made available. The major allergens shellfish and tree nuts were excluded from the table because no WIC foods are provided in these categories. Soy is excluded as a major allergen because the baseline food packages do not contain soy products. The WIC food categories mature legumes, juice, and the CVV were excluded from the table because they are suitable for all cases covered in this table.
SOURCES: USDA/FNS, 2014, 2015a.

to be a medical condition for which food package III should be prescribed by the health care provider. Importantly, WIC offers participants with food allergies a number of educational resources to support adherence to dietary restrictions (USDA/FNS, 2015b).

Celiac disease Approximately 1 in 200 individuals living in the United States has celiac disease, an immune-mediated inflammation of the small bowel caused by sensitivity to dietary gluten (a protein found in wheat and other grains) and related proteins (Guandalini and Assiri, 2014; Mooney et al., 2014). Women with celiac disease may have an increased risk of obstetrical complications and adverse birth outcomes (AND, 2006; Saccone et al., 2016). An Academy of Nutrition and Dietetics (AND) systematic review indicated that women with undiagnosed or untreated celiac disease have an increased risk of several adverse pregnancy outcomes (evidence graded as fair) (AND, 2006).

Treatment for celiac disease includes lifelong avoidance of wheat, barley, and rye. Individuals with symptoms for celiac disease should be tested and, if positive, receive detailed nutritional counseling on gluten avoidance, because even milligram levels in the diet can have severe long-term health consequences (Rubio-Tapia et al., 2013). Because gluten-free grains (e.g., rice, potato flour, tapioca flour, corn) are not typically fortified, gluten-free diets may be low in iron and folate, as well as dietary fiber (Thompson, 2000). Nutrients of particular concern for pregnant women who follow a gluten-free diet include carbohydrates, iron, folic acid, niacin, calcium, phosphorus, zinc, and fiber (AND, 2014).

All state agencies now offer a nonwheat option for the "whole grain bread" food category (USDA/FNS, 2016b). These are suitable for gluten-free diets if the state-approved products are certified gluten-free. The Final Rule for the WIC food packages does not require that states provide a gluten-free option for cereals, although the provision allows state agencies to offer oat, corn, or rice-based cereals that may be appropriate for participants who must avoid gluten (USDA/FNS, 2014). However, such cereals are not necessarily certified as gluten-free and, thus, the gluten content of state-approved products may not fall under the FDA limit of 20 parts per million of gluten (an amount tolerated by most individuals with celiac disease) (21 C.F.R. § 101). Individuals with non-celiac gluten sensitivity (NCGS)[12] may

[12] NCGS is defined as the occurrence of gastrointestinal symptoms after the ingestion of wheat-containing foods in the absence of celiac disease or wheat allergy. Because there is no biomarker for gluten sensitivity, NCGS is not clinically diagnosable and is generally self-diagnosed (Branchi et al., 2015; Elli et al., 2015; Lebwohl et al., 2015). DiGiacomo et al. (2013) reported a 0.55 percent prevalence of NCGS in NHANES 2009–2010, although gluten-free diets may have become more prevalent since then. Additional studies are needed to understand the etiology and underlying physiology of NCGS (Husby and Murray, 2015).

also benefit from these non-wheat options. Table 3-15 indicates the currently available WIC foods and substitutions that meet the dietary needs of individuals who must or choose to avoid gluten.

Lactose intolerance Lactose intolerance is a set of symptoms caused by lactase deficiency. Individuals with lactose intolerance may be able to consume small amounts of dairy products (up to 8 ounces of milk or yogurt at one time) (Suarez et al., 1995, 1997; Lomer et al., 2008) or dairy products in specific forms. For example, natural cheddar cheese contains 0.18 percent lactose, whereas nonfat milk contains 5.09 percent lactose (USDA/ARS, 2016). For lactose-intolerant individuals, nutrition education might be necessary to ensure adequate calcium intake. A 2013 consensus statement issued by the National Medical Association and the National Hispanic Medical Association indicates that dairy intake may be low among African Americans and Hispanic Americans because of either perceived or actual lactose intolerance. In these cases, consumption of yogurt containing live and active cultures was suggested as a strategy for including dairy in the diet (Bailey et al., 2013).

Table 3-15 also indicates the currently available WIC foods and substitutions that meet the dietary needs of individuals who choose to avoid lactose. Soy products (soy beverages and tofu) are available as substitution options for cow's milk. Although there is no substitution for cheese for fully breastfeeding women, most individuals with lactose intolerance are able to consume cheese in small quantities.

Alignment of Foods with Specific Preferences and Dietary Practices

The committee considered how WIC food packages accommodate preferences for vegetarian and vegan diets and food-related religious practices (e.g., Kosher and Halal diets). This section summarizes the committee's evaluation of evidence supporting inclusion of foods in the packages that comply with these practices.

Vegetarian or Vegan Diets

Plant-based diets can be nutritionally adequate for infants, children, and adults (AND, 2009; AAP, 2014; USDA/HHS, 2016). A vegetarian diet does not include animal flesh foods (i.e., meat, fish, seafood), but it does include other animal products (e.g., eggs, milk, cheese, yogurt), whereas a vegan diet excludes all animal foods and products. Individuals who consume a vegan diet should pay particular attention to their intakes of vitamins B12, calcium (AND, 2009), and vitamin D (AND, 2009; Craig, 2009), but their requirement for these nutrients can be met by consuming fortified foods (AND, 2009). An additional concern exists for intakes of choline by pregnant women consuming vegan diets, but no research to date has assessed the intakes of choline by vegans. Individuals following a vegan diet may also have low intakes of eicosapentaenoic (EPA) and docosahexaenoic acids (DHA) (AND, 2009). The position of AND is that both vegetarian and vegan diets are not only adequate, but they may promote the prevention or aid in the treatment of certain health conditions (AND, 2009).

In cases where an infant's caretaker prefers to provide a vegetarian or vegan diet (as well as in cases where an infant does not tolerate cow's milk formula), the AAP supports the provision of soy protein–based formulas (Bhatia et al., 2008; AAP, 2014). A nutrition-related health challenge for breastfed infants adhering to a vegetarian or vegan diet is ensuring adequate iron intake. The introduction of complementary foods to infants at approximately 6 months of age is recommended, in part, to ensure adequate iron intake, and the AAP (2014) encourages early introduction of red meats and other foods rich in iron. AAP (2014) further indicates that oral iron supplementation may be needed for infants 6 to 12 months of age who are not consuming the recommended amount of iron from formula and complementary foods.

Soy formula is an option in all WIC packages for formula-fed infants. The WIC food packages include several foods that by nature are compliant with vegetarian and vegan diets, including fruits, vegetables, legumes, peanut butter, and grains. However, there are currently no vegetarian/vegan substitutions for fish and no vegan substitutions for eggs or cheese (see Table 3-2). A vegetarian or vegan substitution for infant meat is not permitted in the current WIC food packages.

Kosher or Halal Diets

Although federal regulations do not require foods that meet the needs of individuals who follow Kosher or Halal diets (in accordance with Jewish and Islamic dietary laws, respectively),[13] states have the option to accommodate these individuals (USDA/FNS, 2014). At least 53 percent of WIC participants are served by WIC agencies that allow either Kosher or Halal, or both Kosher and Halal substitutions (USDA/FNS, 2011; personal communication, N. Cole, Mathematica, March 17, 2015) (see Appendix H, Table H-1). A 2015 update of state options indicated that 7 percent of

[13] Eliasi and Dwyer (2002) provide a detailed description of Kosher and Halal diets. Very generally, for Kosher diets, meats must be prepared a certain way, animal products must come from Kosher-prepared animals, and packaged foods must be Kosher-certified. Fruits and vegetables are considered inherently Kosher. To be considered Halal, meats must be prepared in a particular way and milk and foods prepared from milk must come from Halal animals.

state agencies allowed Kosher milk, no state agencies specified whether they allowed Kosher eggs, 92 percent did not specify whether Kosher juice was allowed, and 8 percent did not allow Kosher juice. No additional data were available for other Kosher options, and an update of the national availability of Halal options was not presented (USDA/FNS, 2016b).

Only limited data are available to assess the proportion of WIC participants who observe Kosher or Halal practices, and these data indicate that such individuals are rare in the WIC-participating population. In a nationally representative study in which 2,649 WIC-participating mothers were interviewed, less than 1 percent were found to observe Kosher or Halal feeding practices (see Appendix H, Table H-2). In the same study, 0.4 percent of mothers were found to be vegetarian, and less than 0.1 percent reported following a vegan diet (personal communication, K. Castellanos-Brown, USDA/FNS, April 27, 2016).

Alignment with Other Cultural Needs, Preferences, and Practices

Given the culturally diverse populations served by WIC, it is important to consider the appropriateness of WIC foods in meeting the food preferences of its varied racial and ethnic subgroups. The AAP acknowledges the strong influence of culture on parental behaviors related to food choice, preparation, and consumption (AAP, 2014). However, cultural eating practices, and feeding styles of WIC participants in particular have been examined in only a few studies. What studies do exist have reported cultural differences in breastfeeding initiation and duration, foods available and accessible to young children in the home, parent modeling, parent encouragement, and family rules (Bonuck et al., 2005; Kasemsup and Reicks, 2006; Hurley et al., 2008; Mistry et al., 2008; Arthur, 2010; Evans et al., 2011; Skala et al., 2012; Marshall et al., 2013; Odoms-Young et al., 2014; St. Fleur and Petrova, 2014). In addition, one study indicated that vegetable and fruit consumption differs depending upon the race/ethnicity of WIC participants (Di Noia et al., 2016).

These varying parental styles and practices for infant and child feeding may shape early food preferences and eating patterns that, in turn, have been associated with the risk of overweight or obesity (Adair, 2008; Weng et al. 2012), although no connection has been established with specific foods or food groups (Grote and Theurich, 2014).

Cultural variations in infant and child feeding practices may also affect the use of specific WIC foods. Kim et al. (2013) reported that satisfaction with jarred baby foods varied across ethnic groups, with about half of whites and African Americans preferring cash value vouchers (CVVs) for fruits and vegetables over jarred baby foods compared to more than two-thirds of Latinos and those identifying as "Other" preferring CVVs for vegetables and fruits. However, redemption of jarred infant foods declined at similar rates with increasing infant age across all ethnic groups. Redemption data reviewed by the committee indicate that overall use of jarred infant vegetables and fruits may be poor. The committee also received many public comments requesting that the CVV replace jarred infant foods. This information suggests that in general, the CVV would allow the infant food packages to meet cultural needs and preferences for vegetables and fruits.

Other foods currently in the WIC food packages may also be more or less preferred by certain cultural groups. In the March 31, 2016, workshop convened by the committee,[14] panelists who were asked to speak about cultural preferences of WIC participants shared the following:

- There is variation within broader cultural groups. For example, Latin American diets vary by region. In Mexico, corn and beans are core foods; in South America, potato, rice, and corn are staples; and in the Caribbean, preferences are for starchy root vegetables in addition to rice and beans.
- Dairy, legumes, and peanut butter are not part of most traditional Asian diets.
- WIC staff should avoid making assumptions about the stage of clients in the acculturation process, but instead should ask clients what foods are acceptable to them.
- Several whole grain options offered by WIC, such as whole wheat pasta, brown rice, and whole wheat bread, are not widely accepted by many cultural groups.
- Dry breakfast cereals are popular and often seen as status symbols, but people from porridge-based cultures may prefer hot cereals or boiled root vegetables.

FINDINGS AND CONCLUSIONS: POTENTIAL AREAS FOR FOOD PACKAGE MODIFICATIONS

In this chapter, the alignment of the current food packages with the most recent dietary guidance and the suitability of WIC foods for particular medical conditions and to meet dietary preferences and practices are reviewed. Table 3-16 summarizes the committee's findings on key aspects of the food package as well as the conclusions the committee drew from these findings.

---

[14] See Appendix D for workshop agendas.

TABLE 3-16 Alignment of the Current Food Packages with Dietary Guidance, Special Dietary Needs, and Cultural Eating Practices or Food Preferences

Aspect of the Food Packages Evaluated	Findings and Conclusions
Contribution to recommended intakes of food groups	The food packages provide a more-than-supplemental amount of infant cereal, jarred infant food meats, dairy foods, juice, and peanut butter across food packages for women and children. The amounts of legumes in the food packages for children were also greater than supplemental. Reductions in the foods provided in greater-than-supplemental amounts may be warranted.
Contributions to recommended intakes of nutrients	The quantities of many nutrients in the food packages could be reduced and still provide a significant proportion of the DRI. Although food packages are particularly low in vitamin E, choline, and potassium, it is difficult to increase amounts of these nutrients while still contributing to intakes of other nutrients of concern. Reductions in the foods that provide nutrients in greater-than-supplemental amounts may be warranted.
Alignment with dietary guidance for specific forms of foods	Foods in the WIC packages are generally aligned with dietary guidance. Two exceptions were identified. • Fish high in omega-3 fatty acids is provided only to fully breastfeeding women, although it is considered beneficial during all stages of growth and development. Consideration of the addition of seafood to food packages for other women and children is warranted. • The amount of juice provided to children is 100 percent of the lower end of the AAP limit; the AAP recommends whole fruit over juice. Therefore, replacement of some juice with whole fruit (in the form of increased CVV) is warranted.
Alignment with dietary guidance for calories for other uses (COU)	The percent of calories from COU in the food package for children (specifically, percent of calories from saturated fat and added sugars) exceeded the recommended daily proportions based on the energy content of the package. The food packages for women provided a generally proportional amount of COU based on the proportion of energy provided in these packages. For all food packages, however, the absolute contribution to COU was less than the total daily limit. Dairy was the primary contributor to COU. Based on a serving-equivalent contribution of specific foods to a daily diet, the committee identified some foods with the potential to contribute significant amounts of added sugars. For example, an 8-oz serving of yogurt with 40 g of total sugars would contribute over 100 percent of the recommended daily limit of added sugars for a child participating in WIC. Reductions in foods that contribute disproportionately to COU could be considered.

continued

TABLE 3-16 Continued

Aspect of the Food Packages Evaluated	Findings and Conclusions
Foods for medical needs	The required issuance of WIC formulas (for example, when jarred infant foods are prescribed for participants over age 1) may result in the issuance of excessive supplemental food. This requirement merits re-evaluation.
Foods for allergies, lactose intolerance, or celiac disease	The current food packages generally provide substitution options for individuals with the most common allergies, lactose intolerance, and celiac disease, with a few exceptions. The committee was unable to identify suitable substitution options for individuals with allergies to eggs or fish. It is appropriate that individuals with both cow's milk and soy allergies be referred to food package III and be followed by a health care provider.
Foods for individuals following vegetarian, vegan, Kosher, or Halal diets	The current food packages lack vegetarian or vegan substitutions for eggs, fish, and cheese. Options for individuals who follow Kosher or Halal diets are limited. Possibilities for expanding options to meet these preferences and practices merits consideration.
Alignment with cultural eating preferences of the WIC-participating population	Redemption data, published reports, and public comments suggest that the CVV may provide more culturally suitable options for infant feeding than jarred infant foods. Some foods provided in the WIC packages are not typically consumed by specific racial and ethnic groups served by WIC; these foods include peanut butter, milk, and ready-to-eat cereals. Expanding to allow more culturally suitable options merits consideration. The proportion of women who choose to breastfeed differs by racial and ethnic group and is lowest for African-American women. Breastfeeding promotion and support activities may be particularly critical for African-American women.

NOTES: COU = calories for other uses; CVV = cash value voucher; DRI = Dietary Reference Intake.

REFERENCES

AAP (American Academy of Pediatrics). 2012. Breastfeeding and the use of human milk. *Pediatrics* 129(3):e827–e841.

AAP. 2014. *Pediatric nutrition*. 7th ed. Edited by R. E. Kleinman and F. R. Greer. Elk Grove Village, IL: American Academy of Pediatrics.

AAP Committee on Nutrition. 2000. Hypoallergenic infant formulas. *Pediatrics* 106(2):346–349.

AAP Committee on Nutrition. 2008. Lipid screening and cardiovascular health in childhood. *Pediatrics* 122(1):198–208.

AAP Committee on Nutrition. 2010. Diagnosis and prevention of iron deficiency and iron-deficiency anemia in infants and young children (0–3 years of age). *Pediatrics* 126(5):1040–1050.

AAP Committee on Injury, Violence, and Poison Prevention. 2010. Policy statement—prevention of choking among children. *Pediatrics* 125(3):601–607.

Adair, L. S. 2008. Child and adolescent obesity: Epidemiology and developmental perspectives. *Physiology & Behavior* 94(1):8–16.

AHA (American Heart Association). 2015. *Fish and omega-3 fatty acids*. http://www.heart.org/HEARTORG/HealthyLiving/HealthyEating/HealthyDietGoals/Fish-and-Omega-3-Fatty-Acids_UCM_303248_Article.jsp (accessed August 30, 2016).

AND (Academy of Nutrition and Dietetics). 2006. Pregnancy and nutrition—gluten-free diet. http://andevidencelibrary.com/conclusion.cfm?conclusion_statement_id=250329 (accessed October 18, 2016).

AND. 2009. Position of the Academy of Nutrition and Dietetics: Vegetarian diets. *Journal of the Academy of Nutrition and Dietetics* 109:1266–1282.

AND. 2014. Position of the Academy of Nutrition and Dietetics: Nutrition and lifestyle for a healthy pregnancy outcome. *Journal of the Academy of Nutrition and Dietetics* 114(7):1099–1103.

AND. 2015. Position of the Academy of Nutrition and Dietetics: Promoting and supporting breastfeeding. *Journal of the Academy of Nutrition and Dietetics* 115(3):444–449.

Arthur, T. M. 2010. *An examination of household environmental influences on healthy eating behaviors among African American primary caregivers and children*. College Station: Texas A&M University. http://hdl.handle.net/1969.1/ETD-TAMU-2010-12-9028 (accessed October 18, 2016).

Bailey, R. K., C. P. Fileti, J. Keith, S. Tropez-Sims, W. Price, and S. D. Allison-Ottey. 2013. Lactose intolerance and health disparities among African Americans and Hispanic Americans: An updated consensus statement. *Journal of the National Medical Association* 105(2):112–127.

Bhatia, J., F. Greer, and American Academy of Pediatrics Committee on Nutrition. 2008. Use of soy protein-based formulas in infant feeding. *Pediatrics* 121(5):1062–1068.

Bonuck, K. A., K. Freeman, and M. Trombley. 2005. Country of origin and race/ethnicity: Impact on breastfeeding intentions. *Journal of Human Lactation* 21(3):320–326.

Branchi, F., I. Aziz, D. Conte, and D. S. Sanders. 2015. Noncoeliac gluten sensitivity: A diagnostic dilemma. *Current Opinion in Clinical Nutrition and Metabolic Care* 18(5):508–514.

CDC (Centers for Disease Control and Prevention). 2013. Trends in allergic conditions among children: United States, 1997–2011. *NCHS Data Brief* (121):1–8.

Chafen, J. S., S. Newberry, M. Riedl, D. M. Bravata, M. Maglione, M. Suttorp, V. Sundaram, N. M. Paige, A. Towfigh, B. J. Hulley, and P. G. Shekelle. 2010. Prevalence, natural history, diagnosis, and treatment of food allergy: A systematic review of the evidence. Santa Monica, CA: RAND. http://www.rand.org/content/dam/rand/pubs/working_papers/2010/RAND_WR757-1.pdf (accessed October 18, 2016).

Craig, W. J. 2009. Health effects of vegan diets. *American Journal of Clinical Nutrition* 89(5):1627S–1633S.

Di Noia, J., D. Monica, K. W. Cullen, R. Pérez-Escamilla, H. L. Gray, A. Sikorskii. 2016. Differences in fruit and vegetable intake by race/ethnicity and by Hispanic origin and nativity among women in the Special Supplemental Nutrition Program for Women, Infants, and Children. *Preventing Chronic Disease* 13(E115). doi: 10.5888/pcd13.160130.

DiGiacomo, D. V., C. A. Tennyson, P. H. Green, and R. T. Demmer. 2013. Prevalence of gluten-free diet adherence among individuals without celiac disease in the USA: Results from the continuous National Health and Nutrition Examination Survey 2009–2010. *Scandinavian Journal of Gastroenterology* 48(8):921–925.

Du Toit, G., Y. Katz, P. Sasieni, D. Mesher, S. J. Maleki, H. R. Fisher, A. T. Fox, V. Turcanu, T. Amir, G. Zadik-Mnuhin, A. Cohen, I. Livne, and G. Lack. 2008. Early consumption of peanuts in infancy is associated with a low prevalence of peanut allergy. *Journal of Allergy and Clinical Immunology* 122(5):984–991.

Du Toit, G., G. Roberts, P. H. Sayre, H. T. Bahnson, S. Radulovic, A. F. Santos, H. A. Brough, D. Phippard, M. Basting, M. Feeney, V. Turcanu, M. L. Sever, M. Gomez Lorenzo, M. Plaut, G. Lack, and L. S. Team. 2015. Randomized trial of peanut consumption in infants at risk for peanut allergy. *New England Journal of Medicine* 372(9):803–813.

Eliasi, J. R., and J. T. Dwyer. 2002. Kosher and halal. *Journal of the American Dietetic Association* 102(7):911–913.

Elli, L., F. Branchi, C. Tomba, D. Villalta, L. Norsa, F. Ferretti, L. Roncoroni, and M. T. Bardella. 2015. Diagnosis of gluten related disorders: Celiac disease, wheat allergy and non-celiac gluten sensitivity. *World Journal of Gastroenterology* 21(23): 7110–7119.

Evans, A., J. G. Seth, S. Smith, K. K. Harris, J. Loyo, C. Spaulding, M. Van Eck, and N. Gottlieb. 2011. Parental feeding practices and concerns related to child underweight, picky eating, and using food to calm differ according to ethnicity/race, acculturation, and income. *Maternal and Child Health Journal* 15(7):899–909.

FAO/WHO (Food and Agriculture Organization/World Health Organization). 2010. Joint FAO/WHO expert consultation on the risks and benefits of fish consumption. Rome/Geneva: WHO/FAO. http://www.fao.org/docrep/014/ba0136e/ba0136e00.pdf (accessed December 21, 2016).

FDA/EPA (U.S. Food and Drug Administration/Environmental Protection Agency). 2014. *Fish: What pregnant women and parents should know*. Silver Spring, MD: FDA. http://www.fda.gov/food/foodborneillnesscontaminants/metals/ucm393070.htm (accessed December 21, 2016).

Fewtrell, M. S., J. B. Morgan, C. Duggan, G. Gunnlaugsson, P. L. Hibberd, A. Lucas, and R. E. Kleinman. 2007. Optimal duration of exclusive breastfeeding: What is the evidence to support current recommendations? *American Journal of Clinical Nutrition* 85(2):635S–638S.

Fleischer, D. M., J. M. Spergel, A. H. Assa'ad, and J. A. Pongracic. 2013. Primary prevention of allergic disease through nutritional interventions. *Journal of Allergy and Clinical Immunology: In Practice* 1(1):29–36.

Fleischer, D. M., S. Sicherer, M. Greenhawt, D. Campbell, E. Chan, A. Muraro, S. Halken, Y. Katz, M. Ebisawa, L. Eichenfield, H. Sampson, G. Lack, G. Du Toit, G. Roberts, H. Bahnson, M. Feeney, J. Hourihane, J. Spergel, M. Young, A. As'aad, K. Allen, S. Prescott, S. Kapur, H. Saito, I. Agache, C. A. Akdis, H. Arshad, K. Beyer, A. Dubois, P. Eigenmann, M. Fernandez-Rivas, K. Grimshaw, K. Hoffman-Sommergruber, A. Host, S. Lau, L. O'Mahony, C. Mills, N. Papadopoulos, C. Venter, N. Agmon-Levin, A. Kessel, R. Antaya, B. Drolet, and L. Rosenwasser. 2015. Consensus communication on early peanut introduction and the prevention of peanut allergy in high-risk infants. *Journal of Allergy and Clinical Immunology* 136(2):258–261.

Greenhawt, M. 2016. Early allergen introduction for preventing development of food allergy. *Journal of the American Medical Association* 316(11):1157–1159.

Greer, F. R., S. H. Sicherer, A. W. Burks, and American Academy of Pediatrics Committee on Nutrition. 2008. Effects of early nutritional interventions on the development of atopic disease in infants and children: The role of maternal dietary restriction, breastfeeding, timing of introduction of complementary foods, and hydrolyzed formulas. *Pediatrics* 121(1):183–191.

Grote, V., and M. Theurich. 2014. Complementary feeding and obesity risk. *Current Opinion in Clinical Nutrition and Metabolic Care* 17(3):273–277.

Gruchalla, R. S., and H. A. Sampson. 2015. Preventing peanut allergy through early consumption—ready for prime time? *New England Journal of Medicine* 372(9):875–877.

Guandalini, S., and A. Assiri. 2014. Celiac disease: A review. *JAMA Pediatrics* 168(3): 272–278.

Hurley, K. M., M. M. Black, M. A. Papas, and A. M. Quigg. 2008. Variation in breastfeeding behaviours, perceptions, and experiences by race/ethnicity among a low-income statewide sample of Special Supplemental Nutrition Program for Women, Infants, and Children (WIC) participants in the United States. *Maternal and Child Nutrition* 4(2):95–105.

Husby, S., and J. Murray. 2015. Non-celiac gluten hypersensitivity: What is all the fuss about? *F1000Prime Rep* 7:54.

IOM (Institute of Medicine). 1997. *Dietary Reference Intakes for calcium, phosphorus, magnesium, vitamin D, and fluoride*. Washington, DC: National Academy Press.

IOM. 1998. *Dietary Reference Intakes for thiamin, riboflavin, niacin, vitamin B6, folate, vitamin B12, pantothenic acid, biotin, and choline*. Washington, DC: National Academy Press.

IOM. 2000. *Dietary Reference Intakes for vitamin C, vitamin E, selenium, and carotenoids*. Washington, DC: National Academy Press.

IOM. 2001. *Dietary Reference Intakes for vitamin A, vitamin K, arsenic, boron, chromium, copper, iodine, iron, manganese, molybdenum, nickel, silicon, vanadium, and zinc*. Washington, DC: National Academy Press.

IOM. 2002/2005. *Dietary Reference Intakes for energy, carbohydrate, fiber, fat, fatty acids, cholesterol, protein and amino acids*. Washington, DC: The National Academies Press.

IOM. 2005. *Dietary Reference Intakes for water, potassium, sodium, chloride, and sulfate*. Washington, DC: The National Academies Press.

IOM. 2006. *WIC food packages: Time for a change*. Washington, DC: The National Academies Press.

IOM. 2011a. *Dietary Reference Intakes for calcium and vitamin D*. Washington, DC: The National Academies Press.

IOM. 2011b. *Updating the USDA national breastfeeding campaign: Workshop summary*. Washington, DC: The National Academies Press.

Kasemsup, R., and M. Reicks. 2006. The relationship between maternal child-feeding practices and overweight in Hmong preschool children. *Ethnicity & Disease* 16(1):187–193.

Kim, L. P., S. E. Whaley, P. H. Gradziel, N. J. Crocker, L. D. Ritchie, and G. G. Harrison. 2013. Mothers prefer fresh fruits and vegetables over jarred baby fruits and vegetables in the new Special Supplemental Nutrition Program for Women, Infants, and Children food package. *Journal of Nutrition Education and Behavior* 45(6):723–727.

Lebwohl, B., J. F. Ludvigsson, and P. H. Green. 2015. Celiac disease and non-celiac gluten sensitivity. *BMJ* 351:h4347.

Lomer, M. C., G. C. Parkes, and J. D. Sanderson. 2008. Review article: Lactose intolerance in clinical practice—myths and realities. *Alimentary Pharmacology and Therapeutics* 27(2):93–103.

Marshall, C., L. Gavin, C. Bish, A. Winter, L. Williams, M. Wesley, and L. Zhang. 2013. WIC participation and breastfeeding among white and black mothers: Data from Mississippi. *Maternal and Child Health Journal* 17(10):1784–1792.

Mistry, Y., M. Freedman, K. Sweeney, and C. Hollenbeck. 2008. Infant-feeding practices of low-income Vietnamese American women. *Journal of Human Lactation* 24(4):406–414.

Mooney, P. D., M. Hadjivassiliou, and D. S. Sanders. 2014. Coeliac disease. *BMJ* 348:g1561.

NASEM (National Academies of Sciences, Engineering, and Medicine). 2016. *Review of WIC food packages: Proposed framework for revisions: Interim report*. Washington, DC: The National Academies Press. doi: 10.17226/21832.

Netting, M. J., P. F. Middleton, and M. Makrides. 2014. Does maternal diet during pregnancy and lactation affect outcomes in offspring? A systematic review of food-based approaches. *Nutrition* 30(11–12):1225–1241.

NHLBI (National Heart, Lung, and Blood Institute). 2011. Expert panel on integrated guidelines for cardiovascular health and risk reduction in children and adolescents: Summary report. Bethesda, MD: NIH. http://www.nhlbi.nih.gov/health-pro/guidelines/current/cardiovascular-health-pediatric-guidelines/summary (accessed May 24, 2015).

Odoms-Young, A. M., A. Kong, L. A. Schiffer, S. J. Porter, L. Blumstein, S. Bess, M. L. Berbaum, and M. L. Fitzgibbon. 2014. Evaluating the initial impact of the revised Special Supplemental Nutrition Program for Women, Infants, and Children (WIC) food packages on dietary intake and home food availability in African-American and Hispanic families. *Public Health Nutrition* 17(1):83–93.

PAHO/WHO (Pan American Health Organization/World Health Organization). 2003. Guiding principles for complementary feeding of the breastfed child. Geneva: PAHO/WHO. http://www.who.int/maternal_child_adolescent/documents/a85622/en (accessed August 30, 2016).

Rubio-Tapia, A., I. D. Hill, C. P. Kelly, A. H. Calderwood, J. A. Murray, and American College of Gastroenterology. 2013. ACG clinical guidelines: Diagnosis and management of celiac disease. *American Journal of Gastroenterology* 108(5):656–676; quiz 677.

Saccone, G., V. Berghella, L. Sarno, G. M. Maruotti, I. Cetin, L. Greco, A. S. Khashan, F. McCarthy, D. Martinelli, F. Fortunato, and P. Martinelli. 2016. Celiac disease and obstetric complications: A systematic review and metaanalysis. *American Journal of Obstetrics and Gynecology* 214(2):225–234.

Skala, K., R. J. Chuang, A. Evans, A. M. Hedberg, J. Dave, and S. Sharma. 2012. Ethnic differences in the home food environment and parental food practices among families of low-income Hispanic and African-American preschoolers. *Journal of Immigrant and Minority Health* 14(6):1014–1022.

St. Fleur, R., and A. Petrova. 2014. Knowledge and perception of breastfeeding practices in Hispanic mothers in association with their preferred language for communication. *Breastfeeding Medicine* 9(5):261–265.

Suarez, F. L., D. A. Savaiano, and M. D. Levitt. 1995. A comparison of symptoms after the consumption of milk or lactose-hydrolyzed milk by people with self-reported severe lactose intolerance. *New England Journal of Medicine* 333(1):1–4.

Suarez, F. L., D. Savaiano, P. Arbisi, and M. D. Levitt. 1997. Tolerance to the daily ingestion of two cups of milk by individuals claiming lactose intolerance. *American Journal of Clinical Nutrition* 65(5):1502–1506.

Thompson, T. 2000. Folate, iron, and dietary fiber contents of the gluten-free diet. *Journal of the American Dietetic Association* 100(11):1389–1396.

USDA/ARS (U.S. Department of Agriculture/Agricultural Research Service). 2014. *Food patterns equivalents database 2011–12: Methodology and user guide*. Beltsville, MD: USDA/ARS. http://www.ars.usda.gov/SP2UserFiles/Place/80400530/pdf/fped/FPED_1112.pdf (accessed December 21, 2016).

USDA/ARS. 2016. USDA National Nutrient Database for Standard Reference. Release 28. Beltsville, MD: USDA/ARS. https://www.ars.usda.gov/northeast-area/beltsville-md/beltsville-human-nutrition-research-center/nutrient-data-laboratory/docs/usda-national-nutrient-database-for-standard-reference (accessed November 11, 2016).

USDA/FNS (U.S. Department of Agriculture/Food and Nutrition Service). 2011. *WIC food packages policy options study, final report*. Alexandria, VA: USDA/FNS. http://www.fns.usda.gov/sites/default/files/WICFoodPackageOptions.pdf (accessed February 15, 2017).

USDA/FNS. 2012. Nutrition standards in the National School Lunch and School Breakfast Programs. Final Rule. *Federal Register* 77(17):4088–4167.

USDA/FNS. 2014. Special Supplemental Nutrition Program for Women, Infants and Children (WIC): Revisions in the WIC food packages; final rule, 7 *C.F.R.* § 246.

USDA/FNS. 2015a. *WIC food packages policy options II, final report*. Alexandria, VA: USDA/FNS. https://www.fns.usda.gov/sites/default/files/ops/WICFoodPolicyOptions2.pdf (accessed February 15, 2017).

USDA/FNS. 2015b. *Food allergies*. http://wicworks.nal.usda.gov/topics-z/food-allergies (accessed December 21, 2016).

USDA/FNS. 2016a. Policy memorandum CACFP 17-2016: Nutrition requirements for fluid milk and fluid milk substitutions in the Child and Adult Care Food Program, questions and answers. Alexandria, VA.

USDA/FNS. 2016b. WIC participant and program characteristics 2014 food package report. Alexandria, VA: USDA/FNS. http://www.fns.usda.gov/wic-participant-and-program-characteristics-2014-food-package-report (accessed August 30, 2016).

USDA/HHS (U.S. Department of Agriculture/U.S. Department of Health and Human Services). 2015. *The report of the Dietary Guidelines Advisory Committee on the Dietary Guidelines for Americans, 2015, to the Secretary of Agriculture and the Secretary of Health and Human Services*. Washington, DC: USDA/HHS. http://www.health.gov/dietaryguidelines/2015-scientific-report/PDFs/Scientific-Report-of-the-2015-Dietary-Guidelines-Advisory-Committee.pdf (accessed December 21, 2016).

USDA/HHS. 2016. *2015–2020 Dietary Guidelines for Americans*. Washington, DC: U.S. Government Printing Office. https://health.gov/dietaryguidelines/2015 (accessed August 29, 2016).

Weng, S. F., S. A. Redsell, J. A. Swift, M. Yang, and C. P. Glazebrook. 2012. Systematic review and meta-analyses of risk factors for childhood overweight identifiable during infancy. *Archives of Disease in Childhood* 97(12):1019–1026.

WHO (World Health Organization). 2005. Guiding principles for feeding non-breastfed children 6–24 months of age. Geneva, Switzerland: WHO. http://www.who.int/maternal_child_adolescent/documents/9241593431/en (accessed August 30, 2016).

WHO. 2009. *Infant and young child feeding*. Geneva, Switzerland: World Health Organization.

4

Nutrient and Food Group Intakes of WIC Participants

Three criteria for food package revisions required that the committee evaluate nutrient and food intakes of the Special Supplemental Nutrition Program for Women, Infants, and Children (WIC)-eligible population and assess their adequacy relative to dietary guidance: (1) the package contributes to reduction of the prevalences of inadequate nutrient intakes and of excessive nutrient intakes; (2) the package contributes to an overall dietary pattern that is consistent with the 2015–2020 *Dietary Guidelines for Americans* (DGA)[1] for individuals 2 years of age and older, and; (3) the package contributes to an overall diet that is consistent with established dietary recommendations for infants and children less than 2 years of age, including encouragement of and support for breastfeeding. In addition, the committee was tasked with evaluating the health needs of this population.

To address these criteria and requirements of the task, the committee collected and reviewed published evidence on key nutrition-related health priorities of relevance to the WIC population, reviewed published evidence describing WIC participants' nutrient and food intakes, and conducted independent data analyses (examining nutrient intake, food intake, and diet quality) using data from the National Health and Nutrition Examination Survey (NHANES).

This chapter describes the committee's subsequent findings and related challenges. The chapter concludes with a summary of findings from the committee's evaluation. A description of how the committee applied this information to determine priorities for changes to the food packages is presented in Chapter 5.

[1] References to the DGA in this chapter are specific to 2015–2020 unless otherwise noted.

TABLE 4-1 Selected Nutrition-Related Health Risks Relevant to the WIC Population

Nutrient or Food Component	Associated Health Concern by WIC Subgroup	Reference
Iron	**Women:** Iron deficiency and iron-deficiency anemia are associated with fatigue, weakness, and tachycardia; risk of preterm labor, low body weight, and infant mortality are increased; maternal iron status is associated with iron status of the infant	IOM, 2001; AND, 2014; AHRQ, 2015
	Infants: Breastfed infants older than 6 months of age are at risk of low iron intake	IOM, 2006; AAP, 2014
	Children: Iron is important for growth and cognitive development	AAP, 2014; Berglund and Domellöf, 2014
Zinc	**Infants:** Breastfed infants older than 6 months of age are at risk of low zinc intake; risk of intake above the UL from formula or foods	IOM, 2006; Krebs et al., 2006; AAP, 2014
Folate	**Women:** Inadequate folate intake can cause birth defects including neural tube defects; may be particularly important for Hispanic women who consume nonfortified corn masa flour	CDC, 2010a; Williams et al., 2015
Vitamin D	**Women and infants:** Low serum 25(OH)D has been inconsistently associated with several pregnancy and birth outcomes; vitamin D is important for calcium homeostasis and bone health in infants	IOM, 2011; AHRQ, 2014
Choline	**Women and infants:** Low maternal choline intake is associated with the risk of neural tube defects and orofacial cleft in infants	Zeisel, 2013
Omega-3 fatty acids	**Infants:** Omega-3 fatty acid supplementation may be associated with increased visual acuity	AHRQ, 2016
Food energy	**Women (of reproductive age):** Overweight and obesity before pregnancy is associated with poor birth outcomes including higher risk of fetal death, stillbirth, and infant death; higher birthweight; and reduced breastfeeding rates	AND, 2014; Aune et al., 2014; Shin and Song, 2014; Marchi et al., 2015; Vinturache et al., 2015; Yan, 2015
	Women (pregnant): Excessive gestational weight gain is associated with gestational diabetes, pregnancy-induced hypertension, and preeclampsia	IOM, 2009
	Women (postpartum): Excessive weight retention increases the risk of obesity; postpartum obesity is associated with a less adequate breastmilk supply	Rasmussen and Kjolhede, 2004; Turcksin et al., 2014; Endres et al., 2015
	Children: Childhood obesity increases risk of adult obesity, cardiovascular disease, and type 2 diabetes	Sabin and Kiess, 2015

TABLE 4-1 Continued

Nutrient or Food Component	Associated Health Concern by WIC Subgroup	Reference
Sugar	**Children:** Dental caries in early childhood are associated with intake of dietary carbohydrates, especially sugars	AAPD, 2012

NOTES: Relevant findings of the *Dietary Guidelines for Americans*, including shortfall nutrients identified for individuals 2 years of age and older, are reviewed in Chapter 3.
SOURCES: As noted in the Reference column.

LITERATURE AND REPORT REVIEW RELATED TO THE WIC POPULATION AND WIC PARTICIPANTS' NUTRIENT AND FOOD GROUP INTAKES

Nutrition-Related Health Priorities Relevant to the WIC Population

The committee's review of nutrition-related health risks and the corresponding prevalence of these risks among WIC participants (as available) was part of the phase I review (see Chapter 6 of NASEM, 2016). The review focused on health risks of population groups relevant to the WIC program that are not covered comprehensively in the DGA, namely pregnant women, breastfeeding women, infants, and children less than 2 years of age. The key findings of this review are summarized in Table 4-1. Relevant findings in the DGA, including shortfall nutrients identified for individuals 2 years of age and older (i.e., children and women who are not pregnant or breastfeeding), are reviewed in Chapter 2.

Food Safety Considerations Relevant to the WIC Population

In addition to reviewing nutrition-related health risks as part of its phase I study, the committee also reviewed health risks related to food safety that were relevant to the WIC-eligible population (see Chapter 6 of NASEM, 2016). This review was conducted with the understanding that the safety of the U.S. food supply is ensured by the U.S. Food and Drug Administration (FDA). Table 4-2 presents a summary of the key findings and recommended actions related to food-borne illness, pharmaceutical residues, and environmental contaminants (i.e., recommended not by this committee, but instead by referenced authorities or experts listed in the table).

Since the release of the phase I report, the FDA proposed an action level for inorganic rice in infant cereal (FDA, 2016). The announcement stated that "the majority of infant rice cereal currently on the market either meets, or is close to, the proposed action level" and offered guidance for parents

TABLE 4-2 Summary of Food Safety-Related Health Risks Relevant to the WIC Population

Food	Associated Food Safety Consideration by WIC Subgroup	Recommended* Action to Reduce Risks	Reference
Vegetables and fruits	**Women, infants, and children:** Raw and unwashed vegetables and fruits linked to foodborne illness or pesticide exposure	Thorough washing or cooking; provide children with a wide variety of produce	AAP 2014; USDA/FNS, 2014; USDA/HHS, 2016
Fish	**Pregnant and breastfeeding women and young children:** Methylated mercury in larger fish such as shark, swordfish, and king mackerel associated with adverse effects on nervous system	Avoid consumption of high-mercury varieties of fish	FAO/WHO, 2011
Full-fat dairy food	**Women (also has implications for breastfeeding infants) and children:** Chronic exposure to high level of dioxins in full-fat dairy linked to impaired immune, nervous, endocrine, and reproductive functions	Limit dairy to low-fat products	Geyer et al., 2002; IOM, 2003; WHO, 2014
Rice	**Women, infants, and children:** Arsenic, which is found in rice, is classified as a human carcinogen	Pregnant women should consume a variety of grains; adhere to FDA guidance for providing rice cereals to infants (Box 4-1)	EPA, 1994; IARC, 1998; FDA, 2016

* Recommended not by this committee, but by referenced authorities or experts listed in the table.
SOURCE: As noted in the Reference column. See Chapter 6 of NASEM, 2016, for additional details of the committee's health risk review.

and caregivers of infants (see Box 4-1). This guidance supports varying grain intake for both infants and pregnant women.

Nutrient Intakes of WIC Participants Before and After the 2009 Food Package Changes

As part of its first step toward evaluating whether the food packages meet the three criteria outlined in the introduction of this chapter, the committee evaluated the scientific literature and reports on nutrient intakes

BOX 4-1

U.S. Food and Drug Administration Dietary Guidance Related to Arsenic

- Feed your baby iron-fortified cereals to be sure she or he is receiving enough of this important nutrient.
- Rice cereal fortified with iron is a good source of nutrients for your baby, but it should not be the only source, and it does not need to be the first source. Other fortified infant cereals include oat, barley, and multigrain options.
- For toddlers, provide a well-balanced diet, which includes a variety of grains.
- It would be prudent for pregnant women to consume a variety of foods, including varied grains (such as wheat, oats, and barley), for good nutrition. This advice is consistent with long-standing nutrition guidance to pregnant women from the American Congress of Obstetricians and Gynecologists to have half of their grains consist of whole grains.
- Published studies, including new research by the FDA, indicate that cooking rice in excess water (from 6 to 10 parts water to one part rice), and draining the excess water, can reduce from 40 to 60 percent of the inorganic arsenic content, depending on the type of rice—although this method may also remove some key nutrients.

SOURCE: FDA, 2016.

among WIC participants. The committee identified three reports comparing nutrient intakes by infants or children before versus after the 2009 WIC food package revisions (see Table 4-3). Together, these studies indicate that there were some beneficial changes in food intake after the introduction of the new food packages, but specific findings were inconsistent from study to study. It is noteworthy that the committee was unable to identify any nationally representative "pre-post" (before and after the 2009 food package changes) studies of nutrient intake by WIC-participating women apart from the Diet Quality of Young American Children study (USDA/FNS, 2015a), for which sample sizes for both women and infants were too small to be reliable. As described later in this chapter, there are several challenges with collecting and comparing pre-post data in this context.

TABLE 4-3 Pre/Post Studies of 2009 Food Package Revision Effects on Nutrient Intake of WIC Participants

Reference	Study Location and Population	Study Design	Findings
Odoms-Young et al., 2014	Chicago, mother–child pairs, 143 Hispanic and 130 African American	Natural experiment, survey before package changes and 6, 12, and 18 months after revisions were implemented	Hispanic children had reduced saturated fat and increased fiber intakes following the food package changes. African-American children significantly increased their caloric intake
Kong et al., 2014	Chicago, mother–child pairs, including 209 mothers (112 Hispanic and 97 African American) and 164 children (94 Hispanic and 70 African American)	Natural experiment, 24-hour recalls immediately before package changes and 18 months after revisions were implemented	In Hispanic children only: decreases in total and saturated fat and increases in dietary fiber and overall diet quality; no significant changes in nutrient intake in other groups
Thornton et al., 2014	Central Texas, 84 (pre), 120 (post) infants and toddlers, majority Hispanic	Natural experiment, "pre" cross-section in 2009 and "post" cross-section in 2011	Decreased energy intakes; mean usual intakes of retinol and zinc exceeded the UL, although the proportion of individuals exceeding the UL for zinc decreased after the package changes

NOTES: Nationally representative data examining the effects of food package changes on nutrient intakes of WIC participants were not identified.
SOURCES: As noted in the Reference column.

Food Group Intakes of Women and Children Participating in WIC

The Effect of the 2009 Food Package Revisions on Food Group Intakes

Except for studies on breastfeeding, data characterizing the effect of the 2009 WIC food package changes on participants' food intake or health are sparse. The data that do exist are from pre-post regional studies, and the outcomes are summarized in Table 4-4. These data indicate that the food package revisions were generally associated with improved intake of key food groups. In their systematic review, Schultz et al. (2015) examined the same studies and reported that there was an overall improvement in dietary intake after the 2009 food package changes, although the body of evidence was limited. The WIC food package changes were associated

TABLE 4-4 Regional Pre/Post Studies of 2009 Food Package Revision Effects on Food Intake of WIC Participants

Reference	Study Location and Population	Study Design	Findings
Odoms-Young et al., 2014	Chicago, mother–child pairs, 143 Hispanic and 130 African American	Natural experiment, survey before package changes and 6, 12, and 18 months after revisions were implemented	Fruit consumption increased among Hispanic mothers; low-fat dairy consumption increased among Hispanic mothers, Hispanic children and African-American children; and whole milk consumption decreased among all groups
Kong et al., 2014	Chicago, mother–child pairs, including 209 mothers (112 Hispanic and 97 African American) and 164 children (94 Hispanic and 70 African American)	Natural experiment, 24-hour recalls immediately before package changes and 18 months after revisions were implemented	Reduced-fat milk intake increased for African-American and Hispanic children and whole milk intake decreased for all groups
Chiasson et al., 2013	New York state, 3.5 million children (administrative records)	Secondary analysis of administrative records, compares July to December in 2008 versus 2011	Delayed introduction of solids and increased consumption of fruits, vegetables, and whole grains and reduced-fat milk, increase in breastfeeding
Ishdorj and Capps, 2013	Indian Tribal Organizations across multiple states, 1,642 Native American children	Secondary analysis of National Food and Nutrition Survey for WIC (NATFAN) data, two repeated cross-sections before and after revisions	Increased low-fat and reduced-fat milk, fruit, vegetable, and whole grain intake, decreased consumption of whole milk
Whaley et al., 2012	California, approximately 3,000 pregnant or postpartum women and caregivers of children	Telephone surveys of randomly sampled WIC families in September 2009 and March 2010	Increases in consumption of fruits, vegetables, and whole grains and increased consumption of reduced-fat milk, decreased consumption of whole milk
Meiqari et al., 2015	Atlanta, Georgia, African-American mothers and eldest child, 46 children and 38 mothers	Questionnaires before package changes and 1 and 4 weeks after	Children, but not mothers, significantly increased their intake of low-fat milk

SOURCES: As noted in the Reference column.

with a positive effect on the purchase of healthful foods targeted by WIC in WIC-participating households compared to WIC-eligible, nonparticipating households in two studies (Andreyeva and Tripp, 2016; Oh et al., 2016). Oh et al. (2016) reported an increase in household purchases of whole grain products using a national dataset. Andreyeva and Tripp (2016) reported an increase in purchases of healthful foods (categorized by sodium, saturated fat, and added sugars content) in two states. These two studies suggest potential positive effects of the food package changes. After its own independent review, the committee likewise concluded that the 2009 food package changes likely had some positive effects on intake.

The Effect of Racial and Ethnic Differences on Food Purchasing and Consumption Among WIC Participants

Findings from several reports suggest that food purchasing and consumption patterns may be strongly connected to culture, race, or ethnicity (Dubowitz et al., 2007, 2008; Bermúdez-Millán et al., 2009; Kong et al., 2013; Pooler and Gleason, 2014; Chaparro et al., 2015; Di Noia et al., 2016). This is evident in the WIC population. For example, Kong et al. (2013) reported that the diets of Hispanic mothers and children who participated in WIC were lower in the proportion of calories from fat, added sugars, sodium, and sweetened beverages and higher in whole grains, fruits, and dairy foods compared to their African-American counterparts. Reported differences in intake among and between racial and ethnic groups, however, are not always consistent (Faith et al., 2006; Odoms-Young et al., 2014; Chaparro et al., 2015; Cho et al., 2015).

Geographical Differences in Food Intakes Among WIC Participants

The committee identified one cross-sectional study on geographic differences in food intake. In a comparison of fruit and vegetable consumption between urban and rural African-American WIC participants in Texas, Ettienne-Gittens et al. (2013) found that urban African-American women consumed a wider variety of fruits compared to their rural counterparts. Urban children were provided with a wider variety of vegetables and consumed them more frequently than rural children.

Complementary Food Intakes of Infants Participating in WIC

It is recommended that the transition to intake of food begin at around 6 months of age (AAP, 2014), although parents often offer solid foods earlier than this time. The transition to the family diet lasts until a child is about 24 months of age (AAP, 2014).

As part of its phase I review (NASEM, 2016), the committee relied on food intake data from three large contemporary datasets for its evaluation of complementary food intakes among WIC-participating infants: (1) Infant Feeding Practices Study II (IFPS II) (Grummer-Strawn et al., 2008; CDC, 2014),[2] (2) 2008 Feeding Infants and Toddlers Study (FITS 2008)[1] (Briefel et al., 2010; Deming et al., 2014), and (3) NHANES (Grimes et al., 2015). A summary of the study designs and key results of these three studies are outlined in Appendix I, Tables I-1 through I-3.[3] Details of the committee's review are available in the phase I report (NASEM, 2016), and a summary of key findings is presented here. Additionally, for this report, the committee reviewed limited results from the currently underway WIC Infant and Toddler Feeding Practices Study (WIC ITFPS-2) (Personal communication, K. Castellanos-Brown, USDA-FNS, April 27, 2016).

Areas of Concern for Complementary Feeding

The committee's review of these studies led to the identification of four areas of concern about complementary feeding: (1) early introduction of complementary foods; (2) insufficient intake of iron-fortified foods and supplements among older infants; (3) early introduction of cow's milk; and (4) consumption of foods of poor nutritional value. Details of the committee's evaluation leading to these areas of concern are provided in the phase I report (NASEM, 2016).

It should be reiterated that data collection for IFPS II, FITS 2008, and most of the NHANES analysis in Grimes et al. (2015) occurred before full implementation of the 2009 WIC food package revisions. Some of the changes in the food packages, such as not issuing complementary foods before an infant reached 6 months of age, have the potential to affect some of these areas of concern.

ANALYSIS OF THE NATIONAL HEALTH AND NUTRITION EXAMINATION SURVEY DATA: NUTRIENT ADEQUACY

As a second step toward assessing the adequacy of nutrient and food intakes of the WIC-eligible population, the committee estimated nutrient intake adequacy based on recommended Dietary Reference Intakes (DRIs)

[2] These data were collected prior to the 2009 food package changes.

[3] The IFPS II analysis combined WIC with WIC-eligible, nonparticipating infants, and the results reflect all consumption in the 7 days before the survey. The FITS 2008 analysis described in this section, in contrast, compared WIC participants and eligible, non-WIC participants, and the data collected were for food intake only during the 24 hours before the interview.

(IOM, 1997, 1998, 2000a, 2001, 2002/2005, 2005, 2011). This section describes the methods and results of this analysis.

Analytical Methods in Brief

The U.S. Department of Agriculture's Food and Nutrition Service (USDA-FNS) tasked the committee with two comparisons: (1) nutrient and food group intake of WIC participants compared to WIC-eligible nonparticipants and (2) nutrient and food group intake of WIC participants before the 2009 food package changes compared to after the 2009 food package changes. For this task, the committee analyzed the 2005–2012 data from the NHANES (USDA/ARS, 2005–2012). NHANES was used because it is the most comprehensive national nutrition survey and also because it captures reported household income and WIC participation. Portions of these data were used depending on the subgroup and comparisons of interest to this review (see Table 4-5). Full details on the methodology applied are described in Appendix J, and a description of the portion of data presented in this chapter can be found below in the section titled, "Nutrient and Food Group Intake Data Presented in This Chapter."

This section highlights the following:

- The committee's rationale for including in this chapter only nutrient and food intake data for WIC participants after the 2009 food package changes (other results are available in Appendix J);
- The analytical subgroups and NHANES survey years used for each subgroup analysis;
- The challenge of assessing nutrient intake of women who are breastfeeding at unknown intensity;
- The committee's relaxed 5 percent threshold for identifying nutrient intake as being either inadequate or excessive.

Nutrient and Food Group Intake Data Presented in This Chapter

Results presented in this chapter are limited to the dietary intakes of WIC participants.[4] Although intake estimates were generated for both WIC participants and WIC-eligible nonparticipants, interpretation of any differences is complicated by the potential for underlying differences between the two groups or selection bias. Selection bias results from the likelihood that differences in intake, even if statistically significant, result not from WIC participation, but from factors that caused an individual to participate in WIC. These comparisons could also be affected by challenges that the

[4] Dietary supplement intake was not included in the analysis.

TABLE 4-5 NHANES Survey Years Applied for Each Analytical Subgroup

Population Subgroup	Survey Years Analyzed	Rationale
Women	2005–2012	Survey years were combined to increase sample size and allow for separation by physiological state; no postpartum variable is available in NHANES 2005–2006, so for women categorized as postpartum, the data span NHANES 2007–2012
Formula-fed infants	2005–2008;[a] 2011–2012	Sample size allows for examination of pre- and post-2009 food package changes
Breastfed infants	2009–2012[b]	Survey years were combined to increase sample size; the starting year of 2009 was chosen because sometime during this year, states issued jarred infant food meats
Children	2005–2008;[a] 2011–2012	Sample size allows for examination of pre- and post-2009 food package changes

NOTES: NHANES = National Health and Nutrition Examination Survey.

[a] The pre-2009 food package change results (NHANES 2005–2008) are available in Appendix J.

[b] This group includes some WIC participants receiving the pre-2009 food package because the committee was unable to divide the 2009–2010 NHANES survey data set. As a result, the 2009–2010 NHANES release was included in the post-2009 food package change analysis to ensure adequacy of sample sizes.

committee experienced with correct identification of survey respondents as participating in WIC. Challenges related to selection bias are described in more detail later in this chapter.

Similarly, statistical comparisons of pre- to post-2009 intake data were considered inappropriate. For women and breastfed infants, small sample sizes required the committee to collapse multiple survey years (see Table 4-5); therefore, presented results do not uniquely represent pre- or post-2009 intake data. For other subgroups, results presented in this chapter are limited to nutrient intakes after the 2009 food package changes (that is, NHANES 2011–2012 data) because any detected differences before and after 2009 cannot necessarily be attributed to changes in the food packages. For example, as discussed in more depth in Chapter 2, adoption of the new food package in 2009 took place at the end of a recession and at a time when families were facing the worst labor market since the recession of the early 1980s. The American Recovery and Reinvestment Act of 2009 provided the funds necessary to increase the maximum benefit level of the Supplemental Nutrition Assistance Program (SNAP) by about 15 percent (EOPUS, 2014). SNAP recipients who meet the requirements for age and physiological state for WIC are automatically income-eligible for WIC. As a result, because many WIC participants also receive SNAP benefits, food expenditures and consumption may have changed among those who were receiving both benefits. Additionally, the NHANES design is a repeated cross-sectional survey that does not allow for longitudinal analysis at any level (i.e., individual, state, or locality).

NHANES Analytical Subgroups

Using information available in NHANES, population subgroups were defined based on income, age, and physiological state required for WIC eligibility (i.e., women must be pregnant, breastfeeding, or postpartum). The committee finalized the subgroups as follows:

1. Women 19 to 50 years of age
   a. WIC participants[5]
   b. WIC-eligible (income ≤185 percent of poverty, pregnant, breastfeeding or postpartum) nonparticipants
   c. Low-income, WIC-ineligible (income ≤185 percent of poverty but neither pregnant, nor breastfeeding, nor postpartum) nonparticipants[6]
2. Formula-fed infants 0 to less than 6 months of age
   a. WIC participants
   b. WIC-eligible (income ≤185 percent of poverty) nonparticipants
3. Formula-fed infants 6 to less than 12 months of age
   a. WIC participants
   b. WIC-eligible (income ≤185 percent of poverty) nonparticipants
4. Breastfed infants[7] 6 to less than 12 months of age
   a. WIC participants
   b. WIC-eligible (income ≤185 percent of poverty) nonparticipants
5. Children 1 to less than 2 years of age
   a. WIC participants
   b. WIC-eligible (income ≤185 percent of poverty) nonparticipants
6. Children 2 to less than 5 years of age
   a. WIC participants
   b. WIC-eligible (income ≤185 percent of poverty) nonparticipants

[5] Survey respondents for which current WIC participation was reported in the NHANES survey.

[6] The purpose of this subgroup is to anticipate needs of women who might become eligible at a later time with a change in physiological status, and therefore are potential WIC participants.

[7] In the NHANES datasets, only intakes of formula and foods were quantified. Breastmilk intakes were not quantified for infants coded as breastfed, which posed a challenge for assessment of total nutrient intakes for these infants. Given that iron and zinc intakes are a concern for breastfed infants over 6 months of age, the committee analyzed intakes of these nutrients only for infants coded as breastfed.

NHANES Survey Years Applied

Table 4-5 summarizes the survey year data analyzed for each population subgroup and provides the rationale for each decision. All results from the analyses outlined in Table 4-5, including mean usual intakes and intake distributions of all subgroups, both before and after the 2009 food package changes (when possible) for both WIC and WIC-eligible subgroups, are available in Appendix J.

Challenges with Dietary Intake Assessment of Pregnant and Breastfeeding Women

For this report, nutrient intakes of all women coded as "pregnant" in NHANES were compared to the DRIs for pregnant women and to a 2,600-kcal food pattern.[8] This corresponds to the energy needs of a pregnant woman in the second trimester of pregnancy and, thus, overestimates the needs of some pregnant women and underestimates the needs of others. The WIC pregnant women in NHANES were distributed among the trimesters of gestation. As a result, the estimates of food intakes below that recommended for pregnant women are not biased in one direction or another, but they are more imprecise than if trimester-specific estimates could have been generated. Unfortunately, the available sample sizes were inadequate for this purpose.

Intakes of all women coded as "breastfeeding" in NHANES were compared to the DRIs for exclusively breastfeeding women and to a 2,600-kcal food pattern. For breastfeeding women, NHANES identifies which women are breastfeeding, but not the intensity of their breastfeeding or the amount of milk they are producing. Therefore, in the tables in this report, the "BF" subgroup includes a mix of women who are exclusively and partially breastfeeding. For women who are partially breastfeeding and producing less milk than exclusively breastfeeding women, a 2,600-kcal diet is likely to be an overestimate of their caloric need. Given that only a minority of breastfeeding women in WIC are exclusively breastfeeding, the proportion of breastfeeding women whose nutrient intakes are inadequate and the proportion with food group intakes below that recommended are both overestimated.

---

[8] The food patterns were selected because they most closely matched the estimated energy expenditure (EER) for the corresponding subgroups. To calculate the EER in this report, a "low-active" physical activity level was assumed. Additional details on the methodology applied for all NHANES analyses are presented in Appendix J.

Estimates of Inadequate and Excessive Nutrient Intakes: Using a Relaxed 5 Percent Threshold

The tables in this chapter show both the estimated prevalence of inadequate nutrient intakes and the estimated prevalence of excessive nutrient intakes for WIC subpopulations. As described in Appendix J (detailed methodology), the prevalence of dietary nutrient inadequacy is the estimated proportion of reported intakes below the Estimated Average Requirement (EAR); the prevalence of excessive intakes[9] is the estimated proportion of the population with intakes above the Tolerable Upper Intake Level (UL) (IOM, 2000b). Inadequate or excessive intake of a nutrient typically becomes a concern when it occurs in 2.5 percent or more of the population of interest (IOM, 2003). However, for this report, a 5 percent threshold was applied. This slightly relaxed standard accounts for some of the uncertainty in setting the EARs as well as some of the generally accepted errors associated with dietary assessment. Inasmuch as inadequacy was 5 percent or greater for many nutrients, the committee considered two additional levels of inadequacy: (1) 10 to less than 50 percent and (2) inadequacy of 50 percent or greater. Nutrients with proportions of inadequacy in the latter category were considered of greatest concern.

Nutrient Intake Adequacy of Women Participating in WIC

Micronutrient Adequacy

As shown in Table 4-6, vitamin E intakes were inadequate in between 96 and 100 percent of women across subgroups. Additional inadequacies are noted below by physiological stage.

More than 50 percent of pregnant women participating in WIC reported intakes below the EAR for iron. The prevalence of inadequacy was between 10 and 50 percent for magnesium, folate, zinc, and vitamins A, C, and B6. Calcium intakes were below the EAR in only 6 percent of pregnant women.

More than 50 percent of breastfeeding women participating in WIC had intakes below the EAR for vitamin A. Inadequacy was between 10 and 50 percent for magnesium, zinc, vitamin C, vitamin B6, folate, copper, and calcium. Thiamin intakes were also below the EAR in approximately 10 percent of breastfeeding women.

---

[9] Not all nutrients have ULs and, for four nutrients (folate, vitamin E, niacin, and magnesium), the UL is based on intake from supplements, fortificants, or pharmacological agents only (IOM, 1997, 1998, 2000a). Thus, the probability of exceeding the UL was determined only for retinol, vitamins C and B6, calcium, iron, phosphorous, zinc, copper, choline, and selenium in this report.

TABLE 4-6 Estimated Prevalence of Inadequacy of Selected Nutrients, WIC-Participating Women 19 to 50 Years of Age, NHANES 2005–2012

		Inadequacy, % (SE)[a]		
Nutrient	EAR per Day (P/BF/PP)[b]	P (N = 165)[c]	Any BF (N = 27)[d]	PP (N = 62)[e]
Calcium	800 mg	6.1 (5.5)	15.8 (19.9)	51.7 (9.7)
Copper	0.8/1.0/0.7 mg	0.2 (0.8)	21.8 (19.9)	32.4 (11.0)
Iron	22.0/6.5/8.1 mg	82.0 (8.6)	0	13.3 (11.9)
Magnesium	255/290/255 mg	32.2 (6.7)	38.7 (15.4)	77.6 (12.6)
Phosphorus	580 mg	0	0	2.2 (5.2)
Selenium	49/59/45 µg	0	0.1 (0.9)	2.1 (5.1)
Zinc	9.5/10.4/6.8 mg	19.5 (8.0)	38.5 (15.9)	30.2 (11.5)
Vitamin A	550/900/500 µg RAE	20.1 (9.0)	75.0 (19.7)	69.4 (11.7)
Vitamin E	12/16/12 mg αTOC	95.8 (4.9)	99.4 (3.4)	99.8 (0.9)
Vitamin C	70/100/60 mg	17.1 (7.1)	32.8 (18.5)	37.5 (10.7)
Thiamin	1.2/1.2/0.9 mg	4.7 (5.9)	9.8 (17.7)	20.3 (12.5)
Riboflavin	1.2/1.2/0.9 mg	0.4 (1.0)	1.4 (6.0)	10.8 (11.4)
Niacin	14/13/11 mg	2.2 (3.2)	4.1 (11.7)	6.3 (9.4)
Vitamin B6	1.6/1.7/1.1 mg	12.2 (6.7)	29.7 (18.3)	19.7 (12.7)
Folate	520/450/320 µg DFE	22.4 (8.9)	26.8 (19.4)	32.6 (11.6)
Vitamin B12	2.2/2.4/2.0 mg	0.3 (0.8)	2.0 (7.6)	14.3 (12.3)

NOTES: αTOC = α-tocopherol; DFE = dietary folate equivalents; EAR = Estimated Average Requirement; N = sample size; RAE = retinol activity equivalents; SE = standard error.

[a] Inadequacy, % = percentage of individuals with usual intake below the EAR.

[b] Values represent the P/BF/PP groups. One value indicates that the EAR is the same across groups.

Subgroup definitions are as follows:

[c] P = Pregnant WIC-participating women.

[d] BF = Breastfeeding (any intensity), nonpregnant WIC-participating women.

[e] PP = WIC-participating women who are 6 months postpartum, not pregnant, and not breastfeeding; data were sourced only from 2007–2012 NHANES because no postpartum variable is available in the 2005–2006 dataset.

SOURCES: IOM, 1997, 1998, 2000a, 2001, 2002/2005, 2005, 2011; USDA/ARS, 2005–2012.

More than 50 percent of postpartum women in WIC had intakes of magnesium, vitamin A, and calcium below the EAR. Intakes were inadequate for between 10 and 50 percent of postpartum women for many nutrients: vitamin C, folate, copper, zinc, thiamin, vitamin B6, vitamin B12, iron, and riboflavin.

Serum vitamin D concentrations are discussed later in this chapter and presented in Table 4-22.

Intakes of Micronutrients with an AI

For nutrients with only an Adequate Intake (AI) value, although the proportion of individuals with an inadequate intake cannot be determined, mean intakes at or above the AI imply that there is a low probability of inadequacy in the group (IOM, 2000b). As shown in Table 4-7, mean usual intakes of potassium and choline fell below the AI for all three subgroups of women. Intakes of sodium were far above the AI.

Macronutrients and Energy

The prevalence of inadequate dietary protein intakes ranged from 21.1 percent to 42.6 percent across the three groups of women (see Table 4-8). Mean intakes of fiber were below the AI in all subgroups of women. Approximately 68 to 78 percent of women had intakes of added sugars above recommended limits, whereas 50 to 79 percent of women had intakes of saturated fat above recommended limits.

Mean reported energy intake was below the median Estimated Energy Requirement (EER) by 10, 15, and 22 percent for pregnant, breastfeeding, and postpartum women, respectively (see Table 4-9).

TABLE 4-7 Reported Mean Usual Intakes of Selected Nutrients Compared to the Adequate Intake (AI) Value, WIC-Participating Women 19 to 50 Years of Age, NHANES 2005–2012

		Mean Intakes, mg/d (SE)		
Nutrient	AI (P/BF/PP), mg/d[a]	P (N = 165)[b]	Any BF (N = 27)[c]	PP (N = 62)[d]
Potassium	4,700/5,100/4,700	2,997 (52)	2,885 (130)	1,940 (71)
Sodium	1,500	3,603 (59)	3,266 (124)	2,855 (87)
Choline	450/550/425	362 (5)	356 (10)	247 (11)

NOTES: AI = Adequate Intake; N = sample size; SE = standard error.

[a] Values represent the AI for P/BF/PP groups. One value indicates that the AI is the same across groups.

Subgroup definitions are as follows:

[b] P = Pregnant WIC-participating women.

[c] BF = Breastfeeding (any intensity), nonpregnant WIC-participating women.

[d] PP = WIC-participating women who are 6 months postpartum, not pregnant, and not breastfeeding; data were sourced only from 2007–2012 NHANES because no postpartum variable is available in the 2005–2006 dataset.

SOURCES: IOM, 1998, 2005; USDA/ARS, 2005–2012.

TABLE 4-8 Reported Intakes of Selected Macronutrients Compared to Recommended Intakes, WIC-Participating Women, 19 to 50 Years of Age, NHANES 2005–2012

Nutrient and DRI or Recommended Daily Limits (P/BF/PP)[a]	Units for Comparison to DRI or Recommended Limit per Day	Comparison to DRI or Recommended Limit (SE)		
		P (N = 165)[b]	Any BF (N = 27)[c]	PP (N = 62)[d]
Protein (EAR)				
0.88/1.05/0.66 g/kg	% below EAR	21.1 (6.2)	42.6 (12.6)	31.2 (9.7)
Fiber (AI)				
28/29/25 g	Mean, g	18.9 (0.5)	16.2 (0.8)	12.2 (0.6)
Added sugars (limit)[e,f]				
15.5/15.5/13.7 tsp-eq	Mean, tsp-eq	23.8 (1.5)	24.0 (2.7)	23.8 (1.8)
10% of kcal	% above 10% of energy	68.3 (5.1)	73.6 (7.1)	78.0 (13.2)
Saturated fat (limit)[f]				
28.9/28.9/25.6 g	Mean, g	30.1 (0.6)	28.6 (1.8)	20.5 (0.9)
10% of kcal	Mean, % of kcal	11.1 (0.1)	11.6 (0.4)	10.0 (0.3)
	% above 10% of energy	74.6 (8.7)	78.5 (15.9)	49.4 (8.5)

NOTES: AI = Adequate Intake; DRI = Dietary Reference Intake; EAR = Estimated Average Requirement; g/d = grams per day; g/kg/d = grams per kilogram of body weight per day; kcal = kilocalories; SE = standard error; tsp-eq = teaspoon-equivalents.

[a] Values represent a DRI. One value indicates recommendation is the same across P/BF/PP groups.

Subgroup definitions are as follows:

[b] P = Pregnant WIC-participating women.

[c] BF = Breastfeeding (any intensity), nonpregnant WIC-participating women.

[d] PP = WIC-participating women who are 6 months postpartum, not pregnant, and not breastfeeding; data were sourced only from 2007–2012 NHANES because no postpartum variable is available in the 2005–2006 dataset.

[e] Added sugars data were generated as part of the food group analysis. See methodology in Appendix J.

[f] Tsp-eq and gram limits shown for added sugars and saturated fat, respectively, are based on energy intakes of 2,600 (pregnant and breastfeeding) and 2,300 (postpartum) kcals. The percent above 10 percent of energy is based on the limits corresponding to the actual energy intake reported in NHANES.

SOURCES: IOM, 2002/2005; USDA/ARS, 2005–2012; USDA/HHS, 2016.

TABLE 4-9 Estimated Energy Requirement and Reported Energy Intake, WIC-Participating Women, 19 to 50 Years of Age, NHANES 2005–2012

	Mean kcal/d (SE)		
Estimated Energy Requirement and Energy Intake	P (N = 165)[a]	Any BF (N = 27)[b]	PP (N = 62)[c]
Estimated Energy Requirement[d]			
Median	2,612 (22)	2,530 (36)	2,350 (23)
Mean	2,679 (24)	2,557 (38)	2,379 (33)
Food pattern applied in the report	2,600	2,600	2,300
Usual Energy Intake			
Median	2,333 (67)	2,088 (143)	1,788 (95)
Mean	2,360 (43)	2,129 (92)	1,832 (62)

NOTES: kcal = kilocalories; N = sample size; SE = standard error.
Subgroup definitions are as follows:
[a] P = Pregnant WIC-participating women.
[b] BF = Breastfeeding (any intensity), nonpregnant WIC-participating women.
[c] PP = WIC-participating women who are 6 months postpartum, not pregnant, and not breastfeeding; data were sourced only from 2007–2012 NHANES because no postpartum variable is available in the 2005–2006 dataset.
[d] EERs were calculated assuming a low-active physical activity level. For pregnant women, EER calculations assumed the second trimester. For breastfeeding women, EER calculations assumed the first 6 month period postpartum.
SOURCES: USDA/ARS, 2005–2012; EERs calculated according to the method in IOM, 2002/2005.

Micronutrient Excess

The prevalence of excessive sodium intakes was greater than 50 percent across all three subgroups of women. Nearly all pregnant and breastfeeding women had excessive sodium intakes (see Table 4-10). Prevalences of intakes above the UL were less than 0.01 across subgroups for calcium, copper, iron, phosphorus, zinc, selenium, vitamin C, vitamin B6, retinol, and choline, and, thus, are not included in the table.

Nutrient Intake Adequacy of Formula-Fed WIC-Participating Infants

This section applies exclusively to infants in WIC who were coded as "formula-fed" in the NHANES datasets. This designation means that they received infant formula but is uninformative about the amount of breast milk that they may also have received. No infants in the dataset were characterized as "partially breastfed" even though this behavior is sufficiently common to have detected. As a result, the amount of breast milk that these

TABLE 4-10 Estimated Prevalence of Micronutrient Excess Compared to Tolerable Upper Intake Level (UL), WIC-Participating Women, 19 to 50 Years of Age, NHANES 2005–2012

		% of Population Above the UL (SE)		
Nutrient	UL per Day	P (N = 165)[a]	Any BF (N = 27)[b]	PP (N = 62)[c]
Sodium	2,300 mg	96.9 (4.0)	96.1 (11.5)	78.7 (13.3)

NOTES: N = sample size; SE = standard error; UL = Tolerable Upper Intake Level.
Subgroup definitions are as follows:
[a] P = Pregnant WIC-participating women.
[b] BF = Breastfeeding (any intensity), nonpregnant WIC-participating women.
[c] PP = WIC-participating women who are 6 months postpartum, not pregnant, and not breastfeeding.
SOURCES: IOM, 2005; USDA/ARS, 2005–2012.

infants may have received in addition to formula is unknown. The nutrient intakes of formula-fed infants were analyzed in two age groups: (1) from birth to less than 6 months of age and (2) from 6 to less than 12 months of age. These groups align with the recommended age for introduction of complementary feeding (about 6 months [AAP, 2014]) and also the current age categories for the WIC food packages for infants (see Chapter 1, Tables 1-2 and 1-3).

Formula-Fed Infants 0 to Less Than 6 Months of Age

Micronutrient intake compared to AIs Only AI levels (no EARs) are available for infants from birth to less than 6 months of age. These AIs are presented in Table 4-11 along with mean usual intakes for each nutrient. With the exception of choline, mean usual intakes for all nutrients exceeded these AIs.

Macronutrient and energy intake Macronutrient and energy intakes of infants up to 6 months of age are presented in Tables 4-12 and 4-13. Mean protein intakes exceeded the AI for this nutrient. Fiber, saturated fat, and added sugars were not evaluated for infants.[10]

[10] There are no DRIs or dietary guidance for intake of fiber, added sugars, or saturated fat by infants. In addition, the AAP (2014) advises whole fat dairy products for children 1 to less than 2 years of age, and restriction of saturated fat generally begins at 2 years of age. Therefore, it would be difficult to assess intake adequacy or excess for these nutrients. In addition, infants begin complementary feeding at 4 to 6 months of age; it would be difficult to evaluate "mean" intake of nutrients from foods for a population subgroup that spans 0 to less than 6 months of age since some of these infants are not yet consuming any solid foods.

TABLE 4-11 Reported Mean Usual Intakes of Selected Micronutrients Compared to Adequate Intake (AI) Values, Formula-Fed, WIC-Participating Infants 0 to 12 Months of Age, NHANES 2011–2012

		Mean Usual Intake (SE)	
Nutrient	AI or EAR[a] per Day (<6 Months/6 to <12 Months)	<6 Months (N = 93)	6 to <12 Months (N = 98)
Calcium	200/260 mg	690 (26)	789 (22)
Copper	0.2/0.22 mg	0.62 (0.02)	0.73 (0.02)
Iron	0.27/6.9 mg	14.8 (0.6)	17.6 (0.8)[b]
Magnesium	30/75 mg	78 (3)	127 (4)
Phosphorus	100/275 mg	401 (20)	595 (22)
Selenium	15/20 μg	16.9 (0.6)	32.9 (1.5)
Zinc	2/2.5 mg	5.7 (0.2)	6.8 (0.2)[c]
Potassium	400/700 mg	806 (25)	1,276 (37)
Sodium	120/370 mg	237 (8)	656 (43)
Vitamin A	400/500 μg RAE	620 (17)	698 (24)
Vitamin E	4/5 mg αTOC	7.5 (0.2)	8.1 (0.3)
Vitamin C	40/50 mg	75.4 (2.5)	102.4 (3.0)
Thiamin	0.2/0.3 mg	0.74 (0.04)	1.07 (0.04)
Riboflavin	0.3/0.4 mg	1.06 (0.04)	1.50 (0.05)
Niacin	2/4 mg	9.1 (0.4)	12.9 (0.5)
Vitamin B6	0.1/0.3 mg	0.47 (0.02)	0.81 (0.03)
Folate	65/80 μg DFE	172 (4)	237 (8)
Vitamin B12	0.4/0.5 mg	1.9 (0.1)	2.30 (0.09)
Choline	125/150 mg	109 (5)	138 (5)

NOTES: αTOC = α-tocopherol; AI = Adequate Intake; DFE = dietary folate equivalents; EAR = Estimated Average Requirement; N = sample size; RAE = retinol activity equivalents; SE = standard error.

[a] Values represent AI or EAR for infants <6 months and 6 to <12 months; iron and zinc values for infants 6 to <12 months are EARs; all other values are AIs.

[b] Iron inadequacy was 4.2 percent.

[c] Zinc inadequacy was less than 1 percent.

SOURCES: IOM, 1997, 1998, 2000a, 2001, 2002/2005, 2005, 2011; USDA/ARS, 2011–2012.

TABLE 4-12 Reported Mean Intakes of Macronutrients, Formula-Fed, WIC-Participating Infants 0 to 12 Months of Age, NHANES 2011–2012

Nutrient	DRI per Day (<6 Months/6 to <12 Months)*	Units per Day	Mean Usual Intake (SE) <6 Months (N = 93)	6 to <12 Months (N = 98)	Inadequacy, % (SE), 6 to <12 Months (N = 98)
Protein	1.52 g/kg (AI)/1.0 g/kg (EAR)	g/kg	2.4 (0.1)	2.8 (0.1)	0.3 (0.5)
Carbohydrate, total	60/95 g (AI)	g	79.2 (2.2)	122.9 (2.8)	NA

NOTES: AI = Adequate Intake; EAR = Estimated Average Requirement; g/kg = grams per kilogram of body weight; kcal = kilocalories; N = sample size; NA = not applicable; SE = standard error.

* Values represent AI/EAR for infants <6 months and 6 to <12 months.

SOURCES: IOM, 2002/2005; USDA/ARS, 2011–2012.

TABLE 4-13 Estimated Energy Requirement and Reported Energy Intake, Formula-Fed, WIC-Participating Infants 0 to 12 Months of Age, NHANES 2011–2012

Estimated Energy Requirement and Energy Intake	Mean kcal/d (SE) <6 Months (N = 93)	6 to <12 Months (N = 98)
Estimated Energy Requirement		
Median	617 (10)	727 (10)
Mean	623 (10)	734 (8)
Usual Energy Intake		
Median	677 (21)	910 (34)
Mean	692 (17)	928 (22)

NOTES: kcal = kilocalories; N = sample size; SE = standard error.

SOURCES: USDA/ARS, 2011–2012; EERs calculated according to the method in IOM, 2002/2005.

Mean usual energy intake of WIC-participating infants less than 6 months of age was 692 kcal per day, which is slightly higher than the median EER of 617 kcal per day (see Table 4-13).

Micronutrient excess The prevalence of excessive micronutrient intakes compared to the UL for formula-fed infants are presented in Table 4-14. UL values for this age group have been defined only for calcium, iron, selenium, retinol, and zinc. Excess zinc intakes occurred in 88 percent and

TABLE 4-14 Estimated Prevalence of Micronutrient Excess Compared to the Tolerable Upper Intake Level (UL), Formula-Fed, WIC-Participating Infants 0 to 12 Months of Age, NHANES 2011–2012

Nutrient	UL per Day (<6 Months/ 6 to <12 Months)*	% of Population Above the UL (SE)	
		<6 Months (N = 93)	6 to <12 Months (N = 98)
Calcium	1,000/1,500 mg	10.8 (4.9)	0.5 (0.9)
Iron	40 mg	0.6 (0.9)	1.5 (1.7)
Zinc	4/5 mg	87.6 (5.1)	84.5 (7.4)
Retinol	600 μg	39.7 (5.2)	28.1 (6.0)
Selenium	45/60 μg	0.07 (0.2)	5.4 (4.1)

NOTES: N = sample size; SE = standard error; UL = Tolerable Upper Intake Level.
* Values represent UL for infants <6 months and 6 to <12 months. One value indicates that the UL is the same across groups.
SOURCES: IOM, 1998, 2001, 2011; USDA/ARS, 2011–2012.

excess retinol intake in 40 percent of the formula-fed infants in this analysis. However, zinc and retinol intakes above the established ULs are not considered of concern because the method used to set the UL resulted in a narrow margin between the RDA and the UL and because retinol toxicity is rare unless from supplemental sources (IOM, 2001). Infant formula (and the zinc and other nutrients provided in it) is tightly regulated for safety by the Food and Drug Administration.

Formula-Fed Infants 6 to Less Than 12 Months of Age

Micronutrient adequacy Micronutrient EARs for this age group have been established only for zinc and iron (see Table 4-11). The prevalence of inadequate zinc and iron intake was low in formula-fed infants of this age group.

Intake of nutrients with an AI Mean usual intakes fell below the AI for choline but above the respective AIs for all other nutrients (see Table 4-11).

Macronutrient and energy intake Nearly 100 percent of the infants in this age group exceeded the EAR for protein (see Table 4-12). For other macronutrients, no DRI value (fiber, saturated fat) or only an AI value (i.e. carbohydrate) is published, and therefore the basis for evaluation of intakes is limited. As noted above, fiber, saturated fat, and added sugars were not evaluated for infants.

The mean energy intake of WIC-participating infants 6 to less than 12 months of age was 928 kcal per day, which is 28 percent higher than the median EER of 727 kcal per day for this population subgroup (see Table 4-13).

Micronutrient excess The prevalence of excessive micronutrient intakes compared to the UL for infants in this age subgroup are presented in Table 4-14. Excess zinc intakes occurred in 85 percent and excess retinol intake in 28 percent of formula-fed infants 6 months and older. However, zinc and retinol intakes above the UL are not considered of concern for formula-fed infants for the reasons noted previously.

Evaluation of Energy and Iron Provided in the WIC Food Packages for Fully Formula-Fed Infants

Formula-fed infants ages 0 to 3 months of age receive 806 fluid ounces per month (537 kcal per day) as the full nutrition benefit[11] or, if the powder form is provided, 870 fluid ounces as the maximum monthly allowance (MMA).[12] Infants 4 to less than 6 months of age receive 884 fluid ounces per month (589 kcal per day) as the full nutrition benefit. These quantities of formula provide slightly less energy than the median EER determined for the WIC subgroup of infants ages 0 to less than 6 months (617 kcal per day [see Table 4-15]). WIC-participating infants 0 to less than 6 months of age who consume infant formula as their sole source of nutrition would be provided with 9.5 to 10.5 mg of iron per day, a quantity that is above the AI (0.27 mg per day)[13] but below the UL (40 mg per day) for this population subgroup. WIC formula provided to infants ages 6 to less than 12 months provides 57 percent of energy needs, based on the EER for children participating in WIC, and slightly more than the EAR for iron. The committee presumed that infants begin to receive complementary foods between 4 and 6 months of age and that those complementary foods meet the balance of their needs for both energy and nutrients. Some additional detail related to the committee's consideration of iron and energy provided by infant formulas is presented in Appendix Q.

---

[11] The full nutrition benefit (FNB) is the minimum amount of reconstituted fluid ounces of amounts for infant formula (based on a 13-ounce can), which formed the basis of substitution rates for other physical forms of infant formula (i.e., powder and ready-to-feed infant formula). The FNB is defined to ensure that participants receive a comparable nutritional benefit no matter which physical form of infant formula they receive.

[12] Formula provided to infants in any form may not exceed the maximum monthly allowance.

[13] The Adequate Intake (AI) was set based on iron intake of fully breastfed infants. The iron bioavailability from human milk differs from that of formula. Healthy infants born to iron-sufficient mothers have iron stores adequate to meet their needs in the first 6 months of life.

Iron and Zinc Intakes of Breastfed Infants Participating in WIC

For older breastfed infants (6 to less than 12 months of age) only zinc and iron intake were examined because human milk contains low levels of these nutrients and, thus, they are of particular concern. This fact is recognized by the American Academy of Pediatrics (AAP), which indicates that breastfed infants 6 to 12 months of age who are not consuming the recommended amount of iron from formula and complementary foods may benefit from oral iron supplementation (AAP, 2014). To increase the sample sizes, data for breastfeeding infants were merged across NHANES 2009–2012 (see Table 4-5). As shown in Table 4-16, at least 10 percent of these infants had inadequate intakes of iron and zinc.

Nutrient Intake Adequacy of Children Participating in WIC, Ages 1 to Less Than 2 Years

Micronutrient Adequacy

For WIC-participating children 1 to less than 2 years of age, the estimated prevalence of inadequacy was less than 5 percent for all nutrients, with the exception of vitamin E (see Table 4-17).

Intakes of Micronutrients with an AI

Mean potassium intakes were below the AI for children 1 to less than 2 years of age (see Table 4-18). Mean intakes of sodium and choline were above the AI values.

Macronutrient and Energy Intake

Selected macronutrient intakes for this age group are summarized in Table 4-19. Protein intakes were adequate for all children, but fiber intakes fell below the AI. Added sugars and saturated fat intakes are not reported for children ages 1 to less than 2 years because the DGA limits for these nutrients apply only to children 2 years of age and older. Eighty percent of children ages 2 to less than 5 years of age exceeded the DGA limit of 10 percent of kilocalories from added sugars. Intake of saturated fat averaged 10.9 percent of kilocalories for children 2 to less than 5 years of age. Seventy percent of these children had saturated fat intakes above the recommended limit of 10 percent of kilocalories.

Mean usual energy intakes and the corresponding EER values are presented in Table 4-20. Estimated mean energy intake of children participating

TABLE 4-15 Energy and Iron Provided to Fully Formula-Fed WIC-Participating Infants in the Current WIC Food Packages, Compared to the EER and DRI

		Infant Age (months)			
Formula Volume or Component[a]	Units	0–3	0–3 (powder)	4–5	6–11
FNB[b]	fl oz/month	806	870[g]	884	624
FNB, formula only[c]	kcal/d	537	580	589	416
FNB, formula[b] + foods[d]	kcal/d	NA	NA	NA	583
median EER[e]	kcal/d	617[h]	617[h]	617[h]	727[i]
% of EER in the food package, formula only	%	87	94	96	57
% of EER in the food package, food only	%	NA	NA	NA	23
% of EER in the food package, formula + foods	%	NA	NA	NA	80
Iron provided in FNB of formula[f]	mg/d	9.5	10.4	10.5	7.4
DRI Values					
AI or EAR for iron	mg/d	0.27[j]	0.27[j]	0.27[j]	6.9[k]
UL for iron	mg/d	40	40	40	40

NOTES: AI = Adequate Intake Level; DRI = Dietary Reference Intake; EAR = Estimated Average Requirement; EER = Estimated Energy Requirement; FNB = full nutrition benefit; NA = not applicable; UL = Tolerable Upper Intake Level.

[a] Unless otherwise indicated.

[b] Based on the USDA-FNS Final Rule.

[c] Values were based on reconstituted powdered formula, which is the most commonly issued formula in the WIC program; total energy therefore differs slightly from those presented in the phase I report.

[d] Based on the baseline nutrient profile calculations, as detailed in Appendix R.

[e] EER was calculated for WIC-participating infants using NHANES 2011–2012.

[f] Based on the average amount of iron across formulas from the three major manufacturers that contain 20 kcal/oz: 1.76 mg iron per 100 kcal.

[g] This volume is the maximum monthly allowance, which aligns with available sizes of powdered formula. Powdered formula is the form most commonly provided for infants ages 0 to 3 months.

[h] Based on formula-fed infants ages 0 to less than 6 months in NHANES 2011–2012, n = 93.

[i] Based on formula-fed infants ages 6 to less than 12 months in NHANES 2011–2012, n = 98.

[j] An Adequate Intake value (a population mean intake exceeding this value implies a low prevalence of inadequacy).

[k] An Estimated Average Requirement value (used to estimate the prevalence of inadequacy).

SOURCES: USDA/ARS, 2011–2012; USDA/FNS, 2014; EERs calculated according to method in IOM, 2002/2005.

TABLE 4-16 Iron and Zinc Intake of Breastfed WIC-Participating Infants 6 to Less Than 12 Months of Age, NHANES 2009–2012

		Inadequacy, % (SE)*	
Subgroup and EAR	N	Iron (mg)	Zinc (mg)
Breastfed infants	39	38 (9.5)	44 (8.3)
EAR (mg)		6.9	2.5

NOTES: N = sample size; SE = standard error.
* Inadequacy, % = percentage of individuals with usual intake below the EAR.
SOURCES: IOM, 2001; USDA/ARS, 2009–2012.

TABLE 4-17 Estimated Prevalence of Inadequacy of Selected Nutrients, WIC-Participating Children, NHANES 2011–2012

Nutrient	EAR per Day (Ages 1–3/Age 4)[b]	Inadequacy, % (SE)[a]	
		1 to <2 Years (N = 96)	2 to <5 Years (N = 263)
Calcium	500/800 mg	3.2 (4.2)	2.0 (1.4)
Iron	3 mg	1.7 (2.0)	0
Copper	0.26/0.34 mg	0.7 (1.1)	0
Magnesium	65/110 mg	0.07 (0.2)	0
Phosphorus	380/405 mg	0.1 (0.4)	0.02 (0.04)
Zinc	2.5/4.0 mg	0.09 (0.3)	0
Selenium	17 μg	0	0
Vitamin A	210/275 μg RAE	1.2 (2.3)	0.9 (1.0)
Vitamin E	5/6 mg αTOC	76.1 (6.8)	34.9 (4.5)
Vitamin C	13/22 mg	0.5 (1.1)	0
Thiamin	0.4/0.5 mg	1.1 (1.5)	0
Niacin	5/6 mg	2.5 (3.1)	0
Vitamin B6	0.4/0.5 mg	0.2 (0.5)	0
Folate	120 μg DFE	2.0 (2.7)	0
Vitamin B12	0.7 mg	0.02 (0.06)	0

NOTES: αTOC = α-tocopherol; DFE = dietary folate equivalents; EAR = Estimated Average Requirement; N = sample size; RAE = retinol activity equivalents; SE = standard error.
[a] Inadequacy, % = percentage of individuals with usual intake below the EAR.
[b] Values represent EAR for children 1 to 3 years and 4 to <5 years of age. One value indicates that the EAR is the same across groups.
SOURCES: IOM, 1997, 1998, 2000a, 2001, 2002/2005, 2005, 2011; USDA/ARS, 2011–2012.

TABLE 4-18 Reported Mean Intakes of Selected Micronutrients Compared to the Adequate Intake (AI) Value, WIC-Participating Children 1 to Less Than 5 Years of Age, NHANES 2011–2012

		Mean Intake, mg/d (SE)	
Nutrient	AI (Ages 1–3/Age 4) (mg/d)*	1 to <2 Years (N = 96)	2 to <5 Years (N = 263)
Potassium	3,000/3,800	1,881 (41)	2,110 (29)
Sodium	1,000/1,200	1,660 (50)	2,190 (38)
Choline	200/250	211 (6)	228 (40)

NOTES: AI = Adequate Intake; N = sample size; SE = standard error.

* Values represent AI for children 1 to 3 years and 4 to <5 years of age. One value indicates that the AI is the same across groups.

SOURCES: IOM, 1998, 2005; USDA/ARS, 2011–2012.

in WIC (1,314 kcal per day) was 43 percent higher than the median EER for WIC participants of this age group (917 kcal per day).

Micronutrient Excess

Among WIC-participating children 1 to less than 2 years of age, the prevalence of nutrient intakes exceeding the UL was more than 5 percent for sodium, zinc, copper, and retinol (see Table 4-21). As is the case with infants, zinc and retinol intakes above the UL are not of concern for children in this age group because of the way these values were derived. The UL for copper is an extrapolation of the UL for adults, and adult intakes of up to 12 mg of copper per day from food have not resulted in adverse effects (IOM, 2001). Therefore, copper intakes above the UL in this age group are likewise not considered to be of concern. Fewer than 0.01 percent of children ages 1 to less than 2 years exceeded the UL for iron, phosphorus, vitamin B6, and choline.

Nutrient Adequacy of WIC-Participating Children, Ages 2 to Less Than 5 Years

Micronutrient Adequacy

For children 2 to less than 5 years of age, there was a high prevalence of inadequate vitamin E intake (see Table 4-17). Intake inadequacy of other nutrients was below the threshold of 5 percent.

TABLE 4-19 Reported Intakes of Selected Macronutrients Compared to Recommended Intakes, WIC-Participating Children 1 to Less Than 5 Years of Age, NHANES 2011–2012

Nutrient and DRI or Recommended Daily Limit	Units for Comparison to DRI or Recommended Limit per Day	Comparison to DRI or Recommended Limit (SE)	
		1 to <2 Years (N = 96)	2 to <5 Years (N = 263)
Protein (EAR)			
0.87/0.76 g/kg[a]	% below EAR	0	0
Fiber (AI)			
19/25 g[a]	Mean, g	8.5 (0.3)	12.0 (0.2)
Added sugars (limit)[b,c]			
7.7 tsp-eq	Mean, tsp-eq	NA	12.2 (0.4)
10% of kcal	% above 10% of energy	NA	80.1 (3.0)
Saturated fat (limit)[c]			
14.4 g	Mean, g	NA	18.6 (0.4)
10% of kcal	Mean, % of kcal	NA	10.9 (0.1)
	% above 10% of energy	NA	70.4 (6.3)

NOTES: AI = Adequate Intake; g/kg = grams per kilogram of body weight; kcal = kilocalories; N = sample size; NA = not applicable; SE = standard error; tsp-eq = teaspoon equivalents.

[a] Numbers represent an EAR, AI, or upper limit as noted, for ages 1–3/age 4.

[b] Added sugars data were generated as part of the food group analysis. See methodology in Appendix J.

[c] The DGA limits for added sugars and saturated fat apply only to children 2 years of age and older. Tsp-eq and gram limits shown for added sugars and saturated fat, respectively, are based on an energy intake of 1,300 kcal. The percent above 10 percent of energy is based on the limits corresponding to the actual energy intake reported.

SOURCES: IOM, 2002/2005; USDA/ARS, 2011–2012; USDA/HHS, 2016.

Intakes of Micronutrients with an AI

For children ages 2 to less than 5 years of age, mean potassium and choline intakes were below the AI (see Table 4-18).

Macronutrient and Energy Intakes

Protein intakes were adequate for all children in this age group (see Table 4-19). Mean fiber intake was approximately half the AI. Usual mean energy intakes and the corresponding EER values are presented in Table 4-20. Reported mean energy intake (1,509 kcal) was comparable to the median EER (1,517 kcal).

TABLE 4-20 Estimated Energy Requirement and Reported Energy Intake, WIC-Participating Children 1 to Less Than 5 Years of Age, NHANES 2011–2012

Estimated Energy Requirement and Energy Intake	Mean kcal/d (SE)	
	1 to <2 Years (N = 96)	2 to <5 Years (N = 263)
Estimated Energy Requirement*		
Median	917 (11)	1,517 (9)
Mean	925 (9)	1,532 (9)
Usual Energy Intake		
Median	1,284 (26)	1,479 (27)
Mean	1,314 (17)	1,509 (21)

NOTES: kcal = kilocalories; N = sample size; SE = standard error.
* EERs were calculated assuming a low-active physical activity level.
SOURCES: USDA/ARS, 2011–2012; estimated energy requirements calculated according to IOM, 2002/2005.

Micronutrient Excess

More than 5 percent of children in this age category exceeded the UL for a number of micronutrients evaluated for this report: retinol, zinc, copper, selenium, and sodium (see Table 4-21). As noted previously, intakes above the UL for retinol, zinc, or copper are not of concern for children. Similar to copper, the UL for selenium is extrapolated from the selenium UL for adults (IOM, 2000a). In addition, no cases of selenosis have been reported even in high-selenium areas of the United States (IOM, 2000a). For these reasons, intakes of selenium above the UL were not considered of concern. Fewer than 0.01 percent of children ages 2 to less than 5 years exceeded the UL for iron, phosphorus, vitamin B6, and choline.

Special Case: Vitamin D Status Across Age Categories

As described in Appendix J, because an individual's vitamin D status is determined by both dietary intake and sun exposure, serum 25(OH)D concentrations were used to assess vitamin D status of all population subgroups, except infants.

The data presented in Table 4-22 indicate a low prevalence of inadequacy (less than 5 percent) for both subgroups of children when compared to the serum value linked to the EAR (40 nmol/L [IOM, 2011]). However,

TABLE 4-21 Estimated Prevalence of Micronutrient Excess, WIC-Participating Children 1 to Less Than 5 Years of Age, NHANES 2011–2012

Nutrient	UL per Day (Ages 1–3/Age 4)*	% of Population Above the UL (SE)	
		1 to <2 Years (N = 96)	2 to <5 Years (N = 263)
Calcium	2,500/2,500 mg	0	4.8 (2.5)
Copper	1/3 mg	8.6 (5.3)	9.8 (5.4)
Selenium	90/150 μg	3.4 (4.2)	11.0 (5.8)
Zinc	7/12 mg	39.2 (6.8)	95.0 (3.5)
Sodium	1,500/1,900 mg	58.6 (6.0)	65.2 (4.0)
Retinol	600/900 μg	18.5 (7.5)	15.1 (4.9)
Vitamin C	400/650 mg	0	0.1 (0.3)

NOTES: N = sample size; SE = standard error; UL = Tolerable Upper Intake Level.
* Values represent the UL for children 1 to 3 years/4 to <5 years of age.
SOURCES: IOM, 1997, 1998, 2000a, 2001, 2002/2005, 2005, 2011; USDA/ARS, 2011–2012.

TABLE 4-22 Serum 25-Hydroxy Vitamin D of WIC Participants, NHANES 2005–2006

WIC Participant Category	% <40 nmol/L*
Women, P	8.6 (3.6)
Women, Any BF	21.2 (12.2)
Women, PP	12.6 (7.6)
Children, 1 to <2 Years	1.1 (1.2)
Children, 2 to <5 Years	2.1 (1.3)

NOTES: 25(OH)D = 25-hydroxy-vitamin D; BF = breastfeeding (any intensity), nonpregnant WIC-participating women; N = sample size; P = pregnant WIC-participating women; PP = WIC-participating women who are 6 months postpartum, not pregnant, and not breastfeeding. Serum data for 25-hydroxy vitamin D were only available in NHANES 2005–2006.
* A serum 25(OH)D level of 40 nmol/L was established by the Institute of Medicine (2011) as an average requirement that meets the needs of approximately half the population, used to establish EARs for dietary intake of vitamin D.
SOURCE: USDA/ARS, 2005–2006.

the prevalence of inadequacy was greater than 5 percent among pregnant women and greater than 10 percent among breastfeeding and postpartum women. Percentile data are presented in Appendix J.

Dietary vitamin D intakes of infants are presented separately in Table 4-23. The AI for vitamin D in infants is 10 μg per day. Mean intake

TABLE 4-23 Mean Vitamin D Intakes of Formula-Fed WIC-Participating Infants 0 to Less Than 12 Months of Age, NHANES 2011–2012

Participant Age	AI per Day	Mean Intake (SE)
Infants 0 to <6 months (N = 93)	10 µg	9.7 (0.2)
Infants 6 to <12 months (N = 98)	10 µg	8.5 (0.2)

NOTES: AI = Adequate Intake; N = sample size; SE = standard error.
SOURCES: IOM, 2011; USDA/ARS, 2011–2012.

among formula-fed WIC-participating infants less than 12 months of age falls slightly below the AI.

ANALYSIS OF THE NATIONAL HEALTH AND NUTRITION EXAMINATION SURVEY DATA: FOOD GROUP INTAKES COMPARED TO RECOMMENDATIONS

In addition to evaluating NHANES findings reported in the literature (described earlier in this chapter), the committee conducted its own analysis of food intake among WIC-eligible individuals using the same NHANES dataset, analytical subgroups, and survey years used for its nutrient intake analysis. Because dietary intakes were evaluated relative to the DGA food patterns, which are available only for adults and children 2 years of age and older, the committee's analysis of food intake by infants was limited to an assessment of intake of "meat, poultry, and seafood" (as a key source of the key nutrients iron and zinc) among older breastfed infants. The analysis of food intake in children ages 1 to less than 2 years was limited to mean intakes (i.e., did not include assessment of the percent of the population below recommended intakes). For women and children 2 years of ages and older, priority concern was given to food groups for which the prevalence of intakes below recommended amounts was 75 percent or greater, followed by food groups for which the prevalence of intakes below recommended amounts was 50 to less than 75 percent.

As was done with nutrients, this section presents data for WIC participant subgroups only, with pre- and post-2009 survey years for women and breastfed infants collapsed into a single analysis and only post-2009 data presented for the other subgroups. Detailed methodology, mean usual intake data, and intake distributions for all of the analyzed population subgroups are presented in Appendix J.

Food Group Intake of Women Participating in WIC

Intakes of food groups and subgroups for women compared to recommendations are presented in Table 4-24. For all food groups except refined grains, approximately 50 percent or more of women participating in WIC had intakes below recommended amounts. For total vegetables, nearly 100 percent of pregnant or postpartum women had intakes lower than the recommended amount and 50 percent of breastfeeding women had intakes lower than the recommended amount. Too few women reported intake of several food subgroups to produce estimates of those foods.

Intake of whole fruit was less than half of recommended fruit intakes in 69 to 90 percent of women. The 1 cup-equivalent of fruit juice included in Table 4-24 represents the DGA recommendation that not more than 50 percent of fruit intake come from juice and is, therefore, an upper limit rather than a target (USDA/HHS, 2016).

Between 70 and 77 percent of women had intakes of solid fat[14] exceeding 10 percent of energy. Data in Table 4-8 indicate that women consume approximately 15 (pregnant and breastfeeding) to 17 (postpartum) percent of energy from added sugars. On average, women consume 13 (postpartum) to 14 (pregnant and breastfeeding) percent of energy from solid fat. Together, this equates to 29 to 30 percent of total energy as "calories for other uses" apart from any other dietary contributions (i.e., excesses of other food groups such as refined grains) to this value.[15] The DGA recommend a limit of 14 and 15 percent of energy be allotted to these calories for a 2,300- or a 2,600-kcal diet, respectively.

Food Group Intake of Breastfed WIC-Participating Infants

Because there are no recommended food group patterns by which to assess the adequacy of infants' intake, the committee did not assess overall food intake in the infant subgroups. The AAP generally recommends introduction of a variety of complementary foods at approximately 6 months of age (while also recommending exclusive breastfeeding for the first 6 months of life). Inasmuch as iron and zinc intake are of concern for breastfed infants who begin complementary feeding, intake of meat (a source of bioavailable iron as well as zinc) was assessed for older breastfed infants only (6 to 12 months of age). Of the 39 identified infants participating in WIC who were breastfed in NHANES 2009–2012, 10 percent consumed infant

[14] Most solid fats are high in saturated fats and/or trans fats and have less monounsaturated or polyunsaturated fats.

[15] Calories for other uses (COU) includes added sugars, added refined starches, solid fats, alcohol, or calories from consuming more than the recommended amount of food in a food group (USDA/HHS, 2016). Chapter 2 includes a more detailed discussion of COU.

TABLE 4-24 Food Group Intakes Compared to the DGA Recommendations: Pregnant, Breastfeeding, or Postpartum WIC-Participating Women 19 to 50 Years, NHANES 2005–2012

Food Group	Recommended Intake (P and BF/PP)	% of Population Below Recommended Intake (SE)		
		P (N = 139)[a]	Any BF (N = 25)[b]	PP (N = 54)[c]
Total fruit	2 c-eq/d	69.1 (6.6)	78.7 (6.2)	89.9 (6.7)
Whole fruit	1 c-eq/d	64.4 (12.1)	74.2 (9.3)	96.1 (NA)
Fruit juice	1 c-eq/d[d]	75.8 (7.1)	53.1 (12.9)	84.6 (8.9)
Total vegetables	3.5/3 c-eq/d	98.9 (0.3)	50.0 (16.1)	99.9 (25.1)
Dark green vegetables	2.5/2 c-eq/wk	97.4 (3.7)	NA	89.2 (NA)
Total red and orange vegetables	7/6 c-eq/wk	97.0 (1.5)	97.4 (9.8)	93.9 (7.1)
Beans and peas computed as vegetables	2.5/2 c-eq/wk	NA	NA	NA
Total starchy vegetables	7/6 c-eq/wk	65.2 (8.0)	83.8 (6.8)	98.8 (1.7)
Other vegetables	5.5/5 c-eq/wk	83.1 (4.8)	92.1 (10.2)	85.4 (9.3)
Total grains	9/7.5 oz-eq/d	71.0 (5.6)	87.6 (16.0)	57.6 (9.8)
Whole grains	4.5/3.75 oz-eq/d	100.0 (0.0)	100.0 (0.0)	100.0 (0.3)
Refined grains	4.5/3.75 oz-eq/d	10.4 (3.9)	14.4 (16.8)	13.2 (9.7)
Total protein foods	6.5/6.25 oz-eq/d	75.3 (5.1)	76.0 (12.4)	74.7 (7.8)
Meat, poultry, and eggs (not seafood)	31/29.5 oz-eq/wk	56.1 (5.4)	48.6 (12.6)	54.0 (13.0)
Seafood	10/9.5 oz-eq/wk	82.1 (8.7)	NA	NA
Nuts, seeds, and soy	5 oz-eq/wk	87.2 (6.6)	NA	90.7 (6.5)
Total dairy	3 c-eq/d	82.5 (6.9)	72.9 (13.1)	96.0 (10.3)
Oils	34/39 g-eq/d	87.6 (3.7)	50.0 (15.8)	87.6 (22.5)
		% of Population Above Recommended Intake (SE)		
Solid fats	<28.9/25.6 g-eq/d[e]	76.9 (6.2)	71.5 (8.3)	70.4 (11.8)
Added sugars	<15.5/13.7 tsp-eq/d[d]	68.3 (5.1)	73.6 (7.1)	78.0 (13.2)

TABLE 4-24 Continued

NOTES: c-eq = cup-equivalents; d = day; g-eq = gram-equivalents; N = sample size; NA = data not available because an inadequate number of individuals reported intake; oz-eq = ounce-equivalents; SE = standard error; tsp-eq = teaspoon-equivalents; wk = week. Kilocalorie (kcal) patterns determined from NHANES assessment of usual intake for each group. Recommended intakes are indicated for P and BF/PP women; one value indicates that the recommendation is the same across groups. See Appendix J, Table J-4, for a description of the foods that compose each food group.

Population subgroups are as follows:

[a] P = Pregnant WIC-participating women; kcal pattern = 2,600 kcal.

[b] BF = Breastfeeding (any intensity), nonpregnant WIC-participating women; kcal pattern = 2,600 kcal.

[c] PP = WIC-participating women who are 6 months postpartum, not pregnant, and not breastfeeding; data were sourced only from 2007–2012 NHANES because no postpartum variable is available in the 2005–2006 dataset.; kcal pattern = 2,300 kcal.

[d] The DGA include the recommendation that not more than 50 percent of fruit intake should come from juice.

[e] Limits for solid fats and added sugars are based on an upper limit of 10 percent of energy for the 2,600 and 2,300 kcal patterns.

SOURCES: USDA/ARS, 2005–2012; USDA/HHS, 2016.

food meats (specifically, meat, poultry or seafood) over the two survey days (see Table 4-25). For the few who consumed infant meats alone (not as a component of mixed dinners), intake was reported to be 1.9 ounces on the first day observed, an amount that is close to the AAP recommended maximum intake per day of 2 ounces per day (AAP, 2014), though only for the 10 percent of infants who consumed the infant food meats.

Food Group Intake of Children Ages 1 to Less Than 2 Years Participating in WIC

As was the case for infants, the DGA do not include recommended food patterns for children 1 to less than 2 years of age. Inasmuch as there is no comparator for adequacy, mean usual food group and subgroup intakes for children of these ages are presented in Table 4-26. Intake of juice was 0.83 cup-equivalents per day (6.3 ounces), which exceeds the AAP recommended maximum of 6 ounces per day. Solid fat intake in this subgroup was estimated to be 26.5 g-equivalents per day, whereas reported added sugars intake was 9.59 tsp-equivalents per day.

TABLE 4-25 Consumption of Infant Food Meat and Other Sources of Meat by WIC-Participating Breastfed Infants Ages 6 to Less Than 12 Months, NHANES 2009–2012

Food Type	N	Percent of All WIC-Participating Breastfed Infants That Consumed the Food Type	Percent of All Breastfed Infants That Consumed the Food Type[a]	Average Amount of Meat Consumed on Day 1 by WIC-Participating Breastfed Infants Reporting Meat Intake (oz)
Infant food meat (meat, poultry, or seafood)	4[b]	10	6	1.9
Infant food dinner with meat	3[b]	8	12	0.3
Meat (not infant food)	39	100	100	0.2

NOTES: Population weights were applied. N = sample size for WIC-participating breastfed infants. Data from two days of reported intakes.

[a] A total of 68 breastfed infants were identified in NHANES 2009–2012.

[b] Includes 3 infants with reported intake on day 1.

SOURCE: USDA/ARS 2009–2012.

Food Group Intake of WIC-Participating Children Ages 2 to Less Than 5 Years

The proportions of children ages 2 to less than 5 years with food group and subgroup intakes below the DGA food pattern recommendations are presented in Table 4-27. (As with the other age groups, mean intakes and intake distributions are presented in Appendix J.) The prevalence of inadequate intake was greater than 75 percent of this population subgroup for total vegetables (including dark green and total red and orange); whole grains; seafood; and nuts, seeds, and soy. It was between 50 and 75 percent for beans and peas, total starchy vegetables, other vegetables, total protein foods, and total dairy. The prevalence of excess intake was greater than 75 percent for added sugars and solid fats. Only intakes of total fruit and whole fruit; total grains; refined grains; and meat, poultry, and eggs met or exceeded the DGA recommended amounts in more than 50 percent of these children.

As with WIC-participating women (see Table 4-24), the recommended 0.63 cup-equivalent of fruit juice included in Table 4-27 is an upper limit rather than a target amount (USDA/HHS, 2016). Juice intake among these children averaged 0.71 cup-equivalents per day.

TABLE 4-26 Mean Usual Food Group Intakes of WIC-Participating Children 1 to Less Than 2 Years, NHANES 2011–2012

Food Group	Units	Mean Usual Intake (SE) (N = 81)
Total fruit	c-eq/d	1.36 (0.12)
Whole fruit	c-eq/d	0.62 (0.07)
Fruit juice	c-eq/d	0.83 (0.10)
Total vegetables	c-eq/d	0.47 (0.04)
Dark green vegetables	c-eq/wk	0.14 (NA)
Total red and orange vegetables	c-eq/wk	1.57 (0.30)
Beans and peas computed as vegetables	c-eq/wk	1.11 (0.14)
Total starchy vegetables	c-eq/wk	0.45 (0.12)
Other vegetables	c-eq/wk	0.78 (0.15)
Total grains	oz-eq/d	3.36 (0.18)
Whole grains	oz-eq/d	0.83 (0.20)
Refined grains	oz-eq/d	2.83 (0.14)
Total protein foods	oz-eq/d	2.05 (0.13)
Meat, poultry, and eggs (not seafood)	oz-eq/wk	12.98 (0.83)
Seafood	oz-eq/wk	NA (NA)
Nuts, seeds, and soy	oz-eq/wk	0.81 (0.27)
Total dairy	c-eq/d	2.48 (0.12)
Oils	g-eq/d	8.62 (0.60)
Food Groups to Limit		
Solid fats	g-eq/d	26.37 (1.72)
Added sugars	tsp-eq/d	9.59 (0.67)

NOTES: c-eq = cup-equivalents; d = day; g-eq = gram-equivalents; N = sample size; NA = data not available because an inadequate number of individuals reported intake; oz-eq = ounce-equivalents; SE = standard error; tsp-eq = teaspoon-equivalents; wk = week. There is no recommended food pattern for this age group in the 2015–2020 *Dietary Guidelines for Americans* (USDA/HHS, 2016). See Appendix J, Table J-4, for a description of the foods that comprise each food group.
SOURCE: USDA/ARS, 2011–2012.

Intakes of solid fats and added sugars exceeded 10 percent of energy in over 90 and 80 percent of children in this age group, respectively. On average, children in this age group consume 18 percent of their energy from solid fats and 16 percent of their energy from added sugars. Together, this means that approximately 34 percent of energy is derived from "calories

TABLE 4-27 Food Group Intakes Compared to the DGA Recommendations: WIC-Participating Children 2 to Less Than 5 Years, NHANES 2011–2012

Food Group	Recommended Intake[a]	% of Population Below Recommended Intake (SE) (N = 228)
Total fruit	1.25 c-eq/d	42.6 (7.2)
Whole fruit	0.63 c-eq/d	42.5 (5.8)
Fruit juice	0.63 c-eq/d[b]	53.0 (10.8)
Total vegetables	1.50 c-eq/d	98.7 (1.1)
Dark green vegetables	1.00 c-eq/wk	94.3 (NA)
Total red and orange vegetables	3.00 c-eq/wk	90.5 (2.2)
Beans and peas computed as vegetables	0.50 c-eq/wk	58.8 (3.5)
Total starchy vegetables	3.50 c-eq/wk	73.1 (4.4)
Other vegetables	2.50 c-eq/wk	73.4 (7.5)
Total grains	4.50 oz-eq/d	45.0 (7.1)
Whole grains	2.25 oz-eq/d	93.3 (1.7)
Refined grains	2.25 oz-eq/d	6.6 (5.3)
Total protein foods	3.50 oz-eq/d	68.0 (12.8)
Meat, poultry, and eggs (not seafood)	16.50 oz-eq/wk	45.1 (8.0)
Seafood	5.00 oz-eq/wk	99.5 (1.7)
Nuts, seeds, and soy	2.50 oz-eq/wk	77.3 (7.6)
Total dairy	2.50 c-eq/d	72.8 (5.0)
Oils	16.50 g-eq/d	73.7 (8.4)
		% of Population Above Recommended Intake (SE)
Solid fats	<14.4 g-eq/d[c]	92.0 (1.9)
Added sugars	<7.7 tsp-eq/d[c]	80.1 (3.0)

NOTES: c-eq = cup-equivalents; d = day; g-eq = gram-equivalents; N = sample size; NA = data not available because an inadequate number of individuals reported intake; oz-eq = ounce-equivalents; SE = standard error; tsp-eq = teaspoon-equivalents; wk = week.

[a] Reference values are the USDA food patterns from the 2015–2020 *Dietary Guidelines for Americans* (DGA) for a 1,300 kilocalorie (average of 1,200 and 1,400 kilocalorie) food pattern. See Appendix J, Table J-4, for a description of the foods that comprise each food group.

[b] The DGA include the overall recommendation that not more than 50 percent of fruit intake should come from juice.

[c] Limits for solid fats and added sugars are based on an upper limit of 10 percent of energy for the 1,300-kcal food pattern.

SOURCES: USDA/ARS, 2011–2012; USDA/HHS, 2016.

from other uses" (COU) apart from other dietary contributions (COUs are discussed earlier in this chapter and in Chapter 2). The DGA recommend a limit of 8 percent of energy be allotted to COU for diets ranging between 1,200 and 1,600 kcal.

QUALITY OF WIC PARTICIPANTS' DIETS

The committee was tasked with applying two different indexes to evaluate the diet quality of WIC participants: the healthy eating index–2010 (HEI–2010) and a second index of the committee's choosing. As described in the phase I report (NASEM, 2016), the committee developed a nutrient-based diet quality (NBDQ) index to serve as the second index. Both the HEI–2010 and the NBDQ index have maximum scores of 100. The HEI–2010 measures conformance to the DGA. The NBDQ score is based on the probability of adequacy of the shortfall nutrients, as identified in the DGA. The rationale for development of the NBDQ index and methodologies for generating these two indexes are available in Appendix J. The results of this evaluation are summarized here, beginning with calculated HEI–2010 values.

Healthy Eating Index–2010

Mean HEI–2010 index scores ranged from 52 to 61 for women (Table 4-28). For children 2 to less than 5 years of age, the mean HEI–2010 index score was 65 (see Table 4-29). These scores are comparable to the HEI–score estimates of 54 to 58 for the total U.S. population ages 2 years and older, which were based on data from NHANES 2005 to 2010 (USDA/HHS, 2016). As with the NBDQ results, HEI–2010 scores for the subgroups of women were highest among breastfeeding women and lowest among postpartum women, and the score for children was higher than the score for any subgroup of women. Inasmuch as the HEI–2010 measures conformance to the DGA and because the DGA do not provide recommendations for infants or children less than 2 years of age, the HEI–2010 index scores could not be calculated for children in these age groups.

Nutrient-Based Diet Quality Index

Median nutrient-based diet quality (NBDQ) index scores ranged from 40 to 54 among the three subgroups of WIC-participating women (see Table 4-30); median NBDQ index scores were 66 for children ages 1 to less than 2 years and 69 for children ages 2 to less than 5 years (see Table 4-31). Scores for women were highest among breastfeeding women and lowest among postpartum women. The NBDQ could not be calculated for infants because there are so few nutrient EAR values have been determined.

TABLE 4-28 Healthy Eating Index: Results for WIC-Participating Women, 19–50 Years of Age, NHANES 2005–2012

HEI–2010 Component	Maximum Score	Pregnant (N = 169)	Breastfeeding[i] (N = 54)	Postpartum[j] (N = 62)
		Mean HEI Score (SE)		
Adequacy				
Total vegetables	5	2.7 (0.3)	3.2 (0.4)	2.5 (0.3)
Greens and beans[a]	5	2.1 (0.9)	2.6 (1.1)	2.1 (1.0)
Total fruit[b]	5	4.5 (0.4)	4.6 (0.5)	3.9 (1.2)
Whole fruit[c]	5	3.8 (0.4)	5.0 (0.2)	2.2 (0.5)
Whole grains	10	2.1 (0.3)	2.8 (0.8)	2.3 (0.6)
Dairy[d]	10	7.3 (0.5)	7.9 (0.9)	5.5 (0.8)
Total protein foods[e,f]	5	4.9 (0.2)	5.0 (0.1)	5.0 (0.1)
Seafoods and plant proteins	5	3.6 (0.6)	2.8 (0.8)	2.4 (0.9)
Fatty acid ratio[g]	10	3.6 (0.5)	2.9 (0.6)	4.8 (0.7)
Moderation				
Sodium	10	5.8 (0.7)	5.4 (0.6)	5.2 (0.7)
Refined grains	10	5.8 (0.5)	5.8 (1.0)	5.6 (0.9)
Empty calories[h]	20	10.9 (1.0)	12.7 (1.4)	10.3 (1.5)
Total HEI–2010 Score	100	57.0 (2.4)	60.6 (3.3)	51.8 (3.3)

NOTES: HEI = Healthy Eating Index; SE = standard error. For postpartum women, data were sourced from 2007–2012 NHANES. Sample sizes may differ from the nutrient and food group analyses because the methodology uses reported intake on day 1 only.

[a] Includes any beans and peas not counted as Total Protein Foods.

[b] Includes 100 percent fruit juice.

[c] Includes all forms except juice.

[d] Includes all milk products, such as fluid milk, yogurt, and cheese, as well as fortified soy beverages.

[e] Beans and peas are included here (and not with vegetables) when the Total Protein Foods standard is otherwise not met.

[f] Includes seafood, nuts, seeds, soy products (other than beverages) as well as beans and peas counted as Total Protein Foods.

[g] Ratio of poly- and monounsaturated fatty acids (PUFAs and MUFAs) to saturated fatty acids (SFAs).

[h] Calories from solid fats, alcohol, and added sugars; threshold for counting alcohol is more than 13 grams/1,000 kcal.

[i] Breastfeeding intensity was not known.

[j] WIC-participating women who are 6 months postpartum, not pregnant, and not breastfeeding; data were sourced only from 2007–2012 NHANES because no postpartum variable is available in the 2005–2006 dataset.

SOURCE: USDA/ARS, 2005–2012.

TABLE 4-29 Healthy Eating Index: Results for WIC-Participating Children, 2 to Less Than 5 Years of Age, NHANES 2011–2012

HEI–2010 Component	Maximum Score	Mean HEI Score (SE)
Adequacy		
Total Vegetables	5	2.1 (0.2)
Greens and Beans[a]	5	1.1 (0.8)
Total Fruit[b]	5	5.0 (0.0)
Whole Fruit[c]	5	5.0 (0.1)
Whole Grains	10	3.1 (0.4)
Dairy[d]	10	10.0 (0.1)
Total Protein Foods[e,f]	5	4.4 (0.2)
Seafoods and Plant Proteins	5	3.0 (0.4)
Fatty Acid Ratio[g]	10	3.6 (0.5)
Moderation		
Sodium	10	6.1 (0.2)
Refined Grains	10	6.8 (0.5)
Empty Calories[h]	20	14.7 (0.6)
Total HEI–2010 Score	100	65.0 (0.9)

NOTES: HEI = Healthy Eating Index; SE = standard error. N = 263.

[a] Includes any beans and peas not counted as Total Protein Foods.

[b] Includes 100 percent fruit juice.

[c] Includes all forms except juice.

[d] Includes all milk products, such as fluid milk, yogurt, and cheese, and fortified soy beverages.

[e] Beans and peas are included here (and not with vegetables) when the Total Protein Foods standard is otherwise not met.

[f] Includes seafood, nuts, seeds, soy products (other than beverages) as well as beans and peas counted as Total Protein Foods.

[g] Ratio of poly- and monounsaturated fatty acids (PUFAs and MUFAs) to saturated fatty acids (SFAs).

[h] Calories from solid fats and added sugars.

SOURCE: USDA/ARS, 2011–2012.

CONSIDERATIONS FOR INTERPRETATION OF FINDINGS FROM THE LITERATURE AND THE COMMITTEE'S ANALYSES

The potential limitations to interpreting the data presented in this chapter are summarized here. First, the challenges the committee faced when evaluating WIC-specific data are discussed. Then, the challenges faced by relying on the NHANES dataset are discussed. These limitations

TABLE 4-30 Nutrient-Based Diet Quality Index: Results for WIC-Participating Women, 19–50 Years of Age, NHANES 2005–2012

		Percentile		
Subgroup	N	25th	50th	75th
Pregnant	165	40.5	48.3	56.9
Breastfeeding	27	48.0	53.9	59.4
Postpartum*	62	33.8	40.3	42.0

NOTES: N = sample size. The index is based on nine nutrients considered to be of some concern in the diets of Americans: calcium, fiber, folate, iron, magnesium, potassium, vitamin A, vitamin C, and vitamin E. It is computed as the average percent adequacy of these nine nutrients for each individual (see Appendix J for a description of the methodology).

* Data were sourced only from 2007–2012 NHANES because no postpartum variable is available in the 2005–2006 dataset.

SOURCE: USDA/ARS, 2005–2012.

are linked directly to the recommendations for data collection presented in Chapter 11.

Evaluating WIC-Specific Data: The Challenge of Selection Bias

Since the creation of the WIC program, it has been difficult to evaluate the effect of participation on any outcome. Because random assignment of individuals to study groups that either receive or do not receive WIC benefits is not considered ethical, experimental study design options suitable for causal inference are limited (e.g., random assignment of a WIC service area, delayed start of a new benefit). In the 1980s, David Rush and his colleagues used studies of several different designs (e.g., historical, longitudinal cohort, and cross-sectional), each with different weaknesses, to provide a

TABLE 4-31 Nutrient-Based Diet Quality Index: Results for WIC-Participating Children, 1 to Less Than 5 Years of Age, NHANES 2011–2012

		Percentile		
Subgroup	N	25th	50th	75th
1 to <2 Years	96	61.5	66.1	71.2
2 to <5 Years	263	65.9	69.3	72.8

NOTES: N = sample size. The index is based on nine nutrients considered to be of some concern in the diet of Americans: calcium, fiber, folate, iron, magnesium, potassium, vitamin A, vitamin C, and vitamin E. It is computed as the average percent adequacy of these nine nutrients for each individual (see Appendix J for a description of the methodology).

SOURCE: USDA/ARS, 2011–2012.

comprehensive assessment of the WIC program (Rush et al., 1988a,b,c,d). Such a large and comprehensive set of studies has not been repeated. Nearly all studies reviewed for this report either compare WIC participants to a group of nonparticipants or compare WIC participation before and after the 2009 food package changes. The study designs for these comparisons are not only insufficient for causal inference, but they are likely also confounded by factors that result in the decision to participate in WIC. This phenomenon, known as selection bias, occurs when individuals who choose to participate in a program differ from eligible individuals who choose not to participate.

Differences that contribute to selection bias can be either observable or unobservable. With many social assistance programs, participants are likely to be negatively selected (e.g., participants likely have lower educational achievement or lower wage income than nonparticipants). Negative selection leads to results that make it appear as though the program is not as effective as it really is. Conversely, participants may be positively selected, again for either observable or unobservable characteristics (e.g., parents' motivation or eagerness to keep their children healthy [Besharov and Germanis, 2001]). Positive selection leads to results that make it appear that a program, such as WIC, has more positive effects than it really does. For WIC specifically, positively biased effects could also result from longer-lasting pregnancies which increase the chances that WIC-eligible women will enter the program and also provide for a longer period of time during which women can benefit from the program.[16] However, there is little reason to expect that there is solely a positive bias in reported WIC program effects, given the likely cumulative effect of negative selection on both observable and unobservable factors (Altonji et al., 2005; Altonji and Elder, 2008).There are several examples in the published literature in which WIC participants differed from WIC-eligible nonparticipants based on negatively selected observable factors. And when there is negative selection on observable factors, as shown in Bitler and Currie (2005) and Currie and Rajani (2015), it seems likely that there is also negative selection on at least some unobservable factors (e.g., the woman's propensity to have negative birth outcomes outside of any conditions that can be measured by the researcher).

As a result of selection bias, there are critical problems with any

[16] One important possible source of bias that is prominent in the recent WIC literature is gestational age bias. For example, suppose two women are similar on every dimension, but for idiosyncratic reasons unrelated to WIC use one gives birth at 7.5 months and the other at 9 months. Suppose further that the woman with the premature birth did not enroll in WIC, but would have enrolled at 8 months had her pregnancy lasted to 8 months, and that the second woman does enroll at 8 months. In this case, a comparison of prenatal WIC use and gestation would lead to the mistaken conclusion that WIC participation caused longer gestation.

comparison of WIC participants to nonparticipants. Any observed differences in nutrient or food intake adequacy may misrepresent the intake adequacy of either group. For observed differences in nutrient or food intake to be real, the data cannot be confounded by differences that led to an individuals' participation (or nonparticipation) in WIC.

Methods for Addressing Selection Bias

Researchers have used several approaches to address selection bias. These methods are briefly reviewed in this section. In one example, researchers use variations in state WIC and Medicaid rules as instrumental variables that predict use of WIC but are assumed not to be correlated with any outcomes other than via the changes they induce in participation (e.g., Chatterji et al., 2002). These studies report some negative effect of WIC on breastfeeding. Other studies have used propensity score matching or other propensity score approaches, which ensure that WIC participants and non-participants also are comparable on other dimensions.[17] This allows the comparison to more closely estimate the effect of WIC on breastfeeding and the health of newborns (Foster et al., 2010; Jiang et al., 2010) and food purchases (Oh et al., 2016). A third approach uses variation in the timing of WIC program rollout in specific counties (e.g., Hoynes et al., 2011) to examine its effects on birth weight. These studies generally find positive effects of having WIC implemented in a particular county. The methods used by Kreider et al. (2016) offer another alternative approach. They used nonparametric, partial identification methods to account for selection and measurement problems jointly and evaluated the impacts of WIC on food insecurity in children with NHANES data. Other possible methods include difference-in-differences approaches (interrupted time-series approaches) that leverage changes affecting one group but not another (e.g., a state-level policy change, also in Chatterji et al., 2002, or Hoynes et al., 2011). Some studies have resolved the challenge of selection bias by using a panel-data approach (see, e.g., Odoms-Young et al., 2014). However, this approach may miss effects of the program on new participants.

Strengths and Limitations of NHANES Data for This Analysis

NHANES is the most comprehensive source of national survey data of individuals with information on both food intake and WIC participation

[17] Propensity score matching controls for observed confounding variables that are included in the analysis. It does not address differences in observed factors that are not included nor unobservable factors that cannot be accounted for (Cook et al., 2008; Steiner et al., 2010).

that was available to the committee. It provides consistent data collection over time, so survey rounds can be combined or compared. NHANES is nationally representative of women by age groups, as well as for children less than 5 years of age. Despite these important strengths, it was difficult for the committee to create a sample population that accurately represented the national WIC population with data from NHANES. This was because NHANES is not designed to provide a nationally representative sample of several population subgroups served by the WIC program. For example, the numbers of pregnant, breastfeeding, or postpartum women who are captured in NHANES are relatively small and the number eligible for and served by WIC is smaller still. Major challenges that were experienced by the committee included small sample sizes for some subgroups of the WIC population, limitations imposed by combining NHANES samples, inaccurate reporting of WIC participation and household income as well as caveats to interpreting micronutrient adequacy, energy intake, food intake, and diet quality.

Sampling

As noted above, NHANES was not designed to be representative of the WIC population or some of the committee's key subgroups of interest. As a result, extracting from NHANES only data on low-income individuals of specific ages and in specific physiological states resulted in some sample sizes that were quite small (for women, WIC subgroups ranged between 27 and 165). This problem was exacerbated by restricting the sample to reported WIC participation. These limitations 0required the committee to combine data over several 2-year survey rounds. Although this approach makes the committee's results more robust because of the larger sample sizes achieved, merging older with more recent data compromises inferences to contemporary dietary intakes. As explained earlier, the need to merge survey rounds to achieve adequate sample sizes for its primary analyses made it impossible for the committee to conduct pre-post analyses of the effects of the 2009 food package changes.

Reported WIC Participation in NHANES and Evaluating Pre-Post 2009 Changes

In NHANES, as in most other surveys, there is substantial misclassification of program use, which likely extends to WIC (Bitler et al., 2003; Celhay et al., 2015; Meyer et al., 2015). When WIC use is underreported, data from participants may erroneously be combined with those of nonparticipants. Conversely, some individuals who are income-eligible or of slightly higher incomes and who did not report WIC use may actually be WIC participants. Some women also reported being WIC participants although they did not meet the income (income may have changed since the interview) or physiological criteria. Along with selection bias, this misclassification confounds the challenge of comparing WIC participants and nonparticipants. As noted above, some women reported participation in WIC and also reported not being pregnant, breastfeeding, or postpartum. It is unclear whether these women are actually receiving WIC benefits themselves. Reported WIC participation by these women may indicate instead that they have a child who is receiving WIC benefits.

Income Reporting

Identifying which low-income individuals in NHANES are eligible for WIC poses another challenge. State-level income requirements for WIC eligibility do not correspond to the measure of income reported in NHANES (at the household level and annually). Additionally, some individuals may legitimately participate in WIC if adjunctively or automatically eligible because of their participation in Medicaid, Temporary Assistance for Needy Families, or SNAP. These are programs with different eligibility thresholds, as well as different rules, than what WIC uses regarding how income is calculated and compared to the respective program-specific thresholds. For example, SNAP does not include the fetus in the count of individuals in the household unit, but WIC does in some states. Finally, although the NHANES population weights include an income-adjustment that accounts for the national income distribution with adjustment for low-income persons defined as those at or below 130 percent of the federal poverty level, it does not account for the distribution of income characteristic of the WIC population. The most recently available national data (from 2014) indicate that more than 65 percent of WIC participants have household incomes that are less than 100 percent of the poverty-to-income ratio (CDC, 2013; USDA/FNS, 2015b).

Estimating Micronutrient Adequacy

For certain nutrients, estimates of prevalence of inadequacy based on NHANES data must be interpreted carefully. For iron specifically, requirements are not normally distributed for women, mostly because of menstrual losses of iron. As a result, the EAR cut-point method cannot be used to estimate its prevalence of inadequacy. Inasmuch as most of the women in the NHANES analytical sample were either pregnant or breastfeeding and the sample size was small (for WIC-participating and breastfeeding women, N = 27), the EAR cut-point method was implemented nonetheless. This limitation was considered when interpreting the data.

Several additional micronutrient intake estimates should be interpreted with caution because of small sample sizes. The committee determined that calculating a mean usual intake within 3 percent of the true value (95 percent confidence interval) required a minimum of 25 to 30 individuals, depending on the nutrient and age group. However, this minimum is not adequate for accurate calculation of population-level intake adequacy. Although the statistical method applied by the committee gives relatively reliable numbers around the median and mean even with small sample sizes, it provides less reliable numbers at the tails of distributions. Given that inadequacy is defined by the proportion of individuals in the lower tail of the distribution, this source of unreliability makes it difficult to determine the proportion of individuals with inadequate intakes. Thus, the committee applied a less stringent threshold of 5 percent in the assessment of nutrient intake adequacy and, furthermore, focused its attention on those nutrients with evidence of still higher proportions of inadequate intakes (see Chapter 5).

Estimating Energy Requirements and Energy Intake

The Estimated Energy Requirements (EERs) in this report were calculated based on established equations developed by the IOM (2002/2005). Recently, however, Butte et al. (2014) proposed that these IOM equations overestimate energy expenditure for toddlers because they are based on incorrect physical activity assumptions. This possibility was considered by the committee in the evaluation of the energy expenditure of WIC-participating children.

Self-reported energy intake is of limited value as a measure of true energy intake (Archer et al., 2013; Subar et al., 2015). In general, underreporting is more pervasive than overreporting (Murakami and Livingstone, 2015), especially among overweight and obese women (Briefel et al., 1997; Macdiarmid and Blundell, 1998; McKenzie et al., 2002). CDC data indicate higher levels of obesity in lower-income women (CDC, 2010b), and overweight is commonly reported as a nutritional risk factor in WIC participants. A recent evaluation of reporting accuracy in NHANES 2002–2012 indicated that 25 percent of adults (ages 20 and older) were likely to underreport energy intake and that respondents were more likely to underreport if they were female, non-Hispanic black, had lower education or income, or were overweight or obese (Murakami and Livingstone, 2015). Underreporting could exaggerate the estimated micronutrient inadequacies for women identified in this report. As noted in Subar et al. (2015), even if the discrepancy between reported and recommended intakes is large, concern that actual intakes are low may still be warranted.

Assessing energy (and dietary) intake in any age is challenging (as described in more detail in the phase I report [NASEM, 2016]), but measuring energy (and dietary) intake of infants and young children can be particularly problematic. Overreporting of energy intake for children in NHANES has been documented (Murakami and Livingstone, 2015). The energy intake of infants and children in the NHANES dataset was estimated based on reports given by the caregiver who accompanied the child to the interview. However, given that multiple people may be responsible for the care of the child, collecting an accurate estimate of intake often requires combining parental reports with observations from other caregivers (Foster and Adamson, 2014); such multiple reports are not available in NHANES.

Estimating Food Intake

The sample sizes were smaller in the food intake analysis compared to those for nutrient intake. For example, the sample size for pregnant women was 165 for nutrient intake and 139 for intake of food groups. The already low sample size for breastfeeding women was 27 for nutrients but just 25 for food groups. These smaller samples sizes resulted from the fact that the software used to estimate food intake[18] required 2 days of reported food intake per survey respondent. Reported intake could be zero on one or both days.

Evaluating Diet Quality

Although the reliability and consistency of the HEI–2010 has been validated for prediction of diet quality (Guenther et al., 2014), the index has a few limitations. Specifically, consumers of beans and peas may have lower scores for "seafood and plant proteins" or "total vegetables" because beans and peas are counted towards other groups first, with only "leftovers" contributing to these groups. Additionally, the HEI–2010 does not account for physical activity or the appropriateness of energy intake. Therefore, an individual who consumes too much energy may have a higher HEI–2010 score than one who consumes an appropriate level of energy but who, as a result, has difficulty meeting the recommended food pattern. Moreover, even if the recommended food pattern is met, individuals may have difficulty meeting nutrient requirements. For example, individuals over the age of 8 with energy needs less than 1,600 kcal will have difficulty meeting nutrient requirements (Guenther et al., 2013). Although consuming amounts of food groups according to the 2010 DGA food patterns would

[18] The only software that does not require equal number of observations per person is the National Cancer Institute (NCI) software, but it failed to converge in several cases in these analyses.

result in a perfect score, neither the 2010 food patterns (Guenther et al., 2013) nor the 2015–2020 food patterns (USDA/HHS, 2016) provide the recommended amounts of vitamins D or E, or potassium or choline. However, the HEI–2010 does provide a validated way to compare diet quality among population groups.

Comparison of the Committee's Analyses to Other Published Results

Nutrient Intake

In accordance with the results presented in the DGA (USDA/HHS, 2016), the committee found that intakes of vitamins A, D, E, C, folate, calcium, and magnesium were below recommended amounts and intakes of fiber and potassium were below the AI in more than 5 percent of all subgroups of WIC-participating women. In addition, intakes of iron and zinc, as well as several B vitamins, were below recommended amounts in more than 5 percent of subgroups of women. Saturated fat, sodium, and added sugars intakes exceeded recommended amounts in a high proportion of WIC-participating subgroups, again in accordance with what was reported in the 2015–2020 DGA for the overall U.S. population of individuals ages 2 years and older (USDA/HHS, 2016).

The low prevalence of nutrient inadequacies reported here for infants and young children are similar to those reported by Ahluwalia et al. (2016) using NHANES data from 2009–2012. These authors also reported similarly low intakes of vitamin E, fiber, and potassium, and high intakes of vitamin A in children less than 2 years of age. Breastfed infants participating in WIC showed inadequacies of iron and zinc intake above the committee's threshold of 5 percent, which is commonly the case given the low iron and zinc content of human milk (AAP, 2014).

Food Group Intake

Overall, results from comparisons of actual intakes to recommended food patterns presented in this report are similar to what has been reported in other studies. Most recently, in their comparison of food group intakes of the U.S. population to federal dietary recommendations, Krebs-Smith et al. (2010) applied an approach similar to the committee's approach. They used 2001–2004 NHANES data and found that most individuals in the U.S. population did not meet the recommended intakes for any food group except "total grains" and "meat and beans" (food groups were categorized differently then). Additionally, similar to the findings reported here and in the DGA (USDA/HHS, 2016), Krebs-Smith et al. (2010) found that energy intake from solid (saturated) fats and added sugars was excessive.

Diet Quality

HEI–2010 results for WIC-participating children reported herein are higher than those reported by Tester et al. (2016), who evaluated the HEI–2010 among children ages 2 to 4 years old using NHANES 2011–2012. Tester et al. (2016) identified WIC participants by response to the NHANES question, "In the last 12 months, did you [the child] or any member of the household receive benefits from the WIC program, that is, the Women, Infants and Children program?"; whereas, for the committee's analysis, "Is [child] now receiving benefits from the WIC program" was the determinant for reported WIC participation. The Tester et al. (2016) question is not a robust identifier of WIC participation, because many children do not participate after 1 year of age and therefore may not have been participants at the time the caregiver was surveyed. In addition to reporting lower HEI–2010 results overall, Tester et al. (2016) also found that the HEI–2010 was significantly higher for children participating in WIC after the 2009 food package changes compared to before. However, as discussed earlier in this chapter, the committee found it impossible to use NHANES data to link pre- versus post-2009 nutrient and food intake differences to changes in the WIC food packages.

Considerations for the Design of Studies to Evaluate Effects of the WIC Food Packages

In Appendix K, the committee proposes study designs that would facilitate evaluation of the effects of the WIC program on various outcomes. In its deliberations, the committee considered three common limitations of existing research studies of the WIC program.

Issues of Measurement of Dietary and Nutritional Status Outcomes

Measurement issues related to dietary intake (whether of nutrients or food groups) and nutritional status include identifying the best method to use, deciding on the timing of baseline measure or the reference period, and determining the amount of time required to ensure a measurable effect of the WIC services on outcomes. The methodological challenges and limitations of self-reported dietary assessment instruments are well-recognized. The National Cancer Institute has developed a Dietary Assessment Primer intended to assist researchers with determining the best way to assess the dietary intake of a study group (NIH, 2016). Although biomarkers of nutritional status are generally superior indicators compared to self-reported methods, factors such as genetic variability, lifestyle or physiologic factors (e.g., smoking), biological sample variability, and analytical methodology could affect biomarker measurements (Jenab et al., 2009). Thus, research studies that use biomarkers of nutritional status need to consider these factors in study design or analyses.

Selection Bias

As discussed earlier in this chapter, because the majority of research studies on WIC are observational, selection bias is particularly problematic for research on the WIC program (as it is in evaluations of many other social programs). Several types of observational designs have been used to compare WIC-participants with some set of nonparticipants:

- Regression discontinuity
- Comparison group or comparisons over time (difference in differences or interrupted time series)
- Instrumental variables (an approach that deals with selection bias by finding variables that affect WIC use and that plausibly do not affect the outcomes of interest, such as program rules)
- Fixed effects for families (comparisons among siblings or individuals across time)

These designs are defined in Appendix K. Observational studies will continue to be important for evaluating the differences between WIC participants and nonparticipants on dietary intake or nutrition-related health outcomes as well as for understanding numerous aspects of WIC program implementation.[19]

Lack of Generalizability to the National Level

Most research studies on the WIC program either have small sample sizes or use only regional data because of the lack of comprehensive national data. This is true of both observational studies and the few randomized or nonrandomized quasi-experimental studies that have been conducted (e.g., examinations of the efficacy of breastfeeding support or nutrition education programs in WIC settings). It is likely that experimental studies in

[19] If possible to conduct, randomized controlled trials would be useful because they remove the problem of selection bias. For example, a pilot study in which the CVV for children is increased and effects on child retention are evaluated; or USDA allowing an agency or state to match clinics on demographics and breastfeeding rates and then randomly assign clinics to implement various models of breastfeeding support. If testing of the food packages in this way is prohibited, providing a waiver to states allowing design of the food packages in the first 30 days would provide information about whether the choice to breastfeed is influenced by the food package. Such studies would be conducted in alignment with 7 C.F.R. § 246.26 which states that all participant or applicant information is confidential.

WIC settings will continue to be small in scale and with potentially limited generalizability. Although larger sample size and/or better geographic coverage would increase external validity, large studies are not necessarily better than smaller ones for internal validity (the extent to which causality can be inferred). Pooled analyses of administrative data across regions would enhance generalizability to the national level as long as WIC participation is not affected by program changes currently under consideration.

SUMMARY OF FINDINGS

In this chapter, the committee describes the data sources used for its analyses as well as its strengths and limitations for this purpose. In addition, nutrient- and food safety-related health concerns as well as nutrient, food intake, and diet quality of WIC participants were evaluated. The next chapter describes how the committee used a decision tree to (1) evaluate the data presented here, and (2) develop proposed actions for revising the food packages. Important findings from this chapter's evaluation are summarized here:

- Changes to the current WIC iron specifications for infant formula are not warranted at this time, given that fully formula-fed infants ages 0 to less than 6 months are provided with an amount of iron that falls above the AI but below the UL for this group.
- Both women and children (ages 2 to less than 5 years) had several nutrient inadequacies that potentially could be addressed with changes to the food packages. These inadequacies may be linked to food intakes that were below recommended levels.
- Women, infants, and children also had excessive intakes of several nutrients, including sodium, saturated fat, and added sugars. In some cases, these excessive intakes may be addressed with changes to the food packages.
- Diet quality as measured by the HEI–2010 was similar to HEI–2010 results for the total U.S. population ages 2 years and older.
- There are many challenges to studying the effects of participation in WIC (and other similar programs). Strategies for dealing with selection bias and other methodological challenges were identified and considered by the committee when developing its recommendations for research to enhance future WIC program evaluation (which are outlined in Chapter 11).

REFERENCES

AAP (American Academy of Pediatrics). 2014. *Pediatric nutrition.* 7th ed. Edited by R. E. Kleinman and F. R. Greer. Elk Grove Village, IL: American Academy of Pediatrics.

AAPD (American Academy of Pediatric Dentistry). 2012. Policy on dietary recommendations for infants, children, and adolescents. *Pediatric Dentistry* 30(7 Suppl):47–48.

Ahluwalia, N., K. A. Herrick, L. M. Rossen, D. Rhodes, B. Kit, A. Moshfegh, and K. W. Dodd. 2016. Usual nutrient intakes of U.S. infants and toddlers generally meet or exceed Dietary Reference Intakes: Findings from NHANES 2009–2012. *American Journal of Clinical Nutrition.* doi: 10.3945/ajcn.116.137752.

AHRQ (Agency for Healthcare Research and Quality). 2014. *Vitamin D and calcium: A systematic review of health outcomes (update).* Rockville, MD: U.S. Department of Health and Human Services. http://effectivehealthcare.ahrq.gov/ehc/products/537/1953/vitamin-d-calcium-report-140902.pdf (accessed December 21, 2016).

AHRQ. 2015. *Routine iron supplementation and screening for iron deficiency anemia in pregnant women: A systematic review to update the U.S. Preventive Services Task Force recommendation.* Rockville, MD: U.S. Department of Health and Human Services. http://www.ncbi.nlm.nih.gov/books/NBK285986 (accessed December 21, 2016).

AHRQ. 2016. *Omega-3 fatty acids and maternal and child health: An updated systematic review.* Rockville, MD: U.S. Department of Health and Human Services, https://www.ncbi.nlm.nih.gov/books/NBK395921/pdf/Bookshelf_NBK395921.pdf (accessed August 30, 2016).

Altonji, J. G., and T. E. Elder. 2008. Using selection on observed variables to assess bias from unobservables when evaluating Swan-Ganz catheterization. *American Economic Review* 98(2):345–350.

Altonji, J. G., T. E. Elder, and C. R. Taber. 2005. Selection on observed and unobserved variables: Assessing the effectiveness of catholic schools. *Journal of Political Economy, University of Chicago* 113(1):151–184.

AND (Academy of Nutrition and Dietetics). 2014. Position of the Academy of Nutrition and Dietetics: Nutrition and lifestyle for a healthy pregnancy outcome. *Journal of the Academy of Nutrition and Dietetics* 114:1099–1103.

Andreyeva, T. and A. S. Tripp. 2016. The healthfulness of food and beverage purchases after the federal food package revisions: The case of two New England States. *Preventive Medicine* 91:204–210.

Archer, E., G. A. Hand, and S. N. Blair. 2013. Validity of U.S. nutritional surveillance: National Health and Nutrition Examination Survey caloric energy intake data, 1971–2010. *PLoS One* 8(10):e76632.

Aune, D., O. Saugstad, T. Henriksen, and S. Tonstad. 2014. Maternal body mass index and the risk of fetal death, stillbirth, and infant death: A systematic review and meta-analysis. *Journal of the American Medical Association* 311(15):1536–1546.

Berglund, S., and M. Domellöf. 2014. Meeting iron needs for infants and children. *Current Opinion in Clinical Nutrition and Metabolic Care* 17(3):267–272.

Bermúdez-Millán, Á., A. Hromi-Fiedler, G. Damio, S. Segura-Pérez, and R. Pérez-Escamilla. 2009. Egg contribution towards the diet of pregnant Latinas. *Ecology of Food and Nutrition* 48(5):383–403.

Besharov, D. J., and P. Germanis. 2001. *Rethinking WIC: An evaluation of the women, infants, and children program*: Washington, DC: AEI Press.

Bitler, M. P., and J. Currie. 2005. Does WIC work? The effects of WIC on pregnancy and birth outcomes. *Journal of Policy Analysis and Management* 24(1):73–91.

Bitler, M., J. Currie, and J. K. Scholz. 2003. WIC eligibility and participation. *Journal of Human Resources* 38:1139–1179.

Briefel, R. R., C. T. Sempos, M. A. McDowell, S. Chien, and K. Alaimo. 1997. Dietary methods research in NHANES III: Under-reporting of energy intake. *American Journal of Clinical Nutrition* 65(S):1203S–1209S.

Briefel, R. R., L. M. Kalb, E. Condon, D. M. Deming, N. A. Clusen, M. K. Fox, L. Harnack, E. Gemmill, M. Stevens, and K. C. Reidy. 2010. The Feeding Infants and Toddlers Study 2008: Study design and methods. *Journal of the American Dietetic Association* 110(12, Suppl. 1):S16–S26.

Butte, N. F., W. W. Wong, T. A. Wilson, A. L. Adolph, M. R. Puyau, and I. F. Zakeri. 2014. Revision of dietary reference intakes for energy in preschool-age children. *American Journal of Clinical Nutrition* 100(1):161–167.

CDC (Centers for Disease Control and Prevention). 2010a. CDC grand rounds: Additional opportunities to prevent neural tube defects with folic acid fortification. *Morbidity and Mortality Weekly Report* 59(30):980–984.

CDC. 2010b. *Obesity and socioeconomic status in adults: United States, 2005–2008*. http://www.cdc.gov/nchs/data/databriefs/db50.pdf (accessed December 21, 2016).

CDC. 2013. National Health and Nutrition Examination Survey: Estimation procedures, 2007–2010. http://www.cdc.gov/nchs/data/series/sr_02/sr02_159.pdf (accessed September 27, 2016).

CDC. 2014. *Infant feeding practices study ii and its year six follow-up, chapter 2: Neonatal survey*. http://www.cdc.gov/ifps/pdfs/data/ifps2_tables_ch2.pdf (accessed December 20, 2016).

Celhay, P., B. D. Meyer, and N. Mittag. 2015. *Measurement error in program participation* (forthcoming).

Chaparro, M. P., B. A. Langellier, M. C. Wang, M. Koleilat, and S. E. Whaley. 2015. Effects of parental nativity and length of stay in the US on fruit and vegetable intake among WIC-enrolled preschool-aged children. *Journal of Immigrant and Minority Health* 17(2):333–338.

Chatterji, P., K. Bonuck, S. Dhawan, and N. Deb. 2002. WIC participation and the initiation and duration of breastfeeding. Madison, WI: Institute for Research on Poverty. http://www.ssc.wisc.edu/irpweb/publications/dps/pdfs/dp124602.pdf (accessed August 30, 2016).

Chiasson, M. A., S. E. Findley, J. P. Sekhobo, R. Scheinmann, L. S. Edmunds, A. S. Faly, and N. J. McLeod. 2013. Changing WIC changes what children eat. *Obesity (Silver Spring)* 21(7):1423–1429.

Cho, S. H., K. L. Chang, J. Yeo, L. Wounded Head, M. Zastrow, C. Zdorovtsov, L. Skjonsberg, and S. Stluka. 2015. Comparison of fruit and vegetable consumption among Native and non-Native American populations in rural communities. *International Journal of Consumer Studies* 39(1):67–73.

Cook, T.D., W. R. Shadish, and V. C. Wong. 2008. Three conditions under which experiments and observational studies produce comparable causal estimates: New findings from within study comparisons. *Journal of Policy Analysis and Management* 27(4): 724–750.

Currie, J., and I. Rajani. 2015. Within-mother estimates of the effects of WIC on birth outcomes in New York City. *Economic Inquiry* 53(4):1691–1701.

Deming, D. M., R. R. Briefel, and K. C. Reidy. 2014. Infant feeding practices and food consumption patterns of children participating in WIC. *Journal of Nutrition Education and Behavior* 46(3 Suppl):S29–S37.

Di Noia J., D. Monica, K. W. Cullen, R. Pérez-Escamilla, H. L. Gray, and A. Sikorskii. 2016. Differences in fruit and vegetable intake by race/ethnicity and by Hispanic origin and nativity among women in the Special Supplemental Nutrition Program for Women, Infants, and Children. *Preventing Chronic Disease* 25(13):E115. doi: 10.5888/pcd13.160130.

Dubowitz, T., S. A. Smith-Warner, D. Acevedo-Garcia, S. V. Subramanian, and K. E. Peterson. 2007. Nativity and duration of time in the United States: Differences in fruit and vegetable intake among low-income postpartum women. *American Journal of Public Health* 97(10):1787–1790.

Dubowitz, T., S. V. Subramanian, D. Acevedo-Garcia, T. L. Osypuk, and K. E. Peterson. 2008. Individual and neighborhood differences in diet among low-income foreign and U.S.-born women. *Womens Health Issues* 18(3):181–190.

Endres, L. K., H. Straub, C. McKinney, B. Plunkett, C. S. Minkovitz, C. D. Schetter, S. Ramey, C. Wang, C. Hobel, T. Raju, and M. U. Shalowitz. 2015. Postpartum weight retention risk factors and relationship to obesity at 1 year. *Obstetrics Gynecology* 125(1):144–152.

EOPUS (Executive Office of the President of the United States). 2014. The economic impact of the American Recovery and Reinvestment Act five years later: Final report to Congress. Washington, DC: Executive Office of the President of the United States. https://www.whitehouse.gov/sites/default/files/docs/cea_arra_report.pdf (accessed December 21, 2016).

EPA (U.S. Environmental Protection Agency). 1994. *Arsine*. https://cfpub.epa.gov/ncea/iris2/chemicalLanding.cfm?substance_nmbr=672 (accessed December 21, 2016).

Ettienne-Gittens, R., E. L. McKyer, M. Odum, C. S. Diep, Y. Li, A. Girimaji, and P. S. Murano. 2013. Rural versus urban Texas WIC participants' fruit and vegetable consumption. *American Journal of Health Behavior* 37(1):130–140.

Faith, M. S., B. A. Dennison, L. S. Edmunds, and H. H. Stratton. 2006. Fruit juice intake predicts increased adiposity gain in children from low-income families: Weight status-by-environment interaction. *Pediatrics* 118(5):2066–2075.

FAO/WHO (Food and Agriculture Organization/World Health Organization). 2011. Joint FAO/WHO expert consultation on the risks and benefits of fish consumption. Geneva, Switzerland. http://www.fao.org/docrep/014/ba0136e/ba0136e00.pdf (accessed December 21, 2016).

FDA (U.S. Food and Drug Administration). 2016. *FDA proposes limit for inorganic arsenic in infant rice cereal*. http://www.fda.gov/NewsEvents/Newsroom/PressAnnouncements/ucm493740.htm (accessed August 30, 2016).

Foster, E., and A. Adamson. 2014. Challenges involved in measuring intake in early life: Focus on methods. *Proceedings of the Nutrition Society* 73(2):201–209.

Foster, E. M., M. Jiang, and C. M. Gibson-Davis. 2010. The effect of the WIC program on the health of newborns. *Health Services Research* 45(4):1083–1104.

Geyer, H. J., K. W. Schramm, E. A. Feicht, A. Behechti, C. Steinberg, R. Bruggemann, H. Poiger, B. Henkelmann, and A. Kettrup. 2002. Half-lives of tetra-, penta-, hexa-, hepta-, and octachlorodibenzo-p-dioxin in rats, monkeys, and humans—a critical review. *Chemosphere* 48(6):631–644.

Grimes, C. A., E. A. Szymlek-Gay, K. J. Campbell, and T. A. Nicklas. 2015. Food sources of total energy and nutrients among U.S. infants and toddlers: National Health and Nutrition Examination Survey 2005–2012. *Nutrients* 7(8):6797–6836.

Grummer-Strawn, L. M., K. S. Scanlon, and S. B. Fein. 2008. Infant feeding and feeding transitions during the first year of life. *Pediatrics* 122(Suppl 2):S36–S42.

Guenther, P. M., K. O. Casavale, J. Reedy, S. I. Kirkpatrick, H. A. Hiza, K. J. Kuczynski, L. L. Kahle, and S. M. Krebs-Smith. 2013. Update of the Healthy Eating Index: HEI–2010. *Journal of the Academy of Nutrition and Dietetics* 113(4):569–580.

Guenther, P. M., S. I. Kirkpatrick, J. Reedy, S. M. Krebs-Smith, D. W. Buckman, K. W. Dodd, K. O. Casavale, and R. J. Carroll. 2014. The Healthy Eating Index-2010 is a valid and reliable measure of diet quality according to the 2010 Dietary Guidelines for Americans. *Journal of Nutrition* 144(3):399–407.

Hoynes, H., M. Page, and A. H. Stevens. 2011. Can targeted transfers improve birth outcomes? Evidence from the introduction of the WIC program. *Journal of Public Economics* 95(7–8):813–827.

IARC (International Agency for Research on Cancer). 1998. *Arsenic and arsenic compounds.* http://www.inchem.org/documents/iarc/suppl7/arsenic.html (accessed December 21, 2016).

IOM (Institute of Medicine). 1997. *Dietary Reference Intakes for calcium, phosphorus, magnesium, vitamin D, and fluoride.* Washington, DC: National Academy Press.

IOM. 1998. *Dietary Reference Intakes for thiamin, riboflavin, niacin, vitamin B6, folate, vitamin B12, pantothenic acid, biotin, and choline.* Washington, DC: National Academy Press.

IOM. 2000a. *Dietary Reference Intakes for vitamin C, vitamin E, selenium, and carotenoids.* Washington, DC: National Academy Press.

IOM. 2000b. *Dietary Reference Intakes: Applications in dietary assessment.* Washington, DC: National Academy Press.

IOM. 2001. *Dietary Reference Intakes for vitamin A, vitamin K, arsenic, boron, chromium, copper, iodine, iron, manganese, molybdenum, nickel, silicon, vanadium, and zinc.* Washington, DC: National Academy Press.

IOM. 2002/2005. *Dietary Reference Intakes for energy, carbohydrate, fiber, fat, fatty acids, cholesterol, protein and amino acids.* Washington, DC: The National Academies Press.

IOM. 2003. *Dioxins and dioxin-like compounds in the food supply: Strategies to decrease exposure.* Washington, DC: The National Academies Press.

IOM. 2005. *Dietary Reference Intakes for water, potassium, sodium, chloride, and sulfate.* Washington, DC: The National Academies Press.

IOM. 2006. *WIC food packages: Time for a change.* Washington, DC: The National Academies Press.

IOM. 2009. *Weight gain during pregnancy: Reexamining the guidelines.* Washington, DC: The National Academies Press.

IOM. 2011. *Dietary Reference Intakes for calcium and vitamin D.* Washington, DC: The National Academies Press.

Ishdorj, A., and O. Capps. 2013. The effect of revised WIC food packages on Native American children. *American Journal of Agricultural Economics* 95(5):1266–1272.

Jenab, M., N. Slimani, M. Bictash, P. Ferrari, and S. A. Bingham. 2009. Biomarkers in nutritional epidemiology: Applications, needs and new horizons. *Human Genetics* 125(5–6):507–525.

Jiang, M., E. M. Foster, and C. M. Gibson-Davis. 2010. The effect of WIC on breastfeeding: A new look at an established relationship. *Children and Youth Services Review* 32(2):264–273.

Kong, A., A. M. Odoms-Young, L. A. Schiffer, M. L. Berbaum, S. J. Porter, L. Blumstein, and M. L. Fitzgibbon. 2013. Racial/ethnic differences in dietary intake among WIC families prior to food package revisions. *Journal of Nutrition Education and Behavior* 45(1):39–46.

Kong, A., A. M. Odoms-Young, L. A. Schiffer, Y. Kim, M. L. Berbaum, S. J. Porter, L. B. Blumstein, S. L. Bess, and M. L. Fitzgibbon. 2014. The 18-month impact of Special Supplemental Nutrition Program for Women, Infants, and Children food package revisions on diets of recipient families. *American Journal of Preventive Medicine* 46(6):543–551.

Krebs, N. F., J. E. Westcott, N. Butler, C. Robinson, M. Bell, and K. M. Hambidge. 2006. Meat as a first complementary food for breastfed infants: Feasibility and impact on zinc intake and status. *Journal of Pediatric Gastroenterology Nutrition* 42(2):207–214.

Krebs-Smith, S. M., P. M. Guenther, A. F. Subar, S. I. Kirkpatrick, and K. W. Dodd. 2010. Americans do not meet federal dietary recommendations. *Journal of Nutrition* 140(10):1832–1838.

Kreider, B., J. V. Pepper, and M. Roy. 2016. Identifying the effects of WIC on food insecurity among infants and children. *Southern Economic Journal* 82(4):1106–1122.

Macdiarmid, J., and J. Blundell. 1998. Assessing dietary intake: Who, what and why of under-reporting. *Nutrition Research Reviews* 11(2):231–253.

Marchi, J., M. Berg, A. Dencker, E. K. Olander, and C. Begley. 2015. Risks associated with obesity in pregnancy, for the mother and baby: A systematic review of reviews. *Obesity Reviews* 16(8):621–638.

McKenzie, D. C., R. K. Johnson, J. Harvey-Berino, and B. C. Gold. 2002. Impact of interviewer's body mass index on underreporting energy intake in overweight and obese women. *Obesity Research and Clinical Practice* 10(6):471–477.

Meiqari, L., L. Torre, and J. A. Gazmararian. 2015. Exploring the impact of the new WIC food package on low-fat milk consumption among WIC recipients: A pilot study. *Journal of Health Care for the Poor and Underserved* 26(3):712–725.

Meyer, B. D., W. K. C. Mok, and J. X. Sullivan. 2015. Household surveys in crisis. *National Bureau of Economic Research Working Paper Series* No. 21399. Cambridge, MA: NBER.

Murakami, K., and M. B. Livingstone. 2015. Prevalence and characteristics of misreporting of energy intake in US adults: NHANES 2003–2012. *British Journal of Nutrition* 114(8):1294–1303.

NASEM (National Academies of Sciences, Engineering, and Medicine). 2016. *Review of WIC food packages: Proposed framework for revisions: Interim report.* Washington, DC: The National Academies Press. doi: 10.17226/21832.

NIH (National Institutes of Health). 2016. *Dietary assessment primer.* https://dietassessmentprimer.cancer.gov/citation.html (accessed October 19, 2016).

Odoms-Young, A. M., A. Kong, L. A. Schiffer, S. J. Porter, L. Blumstein, S. Bess, M. L. Berbaum, and M. L. Fitzgibbon. 2014. Evaluating the initial impact of the revised Special Supplemental Nutrition Program for Women, Infants, and Children (WIC) food packages on dietary intake and home food availability in African-American and Hispanic families. *Public Health Nutrition* 17(1):83–93.

Oh, M., H. Jensen, and I. Rahkovsky. 2016. Did revisions to the WIC program affect household expenditures on whole grains? *Applied Economic Perspectives and Policy* 38(4):578–598. doi: 10.1093/aepp/ppw020.

Pooler, J., and S. F. Gleason. 2014. Comparison of WIC benefit redemptions in Michigan indicates higher utilization among Arab American families. *Journal of Nutrition Education and Behavior* 46(3 Suppl):S45–S52.

Rasmussen, K. M., and C. L. Kjolhede. 2004. Prepregnant overweight and obesity diminish the prolactin response to suckling in the first week postpartum. *Pediatrics* 113(5):e465–471.

Rush, D., J. M. Alvir, D. A. Kenny, S. S. Johnson, and D. G. Horvitz. 1988a. The National WIC Evaluation: Evaluation of the Special Supplemental Food Program for Women, Infants, and Children. III. Historical study of pregnancy outcomes. *American Journal of Clinical Nutrition* 48(2 Suppl):412–428.

Rush, D., M. R. Kurzon, W. B. Seaver, and D. S. Shanklin. 1988b. The national WIC evaluation: Evaluation of the Special Supplemental Food Program for Women, Infants, and Children. VII. Study of food expenditures. *American Journal of Clinical Nutrition* 48(2 Suppl):512–519.

Rush, D., J. Leighton, N. L. Sloan, J. M. Alvir, and G. C. Garbowski. 1988c. The National WIC Evaluation: Evaluation of the Special Supplemental Food Program for Women, Infants, and Children. II. Review of past studies of WIC. *American Journal of Clinical Nutrition* 48(2):394–411.

Rush, D., N. L. Sloan, J. Leighton, J. M. Alvir, D. G. Horvitz, W. B. Seaver, G. C. Garbowski, S. S. Johnson, R. A. Kulka, M. Holt, J. W. Devore, J. T. Lynch, M. B. Woodside, D. S. Shanklin. 1988d. The National WIC Evaluation: Evaluation of the Special Supplemental Food Program for Women, Infants, and Children. V. Longitudinal study of pregnant women. *American Journal of Clinical Nutrition* 48(2 Suppl):439–483.

Sabin, M. A., and W. Kiess. 2015. Childhood obesity: Current and novel approaches. *Best Practice & Research Clinical Endocrinology & Metabolism* 29(3):327–338.

Schultz, D. J., C. Byker Shanks, and B. Houghtaling. 2015. The impact of the 2009 Special Supplemental Nutrition Program for Women, Infants, and Children food package revisions on participants: A systematic review. *Journal of the Academy of Nutrition and Dietetics* 115(11):1832–1846.

Shin, D., and W. O. Song. 2014. Prepregnancy body mass index is an independent risk factor for gestational hypertension, gestational diabetes, preterm labor, and small- and large-for-gestational-age infants. *Journal of Maternal-Fetal and Neonatal Medicine*:1–8.

Steiner, P.M., T.D. Cook, W. R. Shadish, M. H. Clark. 2010. The importance of covariate selection in controlling for selection bias in observational studies. *Psychological Methods* 15(3):250.

Subar, A. F., L. S. Freedman, J. A. Tooze, S. I. Kirkpatrick, C. Boushey, M. L. Neuhouser, F. E. Thompson, N. Potischman, P. M. Guenther, V. Tarasuk, J. Reedy, and S. M. Krebs-Smith. 2015. Addressing current criticism regarding the value of self-report dietary data. *Journal of Nutrition* 145(12):2639–2645.

Tester, J. M., C. W. Leung, and P. B. Crawford. 2016. Revised WIC food package and children's diet quality. *Pediatrics* 137(5).

Thornton, H. E., S. H. Crixell, A. M. Reat, and J. A. Von Bank. 2014. Differences in energy and micronutrient intakes among central Texas WIC infants and toddlers after the package change. *Journal of Nutrition Education and Behavior* 46(3 Suppl):S79–S86.

Turcksin, R., S. Bel, S. Galjaard, and R. Devlieger. 2014. Maternal obesity and breastfeeding intention, initiation, intensity and duration: A systematic review. *Maternal and Child Nutrition* 10(2):166–183.

USDA/ARS (U.S. Department of Agriculture/Agricultural Research Service). 2005–2006. *What we eat in America, NHANES 2005–2006*. Beltsville, MD: USDA/ARS. http://www.ars.usda.gov/services/docs.htm?docid=13793 (accessed December 21, 2016).

USDA/ARS. 2005–2012. *What we eat in America, NHANES 2005–2012*. Beltsville, MD: USDA/ARS. http://www.cdc.gov/nchs/nhanes/wweia.htm (accessed December 21, 2016).

USDA/ARS. 2009–2012. *What we eat in America, NHANES 2009–2012*. Beltsville, MD: USDA/ARS. http://www.ars.usda.gov/services/docs.htm?docid=13793 (accessed December 21, 2016).

USDA/ARS. 2011–2012. *What we eat in America, NHANES 2011–2012*. Beltsville, MD: USDA/ARS. http://www.ars.usda.gov/services/docs.htm?docid=13793 (accessed December 21, 2016).

USDA/FNS (U.S. Department of Agriculture/Food and Nutrition Service). 2014. Special Supplemental Nutrition Program for Women, Infants and Children (WIC): Revisions in the WIC food packages; Final Rule, 7 C.F.R. § 246.

USDA/FNS. 2015a. *Diet quality of American young children by WIC participation status: Data from the National Health and Nutrition Examination Survey, 2005–2008*. Alexandria, VA: USDA/FNS. http://www.fns.usda.gov/sites/default/files/ops/NHANES-WIC05-08.pdf (accessed December 21, 2016).

USDA/FNS. 2015b. *WIC participant and program characteristics report*. Alexandria, VA: USDA/FNS. http://www.fns.usda.gov/sites/default/files/ops/WICPC2014.pdf (accessed September 22, 2016).

USDA/HHS (U.S. Department of Agriculture/U.S. Department of Health and Human Services). 2016. *Dietary Guidelines for Americans 2015*. Washington, DC: U.S. Government Printing Office. https://health.gov/dietaryguidelines/2015/ (accessed August 29, 2016).

Vinturache, A. E., S. McDonald, D. Slater, and S. Tough. 2015. Perinatal outcomes of maternal overweight and obesity in term infants: A population-based cohort study in Canada. *Scientific Reports* 5:9334.

Whaley, S. E., L. D. Ritchie, P. Spector, and J. Gomez. 2012. Revised WIC food package improves diets of WIC families. *Journal of Nutrition Education and Behavior* 44(3):204–209.

WHO (World Health Organization). 2014. Dioxins and their effects on human health. Geneva, Switzerland: World Health Organization. http://www.who.int/mediacentre/factsheets/fs225/en (accessed August 30, 2016).

Williams, J., C. T. Mai, J. Mulinare, J. Isenburg, T. J. Flood, M. Ethen, B. Frohnert, and R. S. Kirby. 2015. Updated estimates of neural tube defects prevented by mandatory folic acid fortification—United States, 1995–2011. *Morbidity and Mortality Weekly Report* 64(1):1–5.

Yan, J. 2015. Maternal pre-pregnancy BMI, gestational weight gain, and infant birth weight: A within-family analysis in the United States. *Economics and Human Biology* 18:1–12.

Zeisel, S. H. 2013. Nutrition in pregnancy: The argument for including a source of choline. *International Journal of Women's Health* 5:193–199.

5

Nutrient and Food Group Priorities for the WIC Food Packages

Informed by its evaluation of nutrient-related health priorities, food safety risks, and dietary intake (see Chapter 4), the committee identified nutrient and food group priorities for the Special Supplemental Nutrition Program for Women, Infants, and Children (WIC) food packages. These priorities were then considered along with the committee's charge, that is, to align the food packages with current dietary guidance, take into account the health and cultural needs of participants, support efficient program operations, and allow effective administration of the program. Collectively, this process led to development of a decision tree (see Figure 5-1) for determining potential revisions to the WIC food packages (see Tables 5-2 through 5-10).

As was the case in the previous WIC report (IOM, 2006), overweight and obesity remain a prominent health concern for WIC participants. However, consistent with its charge, the committee did not directly address problems related to excess energy intake. Rather, these outcomes were considered within the context of alignment of WIC program goals with the 2015–2020 *Dietary Guidelines for Americans* (DGA), which encourage the use of foods that are nutrient-dense, and limit the amounts of added sugars and saturated fat in WIC-approved foods.

IDENTIFYING NUTRIENT PRIORITIES

Among some subgroups of WIC-participating women and children, nutrient inadequacies were numerous (see Chapter 4). Here, we describe how the committee decided which of these inadequacies, as well as nutrient excesses, to prioritize when revising the food packages. As illustrated in Figure 5-1, nutrient inadequacies and excesses were determined to be higher-priority, middle-priority, or lower-priority.

Identifying Nutrient Priorities for Women and Children Ages 2 to Less Than 5 Years

Micronutrients with EARs

For nutrients with an Estimated Average Requirement (EAR), the committee ranked nutrients for action by the proportion of each WIC subpopulation with inadequate intakes. Nutrients with the highest proportion of inadequacy (e.g., >50 percent) for a particular population were considered first, followed by nutrients with lower proportions of inadequate intakes. In addition, the committee considered whether a nutrient was linked to a known health consequence for the specific WIC-participating population under review (see Table 5-1 for a compilation of nutrients with known health consequences). Nutrients not linked to known health consequences were considered of lower priority, although all nutrients for which inadequacy was evident in 5 percent or more of a subgroup were considered to some degree.

Special Case: Vitamin E

As was the case with subgroups included in the committee's National Health and Nutrition Examination Survey (NHANES) analyses (see Chapter 4), low vitamin E intake appears to be ubiquitous in the general U.S. population (USDA/HHS, 2016). However, because clinical vitamin E deficiency is uncommon (IOM, 2000a), the DGA do not include it as a nutrient of public health concern (USDA/HHS, 2016). Similarly, despite the very high prevalence of inadequacy across the WIC-participating population, vitamin E was not considered a priority in the food package revisions and was not carried through the decision tree.

Nutrients with an AI

For nutrients with an Adequate Intake (AI) value, the committee first assessed whether mean intake of the nutrient was below the AI. If so, the committee then considered whether or not the nutrient was linked to a known health consequence for the specific WIC-participating population under review. Nutrients not linked to known health consequences were considered lower priority.

TABLE 5-1 Nutrient Inadequacies and Excesses Linked to Adverse Health Consequences Relevant to WIC-Participating Population Subgroups, Based on the Dietary Guidelines, Literature Review, and Other Expert Guidance

	Population Subgroup					
Nutrients to Increase	Women, P	Women, BF	Women, PP	BF Infants 6 to Less Than 12 Months	Children 1 to Less Than 2 Years	Children 2 to Less Than 5 Years
Calcium	✓[a]	✓[a]	✓[a]			✓[a]
Iron	✓[b,c]	✓[b]	✓[b]	✓[c,d]	✓[c]	✓[b]
Zinc				✓[c,e]		
Folate	✓[c]	✓[c]	✓[c]			
Vitamin D	✓[a]	✓[a]	✓[a]			✓[a]
Fiber	✓[a]	✓[a]	✓[a]		✓[f]	✓[a]
Potassium	✓[a]	✓[a]	✓[a]		✓[f]	✓[a]
Choline	✓[c]					
Nutrients to Limit						
Added sugars	✓[a]	✓[a]	✓[a]		✓[h]	✓[a]
Saturated fat	✓[a]	✓[a]	✓[a]			✓[a]
Sodium	✓[a]	✓[a]	✓[a]		✓[g]	✓[a]

NOTES: BF = breastfeeding/breastfed; DGA = *Dietary Guidelines for Americans*; P = pregnant; PP = postpartum. For infants 0 to less than 6 months of age, or formula-fed infants 6 to less than 12 months of age, no nutrients were linked to relevant adverse health consequences. Because the DGA apply only to individuals ages 2 years and older, recommendations from other authoritative groups were applied to determine nutrients linked to adverse health outcomes for children under 2 years of age and infants. Nutrients were linked to adverse health outcomes relevant to the WIC-participating population based on the following evidence:

[a] A DGA nutrient of public health concern (shortfall nutrients for which under consumption has been linked in the scientific literature to adverse health outcomes) or DGA nutrient to limit.

[b] A DGA nutrient of public health concern; heme iron was considered especially important for young children or women who are capable of becoming pregnant or who are pregnant.

[c] Based on the committee's literature review.

[d] The American Academy of Pediatrics (AAP) recommends that complementary foods rich in iron be introduced early to help meet iron demands of BF infants 6 months and older (AAP, 2014).

[e] The AAP emphasizes foods containing zinc for breastfed infants after 6 months of life (AAP, 2014).

[f] Although the DGA apply only to individuals ages 2 years and older, health effects linked to consumption of these nutrients as described in the Dietary Reference Intake (DRI) report (IOM, 2002/2005, 2005) were considered applicable to younger children.

[g] Although the DGA apply only to individuals ages 2 years and older, sodium intakes exceeding the Tolerable Upper Intake Level (UL) were also considered of concern for young children.

[h] Although not limited to added sugars, the American Academy of Pediatric Dentistry reports that early childhood caries have been associated with frequent in-between meal consumption of sugar-containing snacks or drinks (AAPD, 2012).

Energy from Carbohydrate, Protein, and Fat

Lowering or raising the proportion of energy from one dietary macronutrient affects the proportion of energy from the others. However, beyond recommending that intakes be within the acceptable macronutrient distribution range (AMDR), the DGA (USDA/HHS, 2016) did not include recommendations for energy from total fat, carbohydrates, or protein. Therefore, the proportions of these macronutrients in the food packages were not considered in developing the revised food packages. (See below for the committee's consideration of saturated fat.)

Saturated Fat and Added Sugars

Saturated fat and added sugars were evaluated along with other nutrients, not food groups, because they may occur in several different foods. The current food packages already provide foods that are limited in saturated fat (e.g., only low-fat or nonfat milk and yogurt are allowed in packages for participants over 2 years of age) and added sugars (e.g., ready-to-eat cereals, yogurt, and vegetables and fruits purchased with the cash value voucher (CVV) are allowed in the packages only if they do not exceed required limits). Despite these current limitations, the WIC food packages do contribute some of each nutrient to the diet. Therefore, as described below, they were retained as macronutrients possibly linked to adverse health consequences (see Table 5-1).

Nutrients for Which Intakes Were Excessive

When micronutrient intakes were above the Tolerable Upper Intake Level (UL) in more than 5 percent of a WIC subgroup, the approach applied was similar to what was used when intakes were below the EAR except that the upper ends of intake distributions were examined. For example, nutrients for which intakes exceeded the UL in greater than 50 percent of the subgroup were considered to be of higher priority.

For excess consumption of saturated fat and added sugars, the committee prioritized action according to the proportion of the WIC subpopulation exceeding 10 percent of energy from each (e.g., 5 to <10, 10 to <50, and ≥50 percent of the population).

Identifying Nutrient Priorities for Infants

Because of the known risks of low iron and zinc intakes for breastfed infants, these were the only micronutrient intakes (from complementary foods) that were evaluated (see Table 5-1). Vitamin D was not prioritized because information on the vitamin D status of infants is not available in NHANES. Macronutrient intakes were evaluated against the Dietary Reference Intakes (DRIs), as available. The DGA do not apply to infants. Therefore, intake of added sugars or saturated fat was not evaluated.

Identifying Nutrient Priorities for Children 1 to Less Than 2 Years of Age

Micronutrients for children ages 1 to less than 2 years were evaluated in the same way as for women and for children ages 2 to less than 5 years. Although carbohydrate intakes were below the AMDR in more than 5 percent of this age group, very few children reported carbohydrate intakes below the EAR of 100 grams per day. Therefore, carbohydrate intakes were assumed to be adequate. As with infants, because the DGA do not apply to children 1 to less than 2 years of age, added sugars and saturated fat were not evaluated.

IDENTIFYING FOOD GROUP PRIORITIES

Inasmuch as recommended food group intakes are currently available only for individuals ages 2 years and older, the decision tree was applied to identify priority food groups and subgroups only for women and children ages 2 to less than 5 years. As illustrated in Figure 5-1, food group and subgroup intakes were evaluated separately from nutrient intakes.

Similar to what was done with nutrients, prioritization levels were defined by proportions of the population subgroup with intakes below those recommended in the DGA. Priority was given to food groups (or subgroups) for which intake was below the recommended amount in 75 percent or more of the population subgroup. A second level of priority was given to food groups (or subgroups) for which intake was below the recommended amount in 50 to less than 75 percent of the population subgroup. Although intake of oils fell below recommended amounts in more than 50 percent of some subgroups, this food group was not evaluated because oils do not contain nutrients of public health concern for the WIC-participating population.

IDENTIFYING POTENTIAL ACTIONS FOR FOOD PACKAGE REVISIONS

Nutrients with a high proportion of inadequate intakes and food groups (or subgroups) with lower-than-recommended intakes were evaluated further through the systematic process detailed in Figure 5-1. For each nutrient consumed in inadequate amounts relative to its EAR or AI, or for each food group (or subgroup) consumed in lower-than-recommended amounts

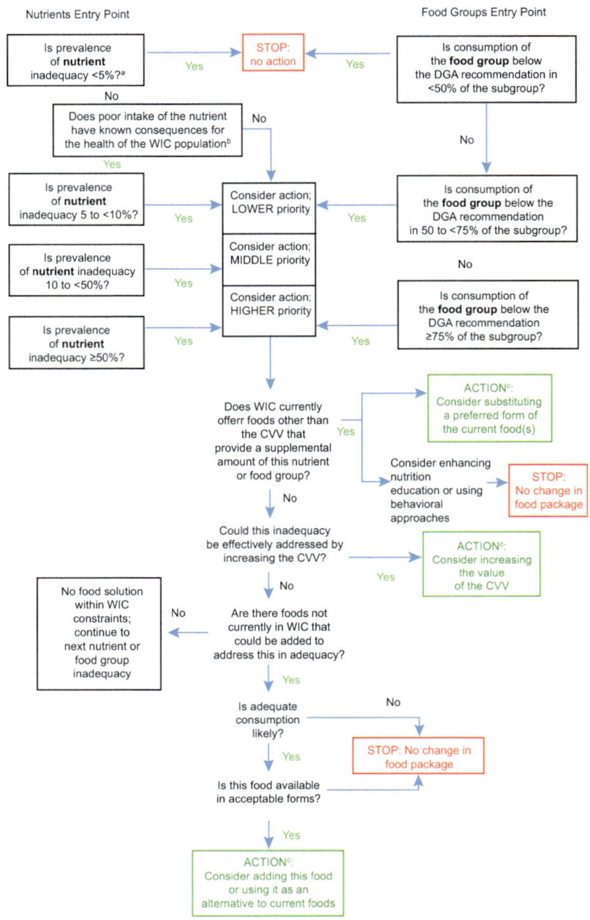

FIGURE 5-1 Decision tree for determining potential food package changes given the prevalence of nutrient inadequacy or food group intake below recommended amounts among WIC-participating women and children.

NOTES: CVV = cash value voucher; DGA = *Dietary Guidelines for Americans*. This figure provides a visual description of the committee's strategy for determining priorities for action and possible solutions to inadequate consumption of nutrients or food group intakes below that recommended for WIC-participating populations. The committee's approach to excess consumption of nutrients, food groups, and calories for other uses is described in the text of this chapter.

[a] For nutrients with an EAR; for nutrients with an AI, mean intakes below the AI value were considered higher-priority.

[b] Assessment based on the DGA where applicable and, where the DGA do not apply, on the committee's literature review and expert guidance (see Table 5-1).

[c] In addition, are the proposed foods culturally suitable for WIC participants? Are more culturally suitable foods available in acceptable forms?

relative to the DGA, the committee evaluated whether or not WIC currently offers foods that provide what it considered a supplemental amount of that nutrient or food group (or subgroup).[1]

In cases where the amount of the nutrient or food group or subgroup in the food package is already more than what is considered supplemental, the committee considered reducing the amount and providing a more preferred form to promote intake. In cases where an appropriate (i.e., supplemental) amount is already included in the food packages and preferred and appropriate forms of the food could not be identified, the committee proposed either enhancing nutrition education or applying behavioral approaches to increase consumption of the currently available foods. Alternatively, if a preferred food could be identified, the committee considered adding that food.

Finally, in cases where WIC does not currently offer foods that provide supplemental amounts of the nutrient or food group (or subgroup) identified as being consumed in lower-than-recommended amounts, the committee considered whether intake of that nutrient or food group (or subgroup) could be improved by increasing the value of the CVV. If not, then the committee considered whether foods could be added to the packages to address this problem. If appropriate foods could not be identified, no further action was considered. If there were foods that could be added, the committee then evaluated whether adequate consumption of such foods was likely (e.g., whether they were commonly consumed) and also whether such foods were available in acceptable forms. Additionally, the committee made an effort to identify changes to the food packages that could address low intakes while also meeting cultural needs and food preferences.

The results of this process are presented in Tables 5-2 through 5-10. Chapter 6 describes how, given cost-neutral constraints, the outcomes presented in these tables were translated into final food package changes.

Strengths and Limitations of the Decision Tree

The decision tree afforded the committee a systematic way to pare down the large body of information into practical actions. Using the tree, each nutrient, food group (and subgroup), and population subgroup was treated with the same degree of attention. The decision tree was used only for nutrients with evidence of inadequate consumption and food groups with evidence of consumption of less-than-recommended amounts.

Additionally, although the committee conducted separate evaluations

---

[1] The committee's application of the term *supplemental* is described in Chapter 6. The committee also evaluated the nutrients provided by the food packages considering the quantities of foods that WIC participants actually redeem (see Appendix R for detail on redemption rates).

for partially breastfeeding and fully breastfeeding women, the evaluation was limited. Because there are no DRI values specifically for partially breastfeeding women, the contribution of the WIC food package for partially breastfeeding women to a set of DRIs could not be evaluated. Additionally, because the intensity of breastfeeding of women coded as "breastfeeding" in NHANES is unknown, the priority nutrients and food groups for these women are presented along with the contents of both food packages V (for partially breastfeeding women) and VII in Tables 5-3 (nutrients) and 5-8 (food groups).

Challenges with Translating the Decision Tree Outcomes into Potential Actions

Although the decision tree used by the committee provides transparency about how nutrient and food groups were prioritized, application of the decision tree outcomes to food package changes was less straightforward. Not only may a prioritized nutrient be provided by several different foods, but those foods may or may not belong to one of the prioritized food groups. In addition, the committee was unable to propose some actions suggested by the decision tree outcomes because of requirements set by the WIC program to provide specific nutrients, ensure that the revised set of food packages are of the same weighted average per-participant cost, ensure cultural suitability, and control administrative burden. The committee considered all of these factors in aggregate when translating the decision tree outcomes into final food package changes.

Nutrition Education as a Potential Action

The nutrition education tools developed by states are one strategy to improve the balance between what is provided in the food packages and participants' nutrient and food intake. As reviewed in Chapter 1, WIC is the only federal supplemental nutrition assistance program to have a nutrition education component required by law (USDA/FNS, 2007). The goals of WIC nutrition education are to

> emphasize the relationship between nutrition, physical activity, and health with special emphasis on the nutritional needs of pregnant, postpartum, and breastfeeding women, infants and children under five years of age; and 2) assist the individual who is at nutritional risk in achieving a positive change in dietary and physical activity habits, resulting in improved nutritional status and in the prevention of nutrition-related problems through optimal use of the WIC supplemental foods and other nutritious foods.[2]

[2] Section 246.11(b) of the federal WIC regulations, p. 392.

One of the ways the U.S. Department of Agriculture's Food and Nutrition Service (USDA-FNS) provides state agencies with guidance and resources for nutrition education through WIC Works (USDA/FNS, 2016).

Behavioral Approaches as a Potential Action

In addition to nutrition education, behavioral approaches are another option for addressing low consumption of nutrients or food groups. Challenges that prevent individuals from making choices that best align with the DGA include treating losses differently than gains, remaining within the status quo, and placing greater value on the present time as opposed to the future (Kahneman and Tversky, 1984; Loewenstein, 1988; Dhar and Wertenbroch, 2000; USDA/ERS, 2007). The phase I report (NASEM, 2016) included a brief review of behavioral economics approaches that may help individuals to overcome these challenges and that could be applied in WIC (see Appendix M for WIC-specific examples).

RESULTS FROM USE OF THE DECISION TREE

The committee's final proposed revisions to the food packages, which are presented in Chapter 6, are based on information in Chapters 1 through 4; considerations described above in the section titled "Challenges with Translating the Decision Tree Outcomes into Potential Actions"; and outcomes of this chapter's decision tree process, as detailed in Tables 5-2 through 5-10. The tables present all nutrient and food groups of lower, middle, and higher priority; a brief discussion of higher-priority nutrients and food groups and preliminary potential actions is provided here.

Evaluation of Priority Nutrients and Potential Actions

Priority Nutrients Across Subgroups of Women and Children

Across subgroups of women (see Tables 5-2 through 5-4) and children (see Table 5-5), fiber, potassium, sodium, and added sugars were considered to be higher priority, with intakes of sodium, and added sugars being excessive. For all women (except for postpartum women) and children, excessive saturated fat intake was also a higher-priority (saturated fat is a middle priority for postpartum women). For breastfeeding women (see Table 5-4) and children ages 1 to less than 5 years (see Table 5-5), there were no additional higher-priority nutrients. Proposed actions to address low fiber and potassium intakes include increasing the CVV or requiring an option for canned legumes as a means of adding convenience and, therefore, promoting intake. Added sugars and sodium are already limited in WIC foods,

TABLE 5-2 Nutrient Priorities and Preliminary Actions, Food Package V for Pregnant Women

Nutrient	Rationale for Prioritization	Amount per Day: Guideline (EAR, AI, UL, or DGA)	Amount per Day: Gap to Reduce Inadequacy or Excess to 5%[b]	Amount per Day: Amount in the Food Package (% of the EAR, AI, or DGA limit)[c]	WIC Foods That Provide a Supplemental Amount of This Nutrient	Potential Action[d]
Higher Priority						
Iron	Inadequacy was 82%; inadequate iron status is associated with health risks in pregnancy and development; heme iron is especially important for women who are capable of becoming pregnant or who are pregnant (as noted in the DGA)	22 mg (EAR)	10.5 mg	13.5 mg (62%)	Breakfast cereal, whole wheat bread, whole wheat pasta, legumes, peanut butter	Retain current sources because iron requirements for this group are higher than can be met by diet alone; foods outside of the food package or dietary supplements are required
Choline	Mean intakes fell below the AI; considered a nutrient linked to adverse health consequences, based on the committee's literature review	450 mg (AI)	102 mg	75 mg (17%)	Milk, eggs	Consider additional eggs
Potassium	Mean intakes fell below the AI; potassium is a DGA nutrient of public health concern	4,700 mg (AI)	1,748 mg	1,837 mg (39%)	Milk, cheese, legumes, CVV	Consider canned legumes to promote intake; additional yogurt to promote intake of dairy; consider increase in the CVV

Fiber	Mean intakes fell below the AI; fiber is a DGA nutrient of public health concern	25 g (AI)	10 g	8.0 g (29%)	Bread (and alternatives), legumes, CVV	Consider increasing whole grains; promote intake of legumes by providing a canned option; consider increase in the CVV
Higher-Priority Nutrients to Limit						
Sodium	Intake exceeded the UL in >90% of the subgroup	2,300 mg (UL)	2,630 mg	727 mg (48%)	Milk, cheese, RTE breakfast cereal, vegetables (canned), legumes (canned), bread	Consider low-sodium choices when possible; nutrition education to reduce sodium in canned foods
Saturated fat[a]	Intake exceeded the DGA limit in 75% of the subgroup	<10% of energy (DGA)	15 g	8.5 g (29%)	Milk (1%), cheese	Consider reducing the key sources of saturated fat or offering lower-fat options
Added sugars[a]	Intake exceeded the DGA limit in 68% of the subgroup	<10% of energy (DGA)	147 g	7.4 g (11%)	Yogurt, soy beverage, peanut butter, breakfast cereal	Consider reducing the maximum allowable amounts of added sugars in yogurt or cereals; propose a maximum for soy beverage and milk

continued

TABLE 5-2 Continued

Nutrient	Rationale for Prioritization	Amount per Day: Guideline (EAR, AI, UL, or DGA)	Amount per Day: Gap to Reduce Inadequacy or Excess to 5%[b]	Amount per Day: Amount in the Food Package (% of the EAR, AI, or DGA limit)[c]	WIC Foods That Provide a Supplemental Amount of This Nutrient	Potential Action[d]
			Middle Priority			
Folate	Inadequacy was 22%; inadequate folate status is associated with health risks in pregnancy	520 μg DFE (EAR)	108 μg DFE	473 μg DFE (91%)	RTE breakfast cereal, legumes, CVV	Consider canned legumes to promote intake; consider increasing the CVV
			Lower Priority			
Magnesium	Inadequacy was 32%; no known health consequence for WIC population	290 mg (EAR)	69 mg	198 mg (68%)	Milk, legumes, RTE breakfast cereal, CVV	Retain RTE breakfast cereals; consider additional options and nutrition education or behavioral interventions to promote intake of milk, legumes, breakfast cereal, and vegetables and fruits already provided
Vitamin A	Inadequacy was 20%; no known health consequence for WIC population	550 μg RAE (EAR)	124 μg RAE	646 μg RAE (117%)	Milk, RTE breakfast cereal, CVV	Consider reducing sources because nutrient amount in the food package is more than supplemental

Zinc	Inadequacy was 20%; no known health consequence for WIC population	9.5 mg (EAR)	1.8 mg	6.6 mg (69%)	Milk, RTE breakfast cereal	Retain RTE breakfast cereals; consider additional options and nutrition education or behavioral interventions to promote intake of milk and breakfast cereal already provided
Vitamin C	Inadequacy was 17%; no known health consequence for WIC population	70 mg (EAR)	24 mg	72.2 mg (103%)	Juice, CVV	Consider reducing sources because nutrient amount in the food package is more than supplemental
Vitamin B6	Inadequacy was 12%; no known health consequence for WIC population	1.6 mg (EAR)	0.2 mg	1.3 mg (79%)	RTE breakfast cereal	Retain RTE breakfast cereals; consider additional options and nutrition education or behavioral interventions to promote intake of cereal already provided
Vitamin D	Serum vitamin D inadequacy was 9%; vitamin D is a DGA nutrient of public health concern	400 IU or 40 nmol/L (EAR)	268 IU	291 IU (73%)	Milk, soy beverage	Consider additional options and nutrition education or behavioral interventions to promote intake of milk already provided
Calcium	Inadequacy was 6%; calcium is a DGA nutrient of public health concern	800 mg (EAR)	27 mg	1,029 mg (129%)	Milk, cheese, tofu, soy milk, lactose-free milk, yogurt, RTE breakfast cereal	Consider reducing sources because nutrient amount in the food package is more than supplemental

continued

TABLE 5-2 Continued

NOTES: AI = Adequate Intake level; CVV = cash value voucher; DFE = dietary folate equivalent; DGA = 2015–2020 *Dietary Guidelines for Americans*; EAR = Estimated Average Requirement; IU = international units; RAE = retinol activity equivalents; RTE = ready-to-eat; UL = Tolerable Upper Intake Level. Vitamin E inadequacy was apparent in nearly 100 percent of WIC subgroups. However, because clinical vitamin E deficiency is uncommon (IOM, 2000a), the DGA do not include it as a nutrient of public health concern (USDA/HHS, 2016). Similarly, despite the very high prevalence of inadequacy across the WIC population, it was not prioritized for action by the committee.

[a] Saturated fat and added sugars intakes were evaluated based on a 2,600-kcal food pattern selected to align with the Estimated Energy Requirement calculated for pregnant women participating in WIC.

[b] For nutrients with an EAR and inadequate intake, the gap is the difference between the EAR and the 5th percentile of intake; for nutrients with an AI and intake below the AI, the gap is the difference between the AI and the median intake; for sodium, saturated, and added sugars, for which there is excess intake, the gap is the difference between the UL and the 95th percentile of intake. Complete results of the gap analysis are presented in Appendix L.

[c] The percent values assume that the food package is fully consumed.

[d] Translation of potential actions into the final food packages depended upon cost and other practical and administrative considerations.

SOURCES: IOM, 1998, 2000a, 2001, 2002/2005, 2005, 2011; USDA/ARS 2005–2012; USDA/HHS, 2016.

TABLE 5-3 Nutrient Priorities and Preliminary Actions, Food Packages for Breastfeeding Women[a]

		Amount per Day					
Nutrient	Rationale for Prioritization	Guideline (EAR, AI, UL, or DGA)	Gap to Reduce Inadequacy or Excess to 5%[c]	Amount in Food Package V	Amount in Food Package VII (% of the EAR, AI, or DGA limit)[d]	WIC Foods That Provide a Supplemental Amount of This Nutrient	Potential Action[e]
				Higher Priority			
Potassium	Mean intakes fell below the AI; potassium is a 2015 DGA nutrient of public health concern	5,100 mg (AI)	2,254 mg	1,836 mg	1,958 (38%)	Milk, cheese, legumes, CVV	Consider increasing the CVV; canned legumes to promote intake; nutrition education or behavioral interventions to promote consumption of dairy that is already provided in the food package
Fiber	Mean intakes fell below the AI; fiber is a DGA nutrient of public health concern	29 g (AI)	13 g	8.0 g	8.0 g (29%)	Bread (and alternatives), legumes, CVV	Consider increasing whole grains; promote intake of legumes by providing a canned option; consider increase in the CVV
				Higher-Priority Nutrients to Limit			
Sodium	Intake exceeded the UL in 96% of the subgroup	2,300 mg (UL)	2,139 mg	727 mg	1,007 mg (67%)	Milk, cheese, RTE breakfast cereal, vegetables (canned),	Consider low-sodium choices when possible; nutrition education to reduce sodium in canned foods

continued

TABLE 5-3 Continued

		Amount per Day					
Nutrient	Rationale for Prioritization	Guideline (EAR, AI, UL, or DGA)	Gap to Reduce Inadequacy or Excess to 5%[c]	Amount in Food Package V	Amount in Food Package VII (% of the EAR, AI, or DGA limit)[d]	WIC Foods That Provide a Supplemental Amount of This Nutrient	Potential Action[e]
						legumes (canned), bread	
Saturated fat[b]	Intakes exceeded the DGA limit in 79% of the subgroup	<10% of energy (DGA)	17 g	8.5 g	12.8 g (44%)	Milk (1%), cheese	Consider reducing the key sources of saturated fat or lower-fat options
Added sugars[b]	Intake exceeded the DGA limit in 24% of subgroups	<10% of energy (DGA)	45 g	7.4 g	6.6 g (10%)	Yogurt, soy beverage, peanut butter, RTE breakfast cereal	Consider reducing the maximum allowable amounts of added sugars in yogurt or cereals; propose a maximum for soy beverage and milk
Middle Priority							
Folate	Inadequacy was 27%; folate is a DGA nutrient of public health concern for premenopausal women	450 µg DFE (EAR)	127 µg DFE	473 µg DFE	489 µg DFE (108%)	RTE breakfast cereal, legumes, CVV	Consider reducing sources because nutrient amount in the food package is more than supplemental

Vitamin D	Serum vitamin D inadequacy was 21%; vitamin D is a DGA nutrient of public health concern	400 IU or 40 nmol/L (EAR)	308 IU	291 IU	371 IU (86%)	Milk, soy beverage, fish	Consider additional options; sun exposure in combination with WIC foods may be required to improve status
Calcium	Inadequacy was 16%; calcium was a DGA nutrient of public health concern	800 mg (EAR)	136 mg	1,029 mg	1,232 mg (154%)	Milk, yogurt, soy beverage, cheese, breakfast cereals	Consider reducing sources because nutrient amount in the food package is more than supplemental
				Lower Priority			
Vitamin A	Inadequacy was 75%; no known health consequence for WIC population	900 μg RAE (EAR)	498 μg RAE	646 μg RAE	754 μg RAE (84%)	Milk, RTE breakfast cereal, CVV	Consider additional options; nutrition education or behavioral interventions to promote intake of milk, breakfast cereal, and vegetables and fruits already provided
Magnesium	Inadequacy was 39%; no known health consequence for WIC population	255 mg (EAR)	73 mg	198 mg	214 mg (81%–84%)	Milk, legumes, RTE breakfast cereal, CVV	Consider additional options and nutrition education or behavioral interventions to promote intake of milk, legumes, breakfast cereal, and vegetables and fruits already provided

continued

TABLE 5-3 Continued

		Amount per Day					
Nutrient	Rationale for Prioritization	Guideline (EAR, AI, UL, or DGA)	Gap to Reduce Inadequacy or Excess to 5%[c]	Amount in Food Package V	Amount in Food Package VII (% of the EAR, AI, or DGA limit)[d]	WIC Foods That Provide a Supplemental Amount of This Nutrient	Potential Action[e]
Zinc	Inadequacy was 39%; no known health consequence for WIC population	10.4 mg (EAR)	3.3 mg	6.6 mg	7.7 mg (74%)	Milk, RTE breakfast cereal	Consider additional options and nutrition education or behavioral interventions to promote intake of milk and breakfast cereal already provided
Vitamin C	Inadequacy was 33%; no known health consequence for WIC population	100 mg (EAR)	47 mg	72.2 mg	72.4 mg (72%)	Juice, CVV	Consider increasing the CVV
Vitamin B6	Inadequacy was 30%; no known health consequence for WIC population	1.7 mg (EAR)	0.5 mg	1.3 mg	1.4 mg (83%)	RTE breakfast cereal	Retain RTE breakfast cereals
Copper	Inadequacy was 22%; no known health	1.0 mg (EAR)	0.2 mg	0.44 mg	0.5 mg (48%)	Milk, legumes, breakfast cereal, CVV	Consider additional options and nutrition education or behavioral

	consequence for WIC population							interventions to promote intake of milk, legumes, breakfast cereal, and vegetables and fruits already provided
Thiamin	Inadequacy was 10%; no known health consequence for WIC population	1.2 mg (EAR)	0.1 mg	0.91 mg	0.9 mg (78%)		RTE breakfast cereal	Retain RTE breakfast cereals

NOTES: AI = Adequate Intake level; CVV = cash value voucher; DFE = dietary folate equivalent; DGA = 2015–2020 *Dietary Guidelines for Americans*; EAR = Estimated Average Requirement; IU = international units; RAE = retinol activity equivalents; RTE = ready-to-eat; UL = Tolerable Upper Intake Level. Vitamin E inadequacy was apparent in nearly 100 percent of WIC subgroups. However, because clinical vitamin E deficiency is uncommon (IOM, 2000a), the 2015 DGA do not include it as a nutrient of public health concern (USDA/HHS, 2016). Similarly, despite the very high prevalence of inadequacy across the WIC-participating population, it was not prioritized for action by the committee.

[a] Inadequacy data in this table are for women coded as "breastfeeding" and participating in WIC in NHANES 2005–2012. The intensity of breastfeeding is not known, but these data represent the best available for evaluation of the degree to which food packages V and VII meet the needs of these women.

[b] Saturated fat and added sugars intakes were evaluated based on a 2,600-kcal food pattern selected to align with the Estimated Energy Requirement calculated for breastfeeding women participating in WIC.

[c] For nutrients with an EAR and inadequate intake, the gap is the difference between the EAR and the 5th percentile of intake; for nutrients with an AI and intake below the AI, the gap is the difference between the AI and the median intake; for sodium, saturated fat, and added sugars, for which there is excess intake, the gap is the difference between the UL and the 95th percentile of intake. Complete results of the gap analysis are presented in Appendix L.

[d] Because DRI values for women that are partially breastfeeding have not been published, no comparison to nutrient intake recommendations is made for food package V.

[e] Translation of potential actions into the final food packages depended upon cost and other practical and administrative considerations.

SOURCES: IOM, 1998, 2000a, 2001, 2002/2005, 2005, 2011; USDA/ARS, 2005–2012; USDA/HHS, 2016.

TABLE 5-4 Nutrient Priorities and Preliminary Actions, Food Package VI, Postpartum Women

Nutrient	Rationale for Prioritization	Amount per Day: Guideline (EAR, AI, UL, or DGA)	Amount per Day: Gap to Reduce Inadequacy or Excess to 5%[b]	Amount per Day: Amount in the Food Package (% of the EAR, AI, or DGA limit)[c]	WIC Foods That Provide a Supplemental Amount of This Nutrient	Potential Action[d]
			Higher Priority			
Calcium	Inadequacy was 52% in postpartum women; calcium is a DGA nutrient of public health concern	800 mg (EAR)	371 mg	739 mg (92%)	Milk, yogurt, soy beverage, cheese, RTE breakfast cereals	Consider reducing sources because nutrient amount in the food package is more than supplemental
Potassium	Mean intakes fell below the AI; potassium is a DGA nutrient of public health concern	4,700 mg (AI)	2,802 mg	1,302 mg (28%)	Milk, cheese, legumes, CVV	Consider increasing the CVV; promote intake of legumes by providing a canned option
Fiber	Mean intakes fell below the AI; fiber is a DGA nutrient of public health concern	25 g (AI)	13 g	5.7 g (23%)	Bread (and alternatives), CVV, legumes	Consider increasing whole grains; consider increase in the CVV; promote intake of legumes by providing a canned option
			Higher-Priority Nutrients to Limit			
Sodium	Intake exceeded the UL in >79% of the subgroup	2,300 mg (UL)	1,771 mg	527 mg (35%)	Milk, cheese, RTE breakfast cereal, vegetables (canned), legumes (canned), bread	Consider low-sodium choices when possible; nutrition education to reduce sodium in canned foods

Added sugars[a]	Intake exceeded the DGA limit in 78% of the subgroup	<10% of energy (DGA)	35 g	6.9 g (12%)	Yogurt, soy beverage, peanut butter, RTE breakfast cereal	Consider reducing the maximum allowable amounts of added sugars in yogurt or cereals; propose a maximum for soy beverage and milk
			Middle Priority			
Folate	Inadequacy was 33%; inadequate folate status is associated with health risks in pregnancy	520 µg DFE (EAR)	131 µg DFE	425 µg DFE (133%)	RTE breakfast cereal, legumes, CVV	Consider canned legumes to promote intake; consider increase in the CVV
Vitamin D	Inadequacy was 13%; vitamin D is a DGA nutrient of public health concern	400 IU or 40 nmol/L (EAR)	364 IU	213 IU (53%)	Milk, soy beverage	Consider additional options; sun exposure in combination with WIC foods may be required to improve status
Iron	Inadequacy was 13%; iron was a DGA nutrient of public health concern for premenopausal females	8.1 mg (EAR)	1.6 mg	12.3 mg (152%)	Breakfast cereal, whole wheat bread, whole wheat pasta, legumes, peanut butter	Consider reducing sources because nutrient amount in the food package is more than supplemental
			Middle Priority Nutrient to Limit			
Saturated fat[a]	Intakes exceeded the DGA limit in 49% of the subgroup	<10% of energy (DGA)	8 g	6.4 g (25%)	Milk, cheese	Consider reducing the key sources of saturated fat (milk, cheese)

continued

TABLE 5-4 Continued

Nutrient	Rationale for Prioritization	Amount per Day: Guideline (EAR, AI, UL, or DGA)	Amount per Day: Gap to Reduce Inadequacy or Excess to 5%[b]	Amount per Day: Amount in the Food Package (% of the EAR, AI, or DGA limit)[c]	WIC Foods That Provide a Supplemental Amount of This Nutrient	Potential Action[d]
			Lower Priority			
Magnesium	Inadequacy was 78%; no known health consequence for WIC population	265 mg (EAR)	144 mg	132 mg (50%–52%)	Milk, legumes, RTE breakfast cereal, CVV	Consider additional options; nutrition education or behavioral interventions to promote intake of milk, legumes, breakfast cereal, and vegetables and fruits already provided in the food package
Vitamin A	Inadequacy was 69%; no known health consequence for WIC population	500 µg RAE (EAR)	355 µg RAE	522 µg RAE (104%)	Milk, RTE breakfast cereal, CVV	Consider reducing sources because nutrient amount in the food package is more than supplemental
Vitamin C	Inadequacy was 38%; no known health consequence for WIC population	60 mg (EAR)	37 mg	57 mg (95%)	Juice, CVV	Consider reducing sources because nutrient amount in the food package is more than supplemental
Copper	Inadequacy was 32%; no known health consequence for WIC population	0.7 mg (EAR)	0.3 mg	0.3 mg (42%)	Milk, legumes, RTE breakfast cereal, CVV	Consider additional options; nutrition education or behavioral interventions to promote intake of milk, legumes,

						breakfast cereal, and vegetables and fruits already provided in the food package
Zinc	Inadequacy was 30%; no known health consequence for WIC population	6.8 mg (EAR)	2.5 mg	5.2 mg (76%)	Milk, RTE breakfast cereal	Consider additional options; nutrition education or behavioral interventions to promote intake of milk and breakfast cereal already provided in the food package
Thiamin	Inadequacy was 20%; no known health consequence for WIC population	0.9 mg (EAR)	0.2 mg	0.7 mg (81%)	RTE breakfast cereal	Retain RTE breakfast cereals
Vitamin B6	Inadequacy was 20%; no known health consequence for WIC population	1.1 mg (EAR)	0.3 mg	1.1 mg (97%)	RTE breakfast cereal	Consider reducing sources because nutrient amount in the food package is more than supplemental
Vitamin B12	Inadequacy was 14%; no known health consequence for WIC population	2.0 μg (EAR)	0.6 μg	3.6 μg (180%)	RTE breakfast cereal	Consider reducing sources because nutrient amount in the food package is more than supplemental
Riboflavin	Inadequacy was 11%; no known health consequence for WIC population	0.9 mg (EAR)	0.2 mg	1.4 mg (153%)	Milk, RTE breakfast cereal	Consider reducing sources because nutrient amount in the food package is more than supplemental

continued

TABLE 5-4 Continued

Nutrient	Rationale for Prioritization	Amount per Day: Guideline (EAR, AI, UL, or DGA)	Amount per Day: Gap to Reduce Inadequacy or Excess to 5%[b]	Amount per Day: Amount in the Food Package (% of the EAR, AI, or DGA limit)[c]	WIC Foods That Provide a Supplemental Amount of This Nutrient	Potential Action[d]
Niacin	Inadequacy was 6%; no known health consequence for WIC population	11 mg (EAR)	0.4 mg	8.0 mg (72%)	RTE breakfast cereal	Retain RTE breakfast cereals

NOTES: AI = Adequate Intake level; CVV = cash value voucher; DFE = dietary folate equivalent; DGA = 2015–2020 *Dietary Guidelines for Americans*; EAR = Estimated Average Requirement; IU = international units; RAE = retinol activity equivalents; RTE = ready-to-eat; UL = Tolerable Upper Intake Level. Vitamin E inadequacy was apparent in nearly 100 percent of WIC subgroups. However, because clinical vitamin E deficiency is uncommon (IOM, 2000a), the 2015 DGA do not include it as a nutrient of public health concern (USDA/HHS, 2016). Similarly, despite the very high prevalence of inadequacy across the WIC-participating population, it was not prioritized for action by the committee.

[a] Values are based on the DGA recommended limits for a 2,300-kcal food pattern selected to align with the estimated energy requirement calculated for postpartum women participating in WIC.

[b] For nutrients with an EAR and inadequate intake, the gap is the difference between the EAR and the 5th percentile of intake; for nutrients with an AI and intake below the AI, the gap is the difference between the AI and the median intake; for sodium, saturated fat, and added sugars, for which there is excess intake, the gap is the difference between the UL and the 95th percentile of intake. Complete results of the gap analysis are presented in Appendix L.

[c] The percent values assume that the food package is fully consumed.

[d] Translation of potential actions into the final food packages depended upon cost and other practical and administrative considerations.

SOURCES: IOM, 1998, 2000a, 2001, 2002/2005, 2005, 2011; USDA/ARS, 2005–2012; USDA/HHS, 2016.

TABLE 5-5 Nutrient Priorities and Preliminary Actions, Food Package IV, Children Ages 1 to Less Than 5 Years of Age

Nutrient	Rationale for Prioritization	Amount per Day (Ages 1–3 y/Age 4 y): Guideline (EAR, AI, UL, or DGA)	Amount per Day: Gap to Reduce Inadequacy or Excess to 5%[b]	Amount per Day: Amount in the Food Package (% of the EAR, AI, or DGA limit)[c]	WIC Foods That Provide a Supplemental Amount of This Nutrient	Potential Action[d]
			Higher Priority			
Fiber	Mean intakes fell below the AI; fiber is a DGA nutrient of public health concern	19/25 g (AI)	7/13 g	7.1 g (38/29%)	Bread (and alternatives), legumes, CVV	Consider increasing the CVV; promote intake of legumes by providing a canned option
Potassium	Mean intakes fell below the AI; potassium is a DGA nutrient of public health concern	3,000/ 3,800 mg (AI)	929/1,729 mg	1,267/ 1,357 mg (42/36%)	Milk, cheese, CVV, legumes	Consider increasing the CVV; promote intake of legumes by providing a canned option
			Higher-Priority Nutrients to Limit			
Sodium	Intake exceeded the UL in 59 to 65% of the subgroups	1,500/ 1,900 mg (UL)	806/1,495/ 1,095[e] mg	587/639 (59/53%)	Milk, cheese, RTE breakfast cereal, vegetables (canned), legumes (canned), bread	Consider low-sodium choices when possible; nutrition education to reduce sodium in canned foods

continued

TABLE 5-5 Continued

		Amount per Day (Ages 1–3 y/Age 4 y)				
Nutrient	Rationale for Prioritization	Guideline (EAR, AI, UL, or DGA)	Gap to Reduce Inadequacy or Excess to 5%[b]	Amount in the Food Package (% of the EAR, AI, or DGA limit)[c]	WIC Foods That Provide a Supplemental Amount of This Nutrient	Potential Action[d]
Saturated fat[a]	Intakes exceeded the DGA limit in 70% of the subgroup (children 2 to less than 5 years)	<10% of energy (DGA)	15 g	6.6 g (46%)	1% milk, cheese	Consider reducing the key sources of saturated fat
Added sugars[a]	Intake exceeded the DGA limit in 80% of subgroups (children 2 to less than 5 years)	<10% of energy (DGA)	59 g	6.9 g (21%)	Yogurt, soy beverage, peanut butter, RTE breakfast cereal	Consider reducing the maximum allowable amounts of added sugars in yogurt or cereals; propose a maximum level for soy beverage and milk

NOTES: AI = Adequate Intake level; CVV = cash value voucher; DFE = dietary folate equivalent; DGA = 2015–2020 *Dietary Guidelines for Americans*; EAR = Estimated Average Requirement; IU = international units; RAE = retinol activity equivalents; RTE = ready-to-eat; UL = Tolerable Upper Intake Level. There were no nutrients linked to adverse health outcomes for which intakes were inadequate in 5 to 50 percent of the subgroup. Vitamin E inadequacy was apparent in nearly 100 percent of WIC subgroups. However, because clinical vitamin E deficiency is uncommon (IOM, 2000a), the 2015 DGA do not include it as a nutrient of public health concern (USDA/HHS, 2016). Similarly, despite the very high prevalence of inadequacy across the WIC-participating population, it was not prioritized for action by the committee.

[a] Values are based on the DGA recommended limits for a 1,300-kcal food pattern selected to approximate the estimated energy needs of children ages 2 to less than 5 years. Data for saturated fat and added sugars specifically represent children of these ages because no limits have been defined for children ages 1 to less than 2 years.

[b] For nutrients with an EAR and inadequate intake, the gap is the difference between the EAR and the 5th percentile of intake; for nutrients with an AI and intake below the AI, the gap is the difference between the AI and the median intake; for sodium, saturated fat, and added sugars, for which there is excess intake, the gap is the difference between the UL and the 95th percentile of intake. Complete results of the gap analysis are presented in Appendix L.

[c] The percent values assume that the food package is fully consumed.

[d] Translation of potential actions into the final food packages depended upon cost and other practical and administrative considerations.

[e] UL intake gap from 95th percentile for children 1–2 years, 2–3 years, and 4–5 years.

SOURCES: IOM, 1998, 2000a, 2001, 2002/2005, 2005, 2011; USDA/ARS, 2011–2012; USDA/HHS, 2016.

but the committee reviewed the specifications for WIC foods to identify possibilities for further limiting these nutrients. Additional priority nutrients and potential actions for pregnant and postpartum, nonbreastfeeding women are outlined below.

Pregnant women Higher-, middle-, and lower-priority nutrients for WIC-participating pregnant women are presented in Table 5-2. In addition to the higher-priority nutrients described above, iron and choline were also identified as higher-priority nutrients for pregnant women. Iron requirements during pregnancy are higher than can be met by diet alone. Low choline intakes could be improved by provision of additional eggs or by increasing consumption of the dairy products already provided by the WIC program.

Postpartum women For postpartum women who are not breastfeeding (food package VI), calcium was identified as another higher-priority nutrient in addition to the nutrients mentioned above (see Table 5-4). Women receiving food package VI currently receive a greater-than-supplemental amount of calcium in this package. Therefore, strategies to improve intake of the calcium that is already provided are needed.

Priority Nutrients for Infants

No priorities were identified for younger (0 to less than 6 months of age) infants or for formula-fed older infants because either human milk or formula meets the nutrient needs of these groups. Given that the protein concentrations of infant formulas are regulated and considered safe by the U.S. Food and Drug Administration, excess intake of protein by formula-fed infants was not considered a priority. Both iron and zinc were considered priority nutrients for breastfeeding infants ages 6 to less than 12 months (see Table 5-6). However, because the amounts of these nutrients in the food package exceeded 100 percent of recommendations, the committee considered the need to decrease amounts of foods provided in the current infant packages and provide a more preferred form to promote intake.

Evaluation of Priority Food Groups and Potential Actions

The evaluation of priority food groups was based on DGA food patterns associated with particular calorie levels. Energy levels were selected based on calculated EERs for NHANES subgroups of pregnant, breastfeeding, and postpartum women, and for children as detailed in Appendix J. Inasmuch as the DGA are targeted to individuals ages 2 years and older, the committee provides an evaluation of food priorities for children ages 1 to less than 2 years and infants based on available AAP guidance (as described

TABLE 5-6 Nutrient Priorities and Preliminary Actions, Food Package II, Partially or Fully Breastfed Infants (Ages 6 to Less Than 12 Months)

		Amount per Day				
Nutrient	Rationale for Prioritization	EAR	Gap to Reduce Inadequacy to 5%[a]	Amount in the Food Package (% of the EAR)[b]	WIC Foods That Provide a Supplemental Amount of This Nutrient	Potential Action[c]
Iron	Inadequacy was 38%; Based on the committee's literature review, breastfed infants are at risk for low iron intakes	6.9 mg	4.8 mg	14.1–20.1 mg (204%–303%)	Infant cereal, infant food meat	Consider decreasing the amounts of infant food meat or infant cereals and providing a more preferred alternative
Zinc	Inadequacy was 44%; Based on the committee's literature review, breastfed infants are at risk for low zinc intakes	2.5 mg	2.0 mg	3.3–5.9 mg (132%–236%)	Infant cereal, infant food meat	Consider decreasing the amounts of infant food meat or infant cereals and providing a more preferred alternative

NOTES: EAR = Estimated Average Requirement.

[a] For nutrients with an EAR and inadequate intake, the gap is the difference between the EAR and the 5th percentile of intake; for nutrients with an AI and intake below the AI, the gap is the difference between the AI and the median intake. Complete results of the gap analysis are presented in Appendix L.

[b] Values represent the amounts in the partially and fully breastfed infant packages, respectively. The percent values assume that the food package is fully consumed.

[c] Translation of potential actions into the final food packages depended upon cost and other practical and administrative considerations.

SOURCES: IOM, 2001; USDA/ARS, 2011–2012.

in Chapter 3). Gap analyses were conducted for nutrients (see Tables 5-2 through 5-6), but not for food groups. This was because food pattern recommendations are set to meet the Recommended Dietary Allowance (RDA) values, which are set to meet the nutrient requirements of nearly all healthy individuals (IOM, 2000b). Therefore a gap analysis would result in food group intake gaps that are unnecessarily high relative to the goal to reduce the prevalence of nutrient inadequacies within a population (i.e., measured as intakes below the EAR).

Priority Food Groups Across Subgroups of Women

Across subgroups of women (see Tables 5-7 through 5-9), food groups of higher priority (75 percent or more of women consumed less than the recommended amount) included: dark green vegetables, total red and orange vegetables, beans and peas, other vegetables, whole grains, seafood, as well as nuts, seeds, and soy. The committee considered increasing the value of the CVV as a possible approach to addressing intakes of vegetables, including subgroups of vegetables.[3] Inasmuch as legumes and peanut butter are already provided in greater-than-supplemental amounts in most food packages, the quantities of these foods were a target for reduction along with nutrition education or behavioral approaches to improve intakes. The committee also considered increasing the amounts or types of whole grains and adding fish to food packages where it is not currently provided as possible approaches to addressing lower-than-recommended intakes of these food groups. There were no additional higher-priority food groups identified for pregnant women. Additional higher-priority food groups for partially breastfeeding, fully breastfeeding, and postpartum subgroups of women are described below.

Breastfeeding Women

Additional higher-priority food groups for breastfeeding women included total fruits, total starchy vegetables, total grains, and total protein foods (see Table 5-8). The committee considered increasing the value of the CVV as a means to increase intakes of fruits and providing a greater quantity and wider variety of grain options to increase intake of grains. For partially breastfeeding women, protein intake could be addressed by providing canned fish. For fully breastfeeding women, low total protein foods intakes could be addressed by including more preferred options or

[3] As described in Appendix U, it was not considered administratively feasible to provide a separate voucher for vegetables and for fruits.

TABLE 5-7 Food Group Priorities and Preliminary Actions, Food Package V, Pregnant Women

DGA Food Group	Identification in the DGA as a Food Group or Subgroup	Amount per Day: Rationale for Prioritization (% of WIC Women Consuming Less Than the Recommended Intake)	Amount per Day: DGA Recommendation[a]	Amount per Day: Food Package Contribution to the DGA Recommendation (%)[b]	WIC Foods That Provide a Supplemental Amount of This Food Group	Potential Action[d]
Higher Priority						
Whole grains	Subgroup	100	4.5 oz-eq/d	17	Bread and alternatives, breakfast cereal	Consider increasing whole grain allowance or adding grain options
Total vegetables	Group	99	3.5 c-eq/d	13	CVV	Consider increasing the CVV
Dark green vegetables	Subgroup	97	2.5 c-eq/wk	—[c]	CVV	Consider increasing the CVV
Total red and orange vegetables	Subgroup	97	7 c-eq/wk	—[c]	CVV	Consider increasing the CVV
Nuts, seeds, and soy	Subgroup	87	5 oz-eq/wk	168	Peanut butter	Consider reducing amount in the food package because it is more than supplemental
Other vegetables	Subgroup	83	5.5 c-eq/wk	—[c]	CVV	Consider increasing the CVV

continued

TABLE 5-7 Continued

DGA Food Group	Identification in the DGA as a Food Group or Subgroup	Amount per Day: Rationale for Prioritization (% of WIC Women Consuming Less Than the Recommended Intake)	Amount per Day: DGA Recommendation[a]	Amount per Day: Food Package Contribution to the DGA Recommendation (%)[b]	WIC Foods That Provide a Supplemental Amount of This Food Group	Potential Action[d]
Total dairy	Group	82	3 c-eq/d	98	Milk, cheese, yogurt	Consider additional yogurt substitution; amount in the food package is more than supplemental and could be reduced
Seafood	Subgroup	82; authoritative bodies recommend intake of fish varieties high in omega-3 and low in mercury during all life stages that affect development	10 oz-eq/wk	0	None	Consider adding canned fish
Beans and peas computed as vegetables	Subgroup	NA	2.5 c-eq/wk	71	Legumes	Consider providing canned options to promote intake of legumes

Lower Priority						
Total protein foods	Group	75	6.5 oz-eq/d	28	Milk and alternatives, cheese, eggs, legumes, and peanut butter	Consider adding canned fish
Total grains	Group	71	9 oz-eq/d	19	Bread and alternatives, breakfast cereal	Consider increasing whole grain allowance or adding grain options
Total fruit	Group	69	2 c-eq/d	52	CVV	Consider increasing the CVV
Total starchy vegetables	Subgroup	65	7 c-eq/wk	—[c]	CVV	Consider increasing the CVV
Whole fruit	Subgroup	64	1–2 c-eq/d	45	CVV	Consider increasing the CVV
Meat, poultry, and eggs (not seafood)	Subgroup	56	31 oz-eq/wk	9	Eggs	Consider additional eggs

NOTES: c-eq = cup-equivalents; CVV = cash value voucher; DGA = *Dietary Guidelines for Americans*; NA = data not available because too few survey respondents reported intake of the food group or subgroup to generate estimates of intake; oz-eq = ounce-equivalents.

[a] Based on a 2,600-kcal food pattern.

[b] Based on the same assumptions applied to develop Table 3-1 in Chapter 3.

[c] The quantity of vegetable subgroups provided by the CVV depends upon the participants' selection.

[d] Translation of potential actions into the final food packages depended upon cost and other practical and administrative considerations.

SOURCES: USDA/ARS, 2005–2012; USDA/HHS, 2016.

TABLE 5-8 Food Group Priorities and Preliminary Actions, Breastfeeding Women

DGA Food Group	Identification in the DGA as a Food Group or Subgroup	Rationale for Prioritization (% of WIC Women Consuming Less Than the Recommended Intake)	Amount per Day			WIC Foods That Provide a Supplemental Amount of This Food Group	Potential Action[e]
			DGA Recommendation[a]	Food Package V Contribution to the DGA Recommendation (%)[b]	Food Package VII Contribution to the DGA Recommendation (%)[c]		
				Higher Priority			
Whole grains	Subgroup	100	4.5 oz-eq/d	19	19	Bread and alternatives, breakfast cereal	Consider increasing whole grain allowance or adding grain options
Total red and orange vegetables	Subgroup	97	7 c-eq/wk	—[d]	—[d]	CVV	Consider increasing the CVV
Other vegetables	Subgroup	92	5.5 c-eq/wk	—[d]	—[d]	CVV	Consider increasing the CVV
Total grains	Group	88	9 oz-eq/d	19	19	Bread and alternatives, breakfast cereal	Consider increasing whole grain allowance or adding grain options

Total starchy vegetables	Subgroup	84	7 c-eq/wk	—[d]	—[d]	CVV	Consider increasing the CVV
Total fruit	Group	79	2 c-eq/d	52	52	CVV	Consider increasing the CVV
Total Protein foods	Group	76	6.5 oz-eq/d	28	50	Milk and alternatives, cheese, eggs, legumes and peanut butter	Consider additional options; nutrition intervention or behavioral interventions to promote intake of foods already provided
Dark green vegetables	Subgroup	NA	2.5 c-eq/wk	—[d]	—[d]	CVV	Consider increasing the CVV
Beans and peas computed as vegetables	Subgroup	NA	2.5 c-eq/wk	71	71	Legumes	Consider providing a canned option to promote intake of legumes
Seafood	Subgroup	NA	10 oz-eq/wk	0	70	None	Enhance nutrition education or use behavioral approaches
Nuts, seeds, and soy	Subgroup	NA	5 oz-eq/wk	168	168	Peanut butter	Consider reducing amount in the food package because it is more than supplemental

continued

TABLE 5-8 Continued

DGA Food Group	Identification in the DGA as a Food Group or Subgroup	Rationale for Prioritization (% of WIC Women Consuming Less Than the Recommended Intake)	Amount per Day: DGA Recommendation[a]	Amount per Day: Food Package V Contribution to the DGA Recommendation (%)[b]	Amount per Day: Food Package VII Contribution to the DGA Recommendation (%)[c]	WIC Foods That Provide a Supplemental Amount of This Food Group	Potential Action[e]
Lower Priority							
Whole fruit	Subgroup	79	1–2 c-eq/d	45	45	CVV	Consider increasing the CVV
Total dairy	Group	73	3 c-eq/d	98	119	Milk, cheese, yogurt	Consider additional yogurt substitution; amount in the food package is more than supplemental and could be reduced
Total vegetables	Group	50	3.5 c-eq/d	13	13	CVV	Consider increasing the CVV

NOTES: c-eq = cup-equivalents; CVV = cash value voucher; DGA = *Dietary Guidelines for Americans*; NA = data not available because too few survey respondents reported intake of the food group or subgroup to generate estimates of intake; oz-eq = ounce-equivalents.

[a] Based on a 2,600-kcal food pattern. The energy needs of partially breastfeeding women may be less.

[b] Based on the same assumptions applied to develop Table 3-1 in Chapter 3.

[c] Based on the same assumptions applied to develop Table 3-3 in Chapter 3.

[d] The quantity of vegetable subgroups provided by the CVV depends upon the participants' selection.

[e] Translation of potential actions into the final food packages depended upon cost and other practical and administrative considerations.

SOURCES: USDA/ARS, 2005–2012; USDA/HHS, 2016.

TABLE 5-9 Food Group Priorities and Preliminary Actions, Food Package VI, Postpartum Women

DGA Food Group	Identification in the DGA as a Food Group or Subgroup	Rationale for Prioritization (% of WIC Women Consuming Less Than the Recommended Intake)	Amount per Day: DGA Recommendation[a]	Amount per Day: Food Package Contribution to the DGA Recommendation (%)[b]	WIC Foods That Provide a Supplemental Amount of This Food Group	Potential Action[d]
Higher Priority						
Whole grains	Subgroup	100	3.75 oz-eq/d	6	Bread and alternatives, breakfast cereal	Consider increasing whole grain allowance or adding grain options
Total vegetables	Subgroup	100	3 c-eq/d	12	CVV	Consider increasing the CVV
Total starchy vegetables	Subgroup	99	6 c-eq/wk	—[c]	CVV	Consider increasing the CVV
Total dairy	Group	96	3 c-eq/d	71	Milk, cheese, yogurt	Consider additional yogurt substitution; amount in the food package is more than supplemental and could be reduced
Whole fruit	Subgroup	96	1–2 c-eq/d	45	CVV	Consider increasing the CVV
Total red and orange vegetables	Subgroup	94	6 c-eq/wk	—[c]	CVV	Consider increasing the CVV

continued

TABLE 5-9 Continued

DGA Food Group	Identification in the DGA as a Food Group or Subgroup	Rationale for Prioritization (% of WIC Women Consuming Less Than the Recommended Intake)	Amount per Day: DGA Recommendation[a]	Amount per Day: Food Package Contribution to the DGA Recommendation (%)[b]	WIC Foods That Provide a Supplemental Amount of This Food Group	Potential Action[d]
Nuts, seeds, and soy	Subgroup	91	5 oz-eq/wk	84	Peanut butter	Consider reducing amount in the food package because it is more than supplemental
Total fruit	Group	90	2 c-eq/d	42	CVV	Consider increasing the CVV
Dark green vegetables	Subgroup	89	2 c-eq/wk	—[c]	CVV	Consider increasing the CVV
Other vegetables	Subgroup	85	5 c-eq/wk	—[c]	CVV	Consider increasing the CVV
Beans and peas computed as vegetables	Subgroup	NA	2 c-eq/wk	44	Legumes	Consider providing canned option to promote intake of legumes
Seafood	Subgroup	NA	9.5 oz-eq/wk	0	None	Consider adding canned fish

Lower Priority						
Total protein foods	Group	75	6.25 oz-eq/d	20	Milk and alternatives, cheese, eggs, legumes, and peanut butter	Consider additional options (i.e., fish for partially breastfeeding women); nutrition intervention or behavioral interventions to promote intake of foods already provided
Total grains	Group	58	7.5 oz-eq/d	16	Bread and alternatives, breakfast cereal	Consider increasing whole grains or adding grain options
Meat, poultry, and eggs (not seafood)	Subgroup	54	29.5 oz-eq/wk	10	Eggs	Consider additional eggs

NOTES: c-eq = cup-equivalents; CVV = cash value voucher; DGA = *Dietary Guidelines for Americans*; NA = data not available because too few survey respondents reported intake of the food group or subgroup to generate estimates of intake; oz-eq = ounce-equivalents.

[a] Based on a 2,300-kcal food pattern.

[b] Based on the same assumptions applied to develop Table 3-2 in Chapter 3.

[c] The quantity of vegetable subgroups provided by the CVV depends upon the participants' selection.

[d] Translation of potential actions into the final food packages depended upon cost and other practical and administrative considerations.

SOURCES: USDA/ARS, 2005–2012; USDA/HHS, 2016.

through nutrition education or behavioral approaches to improving intake of protein foods currently provided.

Postpartum Women

For postpartum women, the committee also considered total fruit, total vegetable, and total starchy vegetable intakes to be higher-priority food groups (see Table 5-9). Increasing the value of the CVV would likely lead to improved intakes of these food groups. Dairy intakes were also below recommended amounts, which may be addressed by allowing options for more preferred forms of dairy in place of milk.

Children Ages 2 to Less Than 5 Years

Food groups and subgroups for which intakes were below recommended levels in more than 75 percent of children ages 2 to less than 5 years included total vegetables, dark green vegetables, total red and orange vegetables, whole grains, seafood, as well as nuts, seeds, and soy (see Table 5-10). The potential actions to address consumption of foods in these food groups were the same as those identified for subgroups of women.

Children Less Than 2 Years of Age and Infants

Although the DGA do not cover individuals ages 2 years and younger, the committee evaluated foods in the packages for these participants in Chapter 3. The amount of juice provided in food package IV-A (which is provided to children ages 1 to 2 years) exceeds the lower end of the AAP recommended limit 4 to 6 ounces per day (see Table 3-10), and a reduction could be considered. Food package II for fully breastfed infants ages 6 to less than 12 months provides 150 percent of the AAP recommended amount of infant cereal, and 130 percent of the recommended amount of jarred infant food meat. This information suggests that reductions in juice, infant cereal, and jarred infant food meat could be considered.

SUMMARY

This chapter describes the committee's decision tree (see Figure 5-1) and how it was used to identify potential changes to and actions for WIC food package revisions based on the committee's findings related to nutrition-related health risks, food safety, and nutrient and food intake among WIC participants. The current food packages were evaluated against the DRIs and the DGA. Packages for individuals less than 2 years of age were evaluated against the DRIs and guidance from AAP and other authorities. In

TABLE 5-10 Food Group Priorities and Preliminary Actions, Food Package IV, Children Ages 2 to Less Than 5 Years[a]

DGA Food Group	Identification in the DGA as a Food Group or Subgroup	Rationale for Prioritization (% of WIC-Participating Children Consuming Less Than the Recommended Intake)	Amount per Day		WIC Foods That Provide a Supplemental Amount of This Food Group	Potential Action[e]
			DGA Recommendation[b]	Food Package Contribution to the DGA Recommendation (%)[c]		
Higher Priority						
Seafood	Subgroup	100	5 oz-eq/wk	0	None	Consider adding canned fish
Total vegetables	Group	99	1.5 c-eq/d	19	CVV	Consider increasing the CVV
Dark green vegetables	Subgroup	94	1 c-eq/wk	—[d]	CVV	Consider increasing the CVV
Whole grains	Subgroup	93	2.25 oz-eq/d	58	Bread and alternatives, breakfast cereal	Consider increasing whole grain allowance or adding grain options
Total red and orange vegetables	Subgroup	90	3 c-eq/wk	—[d]	CVV	Consider increasing the CVV
Nuts, seeds, and soy	Subgroup	77	2.5 oz-eq/wk	167	Peanut butter	Consider reducing amount in the food package because it is more than supplemental

continued

TABLE 5-10 Continued

DGA Food Group	Identification in the DGA as a Food Group or Subgroup	Rationale for Prioritization (% of WIC-Participating Children Consuming Less Than the Recommended Intake)	Amount per Day		WIC Foods That Provide a Supplemental Amount of This Food Group	Potential Action[e]
			DGA Recommendation[b]	Food Package Contribution to the DGA Recommendation (%)[c]		
			Lower Priority			
Total starchy vegetables	Subgroup	73	3.5 c-eq/wk	—[d]	CVV	Consider increasing the CVV
Other vegetables	Subgroup	73	2.5 c-eq/wk	—[d]	CVV	Consider increasing the CVV
Total dairy	Group	73	2.5 c-eq/d	85	Milk, cheese, yogurt	Consider increasing the yogurt substitution; enhance nutrition education or use behavioral approaches to promote intake of milk already provided in the food package
Total protein foods	Group	68	3.5 oz-eq/d	29	Milk and alternatives, cheese, eggs, legumes and peanut butter	Consider adding canned fish

Beans and peas computed as vegetables	Subgroup	59	0.5 c-eq/wk	177	Legumes	Consider reducing amount in the food package because it is more than supplemental and providing canned option to promote intake of legumes

NOTES: c-eq = cup-equivalents; CVV = cash value voucher; DGA = *Dietary Guidelines for Americans*; oz-eq = ounce-equivalents.
[a] Data are specific to children 2 to less than 5 years of age because the DGA apply only to individuals ages 2 years and older.
[b] Based on a 1,300-kcal food pattern.
[c] Based on the same assumptions applied to develop Table 3-4 in Chapter 3.
[d] The quantity of vegetable subgroups provided by the CVV depends upon the participants' selection.
[e] Translation of potential actions into the final food packages depended upon cost and other practical and administrative considerations.
SOURCES: USDA/ARS, 2011–2012; USDA/HHS, 2016.

many cases, the current food packages provide more than a supplemental amount of a nutrient or food group or even provide more than 100 percent of recommended intakes of a nutrient or food group. As a result of the diversity of nutrients that can be provided through the CVV, the committee considered it important to increase this component of the food packages in cases of nutrient intake shortfalls. In other cases, the committee considered that an alternative form of a food (e.g., yogurt as a substitute for milk, canned legumes instead of dry legumes) could be a useful means of promoting consumption of foods already included in the packages. The committee considered fish as a possible addition to the food packages, both because seafood intakes are below recommended amounts and because fish is currently provided in only one food package. These priorities were considered simultaneously with costs and administrative factors to produce actionable revisions to the food packages. For this reason, not all of the proposed actions identified in this chapter resulted in a corresponding change to a food package. In the next chapter, the committee used the potential actions outlined in Tables 5-2 through 5-10 to develop its recommended revisions to the WIC food packages. Proposed changes and the rationale for each are described in detail.

REFERENCES

AAP (American Academy of Pediatrics). 2014. *Pediatric nutrition*. 7th ed. Edited by R. E. Kleinman and F. R. Greer. Elk Grove Village, IL: American Academy of Pediatrics.

AAPD (American Academy of Pediatric Dentistry). 2012. Policy on dietary recommendations for infants, children, and adolescents. *Pediatric Dentistry* 30(7 Suppl):47–48.

Dhar, R., and K. Wertenbroch. 2000. Consumer choice between hedonic and utilitarian goods. *Journal of Marketing Research* 37(1):60–71.

IOM (Institute of Medicine). 1998. *Dietary Reference Intakes for thiamin, riboflavin, niacin, vitamin B6, folate, vitamin B12, pantothenic acid, biotin, and choline*. Washington, DC: National Academy Press.

IOM. 2000a. *Dietary Reference Intakes for vitamin C, vitamin E, selenium, and carotenoids*. Washington, DC: National Academy Press.

IOM. 2000b. *Dietary Reference Intakes: Applications in dietary assessment*. Washington, DC: National Academy Press.

IOM. 2001. *Dietary Reference Intakes for vitamin A, vitamin K, arsenic, boron, chromium, copper, iodine, iron, manganese, molybdenum, nickel, silicon, vanadium, and zinc*. Washington, DC: National Academy Press.

IOM. 2002/2005. *Dietary Reference Intakes for energy, carbohydrate, fiber, fat, fatty acids, cholesterol, protein and amino acids*. Washington, DC: The National Academies Press.

IOM. 2005. *Dietary Reference Intakes for water, potassium, sodium, chloride, and sulfate*. Washington, DC: The National Academies Press.

IOM. 2006. *WIC food packages: Time for a change*. Washington, DC: The National Academies Press.

IOM. 2011. *Dietary Reference Intakes for calcium and vitamin D*. Washington, DC: The National Academies Press.

Kahneman, D., and A. Tversky. 1984. Choices, values, and frames. *American Psychologist* 39(4):341–350.

Loewenstein, G. F. 1988. Frames of mind in intertemporal choice. *Management Science* 34(2):200–214.

NASEM (National Academies of Sciences, Engineering, and Medicine). 2016. *Review of WIC food packages: Proposed framework for revisions: Interim report.* Washington, DC: The National Academies Press. doi: 10.17226/21832.

USDA/ARS (U.S. Department of Agriculture/Agricultural Research Service). 2005–2012. *What we eat in America, NHANES 2005–2012.* Beltsville, MD: USDA/ARS. http://www.cdc.gov/nchs/nhanes/wweia.htm (accessed December 21, 2016).

USDA/ARS. 2011–2012. *What we eat in America, NHANES 2011–2012.* Beltsville, MD: USDA/ARS. http://www.ars.usda.gov/services/docs.htm?docid=13793 (accessed December 21, 2016).

USDA/ERS (U.S. Department of Agriculture/Economic Research Service). 2007. *Could behavioral economics help improve diet quality for nutrition assistance program participants?* Beltsville, MD: USDA/ERS. http://ben.cornell.edu/pdfs/USDA-BeEcon.pdf (accessed December 21, 2016).

USDA/FNS (U.S. Department of Agriculture/Food and Nutrition Research Service). 2007. *Special Supplemental Nutrition Program for Women, Infants and Children (WIC): Revisions in the WIC food packages.* Interim Rule, 7 C.F.R. § 246.

USDA/FNS. 2016. *WIC works resource system: Nutrition education.* https://wicworks.fns.usda.gov/nutrition-education (accessed August 30, 2016).

USDA/HHS (U.S. Department of Agriculture/U.S. Department of Health and Human Services). 2016. *Dietary Guidelines for Americans 2015.* Washington, DC: U.S. Government Printing Office. https://health.gov/dietaryguidelines/2015 (accessed August 29, 2016).

6

The Revised Food Packages

In this chapter, the committee's recommendations for the Special Supplemental Nutrition Program for Women, Infants, and Children (WIC) food package changes are described. The chapter begins with a review of the committee's overarching strategy for making food package changes. Then, proposed changes to all food packages for women, infants, and children are reviewed along with the rationale for each change. Women and children are covered first, followed by infants, because the rationale for many of the changes is similar for the foods in packages for women and children. Next, a brief discussion on proposed changes to food package III is presented. Finally, proposed changes to specifications for WIC-eligible foods are reviewed. The revised food packages based on all proposed changes are presented in Tables 6-1 and 6-2,[1] and specifications for WIC foods are presented in Table 6-4. The changes proposed herein are evaluated against the committee's seven criteria in Chapter 9 and recommendations for implementation and research to evaluate the changes proposed are described in Chapter 11. Chapter 10 presents the projected cost effects of the revised food packages over the long term.

THE COMMITTEE'S OVERARCHING STRATEGY

The committee's overarching strategy for revisions, as articulated in Chapter 1, combined the iterative process illustrated in Figure 1-1 with

[1] Unless otherwise indicated, use of the word *revised* in this chapter refers to the revisions proposed in this report, not revisions that occurred in 2009.

the criteria included in Box 1-4. In particular, the committee sought to fulfill its task to align the WIC food packages with the 2015–2020 *Dietary Guidelines for Americans* (DGA) by designing packages that were balanced across the food groups and supplemental in amount. Possible revisions to the food packages were identified systematically with the use of the decision tree described in Chapter 5. Within this process, the committee also recognized a number of other factors relevant to the revisions. The factors included the following:

- The value of the food packages to the mother–infant dyad
- The flexibility of the cash value voucher (CVV) and its potential value to participants
- The need for additional seafood in the packages because of the importance of this food subgroup and the nutrients it contains to specific stages of development present in the WIC-participating population
- Participant food preferences (both cultural and personal)
- Constraints to changing foods in the packages related to the foods in the marketplace, the capacity of the vendors who provided foods to participants,[2] and administrative issues at the state level

Final adjustments were made in an iterative fashion within the constraints of cost neutrality. Many comments were submitted to and reviewed by the committee, both supporting the foods in the current packages and requesting a change to the amounts or types of foods. These were considered in conjunction with the evidence presented below.

The Concept of Supplemental

The WIC program is designed to supplement participants' diets without regard to whether these diets contain contributions from other federal (e.g., Supplemental Nutrition Assistance Program [SNAP]) or nonfederal programs (e.g., local food pantries). Determination of what a supplement to the diet should contain requires knowledge of participants' diets and how well their diets meet both nutrient requirements and intakes of recommended food groups, as described in Chapters 4 and 5. The committee began by considering the meaning of the word *supplemental*, which is part of the full name of the WIC program, namely the Special Supplemental Food Program for Women, Infants, and Children. Although the U.S. Department of Agriculture's Food and Nutrition Service (USDA-FNS) adheres to a definition of the term "supplemental," as described in Chapter 1, additional specificity

[2] The term *vendor* in this document refers to stores or retailers.

was needed to guide the committee's actions. To provide this specificity, the committee noted that the current food packages provide widely varying proportions of required nutrients (between 5 and 400 percent of the Dietary Reference Intake [DRI]) and recommended food groups (between 0 and 177 percent of recommended intakes). The committee observed that a better balance among these proportions would permit the committee to align the food packages more adequately with the DGA. Given this observation, the committee developed the following guidance for designing food packages that supplement the diet:

- Inasmuch as WIC participants (other than formula-fed infants in the first 6 months of life for whom 100 percent of needs is provided) consume foods and beverages not supplied by the WIC food packages that meet some portion of their nutrient needs or recommended amounts of food groups, the amounts of nutrients and food groups in the WIC packages should provide a moderate proportion of an individual's requirement for a particular nutrient or recommended amount of a food group.
- The supplementation target (i.e. proportion of requirement or recommended amount in the food package) may differ depending on the prioritization of the nutrient or food group (as described in Chapter 5) and the degree to which foods appropriate for the food packages and available in the marketplace could supply these amounts.
- Some accommodation for food preferences or cultural suitability would be considered acceptable.

Finally, the committee considered that food patterns are intended to be achieved over a period of time, and to serve as a framework from which individuals may choose foods to meet preferences and cultural needs (personal communication, T. E. Schap, USDA Center for Nutrition Policy and Promotion, May 10, 2016). As a result of the constraint to produce a set of cost-neutral food packages and other limitations to this process noted briefly in Chapter 1, the committee was not able to provide a moderate proportion of recommended intakes of all nutrients and food groups and subgroups.

THE REVISED FOOD PACKAGES FOR WOMEN AND CHILDREN

This section summarizes the committee's proposed changes to the food packages for women and children along with the supporting rationale for each change. The revised food packages based on these changes are presented in Table 6-1 (mother–infant dyad) and Table 6-2 (children and pregnant women). Inasmuch as what new mothers need (or do not need)

TABLE 6-1 The Revised WIC Food Packages: Maximum Monthly Allowances[a] Presented as the Benefits to the Mother–Infant Dyad in Food Packages I, II, III, V-B, VI, and VII

	Fully Breastfeeding Dyad		Partially (Mostly) Breastfeeding Dyad		Formula-Feeding Dyad	
WIC Food Categories	Infants 0 to 5 Months (FP I or III[b])	Infants 6 to 11 Months (FP II or III[b])	Infants 0 to 5 Months (FP I or III[b])	Infants 6 to 11 Months (FP II or III[b])	Infants 0 to 5 Months (FP I or III[b])	Infants 6 to 11 Months (FP II or III[b])
For Infants						
Formula[c]	—	—	0 to 3 months: up to 364 fl oz[d,e] 4 to 5 months: up to 442 fl oz[d,e]	Up to 312 fl oz[d,e]	0 to 3 months: up to 806 fl oz[d,e] 4 to 5 months: up to 884 fl oz[d,e]	Up to 624 fl oz[d,e]
Infant cereal	—	16 oz	—	8 oz	—	8 oz
Infant food vegetables and fruits	—	128 oz or 64 oz and $10 CVV or 0 oz and $20 CVV[f]	—	128 oz or 64 oz and $10 CVV or 0 oz and $20 CVV[f]	—	128 oz or 64 oz and $10 CVV or 0 oz and $20 CVV[f]
Infant food meats	—	40 oz[g]	—	—	—	—
For Women	Fully Breastfeeding Women (FP VII)[h,i]		Partially (Mostly) Breastfeeding Women (FP V-B)[j]		Postpartum Women (FP VI)	
Vegetables and fruits[k]	$35 CVV		$25 CVV		$15 CVV	No foods are provided to women after 6 months postpartum

Legumes[l,m]	2 lb every 3 months	2 lb every 3 months	2 lb every 3 months
Juice	64 fl oz[n]	64 fl oz[n]	—
Dairy (milk)	16 qt[o,p,q,r]	16 qt[o,p,q,r]	16 qt[o,p,q,r]
Breakfast cereal[s]	36 oz	36 oz	36 oz
Whole grains[t]	16 to 24 oz	16 to 24 oz	—
Peanut butter[m]	16 to 18 oz every 3 months	16 to 18 oz every 3 months	16 to 18 oz every 3 months
Eggs[u]	2 dozen	1 dozen	1 dozen
Fish	60 oz every 3 months	30 oz every 3 months	10 oz every 3 months

NOTES: — = the WIC food category is not authorized in the corresponding food package; CVV = cash value voucher; FP = food package. See Table 6-4 for details related to WIC food specifications.

[a] Amounts presented are maximum monthly amounts, except where specified and for infant formula. Legumes, peanut butter, and fish are to be provided in a rotation, with states deciding on the best way to program the rotation given the flexibility of their individual Management Information Systems.

[b] Food package III is issued to participants with qualifying medical conditions. A WIC formula is issued to participants receiving food package III under the direction of a health care provider. Women who are issued food package III may receive up to 455 fl oz of a WIC formula, as deemed appropriate by a health care provider. Women who require jarred vegetables and fruits may be issued the following amounts corresponding to the value of the CVV: 94 oz, 23 4-oz jars, or 27 3.5 oz packages for the $15 CVV; 156 oz, 39 4-oz jars, or 45 3.5 oz packages for the $25 CVV; 219 oz, 55 4-oz jars, or 63 3.5 oz packages for the $35 CVV. If the participant chooses to substitute juice with an additional $3 in CVV, 5 additional 4-oz jars or 3.5-oz packages may be issued.

[c] WIC formula means infant formula, exempt infant formula, or WIC-eligible nutritionals. Infant formula may be issued for infants in food packages I, II, and III. In food package III, medical documentation is required for issuance of infant formula, exempt infant formula, WIC-eligible nutritionals, and other foods. Numbers indicate the full nutrition benefit, defined as the minimum amount of reconstituted fluid ounces of liquid concentrate infant formula as specified for each infant food package category and feeding variation.

continued

TABLE 6-1 Continued

[d] Amounts represent the full nutrition benefit, defined as the minimum amount of reconstituted fluid ounces of liquid concentrate infant formula as specified for each infant food package category and feeding variation. The corresponding maximum monthly allowance amounts that account for the form of formula are unchanged from those presented in the Final Rule. Infant formula amounts for all infants should be individually tailored to the amounts that meet their nutritional needs.

[e] Following a detailed assessment of the needs of the dyad by WIC staff, infants may be issued the quantity of formula needed to support any level of breastfeeding, up to the full nutrition benefit.

[f] Depending upon the amount of infant food vegetables and fruits selected for food package II for infants, $0, $10 or $20 can be substituted. The infant CVV may be used to purchase fresh, canned, or frozen vegetables and fruits, meeting the WIC specifications for these foods.

[g] Participants may substitute 10 oz of jarred infant food meat with 10 oz of canned fish meeting WIC specifications for this food category.

[h] Food package VII is issued to three categories of WIC participants: fully breastfeeding women whose infants do not receive formula from the WIC program; women partially (mostly) breastfeeding multiple infants from the same pregnancy; and pregnant women who are also fully or partially (mostly) breastfeeding singleton infants.

[i] Women fully breastfeeding multiple infants from the same pregnancy are prescribed 1.5 times food package VII.

[j] Food package V-B is issued to two categories of WIC participants: breastfeeding women participants whose partially (mostly) breastfed infants receive formula from the WIC program in amounts that do not exceed the maximum formula allowances, as appropriate for the age of the infant as described in this table, and women pregnant with two or more fetuses.

[k] State agencies must authorize fresh and at least one nonfresh (canned fruit, canned vegetables, frozen fruit, frozen vegetables, dried fruit, and/or dried vegetables) variety each of vegetables and fruits. The CVV may be redeemed for any eligible fruit and vegetable. Vendors are required to stock at least three varieties of vegetables and two varieties of fruits.

[l] States are required to offer both dry legumes and canned legumes. Two lb of dry legumes or 128 oz (eight 15–16 oz cans) of canned legumes are provided in food packages V-B, VI, and VII once every 3 months.

[m] Legumes and peanut butter must be provided and are not interchangeable. Participants may be issued legumes in place of peanut butter in the case of a peanut allergy.

[n] Participants may select a $3 addition to the CVV in place of juice.

[o] Low-fat (1%) or nonfat milks are the standard milk for issuance to women. Reduced fat (2%) milk is authorized only for participants with certain conditions, including but not limited to, underweight and maternal weight loss during pregnancy. The need for reduced-fat (2%) milk must be based on an individual nutritional assessment as established by state agency policy.

[p] Evaporated milk may be substituted at the rate of 16 fl oz of evaporated milk per 32 fl oz of fluid milk or a 1:2 fl oz substitution ratio. Dry milk may be substituted at an equal reconstituted rate to fluid milk.

[q] For women receiving food packages V-B and VI, two substitution options are available for milk: (1) 1 lb of cheese and 1 qt of yogurt (30–32 oz are allowed at the discretion of the state agency) may substitute for 4 qt of milk or (2) 2 qt of yogurt may substitute for 2 qt of milk. Women receiving food package VII also have a third option of 2 lb of cheese substituting for 6 qt of milk. Low-fat or nonfat yogurts are the only types of yogurt authorized for women. Soy-based yogurt or soy-based cheese substitutes are authorized yogurt and cheese options for individuals with a milk allergy, lactose intolerance, or who consume a vegan diet.

[r] For women, soy-based beverage may be substituted for milk on a quart-for-quart basis up to the total maximum allowance of milk. Tofu may be substituted for milk at the rate of 1 lb of tofu per 1 qt of milk. Additional amounts of tofu may be substituted, up to the maximum allowances for fluid milk, for lactose intolerance or other reasons, as established by state agency policy.

[s] All breakfast cereals on the state agency's authorized food list must meet the whole grain-rich criteria as described in Table 6-4.

[t] Whole wheat bread must be authorized. State agencies have the option to also authorize brown rice, bulgur, oatmeal, whole grain barley, cornmeal (including blue), corn masa flour, whole wheat macaroni (pasta) products, soft corn or whole wheat tortillas, buckwheat, or teff in the range specified.

[u] A substitution of dry legumes (1 lb) or canned legumes (64 oz or four 15–16 oz cans) for each 1 dozen eggs is permitted for individuals with an egg allergy or who consume a vegan diet.

SOURCE: Modified to reflect the revised food packages from 7 C.F.R. § 246 (USDA/FNS, 2014).

TABLE 6-2 The Revised WIC Food Packages: Maximum Monthly Allowances[a] Presented as the Benefits to Children and Pregnant Women in Food Packages IV, V-A, and III

WIC Food Category	Children 1 to Less Than 2 Years (FP IV-A)	Children 2 to Less Than 5 Years (FP IV-B)	Pregnant Women (FP V-A)[b]	Special Dietary Needs (FP III)[c]
WIC formula	—	—	—	Up to 455 fl oz of liquid concentrate, if appropriate
Vegetables and fruits[d]	$12.00 CVV	$12.00 CVV	$15.00 CVV	Other foods in food packages IV and V-A are provided as appropriate
Legumes[e,f]	1 lb every 3 months	1 lb every 3 months	2 lb every 3 months	
Juice	64 fl oz[g]	64 fl oz[g]	64 fl oz[g]	
Dairy (milk)	12 qt[h,i,j,k,l]	14 qt[i,k,l,m]	16 qt[k,m,n,o]	
Breakfast cereal[p]	36 oz	36 oz	36 oz	
Whole grains[q]	16–24 oz	16–24 oz	16–24 oz	
Peanut butter[f]	16–18 oz every 3 months	16–18 oz every 3 months	16–18 oz every 3 months	
Eggs[r]	1 dozen	1 dozen	1 dozen	
Fish	10 oz every 3 months	10 oz every 3 months	10 oz every 3 months	

NOTES: — = the food is not authorized in the corresponding food package; CVV = cash value voucher; FP = food package. See Table 6-4 for details related to WIC food specifications.

[a] Amounts are monthly except where indicated. Legumes, peanut butter, and fish are to be provided in a rotation, with states deciding on the best way to program the rotation given the flexibility of their individual Management Information Systems.

[b] Food package V-A is issued to women participants with singleton pregnancies.

[c] Food package III is issued to participants with qualifying medical conditions. A WIC formula is issued to participants receiving food package III under the direction of a health care provider. Participants that are issued food package III may receive up to 455 fl oz of a WIC formula (liquid concentrate), as deemed appropriate by a health care provider. WIC formula means infant formula, exempt infant formula, or WIC-eligible nutritionals. Powder and ready-to-feed may be substituted at rates that provide comparable nutritive value. The number of fl oz of formula refers to the amount as prepared according to directions on the container. Children or women who require jarred vegetables and fruits may be issued the following amounts

corresponding to the value of the CVV: 75 oz, 19 4-oz jars, or 21 3.5-oz packages for the $12 CVV, or 94 oz, 23 4-oz jars, or 27 3.5-oz packages for the $15 CVV. If the participant chooses to substitute juice with an additional $3 in CVV, 5 additional 4-oz jars or 3.5-oz packages may be issued.

[d] State agencies must authorize fresh and one nonfresh (canned fruit, canned vegetables, frozen fruit, frozen vegetables, dried fruit, and/or dried vegetables) variety each of vegetables and fruits. The CVV may be redeemed for any eligible vegetable and fruit. Vendors are required to stock at least three varieties of vegetables and two varieties of fruits.

[e] States are required to offer both dry legumes (1-lb) and canned legumes (64 oz or four 15 to 16-oz cans). Legumes are provided once per quarter; 1 lb in food packages IV-A and IV-B and 2 lb in food packages V-A and VI.

[f] Legumes and peanut butter must be provided and are not interchangeable. Participants may be issued legumes in place of peanut butter in the case of a peanut allergy.

[g] Participants may select a $3 addition to the CVV in place of juice.

[h] Whole milk is the standard milk for issuance to 1-year-old children (12 through 23 months). At state agency option, reduced fat milks may be issued to 1-year-old children for whom overweight or obesity is a concern. The need for reduced fat milks for 1-year-old children must be based on an individual nutritional assessment and consultation with the child's health care provider if necessary, as established by state agency policy.

[i] Children receiving food package IV-A or IV-B may substitute 1 lb of cheese and 1 qt of yogurt (30–32 oz are allowed at the discretion of the state agency) for 4 qt of milk, or 2 qt of yogurt for 2 qt of milk.

[j] At state agency option, low-fat or nonfat yogurt may be issued to 1-year-old children for whom overweight and obesity is a concern. The need for low-fat or nonfat yogurt for 1-year-old children must be based on an individual nutritional assessment and consultation with the child's health care provider if necessary, as established by state agency policy.

[k] Evaporated milk may be substituted at the rate of 16 fl oz of evaporated milk per 32 fl oz of fluid milk or a 1:2 fl oz substitution ratio. Dry milk may be substituted at an equal reconstituted rate to fluid milk.

[l] For children, issuance of tofu and soy-based beverage as substitutes for milk must be based on an individual nutritional assessment and consultation with the participant's health care provider if necessary, as established by State agency policy. Such determination can be made for situations that include, but are not limited to, milk allergy, lactose intolerance, and vegan diets. Soy-based beverage may be substituted for milk for children on a quart-for-quart basis up to the total maximum allowance of milk. Tofu may be substituted for milk for children at the rate of 1 lb of tofu per 1 qt of milk.

[m] Low-fat (1%) or nonfat milks are the standard milk for issuance to children ≥24 months of age and women. Reduced fat (2%) milk is authorized only for participants with certain conditions including, but not limited to, underweight and maternal weight loss during pregnancy. The need for reduced fat (2%) milk must be based on an individual nutritional assessment as established by state agency policy. Soy-based yogurt or soy-based cheese substitutes are authorized yogurt and cheese options for individuals with a milk allergy or who consume a vegan diet.

[n] Women receiving food package V-A, may substitute 1 lb of cheese and 1 qt of yogurt for 4 qt of milk or 2 qt of yogurt for 2 qt of milk.

continued

TABLE 6-2 Continued

[o] For women, soy-based beverage may be substituted for milk on a quart-for-quart basis up to the total maximum allowance of milk. Tofu may be substituted for milk at the rate of 1 lb of tofu per 1 qt of milk. Additional amounts of tofu may be substituted, up to the maximum allowances for fluid milk, for lactose intolerance or other reasons, as established by state agency policy.

[p] All breakfast cereals on the state agency's authorized food list must meet the whole grain-rich criteria as described in Table 6-4.

[q] Whole wheat bread must be authorized. State agencies have the option to also authorize brown rice, bulgur, oatmeal, whole grain barley, cornmeal (including blue), corn masa flour, whole wheat macaroni (pasta) products, soft corn or whole-wheat tortillas, buckwheat, or teff in the range specified.

[r] A substitution of dry legumes (1 lb) or canned legumes (64 oz or four 15–16 oz cans) for each 1 dozen eggs is permitted for individuals with an egg allergy or who consume a vegan diet.

SOURCE: Modified to reflect the revised food packages from 7 C.F.R. § 246 (USDA/FNS, 2014).

nutritionally depends on how their infants are fed, the committee concluded that it would be most appropriate to consider the mother–infant dyads (breastfeeding mother and her breastfed infant as well as the postpartum mother and her formula-fed infant) together. In designing these dyadic packages, the committee considered nutritional needs (see Chapter 4, and nutrient comparison tables in Appendix T) and costs (see Chapter 7), as prescribed and as redeemed, in the current packages as well as in the revised packages.

Overall, the structure of the revised food packages is essentially the same, except that currently food package V is now divided to provide foods specifically for pregnant (food package V-A) and partially breastfeeding women (food package V-B). Side-by-side comparisons of the current and revised food packages are presented in Appendix N, Tables N-3 through N-7.

The Cash Value Voucher Is Increased as Much as Possible Within Cost-Neutral Constraints

Overall Increases in the CVV

WIC is a source of access to vegetables and fruits for low-income women. Yet, evidence indicates that WIC and SNAP benefits combined may be inadequate for low-income pregnant women to have a steady supply of vegetables and fruits throughout the month (Hromi-Fiedler et al., 2016).[3] Given the current CVV of $8 for children and $11 for women, there is substantial room to improve the extent to which the food packages provide supplemental amounts of vegetables and whole fruits. These current amounts permit participants to purchase less than one cup-equivalent of vegetables or fruits per day. Based on the committee's composite cost for vegetables and fruits most commonly purchased among WIC participants,[4] $23, $41, or $45 would be required for individuals who consumed a 1,300-, 2,300-, or 2,600-kcal diet, respectively, to meet half of the recommended intakes of vegetables and fruits. The committee increased the CVV across food packages to the extent possible within cost-neutral restrictions (see Tables 6-1 and 6-2).

The CVV not only provides participants with access to two food groups

---

[3] Hromi-Fiedler et al. (2016) reported that of 45 pregnant Latino women surveyed (78 percent and 64 percent of whom benefitted from WIC and SNAP, respectively), some had difficulty maintaining the desired level of vegetables and fruits in the household over the course of the month, considering other food needs, accessibility, and affordability.

[4] The fruit and vegetable composite ($0.55 per cup-equivalent) applied in this report considered the vegetables and fruits most commonly purchased by WIC participants in Massachusetts, Texas, and Wyoming.

(vegetables and fruits) for which intakes were below recommended amounts across several population subgroups (see Chapter 5), but it is also the component of the food packages that offers participants the most flexibility to meet their cultural needs. Evidence indicates that preferences for vegetables and fruits vary among WIC participants depending upon race, ethnicity, and geographic region of origin (Di Noia et al., 2016). Additionally, the CVV may help to increase dietary variety, which has been associated with improved diet quality (Arimond and Ruel, 2004).

The committee recognizes that WIC participants have the option to purchase either vegetables, fruits, or a combination of both. Available redemption data (from two states) indicate that the CVV is more commonly used to purchase fruits (67 percent of voucher dollars) than vegetables (33 percent of voucher dollars). Inasmuch as individuals already purchase both vegetables and fruits, the increase in benefit is predicted to enhance the amount of vegetables purchased and may be more effective in doing so with enhanced attention to nutrition education about the selection and preparation of vegetables (see the discussion on nutrition education in Chapter 11).

At Least Two Forms of Vegetables and Fruits Can Be Purchased with the CVV for Women, Infants, or Children

As outlined in the March 2014 Final Rule, states are currently required to authorize fresh vegetables and fruits and may also authorize canned, frozen, or dried forms (USDA/FNS, 2014). At the time of this writing, 10 states offered only fresh forms of vegetables and fruits (USDA/FNS, 2015a). Given the increase in the CVV across food packages in the revised packages, states must authorize at least two forms of vegetables and two forms of fruits: fresh and at least one additional form (frozen, canned, or dried). Limiting participants' options to fresh-only may compromise available options seasonally and in certain geographic regions. Fresh, frozen, or canned forms of vegetables and fruits offer similar nutritional benefits. In some cases, processing may preserve nutrients that would otherwise be lost (Rickman et al., 2007; USDA/HHS, 2010; HHS, 2011; Miller and Knudsen, 2014; PBHF, 2016). Vegetables and fruits preserved through canning, freezing, or drying are also less perishable, thereby adding convenience. Additionally, in some cases, canned or frozen vegetables and fruits may be more economical than fresh (Miller and Knudsen, 2014; USDA/ERS, 2016), thereby increasing the purchasing power of the CVV. Although the sodium content of canned vegetables may be higher than that of other forms, canned vegetables can be prepared in ways that reduce sodium content (CFA, 2016).

The committee recognizes that state agencies that do not currently allow canned, frozen, or dried vegetables and fruits will need to ensure that vendors have electronic benefit card (EBT)–linked Universal Product Codes (UPCs) (i.e., for new WIC-eligible canned, frozen, or dried vegetables and fruits). The USDA-FNS effort to develop a more comprehensive national UPC database (USDA/FNS, 2016a) should facilitate state efforts to meet requirements to stock new or additional products.

Vendors Are Required to Stock at Least Three Varieties of Vegetables and Two Varieties of Fruits

The current regulations require vendors to stock at least two varieties of vegetables and two varieties of fruits. Given the increased value of the CVV, the higher ratio of fruits (67 percent) that are purchased compared to vegetables (33 percent), and the low intakes of vegetables (particularly in contrast to fruits) in all WIC-participating subgroups, the committee decided that weighting the stocking requirements in favor of vegetables is a strategy that may facilitate participant purchase of vegetables over fruits.

Legumes and Peanut Butter Are Reduced to Supplemental Amounts and Are Not Interchangeable

In the current food packages, children and postpartum women may choose between legumes or peanut butter on a monthly basis. For other participants, both are provided on a monthly basis. In the revised food packages, peanut butter and beans are provided to all participants in a 3-month rotation.[5] The intention of the rotation is to provide a better balance of food groups within cost-constraints. The committee envisions that states would decide on the best way to program the rotation, given the flexibility of their individual Management Information Systems.

Legumes

The amount of legumes in the current food packages for children provides 177 percent of recommended amounts of beans and peas, and for women between 44 and 71 percent of recommended amounts (see Chapter 3, Tables 3-1 through 3-4). Legumes are key sources of several nutrients (i.e., potassium, fiber, and folate) for which intakes were found by the committee to be below recommended amounts in several WIC participant subgroups. Therefore, legumes are a valuable component of the WIC food packages. However, to align with the criterion of supplemental, the committee reduced the amounts provided in the revised food packages for

[5] Fish is the third component in the rotation, as described later in this chapter.

children and equalized the amounts provided for women. The reduction in legumes (which are not highly redeemed) increases the funds available for the CVV, one of the most highly redeemed "foods" in the packages which may also serve as a source of vegetables. For children and postpartum women who currently choose peanut butter over legumes, the revised package provides both foods on a regular basis (therefore, legumes may actually be increased for some individuals). Legumes are now provided once every 3 months to all children and women (food packages IV, V-A, V-B, VI, and VII). Children are issued 1 pound of dry legumes (or four 15–16 ounce cans) and women are issued 2 pounds of dry legumes (or eight 15–16 ounce cans). The revised food packages for children still provide 120 percent of recommended amounts because package sizes prohibit reasonable further reductions (see Appendix T). For women, the revision brings the amount provided closer to what is considered supplemental: between 47 and 59 percent of the DGA recommended amount.

Offering Options for Both Dried and Canned Legumes

At present, states may authorize either dried and/or canned legumes. Although dried legumes are more commonly used in some cultures, they require significantly more preparation time, which may serve as a barrier to consumption of legumes for some WIC participants. In the revised packages, states are required to offer both dried and canned legumes in all packages as a way to promote both redemption and consumption. Canned legumes are more convenient because they are essentially ready-to-eat. Dry legumes should still be offered for those with a preference (cultural or personal) for this product, and to offer an easier-to-carry option.

According to the 2015 Food Policy Options report, 85 percent of WIC state agencies have already authorized canned legumes (USDA/FNS, 2015a). Therefore, the committee considered this change to be administratively feasible. Although the mandates to provide canned legumes (as well as processed vegetables and fruits) increase the administrative burden related to ensuring that vendors have EBT-linked UPCs, the USDA-FNS national UPC database mentioned previously (USDA/FNS, 2016a) should facilitate state efforts to meet requirements to stock canned legumes.

Peanut Butter

The amount of peanut butter in the current food packages provides approximately 84 to 168 percent of recommended amounts of nuts, seeds, and soy (a protein food subgroup) to children and women. In the proposed revisions to the food packages, the same quantities of peanut butter currently provided every month will still be provided, but only once every 3 months. This reduces food package provision of nuts, seeds, and soy to between approximately 56 and 111 percent of recommended amounts. Although the latter amount does not meet the committee's criteria for supplemental, the limited availability of smaller package sizes (at a reasonable cost) prohibited further reduction.

Juice Is Reduced, and a CVV Option Is Allowed

Authoritative Recommendations Related to 100% Fruit Juice

The amount of juice in the current packages for children (food package IV) is equivalent to 107 percent of the lower end of the American Academy of Pediatrics (AAP) recommended range (i.e., 4 ounces per day) (AAP, 2014). The AAP (2014) also states that most fruit intake should be from whole fruit because whole fruit also contributes fiber and other plant-based compounds that are removed during processing. The DGA include a recommendation that at least half of fruit intake should be from whole fruit, and state that most individuals in the United States "would benefit from increasing intakes of fruit, mostly whole fruit" (USDA/HHS, 2016). The food packages for women (with the exception of food package VI) currently provide a disproportionate number of fruit servings from juice compared to fruit servings from whole fruit (see Chapter 3, Tables 3-1 through 3-3).[6] As described in Chapter 3, the committee concluded that the amounts of juice in the current food packages are more than supplemental and not aligned with dietary guidance.

Juice in the Revised Food Packages

Based on these considerations, the amount of juice offered in the revised food packages was reduced by approximately half.[7] Juice now provides approximately 50 percent of the AAP recommendation for juice intake for children and 27 percent of the DGA limit for fruit intake from juice for women. The funds saved by the reduction in juice were reallocated to the CVV, a priority component of the revised food packages. In addition, participants now have the option to substitute the remaining amount of juice with a further increase in their CVV (described later in this chapter).

Moreover, the amounts of juice in the revised packages are aligned

---

[6] This analysis assumes that 67 percent of the CVV is used to redeem fruit, based on redemption data provided to the committee from Texas and Wyoming. These data are available in the public access file (Email: paro@nas.edu).

[7] Juice was also removed from food package VI to achieve cost-neutrality and to increase the relative value of the partially (V-B) and fully (VII) breastfeeding packages.

with sizes available in the marketplace. This provides states and vendors with reasonable stocking options. Results of the small study by Andreyeva et al. (2013) indicated that WIC participants did not compensate for 2009 food package reductions in juice with a comparable increase in purchases of other nonjuice beverages.

Substitution of Juice with the CVV

As mentioned in the previous section about juice, in the revised food packages, participants are permitted to choose an additional $3 CVV in place of the 64 ounces of juice. This option aligns with dietary guidance to encourage intake of whole fruit over juice and is consistent with the committee's goal of increasing choice.

Additional Milk Substitutions Are Allowed, and the Amounts of Milk Are Reduced in Most Packages

The committee concluded that the milk in the current food packages provides more than a supplemental amount of dairy (between 85 and 119 percent of recommended amounts [see Chapter 3, Tables 3-1 through 3-3]). At the same time, intakes of dairy foods are below recommended amounts in several WIC-participating population subgroups (see Chapter 5). Available data indicate that redemption of whole milk is approximately 75 percent and that redemption of low-fat milk is approximately 71 percent for children and 56 percent for women.[8] These data suggest that what is redeemed may not be fully consumed by the intended recipient. The amounts of milk provided in the food packages for both women and children were revised, as described below. Nonfat and low-fat milk were retained as required forms of milk for individuals 2 years of age and older because of the DGA recommendation to consume nonfat or low-fat dairy products (USDA/HHS, 2016). Additional detail on the committee's consideration of dairy fat can be found in Appendix Q.

Additional Milk Substitutions

Inasmuch as dairy intakes are below recommended amounts across participant subgroups, milk, or the substitution options currently permitted, may not be preferred forms of dairy. The revised food packages allow more substitution options for milk in food packages IV, V-A, V-B, VI, and VII as follows: (1) 1 pound of cheese and 1 quart of yogurt for 4 quarts of milk; or (2) 2 quarts of yogurt for 2 quarts of milk. Women who receive

[8] See Chapter 7 for details on redemption rates applied by the committee.

food package VII have a third option of 2 pounds of cheese for 6 quarts of milk. Soy-based yogurt or soy-based cheese substitutes meeting the specifications outlined later in this chapter are also allowed. The yogurt 1-quart substitution may range from 30 to 32 ounces to allow states the option to accommodate the smaller container sizes (approximately 5 ounces) that are commonly available in the marketplace today. These substitution options are also structured to eliminate the need for a single quart ("dangling quart") of milk, which may be more difficult to find in stores and is typically more expensive. These additional choices may improve redemption of milk and milk substitutes.

Milk Amounts in the Food Packages for Women

Inasmuch as the Estimated Average Requirement (EAR) for calcium is the same for all subgroups of WIC-participating women (i.e., 800 milligrams),[9] it is reasonable to provide the same quantity of the key food group for calcium (i.e., dairy) across food packages for women. The DGA recommendation for the intake of dairy for all subgroups of women is 3 cup-equivalents per day. Yet, the current food packages for women provide widely varying amounts of dairy (again, see Tables 3-1 through 3-3.) With these factors in mind, the amounts of dairy provided in food packages for pregnant (V-A), partially breastfeeding (V-B), and fully breastfeeding (VII) women were reduced to match the amount of dairy provided in food package VI for postpartum women. This change includes removal of the additional 1 pound of cheese for fully breastfeeding women (VII).[10] The amount of milk in the revised food packages provides 71 percent of the recommended amount of dairy for women.

Milk Amounts in the Food Packages for Children

The current food package for children ages 2 to less than 5 years (IV-B) provides 85 percent of the DGA recommended amount of dairy. The committee considered this a greater than supplemental amount and reduced the amount of dairy provided in this food package to 75 percent of the DGA recommended amount.

Although the DGA food patterns do not apply to children ages 1 to

[9] The EAR for calcium for women ages 14 to 18 years is 1,100 mg per day (IOM, 2011). The most recent (April 2014) data indicate that the proportion of WIC-participating women under the age of 18 is 3.4 percent (USDA/FNS, 2015b). Given this age distribution, changes to the food packages for women target the EAR for women ages 19 to 50 years of 800 mg per day. The revised food packages are considered to still provide more than a supplemental amount of calcium (72 to 78 percent of the EAR) to women ages 14 to 18 years.

[10] Fully breastfeeding women may substitute up to 6 qt of milk for 2 lb of cheese.

less than 2 years, the amount of dairy suitable for this group is likely to be lower (in proportion to energy and nutrient needs) than those for children ages 2 to less than 5 years. Therefore, in the revised food packages, the amount of dairy in food package IV-A was reduced to provide 2 quarts less milk per month (the equivalent of 71 percent of the recommended amounts of dairy for a 1,300-kcal diet) compared to food package IV-B (for children ages 2 to less than 5 years).

Implications of the Revised Amounts of Milk

Not only are the revised amounts of milk better aligned with the committee's concept of supplemental, but the amounts of milk in the revised food packages are closer to the amounts of milk that are currently redeemed (see Appendix T). Therefore, it is anticipated that the volume of milk redeemed in the revised package will be similar to the amount currently redeemed (with the exception of food package VII), or even slightly higher as a result of the additional yogurt option, which may be preferred to fluid milk in some racial and ethnic groups.

Whole Grains Are Expanded to Accommodate a Wider Range of Package Sizes, and Additional Options Are Allowed

Whole Grains Are Expanded to a Range of 16 to 24 Ounces

The committee's analysis of data from National Health and Nutrition Examination Survey (NHANES) indicated that intakes of whole grains continue to be poor and intakes of refined grains are excessive across the WIC subgroups studied. A recent study found that purchases of whole grain products by WIC households were higher after states introduced the requirement that half of cereals offered meet the Final Rule whole grain requirements (Oh et al., 2016). Increasing the focus on whole grains in the WIC food packages may help to increase whole grain intake and improve acceptability of whole grains for the longer term.[11]

For women, the current food packages provide between 6 and 17 percent of the recommended amounts of whole grains, but 58 percent of recommended amounts of whole grains for children. Whole grains in the revised food packages provide 16 to 31 percent of recommended amounts of whole grains for women and 61 percent of recommended amounts of whole grains for children (see Appendix T). The total grains (which is the sum of whole and refined grains) provided to children is less than what the

[11] As noted in Table 3-10, AAP (2014) recommends repeated and early exposure to new foods and flavors to optimize acceptance and promote the selection of a varied diet later in life.

current package provides because allowing the more commonly available 24-ounce bread size, as explained below, removes the need to provide two 1-pound loaves of bread. The ratio of whole grains to refined grains is improved for all food packages.

In the current food packages, a 1-pound (16-ounce) loaf of bread is permitted, which may be substituted with oatmeal, brown rice, barley, corn tortillas, whole wheat tortillas, or whole wheat pasta of the same weight. As reviewed in the phase I interim report (NASEM, 2016) and in Chapter 2 of this report, the 1-pound size of bread was uncommon in the marketplace when the current food packages were introduced and posed a challenge for vendors and manufacturers. The price per ounce of the more commonly available size of whole grain bread ($0.10 per ounce for a 24-ounce size) is lower than for the 1-pound loaf size ($0.14). Thus, a more economical way to provide whole grains to participants is to increase the size of the whole grain bread to one that is more commonly available. The committee therefore changed the whole grain category to a range of 16 to 24 ounces. This range allows for the purchase of bread in 22- to 24-ounce sizes, thereby reducing the burden for vendors to stock the uncommon 1-pound size. Second, it eliminates the need for manufacturers to create WIC-specific product sizes, reducing overall program costs. Third, additional options for package size may increase availability and promote intake of whole grains, for which intake is inadequate in 100 percent of WIC-participating women and more than 90 percent of WIC-participating children. The lower price per ounce allows for delivery of 50 percent more whole grains to participants at an increased cost of only $0.17 per loaf.[12]

Additional Whole Grain Options Are Allowed

A greater degree of flexibility in size, as described above, is one way that the revised packages will allow states to offer a greater number of grain options. The committee further recommends that the WIC food category of whole grains also include fortified corn masa flour (which is not a whole grain, see further description below), cornmeal, teff, and buckwheat, and that states authorize as many of these options as cost constraints allow. Some options may be more or less suitable to a state's particular WIC-participating population. Of note, with the exception of fortified corn masa flour, these products are generally not fortified and, thus, their primary contribution to the diet is provision of whole grains (see Appendix Q, Table Q-1).

In accordance with the Final Rule, in the current food packages state

[12] Price data in this section obtained from the Information Resources, Inc. (IRI) store scanner dataset.

agencies are encouraged to offer corn tortillas with whole grain corn listed as the primary ingredient (USDA/FNS, 2014). The revised food packages include the additional option of ground corn masa flour, even though this option is not whole grain. The committee concluded that this option should be permitted because (1) tortillas made with corn masa flour are currently permitted to improve the cultural suitability of the packages and, (2) early in 2016, the U.S. Food and Drug Administration (FDA) approved corn masa flour for fortification with folic acid (FDA, 2016a). Data from the Centers for Disease Control and Prevention indicate that only 17 percent of Hispanic women report intake of 400 μg or more of folic acid daily through fortified foods or supplements, compared with 30 percent of non-Hispanic white women (Williams et al., 2015). States are therefore encouraged to offer fortified corn masa flour and tortillas made with fortified corn masa flour once such products become available in the marketplace. The other expanded options must be whole grain.

Fortified Ready-to-Eat Breakfast Cereals Are Retained

Fortified ready-to-eat (RTE) cereals offer higher concentrations of nearly all nutrients compared to other whole grain products, so they were retained as a separate food category, in part to address nutrients of concern. Folate and iron are particularly important to the WIC-participating population and are not required fortificants in whole grain products, but are typically added to ready-to-eat breakfast cereals. Therefore, the committee considered that retention of fortified ready-to-eat cereals would support intake of these nutrients. The committee also recognized that RTE cereals may be important to retain as a delivery mechanism for fluid milk (Song et al., 2006). Additional details related to the folic acid content of RTE cereals can be found in the section on food specifications, and additional data supporting this conclusion are available in Appendix Q.

Fish Is Added to Nearly All Food Packages Within Cost-Neutral Constraints

USDA-FNS tasked the committee with evaluating whether fish should be included in additional food packages. As described in Chapter 3, authoritative groups recommend consumption of 1.0 to 1.7 ounces of lower-mercury fish per day by children ages 1 to 4 years (AAP, 2014; AHA, 2015; USDA/HHS, 2016) and pregnant and breastfeeding women (FDA/EPA, 2004; AHA, 2015; USDA/HHS, 2016). Yet, seafood intake is either low or too uncommon to assess in most subgroups of WIC participants. Only food package VII for fully breastfeeding women currently includes fish (USDA/FNS, 2014). In alignment with dietary guidance, the committee considered it appropriate to include fish in additional food packages. However, due to cost constraints, the amount of fish added to the revised food packages varies, providing between 8 and 47 percent of the recommended intakes of seafood. In alignment with the overall strategy to promote any intensity of breastfeeding (discussed later in the chapter), fish was reduced from 30 to 20 ounces per month in the revised food package VII for fully breastfeeding women to allow partially breastfeeding women to receive 10 ounces per month. The other revised food packages contain a smaller amount (10 ounces, or two 5-ounce cans every 3 months). Although this amount provides only 8 percent of the DGA recommended amount of seafood for postpartum women and 19 percent for children, the committee considered it important to provide some amount of this food group in each package to improve balance across the food groups and consistency with the DGA, and introduce this underconsumed food into the diets of WIC participants. Fish is also now permitted as a partial substitute for infant food meat, as described later in this chapter.

Canned Fish May Be Packed in Water and May Include Sauces and Flavorings

In the current food packages, fish may be packed in water or oil and may include added sauces and flavorings. In the revised food packages, fish may be water-packed (not oil-packed), but may include the same sauces and flavorings that are currently allowed. Water-packed varieties are higher in nutrient density because water-packed fish is lower in energy but contains the same levels of key nutrients per serving (see Appendix O, Table O-3). Currently, approximately 43 percent of WIC participants are allowed to purchase oil-packed varieties (based on state WIC food lists [USDA/FNS, 2015a]). Therefore this specification change will affect less than half of the WIC participating population.

Rotating Fish, Legumes, and Peanut Butter

In the revised food packages, legumes and peanut butter are rotated on a quarterly basis to provide more supplemental amounts, and amounts that better align with participant preferences.[13] In most packages (IV, V-A, and VI), fish is added to the quarterly rotation. For food packages V-B and VII, states may decide how best to provide fish based on the capabilities of their individual Management Information Systems (i.e., quarterly or monthly). Although this may appear to add administrative burden, it is similar to the current rotation allowed between legumes and peanut butter. Although

[13] Data provided to the committee indicate that redemption of legumes and peanut butter is approximately 50 percent.

legumes, peanut butter, and fish are not nutritionally interchangeable, the revised amounts of legumes and peanut butter not only improve their alignment with recommended dietary intake but also help to allow for the cost-neutral inclusion of fish. It is anticipated that states will create food packages that rotate the issuance of legumes, peanut butter, and fish over each 3-month period, eliminating the burden of asking for the participants' preference between legumes and peanut butter and optimizing nutrients available to participants through these nonperishable foods.

ADDITIONAL SUBSTITUTION OPTIONS FOR VEGANS OR VEGETARIANS AND FOR ALLERGIES OR INTOLERANCES

The revised food packages include several additional options for vegans, vegetarians, and individuals with specific types of food-triggered immune-mediated sensitivities (e.g., lactose intolerance, milk allergy, celiac disease). The soy-based cheese and soy-based yogurt products allowed in the revised food packages are suitable substitutes for dairy products for both vegans and individuals with lactose intolerance or a milk allergy. Vegans who wish to substitute for 1 dozen eggs may do so with 1 pound of dry legumes or four 15- to 16-ounce cans of legumes; these options provide the same number of ounce-equivalent servings for their respective food groups and are both nutrient-dense. Several of the new grain options may be available in certified gluten-free forms that would be suitable for individuals with celiac disease (the expansion of whole grain options is discussed earlier this chapter).

As discussed in Chapter 3, individuals with lactose intolerance may be able to tolerate yogurt. The revised food packages allow states to authorize a substitution of 2 quarts of yogurt for 2 quarts of milk (a one to one substitution). Participants with a preference for yogurt over milk may also take advantage of this option. Although yogurt is already offered in most states, it is a recent addition to state agency WIC-approved food lists. As a result, adequate data are not yet available to assess redemption of yogurt by WIC participants. In a study of WIC participants in California, Fung et al. (2010) found that that the majority of respondents wanted to substitute some of their milk with yogurt. This preference for yogurt over milk, coupled with low intakes of calcium in some WIC subgroups (see Chapter 5), suggests that offering yogurt may improve dairy redemption and consumption.

Although peanut butter and legumes are no longer considered interchangeable in the revised food packages, participants with a peanut allergy may be issued 1 pound of dry legumes or four 15- to 16-ounce cans of legumes in place of peanut butter.

SUMMARY OF RECOMMENDED CHANGES TO THE AMOUNTS AND TYPES OF FOOD AND SUBSTITUTION OPTIONS IN THE WIC FOOD PACKAGES FOR WOMEN AND CHILDREN

In the previous sections, the committee provides the rationale for a number of changes to the WIC food packages for women and children in alignment with the statement of task. The overarching recommendations and specific changes are summarized below.

6-1. The U.S. Department of Agriculture's Food and Nutrition Service (USDA-FNS) should increase the dollar amount of the cash value voucher, add fish, and reduce the amounts of juice, milk, legumes, and peanut butter in all food packages for women and children (IV, V-A, V-B, and VII), to improve the balance of food groups in alignment with the 2015–2020 *Dietary Guidelines for Americans*. These changes also apply to food package VI, except that the amounts of milk are unchanged and the amounts of legumes are increased.

The specific changes recommended include

- Increase the CVV to at least $12, $15, $25, and $35 in food packages IV (children), V-A (pregnant women) and VI (postpartum women), V-B (partially breastfeeding women), and VII (fully breastfeeding women), respectively, to align with the DGA for increased intakes of vegetables and fruits.
- Add 10 ounces of fish to food packages IV, V-A, and VI once per quarter (once every 3 months), 10 ounces of fish every month in food package V-B, and modify the amount of fish in food package VII to 20 ounces per month.
- Provide 64 ounces of juice in food packages IV, V-A, V-B, and VII, and remove juice from food package VI.
- Provide 12 quarts of milk in IV-A (children ages 1 to less than 2 years), 14 quarts in food package IV-B (children ages 2 to less than 5 years) and 16 quarts in food packages V-A, V-B, VI, and VII.
- Provide legumes once per quarter (once every 3 months): 1 pound (16 ounces of dry or 64 ounces canned [four 15- to 16-ounce cans]) in food package IV and 2 pounds in food packages V-A, V-B, VI, and VII.
- Provide 16 to 18 ounces of peanut butter to women and children on a quarterly basis (once every 3 months).

In addition, the committee recommends substitution options for individuals with special dietary needs or preferences, and to promote intake of foods that are currently underconsumed:

6-2. USDA-FNS should support the cultural food preferences and special dietary needs of WIC participants by requiring states to offer additional options for the WIC food categories, including substitution of a CVV in place of juice, additional forms and varieties of vegetables and fruits, both canned and dried legumes, and a range of options and sizes for grains and yogurt. A substitution of legumes for peanut butter or for eggs should be allowed for individuals who have a peanut allergy, or who are following a vegan diet, respectively.

The specific substitution options recommended include

- Allow participants the choice to select a CVV option for all remaining juice ($3 may be added to the CVV in place of juice for each participant who chooses this option).
- Require states to offer fresh and one additional form (frozen, canned, or dried) each of vegetables and fruits.
- Require vendors to offer at least three varieties of vegetables and two varieties of fruits.
- Allow states to authorize teff, buckwheat, and cornmeal (including blue) as substitutions for whole-wheat bread. Corn masa flour should also be permitted in alignment with the current FNS allowance of corn tortillas, which may be made from corn masa flour.
- Allow participants a range of 16 to 24 ounces of grains to fulfill the maximum allowance for whole grains and a range of 30 to 32 ounces of yogurt to substitute for 1 quart of milk.
- Require states to offer a choice of 1 pound of dry legumes or 64 ounces (four 15- to 16-ounce cans) of canned legumes in all food packages offering legumes.
- Allow WIC participants to substitute 1 pound of soy-based cheese substitute for 3 quarts of milk, or 2 quarts of yogurt or soy-based yogurt substitute for 2 quarts of milk.
- Allow vegan participants to substitute 1 pound of dry legumes or 64 ounces (four 15- to 16-ounce cans) of canned legumes for 1 dozen eggs.
- Allow participants with a peanut allergy to substitute 1 pound of dry legumes or 64 ounces (four 15- to 16-ounce cans) of canned legumes for 16 to 18 ounces of peanut butter.

THE REVISED FOOD PACKAGES FOR WOMEN AND INFANTS

Currently, there are three WIC food packages available to infants: (1) food package I provides only infant formula (no foods) for infants ages 0 to less than 6 months; (2) food package II provides infant formula and foods for infants ages 6 to 11 months; and (3) food package III provides infant formula and foods that meet special dietary needs for infants of all ages with medically documented, qualifying conditions (proposed revisions to food package III are described later in this chapter). As stated earlier, formula-fed infants in the first 6 months of life were considered an exception to the concept of supplemental. The only proposed change to infant formula is a change in provision during the first 30 days, as described in the below recommendation.

6-3. USDA-FNS, as a means of supporting breastfeeding of any duration and intensity, should allow individual tailoring of the infant food packages to best meet the needs of the mother–infant dyad.

The Committee's Vision for Breastfeeding Support in WIC

The first Institute of Medicine (IOM) committee to review the WIC food packages made an important recommendation that attempted to bolster support of breastfeeding in the first 30 days postpartum by limiting the issuance of formula to breastfeeding women (IOM, 2006). This committee fully supports the intent of the previous committee. It shares the vision for WIC in the future that all women receive adequate counseling and support prenatally through the first month postpartum, and the issuance of formula is individually tailored to the needs of every mother–infant dyad, without routine issuance of formula in the first 30 days after the infant's birth as this practice increases the risk of breastfeeding failure (Walker, 2015).

The evidence reviewed in Chapter 2 indicated that providing no formula to breastfeeding mothers in the first month did not lead to the expected gains in initiation and duration of breastfeeding (with the exception of California [Whaley et al., 2012]). Therefore, the committee recommends that, following a detailed assessment of the needs of the dyad by WIC staff, women should be permitted to receive the quantity of formula that they need to support their desired level of breastfeeding. Consistent with USDA Breastfeeding Policy and Guidance (USDA/FNS, 2016b), exclusive breastfeeding remains the goal for those women able to do so. Tailored issuance of formula in the first month, through adequate counseling and support from WIC staff, is recommended not only to maximize the potential for women to achieve exclusive breastfeeding goals, but also to achieve successful partial breastfeeding when exclusive breastfeeding is not possible or desired. This recommendation is in alignment with the USDA Breastfeeding Policy and Guidance Report with only one exception: In the first 30 days, states may opt to create food packages allowing issuance of formula up to 364 fluid ounces (instead of the current 104 ounces).

Allowing states to increase package diversity in the first month to allow smaller amounts of formula and avoid issuance of the full formula package is intended to increase flexibility in food package options and support more women to breastfeed. This is further supported by the creation of food package V-B for postpartum partially (mostly) breastfeeding women. As shown in Table 6-1, each infant package is aligned with a food package for the mother that supports the level of breastfeeding, allowing three choices for the dyad starting at birth: (1) the fully breastfeeding dyad with no formula provided and food package VII provided for the mother; (2) the partially (mostly) breastfeeding dyad, with a tailored amount of formula up to 364 ounces per month and food package V-B for the mother; and (3) the fully formula feeding dyad with up to 806 fluid ounces/month and food package VI for the mother. These revisions allow more opportunities to tailor the food packages for both the infant and the mother, including during the first 30 days. In addition, they are intended to shift some women from receiving the fully formula-feeding dyadic packages to receiving the partially (mostly) breastfeeding dyadic packages. Furthermore, the three revised packages are more similar in monetary value than the comparable current packages. This creates incentives that are more proximal to the infant's birth and, thus, have greater likelihood of supporting the mother's interest in breastfeeding.

"Up to" Amounts of Formula

Although formula amounts to infants are largely unchanged from the current packages, the committee found it important to include language clarifying that, across all infant food packages, formula amounts should be considered *up to* amounts to emphasize the importance of assessing the actual need for formula and reducing the possibility of interfering with the successful establishment of the mother's desired breastfeeding behavior. This language is well aligned with the USDA-FNS guidance for issuance of formula through the WIC program (USDA/FNS, 2016b),[14] and is intended to offer breastfeeding women in need of infant formula more options in the first month in contrast to the current policy, which requires choosing either

[14] The 2016 USDA-FNS document *WIC Breastfeeding Policy and Guidance* specifies that "WIC staff are expected to individually tailor the amount of infant formula based on the assessed needs of breastfed infants and provide the minimal amount of formula that meets but does not exceed infants' nutritional needs" (USDA/FNS, 2016b, pages 16–17).

the fully breastfeeding or the formula-feeding package in the first 30 days (see Chapter 2 for a discussion of the current policy).

Consistent with the modification allowing *up to* amounts in all infant packages that include infant formula, the revised food package for partially breastfed infants 0 to less than 1 month of age (food package I-A) allows *up to* the full nutrition benefit of 364 fluid ounces of formula per month (the same allowance in the current food package I for partially breastfed infants,[15] and a change from the 104 fluid ounces allowed in the current package). Issuance continues to be based upon an assessment by WIC staff of what is needed to support the breastfeeding mother–infant dyad. This recommendation is not intended to undermine the success of states or local agencies that have identified the resources needed to support breastfeeding through the provision of up to 104 fluid ounces of formula. Rather, it is meant to bolster the importance of the support and counseling needed to support breastfeeding in the immediate postpartum period. Without this support, based on available evidence, the 2009 limitations on choice in the first month have not had the intended effect of supporting breastfeeding. Given the paucity of data on alignment of infant food packages with actual feeding behavior, this committee recommends that WIC staff assess the formula needs of all infants and offer amounts *up to* the full nutrition benefit.

As noted in Chapter 11, USDA-FNS should identify resources to increase breastfeeding support, both within the WIC program (e.g., increases in funds for peer counseling) and outside of WIC (e.g., hospital policies, legislation on family leave, and workplace support of breastfeeding). It is the hope of this committee that these supports can be put into place and evaluated by 2024 so the next committee charged to examine the WIC food packages will have substantial evidence on which to base future changes in policies on issuance of WIC formula.

Aligning the Amounts of Infant Foods with American Academy of Pediatrics Recommendations

The Amounts of Infant Cereals Are Reduced

The current food package II (for infants ages 6 to 11 months) provides approximately 6 tablespoons of infant cereal per day, which is 150 percent of the maximum amount recommended by the AAP (4 tablespoons per day) (AAP, 2014). Although iron-fortified infant cereals are a favored first food and are good sources of iron and zinc, this amount is substantially

[15] The full nutrition benefit of 364 fl oz corresponds to the maximum monthly allowance of 388 fl oz reconstituted liquid concentrate, 384 fl oz ready-to-feed, or 435 fl oz reconstituted powder.

greater than supplemental. Infants who receive formula generally exceed their iron and zinc intake recommendations, so the provision of these nutrients through cereal is not critical for them. Therefore, the committee recommends that the amount of infant cereal provided in food package II to formula-fed or partially breastfed infants be reduced to 8 ounces per month, which provides 50 percent of the AAP-recommended amount of iron-fortified infant cereal (AAP, 2014). Iron and zinc are critical nutrients for fully breastfed infants because human milk contains low levels of these nutrients. Therefore, the revised food package II provides more infant cereal to fully breastfed infants per month: 16 ounces, which is 100 percent of the AAP-recommended amount. As described below, fully breastfed infants also receive jarred infant food meats, which are another good source of iron and zinc.

The Amount of Jarred Infant Food Vegetables and Fruits for Fully Breastfed Infants Is Reduced

The current package II (for infants ages 6 to 11 months) provides fully breastfed infants with 256 ounces of jarred infant food vegetables and fruits. This is more than 1 cup-equivalent per day, which may be appropriate for older infants but is likely to be difficult for younger infants to consume. AAP does not recommend specific intake amounts of vegetables and fruits for infants. Instead, these foods are considered useful as a transition to solid foods (AAP, 2014). The IOM (2006) report also did not provide a nutrient-based rationale for the recommended quantities of these infant foods. Rather, it stated, "To encourage or promote full breastfeeding, the recommended amounts of [infant] food vegetables and fruits are more generous for fully breast-fed infants than other infants" (p. 103). Given that there appears to be no nutritional rationale for providing more vegetables and fruits to fully breastfed infants compared to other infants and that the food packages for formula-fed or partially breastfed infants are distinguished in other ways in this revision, the committee recommends providing the same amount of jarred infant food vegetables and fruits to all infants receiving food package II: 128 ounces per month. The revised amounts provide approximately 0.5 cup-equivalents of vegetables and fruits per day to all infants who receive food package II. This decision allowed the committee to provide further support to the breastfeeding dyad by moving the savings from the jarred infant vegetables and fruits to a significantly enhanced CVV for both partially and fully breastfeeding women. Behavioral economics evidence suggests that shifting the benefit closer in time (to a higher CVV when the infant is born, compared to more jarred infant food vegetables and fruits in 6–12 months in the future), may enhance the probability that women choose the fully breastfeeding package (Loewenstein, 1988).

Infant Food Vegetables and Fruits May Be Substituted with the CVV

In the current food packages, infants ages 9 to 11 months may receive either a $4 (partially breastfed) or $8 (fully breastfed) CVV in place of half of the jarred infant food vegetables and fruits. In the revised food packages, the proposed CVV substitution is $10 plus half of the jarred infant foods or $20 and no jarred infant foods for all infants ages 6 to 11 months. The committee compared the nutrient content of infant fruit and vegetable products to noninfant products and found that nutrients provided to infants with the jarred foods were similar to those provided with a CVV of the same value (see Appendix O, Tables O-1 and O-2). Additionally, the committee compared the cost of 4 ounces of infant jarred fruits or vegetables ($0.64) to the composite average cost of the most popular vegetables and fruits purchased by WIC participants ($0.55 per cup-equivalent serving).[16] Not only are the amounts of the proposed CVV substitution cost-neutral options, but participants may be able to buy more servings (of vegetables or fruits) using the CVV. This option also allows caregivers to prepare foods with developmentally appropriate textures for older infants.

In All Food Packages, the CVV Can Be Used to Purchase All Authorized Forms of Vegetables and Fruits

In the current food packages, the infant CVV may only be used to purchase fresh vegetables or fruits. Limiting the infant CVV to only fresh vegetables and fruits creates a significant burden for participants and local agencies in states whose EBT systems already authorize a voucher allowing multiple forms of vegetables and fruits for women and children (personal communication, public comment submitted by Texas WIC, July 30, 2015). In the revised packages, all forms of vegetables and fruits authorized for purchase with the CVV for women and children must be authorized for the infant CVV.[17] As noted previously, the nutritional value of canned or frozen vegetables and fruits can be comparable to that of fresh forms (see Appendix O). Moreover, this expansion of forms offers the opportunity to create foods of varying textures that are suitable to an infant's developmental stage and meet cultural needs. The AAP's (2014) and USDA's (2016e) guidance for home preparation of infant foods is shown in Box 6-1.

---

[16] Some of the most commonly purchased types may not be suitable for infants (e.g., lettuce), but the price was considered an adequate estimate given that the preferred vegetables and fruits purchased with the infant CVV is not known.

[17] Except dried.

BOX 6-1

Guidance for Home of Infant Foods

- Match texture and consistency to infant's oral motor skills.
- Cook using methods that preserve nutrients.
- Use thickened purees to enhance caloric density.
- Provide healthy "single ingredient" foods, especially while total variety is still limited.
- Avoid added sugar or salt.
- Avoid foods that could be choking or aspiration risks (e.g., hot dogs, nuts, grapes, raisins, raw carrots, popcorn, hard candies).
- Use caution when using microwave to warm foods; check temperature prior to feeding infants.
- Store safely.

SOURCES: AAP, 2014; USDA/FNS, 2016e.

The Amount of Jarred Infant Food Meat for Fully Breastfed Infants Is Reduced

The committee agrees with the IOM (2006) recommendation to provide jarred infant food meat as a key source of iron and zinc for fully breastfed infants. The AAP (2014) recommends 1 to 2 ounces of meat per day (30 to 60 ounces per month). The current WIC food packages provide 130 percent of the maximum of this range, which may be one factor in the low redemption of jarred infant food meat (generally 40 percent or less). Jarred infant food meat is not a common complementary food. In the 2008 Feeding Infants and Toddlers Study (FITS 2008) study, infant food meat was consumed by only 4.6 percent of infants ages 6 to less than 9 months and 1.2 percent of infants ages 9 to less than 12 months (Siega-Riz et al., 2010). In the committee's independent analysis of breastfed infants ages 6 to less than 12 months participating in WIC (NHANES 2009–2012), 10 percent consumed any amount of jarred infant food meat. Although noninfant food meat was consumed by 33 percent of older infants (ages 9 to less than 12 months) in the FITS 2008 study (Siega-Riz et al., 2010), provision of noninfant food meat in the WIC food packages, in amounts and forms appropriate for infants as young as age 6 months, was considered and ruled out as administratively unfeasible. The committee considered potential nutritionally equivalent but preferred alternatives to jarred infant food meat, but was unable to identify any options suitable to the WIC food packages in the marketplace.

Given this evidence and in line with providing supplemental amounts of foods in the WIC food packages, the committee reduced the amount of jarred infant food meat provided to fully breastfed infants to 40 ounces per month (approximately 65 percent of the AAP recommended maximum amount). It is noteworthy that, despite reductions in both jarred infant food meats and infant cereals (see above), the revised food package for fully breastfed infants still provides 130 percent of the EAR for iron and 72 percent of the EAR for zinc.

Fish May Be Substituted for a Portion of Jarred Infant Food Meat

Given that redemption of jarred infant food meat is poor and jarred infant food meat is not a preferred infant food, coupled with the importance of providing a bioavailable source of iron as infants begin complementary feeding (AAP, 2014), the committee considered possible substitutions. Global authorities recommend that infants consume flesh foods, including fish, as early as possible (PAHO/WHO, 2003). Canned fish can provide an amount of iron comparable to that of jarred infant food meats (with similar amounts of highly bioavailable heme iron), some (but less) zinc per ounce, and costs approximately half as much per ounce (see Appendix O, Table O-3). Inasmuch as jarred infants food meats are often sold in packages that contain 12 2.5-ounce jars (30 ounces), substitution of two cans of fish (10 ounces) for four jars of infant food meat (10 ounces) is feasible and well suited to package sizes commonly available in the marketplace.

Given this summary of evidence, the committee recommends the following adjustments to the food packages for infants to (1) improve alignment of the food packages with dietary guidance for individuals less than 2 years of age, (2) better reflect typical eating patterns of infants who are consuming complementary foods, and (3) increase flexibility to align with cultural eating patterns, preferences, and developmental needs:

6-4. USDA-FNS should reduce the amounts of infant cereal across food package II for all infants, and reduce the amounts of jarred infant food vegetables and fruits and jarred infant food meats provided in food package II for fully breastfed infants. Caregivers should be permitted to substitute all or part of the jarred infant food vegetables and fruits with a cash value voucher, and a portion of jarred infant food meat with canned fish.

Specific changes recommended are

- Provide 8 ounces of infant cereals to formula-fed and partially breastfed infants, and 16 ounces to fully breastfed infants in food package II.

- Provide 128 ounces per month of jarred infant food vegetables and fruits to all infants in food package II.
- Allow participants to substitute half or all jarred infant food vegetables and fruits with a CVV of comparable value. Caregivers of infants ages 6 to 11 months should have the option to choose a $10 CVV plus 64 ounces of jarred infant food vegetables and fruits or a $20 CVV in place of all jarred infant food vegetables and fruits.
- Allow the purchase of fresh, frozen, or canned vegetables and fruits that meet other current specifications for these forms with CVVs issued to any participant, including infants.
- Provide 40 ounces per month of jarred infant food meats in food package II for fully breastfed infants.
- Allow caregivers to substitute 10 ounces of jarred infant food meat with 10 ounces of canned fish. Fish options should adhere to the revised WIC specifications for canned fish.

FOOD PACKAGE III

As described in Chapter 2, food package III is issued to WIC participants with particular medical needs. The guidance for issuance of foods in this package may vary by state. Most recipients of this package are infants. The committee agrees with the intent of the previous IOM committee that food package III recipients should be provided with "the foods that they would receive from the package to which they would be assigned if they did not have special dietary needs, *to the extent that is appropriate*" (emphasis added) (IOM, 2006, p. 8). Currently, every participant who receives this package is required to be prescribed a WIC formula (i.e., infant formula, exempt infant formula, and WIC-eligible nutritionals) even if these products do not suit the participant's specific medical need. For example, in the current food packages, a participant who is issued food package III because of a need for jarred infant food vegetables and fruits although the participant is over 1 year of age is also required to be issued a WIC formula. In the revised food package III, if a health care practitioner does not specifically prescribe a WIC formula, but prescribes a conventional food for medical reasons, there is no requirement to provide these products.[18]

The committee made no specific changes to the quantities of WIC formulas or WIC-eligible nutritionals that may be provided in food package III. The way in which special products are issued (by reconstituted fluid ounce amount, protein needs, kilocalories, or other) depends on the particular medical condition. No data were identified to suggest that the types of WIC formulas currently permitted at the federal level, the quantities

[18] Text in this paragraph is updated from the original prepublication version.

provided, or the issuance basis were inadequate for participant needs. In addition to specifically prescribing WIC formula, it is also the health care practitioner's responsibility to determine the amounts and issuance methods (reconstituted fluid ounce amount, protein needs, or kilocalories). As stated in Chapter 11, it is important to note that WIC is not the primary payer for therapeutic formulas (USDA/FNS, 2015c). Collaborations with Medicaid are essential to both lessen the cost burden on WIC and increase support of the WIC participant from the medical professional.

The committee recommends one change to the amounts of jarred infant food fruits and vegetables provided to children and women in food package III. In the current packages, children may receive 128 ounces and women may receive 160 ounces jarred infant food vegetables and fruits in place of the CVV. The rationale for these amounts was not outlined in the Final Rule. The committee translated the value of the CVV into an amount of jarred infant food fruit vegetables and fruits to determine the appropriate amounts to provide in these situations, as indicated in Table 6-3.

Given this evidence, the committee recommends the following change to food package III:

> **6-5. USDA-FNS should no longer require provision of a WIC formula to all participants that are issued food package III. Participants should be permitted access to the foods in the package appropriate for their age, physiological state, and medical condition. The health care provider may refer to the WIC registered dietitian and/or qualified nutritionist for identifying appropriate foods (excluding WIC formula) and their prescribed amounts as well as the length of time the participant requires the foods.**

TABLE 6-3 Recommended Substitution of Jarred Infant Food Vegetables and Fruits in Place of the CVV in Food Package III

Food Package(s) Corresponding to the Participant's Age and Physiological State	CVV ($)	Equivalent Amount of Infant Food Veg/Fr (oz)*	Round Number of 4 oz Jars	Round Number of 3.5-oz Packages
IV-A, IV-B	12	75	19	21
V-A, VI	15	94	23	27
V-B	25	156	39	45
VII	35	219	55	63

NOTES: CVV = cash value voucher; veg/fr = vegetables and fruits.

* Based on the composite cost of jarred infant veg/fr of $0.16 per oz. Participants that opt to replace juice with a $3 CVV may be issued an additional 5 jars or 3.5-ounce packages.

OTHER SPECIAL CASES

Women who are fully breastfeeding multiple infants, pregnant with multiple fetuses, or both pregnant and breastfeeding have higher nutrient and caloric needs than women with singletons. In the absence of any evidence on the additional energy needs for the women fully breastfeeding multiple infants, the committee estimated the additional energy need would be approximately 400 kcal per day for the additional milk produced and assumed no further maternal fat mobilization. This represents approximately 50 percent more energy than is supplied by the fully breastfeeding package, indicating that the current regulation to provide 1.5 times food package VII to these women is appropriate.

Similarly, there is a lack of evidence available to estimate the energy needs for women who are pregnant with multiple fetuses or who are partially breastfeeding multiple infants. Providing food package V-B to women pregnant with multiple fetuses increases the CVV by $10 per month and adds more fish compared to food package V-A for pregnant women with singletons. Issuance of food package VII to women partially breastfeeding multiples provides an additional 1 dozen eggs, $10 in CVV, and 10 ounces of fish per month compared to the revised food package V-B for women who are partially breastfeeding singletons.

Therefore, to meet the additional nutrient needs and provide packages that minimize the burden to state agencies, the committee recommends the following in these special cases:

6-6. USDA-FNS should issue food package V-B to women who are pregnant with multiple fetuses and food package VII to women who are partially breastfeeding multiple infants.

In addition, the following regulations are retained:

- Issue food package VII to women who are breastfeeding and also pregnant.
- Issue 1.5 times food package VII to women who are fully breastfeeding multiple infants.

SPECIFICATIONS FOR WIC-ELIGIBLE FOODS

The previous sections of this chapter reviewed the recommended changes across all food packages. The committee also examined current food specifications and considered modifications to improve the potential for food packages to meet the nutritional needs of participants or improve alignment with dietary guidance while still ensuring availability. Foods for which specifications have been changed are presented in Table 6-4 and this section provides the rationale for each change. (Specifications for canned fish are covered earlier in this chapter). A side-by-side comparison of the current and revised specifications for all foods is presented in Appendix P.

Vegetables and Fruits Authorized for Purchase with the CVV

As stated in the Final Rule, vendors are currently required to offer at least two varieties of fruits and two varieties of vegetables in a fresh, frozen, canned, or dried form depending on forms authorized by the state (USDA/FNS, 2014). The revised packages require that vendors offer at least three vegetable and two fruit varieties. When possible, states could consider increasing vendor stocking requirements further, particularly in light of the increased CVV value across food packages. Published guidance related to optimum stocking for promotion of healthy choices is available (see HER, 2016; USDA/FNS, 2016c). Other specifications for canned, frozen, or dried forms of vegetables and fruits remain unchanged. States are encouraged to authorize low- or reduced-sodium forms of all canned foods.

Limiting Added Sugars in the Food Packages

The 2015–2020 DGA are the first of the DGA to recommend that an individual's intake of added sugars not exceed 10 percent of total calories. The contribution of WIC food packages to the intake of nutrients to limit, including added sugars, was of particular concern to the committee because of this guidance and also because of excessive intakes of added sugars across subgroups of WIC participants (see Chapter 5). The current food packages provide close to or above the limit for "calories for other uses" (COU) recommended in the DGA (see Table 3-9).[19] As a result, it was appropriate to decrease the contribution of the food packages to intakes of added sugars in participants' diets while maintaining the acceptability and palatability of the nutrient-dense foods that are provided by WIC. WIC foods that were targeted for reductions in total sugars are described below. The new food labels[20] will allow WIC staff that make decisions about state food lists to identify qualifying foods by using added sugars amounts. Table 6-5 presents the suggested added sugars limits for WIC foods discussed in this section. The committee reviewed current

---

[19] The DGA food patterns recommend different limits for "calories for other uses" (calories from saturated fat and added sugars) depending on energy level. As explained in Chapter 2, with some food patterns it is not possible to consume 10 percent of energy from added sugars and simultaneously meet nutrient needs (USDA/HHS, 2016).

[20] The earliest compliance date for implementation of new food labels is July 26, 2018.

TABLE 6-4 Proposed Changes to Specifications for Foods in the Revised WIC Food Packages[a]

Category/Food	Food Package and Affected Participant Group, Considering the Proposed Food Package Revisions	Selected Current Specifications	Proposed Change to the Specifications[b]	Rationale
Vegetables and Fruits Purchased with CVV	II Infants	Any variety of fresh, whole, or cut vegetable, without added sugars, starches, or salt Any variety of fresh, whole, or cut fruit without added sugars (as defined in 21 C.F.R. 101.95)	Fresh, frozen, or canned forms of vegetables and fruits meeting other specifications may be purchased	Fresh, frozen, and canned vegetables and fruits are suitable for infants and meet developmental needs when prepared appropriately
Milk and Milk Alternatives				
Cow's milk	IV, V-A, V-B, VI, VII Women and children	Must conform to FDA standard of identity for whole, reduced-fat, low-fat, or nonfat milks (21 C.F.R. 131.110). Must be pasteurized and contain at least 400 IU of vitamin D per quart (100 IU per cup) and 2,000 IU of vitamin A per quart (500 IU per cup) May be flavored or unflavored. May be fluid, shelf stable, evaporated (21 C.F.R. 131.130), or dried (i.e., powder) (21 C.F.R. 131.147)	Only unflavored milk is permitted	Low-fat forms (for children 2 years of age and older, and women) align with CACFP provision of milk and with the DGA; requiring unflavored forms reduces inclusion of added sugars in the WIC food packages

		Cultured milks must conform to FDA standard of identity for cultured milk (21 C.F.R. 131.112—cultured buttermilk, kefir cultured milk, acidophilus cultured milk)		
Soy-based beverage	IV, V-A, V-B, VI, VII Women and children	Must be fortified to meet the following nutrient levels: 276 mg calcium per cup, 8 g protein per cup, 500 IU vitamin A per cup, 100 IU vitamin D per cup, 24 mg magnesium per cup, 222 mg phosphorus per cup, 349 mg potassium per cup, 0.44 mg riboflavin per cup, and 1.1 **μg** vitamin B12 per cup, in accordance with fortification guidelines issued by FDA	In addition, the total sugar content of soy-based beverages should be as low as possible, not to exceed 12 g per 8 oz serving	Soy-based beverages are available in the marketplace that contain 12 g or less of total sugars per serving; sugars in soy-based beverages are 100 percent added; intakes of added sugars are excessive in the WIC population, therefore it is appropriate to apply a limit that considers nationwide availability of these products
Tofu	IV, V-A, V-B, VI, VII Women and children	Calcium-set tofu prepared with calcium salts (e.g., calcium sulfate); may not contain added fats, sugars, oils, or sodium	Must contain a minimum of 200 mg of calcium per 100 g of tofu (calcium-set is no longer part of the specification); retain the specification that tofu may not contain added fats, sugars, oils, or sodium	Tofu in the food packages serves as a milk substitution; as such, the revised specification ensures that tofu in the food packages provides an amount of calcium as close to that in a serving of milk as reasonable, considering marketplace options

continued

TABLE 6-4 Continued

Category/Food	Food Package and Affected Participant Group, Considering the Proposed Food Package Revisions	Selected Current Specifications	Proposed Change to the Specifications[b]	Rationale
Yogurt	IV, V-A, V-B, VI, VII Women and children	Must be pasteurized and conform to standards of identity for yogurt as listed in Table 4 of 7 C.F.R. 246.10(e)(12); may be plain or flavored with ≤40 grams of total sugars per 1 cup of yogurt	Must contain no more than 30 g total sugars per 8 oz serving (≤3.75 g total sugars per oz); soy-based yogurt substitute must contain at least 250 mg of calcium and 6.5 g of protein per 8 oz serving[c]	The availability of yogurts that contain 30 g or less of total sugars per 8 oz serving has expanded substantially; this amount is more closely aligned with the DGA; soy products meet the needs of individuals with a milk allergy or who consume a vegan diet
Cheese	IV, V-A, V-B, VI, VII Women and children	Domestic cheese made from 100 percent pasteurized milk. Must conform to FDA standard of identity (21 C.F.R. Part 133); Monterey Jack, Colby, natural Cheddar, Swiss, Brick, Muenster, Provolone, part skim or whole Mozzarella, pasteurized processed American, or blends of any of these cheeses are authorized Cheeses that are labeled low, free, reduced, less, or light in the nutrients of sodium, fat or cholesterol are WIC eligible	In addition, soy-based cheese substitute (not soy curd cheese) is permitted and must contain at least 250 mg of calcium and 6.5 g of protein per 1.5 ounce serving	Soy products meet the needs of individuals with a milk allergy or who consume a vegan diet

Breakfast cereal	IV, V-A, V-B, VI, VII Women and children	Must contain a minimum of 28 mg iron per 100 g dry cereal Must contain ≤21.2 g sucrose and other sugars per 100 g dry cereal (≤6 g per dry oz) At least half of the cereals authorized on a state agency's food list must have whole grain as the primary ingredient by weight *and* meet labeling requirements for making a health claim as a "whole grain food with moderate fat content": (1) contain a minimum of 51% whole grains (using dietary fiber as the indicator); (2) meet the regulatory definitions for "low saturated fat" at 21 C.F.R. 101.62 (≤1 g saturated fat per RACC) and "low cholesterol" (≤20 mg cholesterol per RACC); (3) bear quantitative trans-fat labeling; and (4) contain ≤6.5 g total fat per RACC and ≤0.5 g trans-fat per RACC	All ready-to-eat cereals on a state agency's authorized food list must adhere to the whole grain-rich criteria[d] and conform to other current specifications (e.g., must be iron-fortified, must not exceed added sugars limitations)	Intake of whole grains is low in the WIC population; whole grain cereal options have expanded substantially since the last review; the same products should qualify while aligning with USDA guidance for CACFP, the National School Lunch Program, and the National Breakfast Program (USDA/FNS, 2016d)

continued

TABLE 6-4 Continued

Category/Food	Food Package and Affected Participant Group, Considering the Proposed Food Package Revisions	Selected Current Specifications	Proposed Change to the Specifications[b]	Rationale
Whole grain options	IV, V-A, V-B, VI, VII Women and children			
Whole grain bread		Whole grain bread must conform to FDA standard of identity (21 C.F.R. 136.110) and meet labeling requirements for making a health claim as a "whole grain food with moderate fat content," as outlined above	Whole grain bread is no longer permitted; only 100 percent whole wheat bread is permitted	Very few states offer whole grain bread options other than 100 percent whole wheat; identification of suitable whole-grain breads (>50% whole grain) is challenging; restricting to 100 percent whole wheat bread aligns with most current state WIC authorized food lists and promotes intake of whole grains by WIC participants
Other whole grain options		Other whole unprocessed grains: Brown rice, bulgur (cracked wheat), oats, whole grain barley, and whole wheat macaroni (pasta) without added sugars, fats, oils, or salt (i.e., sodium)	In addition, teff or buckwheat may be offered; cornmeal (including blue); and corn masa flour meeting specifications outlined below are allowed	Additional options provide culturally suitable alternatives; participants and WIC staff expressed an interest in addition of these grains

Tortillas	Soft corn or whole wheat tortillas may be allowed at the state agency's option. Soft corn tortillas made from ground masa flour (corn flour) using traditional processing methods are WIC eligible, and include whole corn, corn (masa), whole ground corn, corn masa flour, masa harina, and white corn flour. For whole wheat tortillas, "whole wheat flour" must be the only flour listed in the ingredient list	In addition, once available in the marketplace, states are encouraged to offer tortillas made with folic acid–fortified corn masa flour	Folic acid is a nutrient of concern for premenopausal women; consumption of folic acid is lower among Hispanic compared to non-Hispanic women (Williams et al., 2015)
Cornmeal	Not yet permitted	Add whole corn meal (including blue) meeting the FDA standard of identity (21 C.F.R. 137.260) and that is in alignment with USDA specifications for corn meal in School Meal Programs (USDA-CNP-01-2008) to current options	Provides a culturally suitable option; similar in nutritive value to some types of permitted corn tortillas
Corn masa flour	Not yet permitted	Add corn masa flour. Once available in the marketplace, states are encouraged to offer folic acid–fortified corn masa flour	Allowing this flour aligns with the allowance of tortillas made with corn masa flour; participants expressed an interest

continued

TABLE 6-4 Continued

Category/Food	Food Package and Affected Participant Group, Considering the Proposed Food Package Revisions	Selected Current Specifications	Proposed Change to the Specifications[b]	Rationale
Fish	IV, V-A, V-B, VI, VII Women and children	May be packed in water or oil. Pack may include bones or skin. Added sauces and flavorings, such as tomato sauce, mustard, or lemon, are authorized at the state agency's option. May be regular or lower in sodium content	Canned fish may be water-packed (not oil packed) and may contain added sauces and flavorings. All other specifications remain unchanged	Few states currently offer oil-packed fish so there is minimal effect on participant choice; water-packed varieties are higher in nutrient-density because water-packed fish is lower in energy but contains the same levels of key nutrients per serving

NOTES: CACFP = Child and Adult Care Food Program; C.F.R. = *Code of Federal Regulations*; CVV = cash value voucher; FDA = U.S. Food and Drug Administration; IU = International Unit; NA = not applicable; RACC = reference amounts customarily consumed; RTE = ready-to-eat; USDA = U.S. Department of Agriculture.

[a] The table covers only cases in which a change to a food specification was made. See Appendix P, Table P-1, for a more comprehensive list of food specifications and proposed changes.

[b] Details are provided only for the proposed change. Other components of the specification remain the same.

[c] The committee's rationale for not requiring vitamin D fortification of yogurt is available in Appendix Q.

[d] It is anticipated that changes to the whole grain-rich criteria in alignment with the FDA proposed changes to the RACCs used for food labeling would be applied to the WIC food packages.

SOURCE: For current specifications, see USDA/FNS, 2014.

TABLE 6-5 Suggested Added Sugars Limits for WIC-Authorized Foods

	g per Serving*		
WIC Food	Naturally Occurring Sugars	Revised Total Sugars Specification	Suggested Added Sugars Specification (Upper Limit)
Yogurt, whole milk	11.4	30	18
Yogurt, low fat	17.3	30	13
Yogurt, nonfat	18.8	30	11
Soy beverage	—	12	10
Ready-to-eat cereals	—	6	6

NOTES: — = naturally occurring sugars are negligible.
* Based on 8 oz for yogurt and soy beverage, and 1 oz for cereals.
SOURCE: Based on data available in USDA/ARS, 2016.

specifications in light of not only the contribution of the current food packages to the DGA limit on COU, but also products now available in the marketplace, the role of added sugars in improving the palatability of nutritious foods, and the preferences of WIC participants. Specifications for total sugars[21] are outlined for yogurt, ready-to-eat cereals, and soy beverages. When the FDA regulation to include added sugars on food labels is implemented (FDA, 2016b), WIC food specifications could be changed from total sugars to added sugars. The rationale for maintaining the current total sugars limit for breakfast cereals is provided in Appendix Q. The rationales for revising the added sugar limits for yogurt and soy beverages are summarized below.

Total Sugars in Yogurt

The committee proposes reducing sugars in yogurt to 30 grams or less of total sugars per 8 ounces. The current limit for total sugars in yogurt (40 grams per 8 ounces) was set by the IOM (2006) committee and was based on amounts of total sugars in yogurts available in the marketplace at that time (personal communication, S. Murphy, July 6, 2016). Over the past decade, yogurt formulations have changed dramatically. In 2015, 55

[21] Although the FDA has issued a Final Rule, at present manufacturers are not required to include the amount of added sugars on food labels until as late as 2019. For this reason, a total sugars specification is required to limit the amount of added sugars in WIC-approved foods.

percent[22] of name-brand yogurt products sold in the United States that met all other WIC specifications contained 30 grams or less of total sugars per 8 ounces (personal communication, National Yogurt Association, March 3, 2016). These data indicate that yogurts containing less total sugars than the current WIC specification permits are widely available. Because private-label products typically follow the formulation changes of name-brand products (personal communication, National Yogurt Association, March 3, 2016), the availability of private-label yogurts with lower amounts of added sugar will probably expand in coming years.

Not only is the added sugars content of yogurts in the marketplace declining, but the committee's proposed reduction of added sugars in yogurt is aligned with the USDA-FNS Final Rule that requires all yogurt provided in the Child and Adult Care Food Program (CACFP) to contain no more than 23 grams of total sugars per 6 ounces (or 30 grams per 8 ounces) (USDA/FNS, 2016d). Market research conducted by USDA-FNS in support of this rule also indicated that yogurts with this amount of total sugars were widely available (USDA/FNS, 2016d).

At the time of this writing, yogurt had been added to WIC-approved food lists in only a few states. As a result, acceptance of this option by WIC participants could not be determined.

Total Sugars in Soy Beverages

At present, there are no specifications for total sugars in WIC-approved soy beverages. Although most states authorize soy beverages that contain 10 grams or less of total sugars, the committee considered it advisable to provide states with guidance about how to identify appropriate soy beverage choices as the market expands. Soy beverages currently available in the marketplace may contain as much as 20 grams of total sugars per 8-ounce serving (USDA/ARS, 2016). The committee proposes that the limit for total sugars in soy beverages selected by states be as low as possible, but not higher than 12 grams per 8 ounce serving. The level of 12 grams was selected because it is equivalent to the amount of total sugars from naturally occurring lactose in 8 ounces of unsweetened cow's milk.

---

[22] Data were extracted from Information Resources, Inc. (IRI) Total Multi-Outlet (MULO), including the latest 52 weeks, ending December 27, 2015. The percentage represents the proportion of the volume of yogurts sold, excluding private-label brands and yogurts containing artificial sweeteners, but includes all available package sizes.

Only Unflavored Milk Is Permitted

The Final Rule permits provision of flavored milk in the current WIC food packages. However, the CACFP allows only low-fat, unflavored milk and does not permit flavored milk to children up to age 5 (USDA/FNS, 2016d). To align the WIC food packages with CACFP regulations and to limit added sugars in the food packages, only unflavored milk is authorized in the revised WIC food packages. Although nonfat, flavored milk is permitted in the school meals programs (USDA/FNS, 2012), the nonfat, low-added-sugars flavored milk provided to schools is not widely commercially available (personal communication, C. Patey, National Dairy Council, July 16, 2016). The committee considered it appropriate for WIC to not only provide children with an easy transition into CACFP, but also to avoid contributing to early establishment of a preference for sweet taste (Beauchamp and Menella, 2009; Ventura and Worobey, 2013; personal communication, S. Johnson, University of Colorado, shared with the committee at the March 20, 2016 workshop).

At present, flavored milk is offered in 6 percent of states and 40 percent of Indian Tribal Organizations (ITOs), which together cover 3 percent of WIC participants (USDA/FNS, 2015a). At least one ITO is removing flavored milk from its food list to align with CACFP policy (personal communication, D. Tipton, Chickasaw Nation WIC, July 2016). Therefore, the recommendation is not expected to cause a significant disruption in administration of food packages nationally.

Changes to Whole Grain Requirements for WIC Foods

All Breakfast Cereals Must Meet "Whole Grain-Rich" Criteria

The current specifications for WIC-approved breakfast cereals (ready-to-eat and instant and regular hot cereals) require that half of such cereals made available by WIC vendors include whole grain as the primary ingredient by weight and meet the FDA labeling requirement for a "health claim notification for whole grain foods with moderate fat content" (i.e., these foods must also contain ≥51 percent whole grain ingredients by weight, but using dietary fiber as a marker [≥1.6 grams fiber per 28.35 grams of cereal]) (USDA/FNS, 2014). In the revised packages, this specification is changed in two ways: (1) "whole grain" breakfast cereals must meet the "whole grain-rich" criteria that is applied in CACFP,[23] the National School

[23] "Foods that qualify as whole grain-rich are foods that contain a blend of whole grain meal and/or whole grain flour and enriched meal and/or enriched flour of which at least 50 percent is whole grain and the remaining grains in the food, if any, are enriched; or foods that contain 100 percent whole grain." Most of the cereals that qualify as whole grain under the current WIC criteria would also qualify under the "whole grain-rich" criteria.

Lunch Program, and the National Breakfast Program (USDA/FNS, 2016d); and (2) all breakfast cereals offered by the WIC program must meet these criteria. All cereals must still meet current WIC requirements for iron (i.e., 28 milligrams of iron per 100 grams of cereal) and added sugars (not more than 6 grams per ounce serving).

Although the DGA have consistently specified that at least half of grain intake should be from whole grains since 2005, the 2015–2020 DGA additionally state that intake of refined grains should be limited but that individuals (particularly women capable of becoming pregnant) who consume all grains as whole should include in their diets at least some sources that are fortified with folic acid as a means of preventing neural tube defects (USDA/HHS, 2016). Table 6-6 illustrates the folic acid content of commonly redeemed ready-to-eat WIC cereals, including some fortified whole grain cereals. Although there is some variability, the popular whole grain cereals presented in the table provide an average of 160 percent of the EAR for folate for children ages 1 to 4 years and 47, 56, and 70 percent of the EAR for pregnant, breastfeeding, and postpartum women, respectively. These data indicate that whole grain and refined grain breakfast cereals are generally fortified with comparable amounts of folic acid.

TABLE 6-6 Folate Content of Commonly Redeemed Selected Cereals in WIC Food Packages

Categorization on Example State WIC Food Lists	Ready-to-Eat Cereal Type	Folate in 1 oz-eq (µg DFE)*
Whole grain	Honey and oat cereal, WG varieties	168
	Oat O's cereal	340
	Wheat squares with frosting (name brand)	175
	Wheat squares with frosting (store brand)	345
	Corn puffs cereal	375
Nonwhole grain	Honey and oat cereal, non-WG varieties	297–318
	Corn puffs cereal, with cartoon theme	353
	Corn flakes cereal	165
	Crisped rice cereal	293

NOTES: DFE = dietary folate equivalent; oz-eq = ounce-equivalents; WG = whole grain; µg = microgram.

* Based on the Food Patterns Equivalent Database value of 28.35 g cereal per serving equivalent.

SOURCES: USDA/ARS, 2016; redemption data provided to the committee from Texas and Wyoming WIC agencies (2015), available in the public access file for this study (Email: paro@nas.edu).

Although there are no specific regulations about fortification of ready-to-eat breakfast cereals other than enrichment of the refined grain portion with 140 micrograms of folic acid per 100 grams grain, both refined and whole grain cereals are generally fortified with at least 25 percent of micronutrient needs for a 2,000-kcal diet (the current basis for Daily Values on the food label[24]) (USDA/ARS, 2016). Therefore, there is no substantive difference in micronutrient content of refined grain cereals compared to whole grain cereals that meet the revised WIC "whole grain-rich" criteria.

Evaluation of Breakfast Cereal Redemption and Current Marketplace Options

To ensure that a variety of breakfast cereal products that meet the new specifications will be available to WIC state agencies, the committee reviewed product information provided by two large national manufacturers of ready-to-eat breakfast cereals.[25] Together, these manufacturers produce at least 14 different types of ready-to-eat cereals that meet the current WIC whole grain criteria, including 4 gluten-free whole grain varieties. Launches of whole grain products, including cereal (wheat and other grains), doubled between 2006 and 2011 (Oldways, 2015). This information suggests that an adequate number of products are now available to meet state needs for WIC-approved choices for "whole grain-rich" breakfast cereals.

All Breads Are 100 Percent Whole Wheat

At present, WIC-authorized breads include both 100 percent whole wheat bread (i.e., whole grain wheat is the primary ingredient by weight) and whole grain breads that meet the FDA requirement for a "health claim notification for whole grain foods with moderate fat content" (again, these foods must also contain at least 51 percent whole grain ingredients by weight, but using dietary fiber as a marker [at least 1.6 grams fiber per 28.35 grams]) (USDA/FNS, 2014). The committee proposes that this specification be revised such that all bread in the WIC food packages be 100 percent whole wheat and that whole grain bread no longer be permitted. Currently, very few states offer a whole grain bread option, possibly

[24] The committee is aware that the FDA has issued a proposed Final Rule for food label revisions (FDA, 2016b) that may affect ready-to-eat cereal fortification levels for some nutrients. This is not anticipated to adversely affect provision of key nutrients (specifically, iron and folate) to WIC participants consuming these cereals.

[25] This information is available in the public access file for this study (Email: paro@nas.edu). One manufacturer collated and provided data on the whole-grain options produced by the "top four RTE cereal manufacturers."

as a result of the expansive selection of bread products in the marketplace that include the words *whole grain* but that contain various proportions of whole grain and refined grain. Manufacturers are permitted to make factual statements about the amounts of whole grains on the labels of their products (e.g., "this product contains 5 grams of whole grains per serving"), but products for which the labels include the words "whole grain" are not required to contain a minimum amount of this ingredient (FDA, 2006). The committee concluded that WIC-approved breads should be restricted to those that contain 100 percent whole wheat to reduce confusion, align WIC-authorized breads with most current state offerings, and improve WIC participants' overall dietary balance of whole to refined grains. For individuals with celiac disease or gluten intolerance, other grain options are available.

Specifications for Tofu

Tofu is included in the current food packages as a substitute for milk and is required to be calcium-set.[26] To ensure that tofu provides an amount of calcium equivalent to the amount in milk it is intended to replace, the proposed new specification requires that tofu contain at least 200 milligrams of calcium per 100 grams of tofu. Products matching this requirement are anticipated to be readily available in the marketplace. The specification that tofu may not contain added fats, sugars, oils, or sodium is retained.

Specifications for New Substitution Options

Specifications for New Grain Options

The revised food packages offer additional grain options to accommodate cultural eating patterns and other food preferences. Cornmeal (including blue), buckwheat, and teff must be 100 percent whole grain. Cornmeals should align with the USDA-FNS specifications for cornmeal in USDA-FNS child nutrition programs (e.g., CACFP), that is, products must be labeled as "whole corn" (or be labeled with other "whole" corn designations, such as whole grain corn, whole ground corn, whole cornmeal [including blue], and whole corn flour) (USDA-CNP-01-2008). To align with USDA-FNS allowances for tortillas (USDA/FNS, 2014), corn masa flour that is not 100 percent whole grain is permitted. States should be encouraged to offer corn masa flour and tortillas made with corn masa flour that is fortified with folic acid when these products become available.

---

[26] Calcium-set tofu is prepared using calcium salts as a coagulant.

Specifications for New Soy Options

To expand options for WIC participants who are lactose-intolerant or who follow a vegan diet, soy-based cheese and soy-based yogurt substitute products are added to the revised packages as substitutions for milk. These products are required to contain 250 milligram of calcium and 6.5 grams of protein per serving equivalent (1.5 ounces of soy-based cheese substitute or 8 ounces of soy-based yogurt substitute). These specifications ensure that these substitutes supplement the diets of WIC participants with key nutrients that the WIC food packages are intended to provide.

Other Specifications for WIC-Approved Foods

The committee reviewed in detail all food specifications outlined in the Final Rule (USDA/FNS, 2014). Any specifications not addressed in this section remain as currently stated in the Final Rule (see Appendix P for details on additional WIC food specifications). Given the evidence presented, the committee recommends the following changes related to specifications for WIC-approved foods in the food packages:

6-7. USDA-FNS should modify required specifications for some WIC foods to improve their alignment with dietary guidance.

The specific specification changes recommended for WIC foods are

- Yogurt may contain no more than 30 grams of total sugars per 8 ounces (3.75 grams of total sugars per ounce).
- Soy beverages may contain no more than 12 grams of total sugars per 8 ounces.
- Only unflavored milk is permitted.
- All breakfast cereals provided through WIC meet the "whole grain-rich" criterion, as outlined for the USDA-FNS Child and Adult Food Care Program. Other specifications, such as 6 grams or less of total sugars per 28.35 grams (1 cup-equivalent) serving and 28 milligrams iron per 100 grams of dry of cereal, are retained.
- Bread should be 100 percent whole wheat bread.
- Tofu should contain at least 200 milligrams of calcium per 100 grams of tofu.
- Each 1.5 ounces of soy-based cheese substitute or 8 ounces of soy-based yogurt substitute should contain 250 milligrams of calcium and 6.5 grams of protein.

- Fish may be packed in water or the currently allowed sauces and flavorings.

Foods and Food Specifications That Were Reviewed, But Not Changed

The committee deliberated over several possible decisions that did not result in a change to the food packages. In particular, USDA-FNS asked that the committee evaluate currently provided amounts of infant formula and specifications for iron and energy density of infant formulas, and inclusion of additional fish species in the food packages. Following a comprehensive review of available evidence, no changes were recommended in these, and other cases. A description of these topics and the rationale for retaining the status quo is presented in Appendix Q.

SUMMARY

The recommended revisions to the WIC food packages outlined in this chapter are based on the committee's considerations of the health of the WIC-participating population, food safety risks relevant to the WIC-participating population, current dietary guidance (i.e., the DGA and dietary guidance for individuals less than 2 years of age), nationwide availability of foods, and state agency and vendor administrative burden. These recommended changes build upon the successes of the 2009 food package changes by further increasing participant access to vegetables and fruits, increasing the flexibility of options to better meet participant cultural eating patterns and food preferences, and increasing the latitude of participants to make the choice to breastfeed. The revised food packages were designed with the benefit of redemption information that was not available to the 2006 committee as well as firsthand experience through committee site visits and shopping experiences. Although the cost-neutral requirement restricted the committee's ability to make all of the changes they would have preferred to make across all food groups, application of the "supplemental" criterion allowed savings that resulted from reduction in some food groups to support increases in other food groups. Overall, the committee was able to improve the balance of food groups and subgroups to better meet the DGA recommendations. In Chapter 11, recommendations for implementation of these revised food packages, as well as recommendations for evaluation of the revised food packages are provided.

REFERENCES

AAP (American Academy of Pediatrics). 2014. *Pediatric Nutrition*. 7th ed. Edited by R. E. Kleinman and F. R. Greer. Elk Grove Village, IL: American Academy of Pediatrics.

AHA (American Heart Association). 2015. *Fish and omega-3 fatty acids.* http://www.heart.org/HEARTORG/HealthyLiving/HealthyEating/HealthyDietGoals/Fish-and-Omega-3-Fatty-Acids_UCM_303248_Article.jsp (accessed August 30, 2016).

Andreyeva, T., J. Luedicke, A. S. Tripp, and K. E. Henderson. 2013. Effects of reduced juice allowances in food packages for the women, infants, and children program. *Pediatrics* 131(5):919–927.

Arimond, M., and M. T. Ruel. 2004. Dietary diversity is associated with child nutritional status: Evidence from 11 demographic and health surveys. *Journal of Nutrition* 134(10):2579–2585.

Beauchamp, G. K., and J. A. Mennella. 2009. Early flavor learning and its impact on later feeding behavior. *Journal of Pediatric Gastroenterology and Nutrition* 48(Suppl 1):S25–S30.

CFA (Canned Food Alliance). 2016. *Enjoying canned foods: 3 tips to lower sodium intake.* http://www.mealtime.org/~/media/files/fact-sheets/Tips-to-Reduce-Sodium_CFA-Infographic_FINAL.pdf (accessed September 29, 2016).

Di Noia, J., D. Monica, K. W. Cullen, R. Pérez-Escamilla, H. L. Gray, and A. Sikorskii. 2016. Differences in fruit and vegetable intake by race/ethnicity and by Hispanic origin and nativity among women in the Special Supplemental Nutrition Program for Women, Infants, and Children, 2015. *Preventing Chronic Disease* 13:E115.

FDA (U.S. Food and Drug Administration). 2006. Guidance for industry and FDA staff: Whole grain label statements. Silver Spring, MD: FDA. http://www.fda.gov/OHRMS/DOCKETS/98fr/06d-0066-gdl0001.pdf (accessed December 21, 2016).

FDA. 2016a. Food additives permitted for direct addition to food for human consumption; folic acid. https://www.gpo.gov/fdsys/pkg/FR-2016-04-15/pdf/2016-08792.pdf (accessed December 13, 2016).

FDA. 2016b. *Food labeling: Revision of the nutrition and supplement facts labels.* https://www.regulations.gov/document?D=FDA-2012-N-1210-0875 (accessed September 29, 2016).

FDA/EPA (U.S. Food and Drug Administration/U.S. Environmental Protection Agency). 2004. FDA and EPA announce the revised consumer advisory on methylmercury in fish. Silver Spring, MD: FDA. http://www.fda.gov/NewsEvents/Newsroom/PressAnnouncements/2004/ucm108267.htm (accessed December 21, 2016).

Fung, E. B., L. D. Ritchie, B. H. Walker, G. Gildengorin, and P. B. Crawford. 2010. Randomized, controlled trial to examine the impact of providing yogurt to women enrolled in WIC. *Journal of Nutrition Education and Behavior* 42(3 Suppl):S22–S29.

HER (Healthy Eating Research). 2016. *Minimum stocking levels and marketing strategies of healthful foods for small retail food stores.* http://healthyeatingresearch.org/wp-content/uploads/2016/02/her_minimum_stocking_final.pdf (accessed September 29, 2016).

HHS (U.S. Department of Health and Human Services). 2011. *Nutrition: Strategies & Guidelines.* http://www.cdc.gov/nutrition/strategies-guidelines/index.html (accessed September 29, 2016).

Hromi-Fiedler, A., D. Chapman, S. Segura-Pérez, G. Damio, P. Clark, J. Martinez, and R. Pérez-Escamilla. 2016. Barriers and facilitators to improve fruit and vegetable intake among WIC-eligible pregnant Latinas: An application of the health action process approach framework. *Journal of Nutrition Education and Behavior* 48(7):468–477.

IOM (Institute of Medicine). 2006. *WIC food packages: Time for a change.* Washington, DC: The National Academies Press.

IOM. 2011. *Dietary Reference Intakes for calcium and vitamin D.* Washington, DC: The National Academies Press.

Loewenstein, G. F. 1988. Frames of mind in intertemporal choice. *Management Science* 34(2):200–214.

Miller, S. R., and W. A. Knudson. 2014. Nutrition and cost comparisons of select canned, frozen, and fresh fruits and vegetables. *American Journal of Lifestyle Medicine* 8(6): 430–437.

NASEM (National Academies of Sciences, Engineering, and Medicine). 2016. *Review of WIC food packages: Proposed framework for revisions: Interim report.* Washington, DC: The National Academies Press. doi: 10.17226/21832.

Oh, M., H. Jensen, and I. Rahkovsky. 2016. Did revisions to the WIC program affect household expenditures on whole grains? *Applied Economic Perspectives and Policy* 38(4):578–598. doi: 10.1093/aepp/ppw020. Advance access, October 17, 2016.

Oldways Whole Grain Council. 2015. *Whole grain statistics.* http://wholegrainscouncil.org/newsroom/whole-grain-statistics (accessed December 21, 2016).

PAHO/WHO (Pan American Health Organization/World Health Organization). 2003. *Guiding principles for complementary feeding of the breastfed child.* Geneva, Switzerland: PAHO/WHO. http://www.who.int/maternal_child_adolescent/documents/a85622/en (accessed August 30, 2016).

PBHF (Produce for Better Health Foundation). 2016. Produce for Better Health Foundation. http://www.pbhfoundation.org (accessed September 29, 2016).

Rickman, J. C., D. M. Barrett, and C. M. Bruhn. 2007. Nutritional comparison of fresh, frozen and canned fruits and vegetables. Part 1. Vitamins C and B and phenolic compounds. *Journal of the Science of Food and Agriculture* 87(6):930–944.

Siega-Riz, A. M., D. M. Deming, K. C. Reidy, M. K. Fox, E. Condon, and R. R. Briefel. 2010. Food consumption patterns of infants and toddlers: Where are we now? *Journal of the American Dietetic Association* 110(12 Suppl):S38–51.

Song, W. O., O. K. Chun, J. Kerver, S. Cho, C. E. Chung, and S. J. Chung. 2006. Ready-to-eat breakfast cereal consumption enhances milk and calcium intake in the US population. *Journal of the American Dietetic Association* 106(11):1783–1789.

USDA/ARS (U.S. Department of Agriculture/Agricultural Research Service). 2016. *USDA national nutrient database for standard reference.* Release 28. Beltsville, MD: USDA/ARS. https://ndb.nal.usda.gov/ndb (accessed September 14, 2016).

USDA/ERS (U.S. Department of Agriculture/Economic Research Service). 2016. *How much do fruits and vegetables cost?* Washington, DC: USDA/ERS. http://www.ers.usda.gov/data-products/fruit-and-vegetable-prices/ (accessed March 2, 2016).

USDA/FNS (U.S. Department of Agriculture/Food and Nutrition Service). 2012. *Nutrition Standards in the National School Lunch and School Breakfast Programs, Final Rule.* 7 C.F.R. § 210 and 220.

USDA/FNS. 2014. *Special Supplemental Nutrition Program for Women, Infants and Children (WIC): Revisions in the WIC food packages.* Final Rule, 7 C.F.R. § 246.

USDA/FNS. 2015a. *WIC food packages policy options II.* Final report. Alexandria, VA: USDA/FNS. http://www.fns.usda.gov/wic-food-package-policy-options-ii (accessed December 21, 2016).

USDA/FNS. 2015b. *WIC participant and program characteristics 2014.* Final report. http://www.fns.usda.gov/sites/default/files/ops/WICPC2014.pdf (accessed December 21, 2016).

USDA/FNS. 2015c. *WIC policy memorandum #2015-7 to WIC state agency directors: Medicaid primary payer for exempt infant formulas and medical foods.* Alexandria, VA: USDA/FNS.

USDA/FNS. 2016a. *Agency information collection activities: WIC program regulations. Federal Register* 81(40). Alexandria, VA: USDA/FNS. https://www.gpo.gov/fdsys/pkg/FR-2016-03-01/html/2016-04262.htm (accessed July 13, 2016).

USDA/FNS. 2016b. *Breastfeeding policy and guidance.* Alexandria, VA: USDA/FNS. http://www.fns.usda.gov/sites/default/files/wic/WIC-Breastfeeding-Policy-and-Guidance.pdf (accessed November 4, 2016).

USDA/FNS. 2016c. *Healthy corner stores guide*. Alexandria, VA: USDA/FNS. http://www.fns.usda.gov/healthy-corner-stores-guide (accessed November 4, 2016).
USDA/FNS. 2016d. *Child and Adult Care Food Program: Meal pattern revisions related to the healthy, Hunger-Free Kids Act of 2010*; 7 C.F.R. § 210, 215, 220, and 226.
USDA/FNS. 2016e. Home-prepared baby food. Alexandria, VA: USDA/FNS. http://www.fns.usda.gov/sites/default/files/feedinginfants-ch12.pdf (accessed November 4, 2016).
USDA/HHS (U.S. Department of Agriculture/U.S. Department of Health and Human Services). 2010. *Dietary Guidelines for Americans 2010*. Washington, DC: U.S. Government Printing Office. http://www.health.gov/dietaryguidelines/dga2010/dietaryguidelines2010.pdf (accessed December 21, 2016).
USDA/HHS. 2016. *Dietary Guidelines for Americans 2015–2020*. Washington, DC: U.S. Government Printing Office. https://health.gov/dietaryguidelines/2015 (accessed August 29, 2016).
Ventura, A. K., and J. Worobey. 2013. Early influences on the development of food preferences. *Current Biology* 23(9):R401–R408.
Walker, M. 2015. Formula supplementation of breastfed infants: Helpful or hazardous? *ICAN: Infant, Child, & Adolescent Nutrition* 7(4):198–207.
Whaley, E. S., M. Koleilat., M. Whaley, J. Gomez, K. Meehan, and K. Saluja. 2012. Impact of policy changes on infant feeding decisions among low-income women participating in the Special Supplemental Nutrition Program for Women, Infants, and Children. *American Journal of Public Health* 102(12):2269–2273.
Williams, J., C. T. Mai, J. Mulinare, J. Isenburg, T. J. Flood, M. Ethen, B. Frohnert, and R. S. Kirby. 2015. Updated estimates of neural tube defects prevented by mandatory folic acid fortification—United States, 1995–2011. *Morbidly and Mortality Weekly Report* 64(1):1–5.

7

Evaluation of Cost

In this chapter, the methods used to generate cost estimates for both the current and revised food packages and to ensure the cost neutrality of the revised packages are described. As explained in Chapter 1, ensuring cost neutrality was at the crux of the committee's final decisions for food package revisions. As part of the committee's strategy to emphasize consideration of the value of the food packages for the mother–infant dyad (described in Chapter 6), this chapter also presents comparisons of the market value of the current and revised food packages for the three types of mother–infant pairs: fully breastfeeding, partially breastfeeding, and fully formula-feeding. The sensitivity of the results to several of the assumptions used to estimate cost are tested and described in Chapter 8. In Chapter 10 (an abridged version of Appendix U), the projected effects of the food package changes on overall costs to the program are evaluated.

METHODS USED TO ESTIMATE COSTS

Overview

As described in Chapter 1 (see Figure 1-1), the framework for revising the food packages required the committee to consider several sets of food packages in an iterative fashion. In each iteration, adjustments were made to ensure that the revised set of packages met the criteria outlined in Chapter 1, Box 1-4, while also being cost-neutral.

To evaluate cost-neutrality, the committee created spreadsheets for each food package that detailed the costs of each food in the package as well as costs of the total package for both actual redemption (i.e., based on available redemption data) and full redemption. These spreadsheets also detailed the nutrient composition of each food in each package.[1] The spreadsheets were linked to participation numbers so the weighted average per-participant food package costs could be estimated for both the revised and current food packages. The difference in the weighted-average, per-participant cost of a single food package between the committee's final, proposed set of revised food packages and the current set of food packages was required to be cost neutral, specifically no greater or less than $0.10.

As explained in more detail in the sections that follow, the weighted-average, per-participant costs of the food packages were based on the number and distribution of the Special Supplemental Nutrition Program for Women, Infants, and Children (WIC) participants across packages and estimated cost of each food package. The methods used to evaluate cost-neutrality were similar to those described in the previous WIC report (IOM, 2006). However, this committee benefited from the availability of cost data specific to WIC foods as well as redemption data. Estimated food package costs were calculated using these prices and redemption rates.

General Data Considerations

The base year for the comparison of cost neutrality between the sets of revised and current food packages was fiscal year (FY) 2015, the year for which the most complete set of participant data was available. The quantities for food items were based on the maximum allowances specified for the current and revised packages (for current food packages, see Chapter 1, for the revised food packages, see Chapter 6). There was no single data source for any component used in the committee's cost-neutrality analyses (i.e., participation, prices, composition of the WIC food categories for which there are multiple options, and redemption). When possible, the committee used data that were considered the most representative of WIC national trends (i.e., the U.S. Department of Agriculture's Food and Nutrition Service [USDA-FNS] price and redemption dataset [further described below] or data from the WIC Participant and Program Characteristics Series), filling in gaps with supplementary sources (i.e., state-specific data) as needed and as available to the committee.

[1] The nutrient composition of the current packages is presented in Chapter 3, Tables 3-11 through 3-13. The food group and nutrient content of the current compared to the revised packages are presented in Appendix T.

Estimating the WIC Participation Distribution Across Food Packages

To evaluate the cost-neutrality of the proposed set of revised food packages, the committee estimated the food costs to the WIC program based on the estimated costs of each food package and the number and distribution of participants. WIC participant distributions across food packages are presented in Table 7-1. These distributions were based on two sources: (1) *WIC Participant and Program Characteristics 2014: Food Package Report* (USDA/FNS, 2016a) representative of participation in April 2014, and (2) average participation by category for FY2015 from administrative data (USDA/FNS, 2016b). Briefly, the *Food Package Report* provides the distribution of the 27 food package options across six participant categories for all participants certified to receive benefits in the month of April of the assessment year (i.e., for this analysis, 2014). This data source includes all participants certified to receive benefits in April 2014, regardless of whether they were issued or claimed their benefits. As a result, total participation in the *Food Package Report* is higher than actual participation. The distributions reported in the *Food Package Report* were applied to the administrative data,[2] a report of average monthly participation for the entire WIC program for FY2015 (USDA/FNS, 2016c). The regulatory impact analysis (see Appendix U) includes a detailed explanation of how participation for each food package was determined.

For the revised set of packages, it was assumed that neither the revisions nor allowed substitutions had any effect on participation, with one exception. As a result of its proposed option for an infant to be partially breastfed in the first 30 days, the committee anticipates that 5 percent of the formula-fed infants and 5 percent of women who were postpartum for 6 months or less but not breastfeeding were shifted to their respective partially breastfeeding categories.[3] Additionally, in the current food packages, postpartum women who are not breastfeeding no longer receive WIC benefits after 6 months (food package VI). To account for a predicted shift of the latter group to partially breastfeeding (for whom benefits extend for 1 year postpartum), 5 percent of these nonbreastfeeding women were shifted back into the program to the partially breastfeeding package (V-B). The 5-percent shift was selected based on data presented in USDA/FNS (2011) that indicated that the 2009 food package (in which women to choose between formula feeding or fully breastfeeding) resulted in an approximately 7- to 11-percent shift of women out of the partially breastfeeding food package. The shifts were largely to the fully formula-fed package (as discussed

---

[2] Administrative data includes all state agencies, Indian Tribal Organizations, and territories.

[3] An explanation of the committee's recommendation to allow up to 364 fluid ounces of formula in the first month (i.e., the partial breastfeeding option in the infant's first 30 days) is provided in Chapter 6.

TABLE 7-1 Participant Distributions Used to Estimate Costs for Current and Revised Food Packages

Group	Age/Participant Category	Description	Package Notation	Current Package: Percentage Within Category	Current Package: Number of Participants	Revised Package[a]: Percentage Within Category	Revised Package[a]: Number of Participants
Infants	0–3.9 months	Fully formula-fed	I-FF-A	69	341,009	66	323,959
	(0–0.9 months)	Partially breastfed	I-BF/FF-A	4	18,053	4	21,622
	(1–3.9 months)	Partially breastfed	I-BF/FF-B	14	68,202	17	81,684
	0–3.9 months	Fully breastfed	I-BF-A	13	66,196	13	66,196
	Subtotals			**100**	**493,460**	**100**	**493,461**
	4–5.9 months	Fully formula-fed	I-FF-B	72	208,617	69	198,187
		Partially breastfed	I-BF/FF-C	17	48,142	17	58,573
		Fully breastfed	I-BF-B	11	32,095	11	32,095
	Subtotals			**100**	**288,855**	**100**	**288,855**
	6–12 months	Fully formula-fed	II-FF	76	710,344	72	674,827
		Partially breastfed	II-BF/FF	12	108,321	15	143,838
		Fully breastfed	II-BF	12	114,338	12	114,338
	Subtotals			**100**	**933,003**	**100**	**933,003**
	Totals for infants				**1,715,318**		**1,715,319**
Children	1–1.9 years		IV-A	30	1,257,128	30	1,257,128
	2–4.9 years		IV-B	70	2,875,993	70	2,875,993
	Totals for children			**100**	**4,133,121**	**100**	**4,133,121**

Women	Pregnant	V,[c] V-A[d]	41	761,551	41	761,551
	Partially breastfeeding	V,[c] V-B[d]	7	132,032	9	170,362
	Nonbreastfeeding postpartum and minimally breastfeeding women[b]	VI	38	700,393	36	665,374
	Fully breastfeeding	VII	14	261,756	14	261,756
	Totals for women		**100**	**1,855,732**	**100**	**1,859,043**
Participants with Qualifying Conditions						
	Infants	III (I–II)	74	188,558	74	188,558
	Children	III (IV)	25	63,574	25	63,574
	Women	III (V–VII)	0.5	1,224	0.5	1,224
	Totals for participants with qualifying conditions		**100**	**253,356**	**100**	**253,356**
Totals for Program				**7,957,526**		**7,960,838**

NOTES: Participation information derived from the *WIC Participant and Program Characteristics 2014: Food Package Report* (USDA/FNS, 2016a) and WIC administrative data (USDA/FNS, 2016b). A detailed description of the participation distributions is available in Chapter 10.

[a] The participant distribution for the current and revised food packages are the same, with one exception. For the revised food packages, 5 percent of formula-fed infants and postpartum, nonbreastfeeding women were shifted to the partially breastfeeding packages. Five percent of postpartum, nonbreastfeeding women who were no longer receiving a package because their infants were 6 months or older were shifted back onto the program, to receive a partially breastfeeding food package.

[b] This group includes both nonbreastfeeding, postpartum women and minimally breastfeeding women who are less than 6 months postpartum.

[c] Food package V in the current set of food packages is issued to both pregnant and partially breastfeeding women.

[d] In the revised set of packages, food package V is separated into V-A for pregnant women and V-B for partially breastfeeding women.

SOURCES: USDA/FNS, 2016a,b.

further in Chapter 2). The 5-percent value was therefore considered a conservative estimate for the number of participants who would shift back to partial breastfeeding.

Estimating WIC Food Costs

In contrast to the IOM (2006) report, this committee had the benefit of cost data that were specific to WIC foods. USDA-FNS provided the committee with 12 months (August 2013 through July 2014) of price and redemption data from a convenience sample of six WIC state agencies, representing five of the seven regions of the country (hereafter referenced as "FNS redemption dataset"). The states were diverse in terms of size and did not include Indian Tribal Organizations or territories.[4,5] (A discussion of other sources of redemption data used by the committee is provided in the "Use of Redemption Rates" section.) The identity of the agencies was not known to the committee. Data from each state agency included the main category of food (e.g., "legume"); subcategory of food (e.g., "canned beans"); size and measure of the container (e.g., 16 ounces); number of containers redeemed in the month; average price for the container; and the total amount paid by WIC for that specific item in the given month. Some states provided specific food subcategories (e.g., "soft corn tortillas") while others provided broad categorizations (e.g., "whole grains, all types"). USDA-FNS summed all available data across the six states and all months. These composite data were used to calculate average price per unit (e.g., price per ounce), as redeemed by WIC participants.

In three cases (i.e., infant formula, yogurt, and new grain sizes), prices were not available in the FNS redemption dataset. For these, marketing data from the 2014 Information Resources, Inc. (IRI) Consumer Network Database were used instead. Prices from all sources were adjusted to represent FY2015.[6] Adjusted prices are presented in Appendix R, Table R-1. Additional details about infant formula cost estimates are provided below.

The committee had no information on either the costs of medical foods or portions of these costs paid by WIC. Thus, the food package III costs presented here account only for foods in the corresponding age and physiological state food package. They do not account for medical products.

[4] These data are available in the public access file for this study (Email: paro@nas.edu).

[5] As characterized by USDA-FNS.

[6] The two sources of price data encompassed different timeframes. The FNS redemption dataset represented August 2013 through July 2014 and the IRI prices represented calendar year 2014. To create a common base year, prices were inflated to FY2015 prices using Bureau of Labor Statistics Consumer Price Index (CPI) adjustments (see BLS, 2016). To accomplish this, the average item-specific CPI for FY2015 was divided by the average CPI for the timeframe encompassed by the available unit price. Additional detail is available in Appendix R, Table R-1.

Costs for the revised food package III were estimated based on 2015 prices and the numbers and categories of participants who were issued that package in 2015.

Infant Formula Cost and Rebate Assumptions

The retail price of each form of formula (powdered, ready-to-feed, and concentrate) was determined by using a 2014 IRI price, adjusted to reflect a FY2015 price. Per-unit prices for each form of formula were then weighted by the volume of each form issued in the WIC program, as reported by USDA-FNS (USDA/FNS, 2013a), to determine a composite price per unit. Starting with this composite price per unit, the post-rebate cost of formula was determined.

To maintain lower costs, states are required to negotiate rebate contracts with infant formula companies. According to the 2010 WIC Cost of Foods report (USDA/FNS, 2013b), the post-rebate cost for formula was $927 million of $2,615 million (retail). This is equivalent to a rebate of 65 percent. Because this number was from 2010, the committee evaluated the stability of rebates between 2010 and 2015.[7] With the exception of 2011, rebates between 2010 and 2015 were relatively stable. Therefore, the committee multiplied the composite price per unit by a factor of approximately 0.35. All assumptions applied to estimate the costs of formula are presented in Appendix R, Table R-2.

Creating Composites for the WIC Food Categories

Similar to the approach used in the IOM (2006) report, the estimated costs of (and nutrients provided by) the current and revised food packages were based on the unit prices for each food (or food category, i.e., "whole grains"), adjusted to FY2015, and the amounts of each food in each food package. For each of the food categories, the price was a weighted average of several food items, estimated using a series of assumptions. The specific assumptions applied for cost are presented in Appendix R, Tables R-1 and R-2. As mentioned previously, the information used to weight the proportions of particular foods for each WIC food category came from different sources, including the USDA-FNS redemption dataset, the *Food Package Report* series, and/or data from individual states. In this way, available information was used to create food package cost and nutrient profiles that represented WIC redemptions as closely as possible (see Appendix R, Tables R-3 and R-4). As an example, the USDA-FNS redemption dataset

[7] Rebates were reported as "rebates billed" before 2013 and "rebates received" after 2013. These were considered equivalent for the purpose of estimating rebate changes over time.

included prices for both canned and dried beans, as well as peanut butter. To estimate the cost of the "legume" WIC food category, the average cost per unit for each of these options was calculated. For each food package, a composite was developed depending on whether participants are issued both legumes and peanut butter each month or only one of these options. In this example, the ratio of canned to dry legumes typically redeemed was ascertained from the USDA-FNS redemption dataset. For food packages that required participants to choose between beans or peanut butter, a proportion of 50 percent of each was assumed to be issued.

For all foods, except those acquired with the cash value voucher (CVV), the committee's cost (and nutrient) composites accounted only for foods for which the USDA-FNS redemption dataset indicated that redemption was at least 1 percent. For example, tofu was not included in the "milk" WIC food category composite because it represented less than 1 percent of redemptions. Therefore, any price (or nutrient) difference of tofu was considered to have no substantive effect on the composite.

For vegetables and fruits, only the five most commonly redeemed vegetables and six most commonly redeemed fruits were considered in the composite. Redemption data for vegetables and fruit were obtained from Massachusetts, Texas, and Wyoming.[8] They were combined with USDA's Economic Research Service (USDA-ERS) price data to determine the cost of a cup-equivalent serving of a composite vegetable and composite fruit (USDA/ERS, 2013). These composite vegetable and composite fruit values were then weighted by the ratio of vegetables to fruits typically purchased with CVV dollars, as indicated by redemption data. This process resulted in one price per cup-equivalent serving representative of vegetables and fruits commonly redeemed by WIC participants.[9]

Use of Redemption Rates

In contrast to the IOM (2006) report, the committee also benefited from data on redemption rates.[10] The USDA-FNS redemption dataset was

---

[8] Information provided from states is available in the public access file for this study (Email: paro@nas.edu).

[9] The committee assumed that the composite of vegetables and fruit would not change when the CVV is expanded, as the committee had no information to assess quantitatively how the composite might change at higher CVV amounts. To the extent that families shift their choices of vegetables and fruits with a higher CVV as their preference for fruits is progressively satisfied, this might lead to different ratios of fruits to vegetables and might affect nutrients and food group delivery of the food packages.

[10] The overall redemption rate refers to the percentage of the maximum allowance prescribed to WIC participants that is actually obtained by recipients. A full redemption means the person redeemed their entire prescription. A partial redemption means they redeemed some but not all. Some participants redeem none of their prescribed benefits.

the primary source of these data.[11] For food categories without redemption data in the USDA-FNS redemption dataset, the committee applied redemption values provided by a few individual states over the course of the study. Redemption values published in the Altarum electronic benefit transfer (EBT) report were also considered (USDA/ERS, 2014a). For the revised food packages, the committee calculated a revised redemption rate based on equations that considered changes to food amounts, the distribution of redemption (e.g., the degree of nonredemption, partial redemption, or full redemption) for specific foods from the Altarum report, and predicted behavioral changes based on reduced or increased options. A detailed description of the method for estimating redemption rates used in this report is provided in Appendix R.

Cost of Substitutions

The revised set of food packages include the same substitutions that are permitted in the current food packages, plus some additional options. In addition to covering all the foods in the basic WIC food categories (formula, infant foods, milk, cheese, peanut butter, beans, whole wheat bread [grains], eggs, fish, and fruits and vegetables), the committee's cost evaluations also covered substitutions.

Substitution costs were based on data on the substitution rate, when available (see Appendix R, Tables R-3 and R-4). For example, generation of cost (and nutrient) information for the low-fat milk composite was based on ratios of nonfat milk, 1% milk, and soymilk that reflect redemption patterns. The same is true for beans: The composite cost (and nutrient) values account for the proportions of canned to dry beans based on available redemption data. When such data were not available, the substitution rate was based on a likely preference. For example, because there was no information on the amount of milk that is redeemed as cheese or yogurt, the committee assumed full substitution.[12] Inasmuch as this full substitution is of greater monetary value to the recipient (that is, 1 pound of cheese or 1 quart of yogurt are more expensive than the milk that is replaced) it resulted in a conservative cost estimate (the highest possible cost) for both

[11] To keep the state agencies anonymous, USDA-FNS inputted average monthly participation by participant category for each state into a spreadsheet containing the redemption equations created by the committee, and returned the overall unweighted average redemption across the state agencies per food package item. Through this process, USDA-FNS identified one of the six states as a clear outlier, and removed it from the averages (personal communication, K. Castellanos-Brown, USDA-FNS, June 22, 2016). As such, redemption estimates represent five of the six state agencies included in the FNS redemption dataset.

[12] The substitution options differ by food package. A specific ratio of the possible full substitution options was assigned to participants for each food package, as detailed in Appendix R.

the current and revised food packages. For example, as shown in Table 7-2, redeeming 1 quart of whole milk yogurt in place of 1 quart of whole milk costs an additional $2.36.

The effects of other selected substitutions are also presented in Table 7-2. For example, redeeming four 16-ounce cans of beans instead of 1 pound of dry beans costs an additional $2.55. Teff and buckwheat both cost substantially more than whole-wheat bread. Although these two new substitutions may not align with cost-containment strategies of all states, states with WIC-participating populations that use these grains as a staple food have the option to make other modifications to their state food lists to accommodate these choices. New whole grain options were not included in the revised food package grain composite because there is no available information upon which to base an assumption about redemption.

Estimating Per-Participant Program Costs for Food

To estimate weighted-average, per-participant food package costs for the current and revised food packages, the estimated number of participants who received each package in 2015 (see Table 7-1) was multiplied by the estimated cost of the respective package (see Table 7-3) and then divided by the total number of participants. Values for the final, cost-neutral set of food packages are presented in the bottom row of Table 7-3.

RESULTS AND DISCUSSION: PROGRAM COSTS

Estimates of monthly, postrebate, per-participant costs for both the current and revised food packages are presented in Table 7-3. Although prerebate costs are an indication of the market value of the food packages to the recipients (e.g., prerebate costs for mother–infant dyad packages only are presented in Table 7-5), post-rebate costs reflect USDA-FNS's costs for the food packages. There are two important features of Table 7-3. First, for the infant packages, subtotals are presented for each of the various food package I and II subpackages (formula-fed, partially breastfed, and fully breastfed). These values were then weighted by the share of participants who received each subpackage to calculate weighted average monthly cost for both food packages I and II. The second feature of note is that the values presented in columns 1 and 2 are based on calculated redemption rates. The rates used for column 1 were calculated from average amounts redeemed in the current packages; the rates used in column 2 represent the amounts that are projected to be redeemed in the revised packages. Columns 3 and 4 present costs for the fully redeemed packages.

Average weighted per-participant costs of the food packages are provided in the bottom row. The committee's estimate of the per-participant cost of the current food packages is $37.27 (i.e., column 1). The USDA-FNS preliminary estimate for 2015 based on reimbursement to states is $43.37[13] (USDA/FNS, 2016b). USDA-FNS calculated the value based on state-reported, per-participant costs. In contrast, the committee's evaluation of WIC food package costs was based primarily on the USDA-FNS redemption dataset, which was the best available for this purpose at the time of this analysis. Potential reasons for differences between the USDA-FNS value and the committee's value are discussed below.

Possible Reasons for Differences in Average Package Cost Compared to the USDA National Average

Possible reasons for the difference between the USDA-FNS weighted average per-participant cost and the committee's estimate are listed here:

- Inasmuch as price and redemption data used were based primarily on information from six and five unidentified states, respectively, the committee's analysis is not nationally representative. USDA-FNS data indicate that average 2015 food package costs vary among states, ranging between $28.89 (Texas) and $78.62 (Guam), depending on costs of food and distribution of participants by package (USDA/FNS, 2016b). This very wide range suggests that estimates generated using the USDA-FNS redemption dataset could vary widely depending on which six states were included.
- The USDA-FNS redemption dataset may have been sourced from EBT states. The weighted average food package cost for EBT states (not including Indian Tribal Organizations) in 2015 was $34.98, compared to $46.23 across all other (non-EBT) states, suggesting that EBT states have considerably lower food package costs compared to other states.
- The USDA-FNS redemption dataset could have come from states with lower cost of WIC foods compared to average national costs of WIC foods.
- Redemption rates in the five states may be lower than the national average generally.[14]

[13] The average monthly benefit equals total annual food cost divided by average monthly participation, divided by 12.

[14] Only five states were used to generate average redemption rates because the data from one state resulted in very low redemption values that fell outside of what was considered the normal range.

TABLE 7-2 Estimated Costs of Basic Foods, Selected Substitutions, and Net Cost Changes Resulting from Selected Substitutions in WIC Food Packages

Food item Substitution	Quantity	Cost per Quantity	Substitution	Difference in Cost with Substitution
Milk, whole	1 qt	$0.86		
Milk, whole	3 qt	$2.57		
Yogurt	1 qt	$3.22	1 qt yogurt for 1 qt milk	+$2.36
Cheese	1 lb	$5.33	1 lb cheese for 3 qt milk	+$2.75
Tofu	1 lb	$2.26	1 lb tofu for 1 qt milk	+$1.41
Soy beverage	1 qt	$1.82	1 qt soy beverage for 1 qt milk	+$0.96
Milk, low fat	1 qt	$0.82		
Milk, low fat	3 qt	$2.45		
Yogurt	1 qt	$3.22	1 qt yogurt for 1 qt milk	+$2.40
Cheese	1 lb	$5.33	1 lb cheese for 3 qt milk	+$2.87
Tofu	1 lb	$2.26	1 lb tofu for 1 qt milk	+$1.45
Soy beverage	1 qt	$1.82	1 qt soy beverage for 1 qt milk	+$1.00
Beans, dry	1 lb	$1.50		
Beans, canned	4 × 16 oz	$4.06	Four, 16-oz cans of beans for 1 lb dry beans	+$2.55
*Whole wheat bread**	18 to 24 oz	$2.65		
Whole wheat bread	16 oz	$2.35	16 oz whole wheat bread for 18 to 24 oz whole wheat bread	–$0.30
Teff	16 to 24 oz	$6.98	16 to 24 oz teff for 18 to 24 oz whole wheat bread	+$4.33
Buckwheat	16 to 24 oz	$6.89	16 to 24 oz buckwheat for 18 to 24 oz whole wheat bread	+$4.24
Cornmeal	16 to 24 oz	$2.38	16 to 24 oz cornmeal for 18 to 24 oz whole wheat bread	–$0.27

Corn tortillas	16 to 24 oz	$2.26	16 to 24 oz corn tortillas for 18 to 24 oz whole wheat bread	–$0.39
Eggs	1 dozen	$2.17		
Beans, dry	1 lb	$1.50	1 lb dry beans for 1 dozen eggs	–$0.67
Beans, canned	16 oz	$4.06	Four, 16-oz cans of beans for 1 dozen eggs	+$1.89
Juice	64 oz	$3.15		
CVV	$3	$3.00	$3 CVV for 64 oz juice	–$0.15
Jarred infant food meat	40 oz	$16.11		
Jarred infant food meat	30 oz	$12.08	30 oz jarred infant meat plus 10 oz canned fish for 40 oz jarred infant meat	–$2.00
Canned fish	10 oz	$2.02		
Jarred infant veg/fruit	128 oz	$21.07		
Jarred infant veg/fruit	64 oz	$10.53	64 oz jarred veg/fruit plus $10 CVV for 128 oz jarred veg/fruit	–$0.53
CVV	$10	$10.00		
CVV	$20	$20.00	$20 CVV for 128 oz jarred fruit/veg	–$1.07

NOTES: CCV = cash value voucher; veg/fruit = vegetables and fruits.

*Whole wheat bread and whole wheat bread substitutions that are expressed as a range were calculated by multiplying the average 2014 IRI price per ounce for all sizes listed by 24 ounces, assuming 24 ounces will be the most commonly redeemed size. This may be an overestimation of cost for some substitutions, for instance corn tortillas, for which 16 ounces is a commonly available size, however, the average IRI price is automatically weighted by the most common size purchased. Brown rice, barley, and wheat tortillas were not evaluated as substitutions for whole wheat bread as they comprise less than 1 percent of substitutions redeemed, based on redemption data made available to the committee. Costs were from FNS redemption data, CPI-adjusted to 2015, with the exception of yogurt and whole wheat bread, which were from IRI 2014.

SOURCES: Personal communication, K. Castellanos-Brown, USDA-FNS, April 7, 2016, and June 30, 2016; BLS, 2016; 2014 IRI Consumer Network Database.

TABLE 7-3 Comparison of Estimated Costs of Current and Revised Food Packages

		As Redeemed		Assuming Full Redemption	
Food Package	Food Package Description	Current Package Cost (postrebate)	Revised Package Cost (postrebate)	Current Package Cost (postrebate)	Revised Package Cost (postrebate)
Infants					
I-FF-A	Formula fed, 0–3 months	$53.68	$53.68	$57.11	$57.11
I-FF-B	Formula fed, 4–5 months	$59.10	$59.10	$62.88	$62.88
I-BF/FF-A	Partially breastfed, 0–1 months	$6.48	$6.48	$6.90	$6.90
I-BF/FF-B	Partially breastfed, 1–3 months	$26.44	$26.44	$28.12	$28.12
I-BF/FF-C	Partially breastfed, 4–5 months	$31.80	$31.80	$33.83	$33.83
I-BF-A	Fully breastfed, 0–3 months	$0.00	$0.00	$0.00	$0.00
I-BF-B	Fully breastfed, 4–5 months	$0.00	$0.00	$0.00	$0.00
I	FP I average weighted by participation	$43.57	$42.52	$46.35	$45.24
II-FF	Formula fed, 6–11 months	$56.34	$57.48	$72.70	$68.48
II-BF/FF	Partially breastfed, 6–11 months	$36.89	$38.03	$52.01	$47.79
II-BF	Fully breastfed, 6–11 months	$34.23	$22.17	$79.68	$39.39
II	FP II average weighted by participation	$51.37	$50.15	$71.15	$61.72
III-I and III-II	Infants with special dietary needs, nonexempt formula and food, weighted by participation	$26.40	$26.95	$34.20	$32.18

Children[a]					
IV-A	1 year	$34.93	$34.20	$50.26	$46.22
IV-B	2–4 years	$33.88	$33.99	$49.86	$47.42
Women[a]					
V,[b] V-A[c]	Pregnant	$36.68	$35.51	$58.70	$52.96
V,[b] V-B[c]	Partially breastfeeding	$36.68	$43.93	$58.70	$64.31
VI	Postpartum, nonbreastfeeding	$29.76	$30.10	$46.58	$47.14
VII	Fully breastfeeding	$47.41	$55.11	$74.16	$78.71
	Average weighted cost per-participant (per month)	**$37.27**	**$37.32**	**$53.21**	**$50.22**

NOTES: BF = fully breastfed; BF/FF = partially breastfed; FF = formula fed. See Appendix R, Table R-5, for determination of redemption percentages. See Appendix R, Tables R-1 through R-3, for assumptions applied to develop the current and revised food package cost profiles. Prices were from USDA-FNS redemption data, CPI-adjusted to 2015, with the exception of infant formula, revised package whole wheat bread and alternatives, and yogurt, which were from the 2014 IRI Consumer Network Database.

[a] Participants of these ages receiving food package III were folded into the appropriate age-and physiological state category to capture issued foods.

[b] Food package V in the current set of packages is issued to both pregnant and partially breastfeeding women.

[c] In the revised set of packages, food package V is separated into V-A for pregnant women, and V-B for partially breastfeeding women.

SOURCES: Personal communication, K. Castellanos-Brown, USDA-FNS, April 7, 2016, and June 30, 2016; USDA/FNS, 2014a; BLS, 2016; USDA/FNS, 2016a; 2014 IRI Consumer Network Database.

- Redemption rates in the five states may be lower for more expensive foods or for more expensive packages compared to national average redemption rates.
- The committee's analysis assumes that all substitutions in a category are redeemed at the same rate as the default WIC food (e.g., that cheese, when substituted for milk, is redeemed at the same rate as milk). It may be that more expensive substitution options are redeemed at higher rates.
- As explained earlier, because there were no available data, the committee's analysis does not include costs for medical foods. Although recipients of food package III comprise approximately only 6 percent of participants (USDA/FNS, 2016a), excluding costs of exempt formula or WIC-eligible nutritionals (formerly "WIC medical foods") may result in lower average per-participant costs. For example, if the weighted-average cost of medical formula provided to the 6 percent of WIC participants who receive food package III is $300 per month (no rebate), inclusion in the cost analysis would increase the estimated weighted-average, per-participant cost of the food package to approximately $46.
- IRI data indicate that the average costs for foods range widely. The cost for each food depends on many factors (e.g., brand, size, store where purchased, how long the individual has shopped for them) (USDA/ERS, 2005, 2014b, 2015, 2016).

Given the current data limitations, it is impossible to speculate about any possible bias in the committee's estimate of weighted-average, per-participant costs of the food packages. As the EBT system is introduced nationally, future committees should have much more nationally representative data. Although its final estimate of the weighted-average, per-participant cost for the current food package is different than that of USDA-FNS, the committee's methods for estimating costs were applied consistently and in the same manner across all food packages to determine cost-neutrality.

Ensuring Cost Neutrality

The committee was tasked with ensuring that the revised food packages are cost-neutral. For the purposes of this review, cost-neutral means that the weighted-average, per-participant cost of each of the food packages I through VII in the revised set of food packages falls within $0.10 of the weighted-average, per-participant cost of the current set of food packages. As presented in Table 7-3, the weighted-average, per-participant cost of the revised set of food packages is $37.32, which is $0.05 higher than the committee's estimate of the weighted-average, per-participant cost of the current package cost. *The revised set of food packages therefore meets the task requirement for cost neutrality.*

Cost neutrality was achieved by offsetting increases in the costs of particular food packages with decreases in the costs of other food packages. As a result of the cost-neutral requirement, the committee was restricted in the degree to which the CVV could be increased and in the amount of fish that could be added to food packages. Inasmuch as food package cost is weighted by participation, the amount of foods added to the food packages for children had larger effects on the weighted-average food package cost compared to foods added to packages for women.

COMPARING COST INCENTIVES FOR BREASTFEEDING

In accordance with the component of the committee's decision to view the value of the food packages from the perspective of the mother–infant dyad (as described in Chapter 6), both postrebate costs (see Table 7-4) and prerebate market values (see Table 7-5) of the three types of mother–infant pairs (formula-feeding, partially breastfeeding, fully formula feeding) were compared. The postrebate costs presented are those as actually redeemed (i.e., based on available redemption data) or projected to be redeemed. The prerebate market values, in contrast, assume full redemption of the food packages.

The annualized postrebate, as-redeemed cost of the revised fully breastfeeding dyad packages is increased by $20 compared to the current fully breastfeeding dyad packages. For the revised partially breastfeeding dyad packages, this difference is $94. Most of these differences in the costs of the dyad packages come from revisions to the food packages for the breastfeeding mothers. The package for fully breastfeeding women is projected to be redeemed at an annual value $92 higher and for the partially breastfeeding mother $87 higher compared to the current packages, respectively. These increases in the value of the fully and partially breastfeeding mothers' packages reflect the committee's objective to support exclusive breastfeeding as well as breastfeeding of any intensity (see Table 7-4). It is noteworthy that, compared to the current packages, the postrebate market value of the food packages for the breastfeeding dyads are revised to be closer to the value of the packages for the fully formula-feeding dyad. Currently, the redeemed values of the packages for the fully formula-feeding dyad is $39 to $75 more than that of the breastfeeding dyads. In the revision, the redeemed values of the packages for the fully formula-feeding dyad range from $46 less to $64 more than that of the partially and fully breastfeeding dyads, respectively.

The annualized pre-rebate market value (fully redeemed) of the food packages for the fully breastfeeding dyad is $187 lower and for the partially

TABLE 7-4 Comparison of the Food Package Costs with Rebates as Redeemed, Current and Revised Food Packages for Mother–Infant Dyads

	Fully Breastfeeding			Partially Breastfeeding			Fully Formula Feeding		
Participant Category	Cost per Month	Number of Months	Cost per Year 1	Cost per Month	Number of Months	Cost per Year 1	Cost per Month	Number of Months	Cost per Year 1
Current Food Package									
Mother	$47.41	12	$568.94	$36.68	12	$440.20	$29.77	6	$178.58
Infant, 0≤1 months	$0.00	1	$0.00	$6.48	1	$6.48	$53.68	1	$53.68
Infant, 1–3 months	$0.00	3	$0.00	$26.44	3	$79.31	$53.68	3	$161.04
Infant, 4–5 months	$0.00	2	$0.00	$31.80	2	$63.59	$59.10	2	$118.21
Infant, 6–11 months	$34.23	6	$205.38	$36.89	6	$221.33	$56.34	6	$338.04
		Total Cost	**$774.32**			**$810.92**			**$849.56**
Revised Food Package									
Mother	$55.11	12	$661.28	$43.93	12	$527.10	$30.10	6	$180.60
Infant, 0≤1 months	$0.00	1	$0.00	$6.48	1	$6.48	$53.68	1	$53.68
Infant, 1–3 months	$0.00	3	$0.00	$26.44	3	$79.31	$53.68	3	$161.04
Infant, 4–5 months	$0.00	2	$0.00	$31.80	2	$63.59	$59.10	2	$118.21
Infant, 6–11 months	$22.17	6	$132.99	$38.03	6	$228.17	$57.48	6	$344.88
		Total Cost	**$794.28**			**$904.65**			**$858.41**

NOTES: Prices were from the USDA-FNS redemption dataset, with the exception of infant formula, yogurt, and revised package whole wheat bread and alternatives, which were from IRI 2014. All prices were adjusted to FY2015.
SOURCES: Personal communication, K. Castellanos-Brown, USDA-FNS, April 7, 2016, and June 30, 2016; BLS, 2016; 2014 IRI Consumer Network Database.

TABLE 7-5 Comparison of the Market (Prerebate) Value of Maximum Allowances (Full Redemption) for Current and Revised Food Packages for Mother–Infant Dyads

	Fully Breastfeeding			Partially Breastfeeding			Fully Formula Feeding		
Participant Category	Cost per Month	Number of Months	Cost per Year	Cost per Month	Number of Months	Cost per Year	Cost per Month	Number of Months	Cost per Year
Current Food Package									
Mother	$74.16	12	$889.96	$58.70	12	$704.40	$46.58	6	$279.46
Infant, 0≤1 months	$0.00	1	$0.00	$19.47	1	$19.47	$161.21	1	$161.21
Infant, 1–3 months	$0.00	3	$0.00	$79.39	3	$238.16	$161.21	3	$483.62
Infant, 4–5 months	$0.00	2	$0.00	$95.49	2	$190.98	$177.50	2	$354.99
Infant, 6–11 months	$79.68	6	$478.06	$96.86	6	$581.18	$155.28	6	$931.68
	Total Cost:		**$1,368.02**			**$1,734.19**			**$2,210.97**
Revised Food Package									
Mother	$78.71	12	$944.55	$64.31	12	$771.66	$47.14	6	$282.85
Infant, 0≤1 months	$0.00	1	$0.00	$19.47	1	$19.47	$161.21	1	$161.21
Infant, 1–3 months	$0.00	3	$0.00	$79.39	3	$238.16	$161.21	3	$483.62
Infant, 4–5 months	$0.00	2	$0.00	$95.49	2	$190.98	$177.50	2	$354.99
Infant, 6–11 months	$39.39	6	$236.37	$92.64	6	$555.85	$151.06	6	$906.35
	Total Cost:		**$1,180.92**			**$1,776.13**			**$2,189.03**

NOTES: Prices were from the USDA-FNS redemption dataset, with the exception of infant formula, yogurt, and revised package whole wheat bread and alternatives, which were from IRI 2014. All prices were adjusted to FY2015.

SOURCES: Personal communication, K. Castellanos-Brown, USDA-FNS, April 7, 2016, and June 30, 2016; BLS, 2016; 2014 IRI Consumer Network Database.

breastfeeding dyad is $42 higher in the revised compared to the current packages, respectively (see Table 7-5). However, the annualized prerebate market value of the revised food package for the fully breastfeeding mother is $55 higher and for the partially breastfeeding dyad is $67 higher than the value of the current food packages for them, respectively. Here it is striking how much higher the prerebate market values of the food packages for the formula-feeding dyads are compared to those for the breastfeeding dyads. For the current food packages, those for the fully formula-feeding dyad are valued at $843 more than those for the fully breastfeeding dyad and $476 more than those for the partially breastfeeding dyad. In the revised food packages, those for the fully formula-feeding dyad are valued at $1,008 more than those for the fully breastfeeding dyad because amounts of foods in the fully breastfed infant packages were reduced. However, the difference between value of the packages for the fully formula-feeding dyad and the partially breastfeeding dyad is smaller ($413 for the revised, $477 for the current).

As is true of all the WIC food packages, the benefit of the breastfeeding food packages extends beyond the foods provided and includes other WIC services, such as nutrition counseling, health referrals, and nutrition education. WIC-participating breastfeeding mothers may benefit from peer-counseling in particular. Communication of this benefit to participants could increase the perceived value of the breastfeeding packages.

Finally, the annualized prerebate market value of the revised formula-feeding dyad packages is slightly lower than that of the current formula-feeding dyad packages (see Table 7-5). The formula-fed packages provide approximately 100 percent of an infant's needs, and the cost of infant formula is high, so the committee found it difficult, within cost-neutral constraints, to lower the value of the formula-feeding dyad packages without decreasing the amounts of infant formula offered.

SUMMARY

The requirement that the revised food packages be cost-neutral was at the crux of the committee's final decisions for food package revisions. This chapter describes the methods used by the committee to ensure cost-neutrality. These methods were part of an iterative process during which the committee considered several sets of food packages. In each iteration, adjustments were made to ensure that the revised set of packages met the criteria outlined in Box 1-4 (see Chapter 1), while also being cost neutral. To evaluate cost neutrality, the committee used three steps. First, it estimated participation distributions across the packages (see Table 7-1). Next, the committee estimated food package costs for all current and revised food packages (see Table 7-3). Finally, the committee estimated weighted-average, per-participant food package costs for both the current and revised food packages. The weighted-average, per-participant cost of the revised set of food packages is $37.32 which is $0.05 higher than the committee's estimate of the weighted-average, per-participant cost of the current package cost ($37.27). The revised set of food packages therefore meets the task requirement for cost neutrality. The annualized costs of the revised food packages for the breastfeeding dyads, as redeemed, are slightly higher than that of the current breastfeeding dyad packages. Similarly, the annualized costs of the revised food packages for breastfeeding women, as redeemed, are higher compared to the costs of the current food packages for these women. However, the redeemed value of the formula-feeding dyad packages remains higher than either of the breastfeeding packages because of the cost-neutral constraint and because the packages for younger formula-fed infants provide approximately 100 percent of needs.

REFERENCES

BLS (Bureau of Labor Statistics). 2016. *Consumer price index—all urban consumers*. Washington, DC: BLS. http://www.bls.gov/news.release/cpi.t01.htm (accessed September 30, 2016).

IOM (Institute of Medicine). 2006. *WIC food packages: Time for a change*. Washington, DC: The National Academies Press.

USDA/ERS (U.S. Department of Agriculture/Economic Research Service). 2005. *Interstate variation in WIC food package costs: The role of food prices, caseload composition, and cost-containment practices*. Washington, DC: USDA/ERS. https://www.ers.usda.gov/publications/pub-details/?pubid=46844 (accessed December 21, 2016).

USDA/ERS. 2013. *Fruit and vegetable prices*. Washington, DC: USDA/ERS. http://ers.usda.gov/data-products/fruit-and-vegetable-prices.aspx (accessed December 21, 2016).

USDA/ERS. 2014a. *Transition to EBT in WIC: Review of impact and examination of participant redemption patterns: Final report*. Washington, DC: Altarum Institute. http://altarum.org/sites/default/files/uploaded-publication-files/Altarum_Transition%20to%20WIC%20EBT_Final%20Report_071614.pdf (accessed December 21, 2016).

USDA/ERS. 2014b. *Cost containment in the WIC program: Vendor peer groups and reimbursement rates*. Washington, DC: USDA/ERS. https://www.ers.usda.gov/publications/pub-details/?pubid=45254 (accessed December 21, 2016).

USDA/ERS. 2015. *Where do Americans usually shop for food and how do they travel to get there? Initial findings from the National Household Food Acquisition and Purchase Survey*. Washington, DC: USDA/ERS. http://www.ers.usda.gov/publications/pub-details/?pubid=79791 (accessed December 21, 2016).

USDA/ERS. 2016. *WIC household food purchases using WIC benefits or paying out of pocket: A case study of cold cereal purchases*. Washington, DC: USDA/ERS. http://www.ers.usda.gov/publications/pub-details/?pubid=45536 (accessed August 29, 2016).

USDA/FNS (U.S. Department of Agriculture/Food and Nutrition Service). 2011. *Evaluation of the birth month breastfeeding changes to the WIC food packages*. Alexandria, VA: USDA/FNS. http://www.fns.usda.gov/sites/default/files/BirthMonth.pdf (accessed December 21, 2016).

USDA/FNS. 2013a. *WIC participant and program characteristics 2012 final report*. Alexandria, VA: USDA/FNS. http://www.fns.usda.gov/sites/default/files/WICPC2012.pdf (accessed December 21, 2016).

USDA/FNS. 2013b. *Fiscal year 2010: WIC food cost report*. Alexandria, VA: USDA/FNS. http://www.fns.usda.gov/sites/default/files/WICFoodCost2010_0.pdf (accessed December 21, 2016).

USDA/FNS. 2014a. *Special Supplemental Nutrition Program for Women, Infants and Children (WIC): Revisions in the WIC food packages*. Final Rule, 7 C.F.R. § 246.

USDA/FNS. 2016a. *WIC participant and program characteristics 2014 food package report*. Alexandria, VA: USDA/FNS. http://www.fns.usda.gov/wic-participant-and-program-characteristics-2014-food-package-report (accessed August 30, 2016).

USDA/FNS. 2016b. *WIC program*. Alexandria, VA: USDA/FNS. http://www.fns.usda.gov/pd/wic-program (accessed July 13, 2016).

USDA/FNS. 2016c. *Monthly data — state level participation by category and program costs*. Alexandria, VA: USDA/FNS. http://www.fns.usda.gov/pd/wic-program (accessed October 3, 2016).

8

Sensitivity Analysis for Food Package Nutrient, Food Group, and Cost Models

The committee was tasked with conducting a sensitivity analysis to evaluate the sensitivity of recommended changes to the Special Supplemental Nutrition Program for Women, Infants, and Children (WIC) food packages to assumptions used to develop the revised food packages. Specifically, the analysis tested the effects of changes in the food packages on the nutrient level in the packages, availability of the *Dietary Guidelines for Americans* (DGA) food groups and subgroups, and cost of the food packages. This type of analysis will provide the U.S. Department of Agriculture's Food and Nutrition Service (USDA-FNS) with a tool to estimate the relative effect of various assumptions used in developing the food package recommendations, as well as to evaluate the potential effects of additional changes on the food packages.

In carrying out the sensitivity analysis, the committee chose a comprehensive approach and first examined the effects of the proposed revisions on the food packages, followed by tests of the effects of selected variations to these revisions. Changes in food quantities, as well as changes in assumptions regarding redemption rates, substitutions within food categories, and shifts in participation were tested. Including sensitivity analyses of the revised food packages adds to the analyses discussed in Chapters 6 and 7 (the rationale for the revised food packages and the cost analysis) by allowing a more detailed examination of the effects of specific changes on the provision of nutrients and food groups, and costs.

In the discussion below, a description of the analytic methods used is presented, followed by the results for the selected changes. Results related to food categories are described first, followed by results related to shifts in participation. A summary of the projected impact of food package changes on the nutrient and food group profiles of the packages, as well as package costs, is presented. In contrast to the Regulatory Impact Analysis (see Chapter 10) which projects cost effects of the revised food packages for fiscal years 2018 through 2022, the cost effects presented in this chapter reflect the effects of individual food category changes to specific food packages, one at a time, based on 2015 costs only.

PURPOSE, GOALS, AND LIMITATIONS OF SENSITIVITY TESTING

In the analyses presented below, the sensitivity of the predicted outcomes (nutrient and food group profiles of the food packages as well as costs) to various changes in the food packages, as well as to assumptions regarding food item substitutions within a food category (i.e. yogurt in place of milk), redemption rates, and participation rates, are examined. USDA-FNS will be able to use the sensitivity analysis results as a way to evaluate effects of various food package options on the specified outcomes, should different regulatory choices be made, or should participants behave in ways that are different than those that were assumed for the revised package (e.g., what would be the cost implications if the actual redemption rates differ from the calculated redemption rates in particular ways).

The initial task for the committee in conducting its sensitivity analysis included assessing the effects of food package item changes on the nutrient and food group profiles of the different packages and on assumed participant intake. Critical to assessing the effects of package changes on intake is information about how much of the prescribed foods in the individual's package are redeemed and consumed. However, information on consumption of specific WIC foods by package was not available to the committee. It was also clear from the intake analysis (see Chapter 4) that the foods and nutrients available in the packages do not coincide with nutrient intakes reported by WIC participants in the National Health and Nutrition Examination Survey (NHANES), the only source of nationally representative population-wide intake data available. In addition, small sample sizes for pregnant, breastfeeding, or postpartum women necessitated collapsing the NHANES data for the years 2005–2012. As a result, it was not possible to focus on the most recent data for subgroups of women. For children, intake data were more robust for 2011–2012.

Given the difficulty of obtaining data as well as limitations in the available data, as described above, the committee devised a method that was applied in the sensitivity tests to estimate the effects of the food package changes on the nutrients and food groups available in the packages, but not on intakes of the participants. In the case of children only, where the sample size from NHANES was sufficient, the committee used estimates of intake changes to calculate projected Healthy Eating Index–2010 (HEI–2010) scores.

METHODOLOGICAL APPROACH TO SENSITIVITY ANALYSIS

Overview of the Approach

The starting point for the committee's sensitivity analysis was the nutrient profile and cost estimates for the current food packages, and redemption data for WIC foods (see Chapter 7 for a description of the methodology and all assumptions applied). Holding all other components constant in the current food package, the effects of a single change to a given component (e.g., food items and/or amount and/or redemption rate, or participation) on the level of nutrients and food groups, and the cost at the food package level were determined. This approach enabled the committee to estimate how various food package changes might potentially affect recipients' intakes within each package type. In addition, effects of package component changes on the average food cost per person were estimated. All tests in the sensitivity analysis evaluated not only the effect of a change to a given food category in the revised food package, but also included one to three alternatives as additional sensitivity tests. The development of the set of tests that were conducted is described briefly below.

The results of the sensitivity test outcomes were examined for each WIC food category in the following order: dairy; breakfast cereal; the cash value voucher (CVV), separately and combined with juice; fish; the rotation of peanut butter, legumes, and fish; and infant food vegetables and fruits. Several of the food categories (e.g., dairy) examined represent a composite of different substitution options (i.e., fluid milk, which can be substituted with yogurt and cheese). As described in Appendix R, the committee assumed that all participants selected a substitution option for dairy. This was because no information was available regarding the frequency of WIC participant selection of cheese or yogurt in place of milk, and because it was assumed that participants would choose the most valuable (highest cost) food item, if given the option.

When the options for food substitutions are changed in the revised food package, the nutrients provided in that package will likely change as well. For example, in the current food package IV-B for children ages 2 to less than 5 years, the assumption used for the dairy food category was that 1 pound of cheese and 1 quart of yogurt are substituted for 4 quarts of milk. In the revised food packages, children have two options: the option described for the current package, and also an option to substitute 2 quarts of yogurt in place of 2 quarts of milk. These two options were accounted for by allotting one of the two substitution options to half of the children, and the other substitution option to the remaining children. Furthermore, the overall amount of milk available in the children's revised package decreased. Thus, there was a decrease in saturated fat in the revised package compared to the current package because, on average, less cheese was included, and also because the overall quantity of dairy was reduced. This change might result in a decrease in dairy provided, but an increase in the HEI–2010 score due to the reduction in saturated fat.

Analyses Conducted

Most of the sensitivity tests were applied to food packages IV-B (for children ages 2 to less than 5 years), V-A (for pregnant women), and VII (for fully breastfeeding women) because these food packages capture the breadth of possible outcomes. Food package IV-B represents the largest proportion of participants and therefore has the greatest proportional effect on cost. Food package V-A includes a CVV amount that falls within that of other food packages. Food package VII includes the largest CVV and the largest quantity of fish. One test is also included for food package II (infants ages 6 to less than 12 months) to evaluate the option to substitute a CVV in place of infant food vegetables and fruits.

The committee developed a list of sensitivity tests that took into consideration which changes to the revised food packages (or assumptions applied, such as those for redemption rates) might have the greatest effect on the outcomes of interest (i.e., nutrient or food group composition of the packages, HEI–2010 score, and cost). A complete list of the tests conducted is provided in Appendix S, Table S-1. Several tests included a combination of variables, for example, a simultaneous change in the amount of a food and the redemption rate, or a change to both juice amounts and the CVV. All tests were conducted using the revised package food composites and redemption rates, as described in Appendix R, except in cases where the objective of the test was specifically to evaluate changes to these assumptions.

The proposed changes with the greatest impact were hypothesized to be: (1) those in the quantities of foods (e.g., changes to milk amounts) or substitution options (including only fluid milk instead of yogurt and cheese substitutions) offered in the different food packages; (2) changes to assumptions about redemption that were linked to the changes in quantities of foods (i.e., the redemption rate increased as milk quantities decreased, following an algorithm developed by the committee and described in Appendix R); (3) changes to the ratio of vegetables to fruits that are purchased (i.e., assuming fewer fruits and more vegetables are purchased with the CVV); and, (4) changes to participation categories (i.e., population shifts from formula to breastfeeding). By testing shifts in these variables for a sample of food packages, the degree to which the assumptions applied affect outcomes was assessed.

Outcome Measures for the Analyses

As described above, to carry out the sensitivity analyses, the committee identified outcome measures that included changes in the nutrient profiles and food groups in the different food packages, costs, and HEI–2010 scores (only for children ages 2 to less than 5 years). For all analyses, the absolute change in the outcome and the percent change compared to the current food package were calculated.

Changes in food groups and subgroups provided by the packages were evaluated in comparison to the current DGA food groups or food subgroups, applying the redemption rates for WIC foods. To evaluate changes to food groups, the food group corresponding to the food to be tested was identified. If the food was categorized as a DGA food subgroup (e.g., peanut butter is categorized as nuts, seeds, and soy), the effect of a change to the food on the total food group (e.g., total protein foods) was also evaluated. The foods in the food package were then converted to serving-equivalents per day using the USDA Food Patterns Equivalents Database (FPED) 2011–2012 (USDA/ARS, 2014). As was done for the nutrient profiles of the current and revised food packages (initially described in Chapter 3), differences in nutrients provided by the food packages for each food tested were sourced from the USDA Standard Reference Database, Release 28 (USDA/ARS, 2016).

Lastly, changes in the per-participant cost of each of the food packages were evaluated using the price per unit for foods (see Appendix R for price details). In addition, the overall average per-participant cost for a WIC food package was calculated to illustrate the impact of the change in one of the packages on the overall WIC program costs for food. The overall cost is a weighted average that incorporates the relative number of participants that are prescribed each different type of package.

In the cases where the food was a composite of different items (e.g., dairy is a composite of milk, yogurt, and cheese), the price of the food was a composite of the prices for the various substitution options. For some of the sensitivity tests, the composite was revised to reflect a food substitution. For example, the additional yogurt option was removed in some tests. Thus, the dairy composite was changed to replace the quart of yogurt with a quart of milk. Parallel changes in the composite nutrients and prices are also reflected in the test result.

Impact of Food Package Changes on HEI–2010 Scores for Children Ages 2 to Less Than 5 Years

To evaluate changes to HEI–2010 scores for children, the committee calculated the difference between the redeemed amounts of foods in the current food packages and the corresponding redeemed amounts in the revised food package. The test used the assumption that the median intake of participants estimated using NHANES data would increase or decrease by this difference. The resulting intake values were then used to estimate HEI–2010 scores for the given test parameters. Only food package IV-B (for children ages 2 to less than 5 years) is used as an example for the HEI–2010 sensitivity test outcome for several reasons. First, children are the largest population subgroup served by WIC (comprising over 35 percent of the WIC-participating population) so this analysis represents the estimated effect of the food packages on a large proportion of participants.[1] Second, the DGA food patterns (which are used in the calculation of the HEI–2010) apply only to individuals 2 years of age and older and therefore are not applicable to younger children or infants. Finally, median intake estimates for women were generated using data from NHANES 2005–2012 and therefore are less representative of current (2011–2012) intakes, and sample sizes remain small.

Interpretation of the Sensitivity Test Results

The relevance of a sensitivity test to a target population group may depend upon the importance of a specific nutrient or food group to the population group under consideration. For example, a 2 percent change in folate provided in a food package may be more relevant to pregnant women than to children. Thus, it may be necessary to evaluate each sensitivity test and outcome on a case-by-case basis. As applied by USDA-FNS, interpretation of the sensitivity test results may differ depending upon the options available (e.g., budgetary changes) or the question that is asked (e.g., Can changes to a particular food alter provision of a particular nutrient?).

Given that the relevance of a proposed food package change depends on the particular question, the committee chose to highlight changes of plus or minus 8 percent in the outcomes of interest, and offer a qualitative interpretation. The 8 percent value represents a potentially relevant level of change, and served as a means of distinguishing very small changes from others that may be more meaningful. The priority nutrients or food groups (as identified in Chapter 5) for the target population that change by at least

[1] Calculation of the revised HEI–2010 is also carried out in Chapter 9 for food package IV-B to compare the current to the revised food package. The same rationale applies to that calculation. A description of how the HEI–2010 is calculated using NHANES data is available in Appendix J.

8 percent are identified. The complete results of the sensitivity analyses are given in Appendix S.

SENSTIVITY ANALYSIS RESULTS

Overview

A summary of the results of the committee's sensitivity analysis is presented below, organized by WIC food category or food package category (e.g., CVV/juice or the revised rotation of peanut butter/legumes/fish), to which changes were made. The nutrient, food group, and HEI–2010 tests followed similar patterns for each. The summary also describes the rationale for each test, such as USDA-FNS may have less funding and needs to reduce a food quantity, or participants may behave differently than was assumed when food package changes were evaluated. For each WIC food category, a discussion of the test results that evaluate the effect of a revised food package change are presented first, followed by additional tests conducted for the same food category. The potential positive or negative consequences of each test result are described relative to the current food package.

Summary of Sensitivity Analysis Results

Dairy Adjustment

Changes to quantities of dairy and substitution options that are proposed for the revised packages were evaluated. The revised food package includes an option for substituting an additional quart of yogurt, therefore, a 5-percent increase in redemption for dairy was assumed based on the potential participant preference for yogurt (Fung et al., 2010). To test this assumption, another set of tests was conducted to evaluate the outcomes should the substitution options (yogurt and cheese) not be offered (only fluid milk is offered). Further reductions in dairy were also tested as an example of a possible food package change that could be implemented in the case of reduced funding. The latter tests retained the substitution options. As amounts of dairy were reduced, the redemption rate was increased, applying the committee's algorithm explained in Appendix R.

Revised packages compared to the current packages When the quantity of dairy foods in the food packages is changed by including an additional yogurt substitution, levels of added sugars increase but levels of saturated fat decrease because milk amounts are reduced and, for some tests, there is less cheese in the average package (see Table 8-1). Both of these food components were priority nutrients to limit for all WIC population groups.

TABLE 8-1 Impact of Dairy Changes on Nutrient and Food Group Food Package Profiles and on the HEI–2010 Scores Relative to the Current Food Packages for Children Ages 2 to Less Than 5 Years (IV-B), Pregnant Women (V-A), and Fully Breastfeeding Women (VII)[a]

Food Package	Adjustments (Amount and Redemption Rate)[b,c]	Nutrients	Food Group(s)[d]	HEI Score[e]	Package Per-Participant Cost	WIC Average Per-Participant Cost	Appendix S Table Reference
IV-B	Revised: –2 quarts, 80%, additional substitutions[f]	(+) added sugars (–) saturated fat	—	—	+$0.08	+$0.03	S-2
	Test 1: –4 quarts, 86%, additional substitutions[f]	(–) calcium, potassium, riboflavin, vitamin D	(–) dairy	—	–$0.89	–$0.27	S-2
	Test 2: –2 quarts, 76%, no substitutions (only fluid milk)	(+) vitamin D (–) added sugars, saturated fat	—	—	–$4.29	–$2.18	S-2
V-A	Revised: –6 quarts, 66%, additional substitutions[f]	(+) added sugars (–) calcium, vitamin A, vitamin D, saturated fat	(–) dairy	NA	–$1.11	–$0.11	S-3
	Test 1: –10 quarts, 74%, additional substitutions[f]	(+) added sugars (–) energy, protein, total fat, calcium, magnesium, phosphorus, potassium, sodium, zinc, selenium, riboflavin, vitamin B12, vitamin A, vitamin D, saturated fat	(–) dairy	NA	–$2.97	–$0.28	S-3
VII	Revised: –8 quarts, 68%, additional substitutions[f]	(+) added sugars (–) calcium, phosphorous, potassium, riboflavin, vitamin A, vitamin D, saturated fat	(–) dairy	NA	–$1.59	–$0.06	S-4

Test 1: –12 quarts, 77%, additional substitutions[f]	(+) added sugars (–) calcium, magnesium, phosphorus, potassium, sodium, zinc, thiamin, riboflavin, vitamin B12, vitamin A, vitamin D, saturated fat	(–) dairy	NA	–$2.49	–0.12	S-4
Test 2: –8 quarts, 65%, no substitutions (only fluid milk)	(–) calcium, phosphorus, sodium, zinc, added sugars, saturated fat	(–) dairy	NA	–$5.51	–$0.19	S-4

NOTES: — = indicates that no changes were in the range of more than approximately ± 8%; (+) = increased amount (an increased amount for saturated fat, added sugars, and sodium is undesirable); (–) = decreased amount (a decreased amount for saturated fat, added sugars, and sodium is desirable); HEI = Healthy Eating Index–2010; NA = unable to calculate change in HEI score for any but food package IV-B. Weighting of milk substitution options for alternative tests were the same as the weighting of milk substitution options for the revised packages. Nutrient and food group composition of the food packages were based on the assumptions outlined in Appendix R.

[a] Notations for nutrients and food groups in the table represent changes of 8% or greater. Not all nutrients or food groups listed were identified in Chapter 5 as a priority for the target population subgroup. See Appendix S for more details on changes in nutrients and food groups.

[b] The adjustment is in reference to the current food package amounts.

[c] For all quantities of milk tested, the maximum amounts of possible substitutions are assumed as the likely participant behavior (i.e. substitutions are of greater value than fluid milk). Therefore, changes to nutrients reflect changes in these substitutions. Particularly, added sugars and saturated fat in the food package are affected by the amounts of yogurt and cheese that may be substituted.

[d] Food group noted corresponds to the appropriate food group or subgroup from the *Dietary Guidelines for Americans*.

[e] The committee created a tool to estimate the HEI for children ages 2 to less than 5 years considering the revised package change or test. To do this, the difference between the redeemed amounts of the HEI components for the current food package and the redeemed amounts of the HEI components for the test food package were added to the median intake estimated using NHANES 2011–2012.

[f] The tests included the maximum substitutions allowable. The substitution options were allocated evenly, for example, 50 percent of children were allotted the 1 lb cheese, 1 qt yogurt substitution and 50% of children were allotted the 2 qt yogurt substitution option.

Overall, the revisions to food package IV-B (for children) will have a positive effect on the nutritional composition of the package for this group. The HEI–2010 dairy score for food package IV-B does not change appreciably. For women, however, increased redemption will not compensate for the reduced quantities of dairy in their revised food packages because calcium, potassium, phosphorus, riboflavin, vitamin A, and vitamin D all are lower in one or both of the tested packages. The relevance of these changes depends on the needs of target population group and on the foods selected from among the package options. Potassium was a priority nutrient to increase for all subgroups of women; whereas, vitamins A and D were priorities only for some subgroups of women. Fluid milk provides more potassium, but a substitution of cheese in place of milk provides more saturated fat. The monthly cost of the dairy changes to the revised packages ranged from –\$1.59 to +\$0.08 per-participant by package and from –\$0.11 to +\$0.03 per-participant overall.

Alternatives to the revised packages compared to the current packages When the quantities of dairy foods in food package IV-B (for children) were reduced further (to 12 quarts), decreases in the key dairy nutrients (calcium, potassium, vitamin D) were noted, along with riboflavin, and the HEI–2010 score for dairy was reduced. Changes in saturated fat and increases in added sugars are less than 8 percent because of the substitution assumptions applied. If all caretakers of children selected a cheese substitution instead of 2 quarts of yogurt, the changes to these nutrients (which are priorities to reduce) would be more substantial. However, the largest decreases in milk tested (–10 quart for food package V-A and –12 quart for food package VII) result in the reduction of additional nutrients beyond the 8 percent threshold, despite the increased redemption rate.

Removing all substitution options in the packages evaluated decreases the added sugars provided. In most cases the reduction of milk and reduced substitutions with yogurt decreased costs (see Table 8-1).

The cost effects of these tests per package ranged from –\$5.51 to –\$0.89. The effects on the overall average food cost per person are –\$2.18 and –\$0.09.

Evaluation Changes to dairy foods in the packages and the substitution options affected levels of calcium, potassium, vitamin A, vitamin D, saturated fat, and added sugars. Allowing for a variety of substitutions or additional substitution options for milk may promote greater consumption and improve level of essential nutrients from dairy foods in the packages; however, these substitutions can have a substantial impact on the cost of the food packages.

Changing Breakfast Cereal to All Whole Grain-Rich

A sensitivity analysis was used to test the revised package requirement that all breakfast cereals meet the whole grain-rich specifications. The assumed redemption of ready-to-eat (RTE) breakfast cereals was decreased by 10 percent (to 54 percent) to account for participants' potential preference for refined grain varieties and the potentially reduced number of choices. To evaluate this assumption, the first test assumed that no change to redemption would occur for breakfast cereals (i.e., 60 percent, based on the current food package redemption rate). A second test was conducted for the children's food package (IV-B) using the highest (69 percent) of the state redemption rates made available to the committee (see Table 8-2).

Revised packages compared to the current packages Across all food packages that were evaluated, the revised package change to all whole grain-rich cereals resulted in higher levels of zinc. There were also lower levels of several B vitamins and iron. However changes in folic acid levels did not exceed the 8 percent threshold. This finding is in alignment with the information reviewed in Chapter 6, which indicates that most ready-to-eat cereals have similar levels of nutrient fortification. Therefore, nutrients in the food packages were unlikely to be greatly affected by this change in cereal specifications. Although whole grain cereals are more expensive than the refined grain options, this food package change results in a substantial increase in the amounts of whole grains offered across the food packages. The HEI–2010 score for whole grains (a priority food subgroup for all population groups evaluated) increases for all tests conducted on food package IV-B (for children). The change to all whole grain-rich cereals results in a savings of $0.08 (based on reduced redemption) per-participant.

Alternatives to the revised packages compared to the current packages If redemption continues at the current rate (60 percent), the change to whole grain-rich cereals will also provide additional fiber compared to the breakfast cereals in the current food packages, but they also provide less riboflavin and vitamin A. If redemption increases to 69 percent, fiber, iron, magnesium, phosphorus, zinc, and folate would all increase above the 8 percent threshold. The cost, if redemption remains at the current rate, is +$0.43 per food package. Increasing redemption rates further would increase the cost of the children's package by $1.16. The overall average per-participant cost for the change to all whole grains if redemption remains at the current rate would range from +$0.01 to +$0.15 across the three packages tested (food package IV-B, V-A, and VII).

TABLE 8-2 Impact of Changes to All Whole Grain-Rich Breakfast Cereals on Nutrient and Food Group Food Package Profiles and on the HEI–2010 Scores Relative to the Current Food Packages for Children Ages 2 to Less Than 5 Years (IV-B), Pregnant Women (V-A), and Fully Breastfeeding Women (VII)[a]

Food Category	Food Package	Adjustments (Amount and Redemption Rate)[b]	Nutrients	Food Group(s)[c]	HEI Score[d]	Package Per-Participant Cost	WIC Average Per-Participant Cost	Appendix S Table Reference
Breakfast cereal	IV-B	Revised: all WG, 54%	(+) zinc (−) iron, thiamin, riboflavin, niacin, vitamin B12, vitamin A, added sugars	(+) whole grains	(+) whole grain score	−$0.08	−$0.03	S-5
		Test 1: all WG, 60%	(+) fiber, zinc (−) riboflavin, vitamin A	(+) whole grains	(+) whole grain score	+$0.43	+$0.15	S-5
		Test 2: all WG, 69%	(+) fiber, iron, magnesium, phosphorus, zinc, folate	(+) total grains, whole grains	(+) whole grain score	+$1.16	+$0.42	S-5
	V-A	Revised: All WG, 54%	(+) zinc (−) iron, thiamin, riboflavin, niacin, vitamin B12, vitamin A, added sugars	(+) whole grains	NA	−$0.08	−$0.01	S-6

	Test: All WG, 60%	(+) fiber, zinc (–) riboflavin, vitamin A	(+) whole grains	NA	+$0.43	+$0.04	S-6
VII	Revised: All WG, 54%	(+) zinc (–) iron, thiamin, riboflavin, vitamin A, added sugars	(+) whole grains	NA	–$0.08	–$0.01	S-7
	Test: All WG, 60%	(+) fiber, zinc	(+) whole grains	NA	+$0.43	+$0.01	S-7

NOTES: (+) = increased amount (an increased amount for saturated fat, added sugars, and sodium is undesirable); (–) = decreased amount (a decreased amount for saturated fat, added sugars, and sodium is desirable); HEI = Healthy Eating Index–2010; NA = unable to calculate change in HEI score for any but food package IV-B; WG = whole grain-rich. Nutrient and food group composition of the food packages were based on the assumptions outlined in Appendix R.

[a] Notations for nutrients and food groups in the table represent changes of 8% or greater. Not all nutrients or food groups listed were identified in Chapter 5 as a priority for the target population subgroup.

[b] The adjustment is in reference to the current food package amounts.

[c] Food group noted corresponds to the appropriate food group or subgroup from the *Dietary Guidelines for Americans*.

[d] The committee created a tool to estimate the HEI for children ages 2 to less than 5 years considering the revised package change or test. To do this, the difference between the redeemed amounts of the HEI components for the current food package and the redeemed amounts of the HEI components for the test food package were added to the median intake estimated using NHANES 2011–2012.

Evaluation The change to all whole grain-rich breakfast cereals increases the level of zinc in all three packages even if redemption rates drop by 10 percent. If redemption continues at the current rate, whole grain rich cereals included in the food packages will also provide additional fiber. Even with a lower rate of redemption, the whole grain component of the food packages is increased. Whole grain-rich cereals are more expensive than refined grain cereals; therefore, costs increase with the change unless redemption is reduced from the current rate.

Adjusting the Cash Value Voucher

The sensitivity analysis tested the proposed increases to the cash value voucher (CVV) for the revised packages that were evaluated. The redemption rate for the CVV was decreased in the revised packages (from 77 to 75 percent), under the assumption that an increase in value may result in a slightly decreased overall rate of use. Higher redemption rates were also tested to evaluate the effects of increased redemption on the nutrients and food groups offered, as well as the cost effects. Finally, the effects of an increased CVV was tested for food package VII to evaluate the effect of moving the CVV value closer to one that would provide approximately 50 percent of fruit and vegetable recommendations for fully breastfeeding women (see Table 8-3).

Revised packages compared to the current packages Increasing the CVV generally increases the amount of fiber (a higher-priority nutrient for all population subgroups) and vitamin C (a lower-priority nutrient for some women) provided by the food packages. Total vegetables (higher-priority food group for all WIC participants), total fruit (a higher- or middle-priority food group for women), and whole fruit (a higher-priority food subgroup for all population subgroups) all increase under this assumption. For food package IV-B (for children), the HEI–2010 score for total vegetables increased at least 8 percent as long as the redemption rate was 75 percent or higher. Because median intake of total and whole fruit already achieves the maximum HEI–2010 scores for total and whole fruit, no change in these HEI components is expected. The cost for the revised food package CVV ranges from +\$2.76 to +\$17.76. The change in the overall average per-participant cost ranges from +\$0.26 to +\$1.03.

Alternatives to the revised packages compared to the current packages In addition to the nutrients noted above for the revised food package tests, magnesium, potassium, copper, vitamin B6, folate, and choline also increased as the dollar value of the CVV increased beyond that proposed for the revised food package. Increasing the redemption rate for food package IV-B (for children) by 5 percent, however, did not result in a large increase in nutrient level, although cost increased by $1.25 per participant. The results of sensitivity tests that adjust the amounts of the CVV are limited by the vegetables and fruits included in the model and the proportions of each that are selected. Participants who make different selections or choose, for example vegetables over fruits, will be provided with different nutrients and food groups than those indicated in the analysis. The cost change when redemption is increased to 85 percent ranged from +$4.02 to +$21.26, depending on the food package, but the range for the overall change in average per-participant food cost increased from +$0.70 to +$1.47. The set of tests described below evaluates a shift in the ratio of vegetables to fruits that were assumed for the revised package.

Evaluation The CVV in the revised packages increased the level of fiber and vitamin C in all packages tested, compared to the current food packages. Given that the CVV permits participants a large degree of flexibility in selecting vegetables and fruits, the specific nutrients and nutrient levels contributed by the CVV will vary. The effects on food package costs vary with the redemption rate because the total value of the CVV varies across packages. The substantially higher CVV in food package VII (fully breastfeeding women) has a much smaller proportional effect on the average per-participant food cost because only about 3 percent of participants receive food package VII.

Additional Tests on the CVV: Proportions of Vegetables to Fruits

The tests described above assumed a decreased redemption rate with no change in the ratio of vegetables and fruits with the higher CVV provided. Therefore, another set of tests was developed to evaluate the effect of changing the redemption rate, the dollar amounts of the CVV, and the ratio of vegetables to fruits purchased. In the revised packages, the proportion of vegetables to fruits was 33 to 67 percent, based on redemption data that was obtained from two states. For the purposes of the sensitivity analyses, this proportion was shifted to 50 percent vegetables and 50 percent fruits. The revised food package tests, although the same as those presented in Table 8-3, are included in Table 8-4 for reference but are not described.

Alternatives to the revised packages compared to the current packages Shifting the proportion of vegetables to fruits that are redeemed to 50 percent of each increased the copper in food packages IV-B (for children) and V-A (for pregnant women). In food package VII (for fully breastfeeding women), which includes a substantially higher revised CVV, the additional nutrients provided are similar to those provided in the revised package when shifting

TABLE 8-3 Impact of Increasing the CVV on Nutrient and Food Group Food Package Profiles and on the HEI–2010 Scores Relative to the Current Food Packages for Children Ages 2 to Less Than 5 Years (IV-B), Pregnant Women (V-A), and Fully Breastfeeding Women (VII)[a]

Food Package	Adjustments (Amount and Redemption Rate)[b]	Nutrients	Food Group(s)[c]	HEI Score[d]	Package Per-Participant Cost	WIC Average Per-Participant Cost	Appendix S Table Reference
IV-B	Revised: +$4, 75%	(+) fiber, vitamin C	(+) total vegetables, total fruit, whole fruit	(+) total vegetable score	+$2.82	+$1.03	S-8
	Test 1: +$4, 65%	—	(+) total fruit, whole fruit, total vegetables	—	+$1.62	+$0.59	S-8
	Test 2: +$4, 80%	(+) fiber, copper, vitamin C	(+) total vegetables, total fruit, whole fruit	(+) total vegetable score	+$3.24	+$1.25	S-8
	Test 3: +$4, 85%	(+) fiber, potassium, copper, vitamin C	(+) total fruit, whole fruit, total vegetables	(+) total vegetable score	+$4.02	+$1.47	S-8
V-A	Revised: +$4, 75%	(+) fiber, vitamin C	(+) total vegetables, total fruit, whole fruit	NA	+$2.76	+$0.26	S-9
	Test 1: +$4, 65%	—	(+) whole fruit, total vegetables	NA	+$1.26	+$0.12	S-9
	Test 2: +$4, 80%	(+) fiber, vitamin C	(+) total vegetables, total fruit, whole fruit	NA	+$3.51	+$0.34	S-9
	Test 3: +$4, 85%	(+) fiber, copper, vitamin C	(+) total fruit, whole fruit, total vegetables	NA	+$4.26	+$0.41	S-9

VII	Revised: +$24, 75%	(+) fiber, magnesium, potassium, copper, vitamin C, thiamin, niacin, vitamin B6, folate, choline	(+) total vegetables, total fruit, whole fruit	NA	+$17.76	+$0.58	S-10
	Test 1: +$24, 85%	(+) fiber, magnesium, potassium, copper, vitamin C, thiamin, niacin, vitamin B6, folate, choline	(+) total fruit, whole fruit, total vegetables	NA	+$21.26	+$0.70	S-10
	Test 2: +$9, 75%	(+) fiber, potassium, copper, vitamin C, vitamin B6	(+) total vegetables, total fruit, whole fruit	NA	+$6.51	+$0.21	S-10
	Test 3: +$34, 75%	(+) fiber, magnesium, potassium, copper, vitamin C, thiamin, riboflavin, niacin, vitamin B6, folate, choline, vitamin A	(+) total vegetables, total fruit, whole fruit	NA	+$25.26	+$0.83	S-10

NOTES: — = indicates that no changes were in the range of more than approximately ± 8%; (+) = increased amount (an increased amount for saturated fat, added sugars, and sodium is undesirable); CVV = cash value voucher; HEI = Healthy Eating Index–2010; NA = unable to calculate change in HEI score for any but food package IV-B. Changes to nutrients and vegetables/fruits are based on the committee's assumptions applied about participant preferences for specific varieties of vegetables and fruits. Nutrient and food group composition of the food packages were based on the assumptions outlined in Appendix R.

[a] Notations for nutrients and food groups in the table represent changes of 8% or greater. Not all nutrients or food groups listed were identified in Chapter 5 as a priority for the target population subgroup.

[b] The adjustment is in reference to the current food package amounts.

[c] Food group noted corresponds to the appropriate food group or subgroup from the *Dietary Guidelines for Americans*.

[d] The committee created a tool to estimate the HEI for children ages 2 to less than 5 years considering the revised package change or test. To do this, the difference between the redeemed amounts of the HEI components for the current food package and the redeemed amounts of the HEI components for the test food package were added to the median intake estimated using NHANES 2011–2012.

TABLE 8-4 Impact of Changes to Vegetable and Fruit Proportions on Nutrient and Food Group Food Package Profiles and on the HEI–2010 Scores Relative to the Current Food Packages for Children Ages 2 to Less Than 5 Years (IV-B), Pregnant Women (V-A), and Fully Breastfeeding Women (VII)[a]

Food Package	Adjustments (Amount and Redemption Rate)[b]	Nutrients	Food Groups[c]	HEI Score[d]	Package Per-Participant Cost	WIC Average Per-Participant Cost	Appendix S Table Reference
IV-B	Revised: +$4, 75%, 33/67 vegetable/fruit	(+) fiber, vitamin C	(+) total fruit, whole fruit, total vegetables	(+) total vegetable score[e]	+$2.82	+$1.03	S-11
	Test 1: +$4, 75%, 50/50 vegetable/fruit	(+) fiber, copper, vitamin C	(+) whole fruit, total vegetables	(+) total vegetable score[e]	+$2.82	+$1.03	S-11
V-A	Revised: +$4, 75%, 33/67 vegetable/fruit	(+) fiber, vitamin C	(+) total fruit, whole fruit, total vegetables	NA	+$2.76	+$0.26	S-12
	Test 1: +$4, 75%, 50/50 vegetable/fruit	(+) fiber, copper, vitamin C	(+) total vegetables	NA	+$2.76	+$0.26	S-12

VII	Revised: +$24, 75%, 33/67 vegetable/fruit	(+) fiber, magnesium, potassium, copper, vitamin C, thiamin, niacin, vitamin B6, folate, choline	(+) total fruit, whole fruit, total vegetables	NA	+$17.76	+$0.58	S-13
	Test 1: +$24, 75%, 50/50 vegetable/fruit	(+) fiber, magnesium, potassium, copper, vitamin C, thiamin, niacin, vitamin B6, folate, choline	(+) total fruit, whole fruit, total vegetables	NA	+$17.76	+$0.58	S-13

NOTES: (+) = increased amount (an increased amount for saturated fat, added sugars, and sodium is undesirable); HEI = Healthy Eating Index–2010; NA = unable to calculate change in HEI score for any but food package IV-B. Nutrient and food group composition of the food packages were based on the assumptions outlined in Appendix R.

[a] Notations for nutrients and food groups in the table represent changes of 8% or greater. Not all nutrients or food groups listed were identified in Chapter 5 as a priority for the target population subgroup.

[b] The adjustment is in reference to the current food package amounts.

[c] Food group noted corresponds to the appropriate food group or subgroup from the *Dietary Guidelines for Americans*.

[d] The committee created a tool to estimate the HEI for children ages 2 to less than 5 years considering the revised package change or test. To do this, the difference between the redeemed amounts of the HEI components for the current food package and the redeemed amounts of the HEI components for the test food package were added to the median intake estimated using NHANES 2011–2012.

[e] No shifts in fruit scores were observed because the HEI scores for total and whole fruit are at the maximum level based on median intake.

from 67 percent to 50 percent fruit. With a smaller CVV (such as for food packages IV-B and V-A), whole fruit (a higher-priority food subgroup for most WIC participants) increased compared to the current food packages. Similar to the previous tests of the higher CVV, the HEI–2010 score for total vegetables increased for food package IV-B. The shift to 50 percent vegetables does not affect the cost of the food packages because the costs applied for vegetables and fruits are approximately the same.[2] The actual cost, however, will vary if different varieties of vegetables and fruits are selected by participants than those assumed in the analysis.

Evaluation For the higher CVV, shifting CVV redemption to an equal proportion of vegetables and fruits does not result in large shifts in the level of essential nutrients in the revised food packages. However, the food groups contributed by the packages do shift from total fruits to total vegetables with a corresponding increase in the vegetable component of the HEI–2010. Ultimately, the cost difference in shifting from fruits to vegetables depends on the varieties of vegetables and fruits selected by participants.

Trade-offs Between Juice and the Cash Value Voucher

In the model applied to generate the revised food packages in this report, monies saved from reductions in juice were used to increase the CVV in all food packages. Sensitivity tests were designed to determine the effects of changes to the combination of juice and the CVV, because both of these WIC food categories contribute to the total fruit food group (the CVV also contributes to total vegetables), and may provide similar nutrients. Additional tests were applied to lower the redemption rate for juice and to evaluate a scenario of no juice plus a further increase in the CVV (see Table 8-5).

Revised food packages compared to the current packages The trade-off of juice for an increased CVV increases the level of fiber, but decreases vitamin C (a lower-priority nutrient for some women). Total vegetables and whole fruit increase (both are higher-priority food groups for most WIC participants). However, because juice is less expensive than vegetables and whole fruit on a per serving basis, transferring the savings from a reduction in juice to an increase in the CVV results in an overall decrease in the amount of total fruit in the packages, although within food package VII ($35, for fully breastfeeding women) both total fruit and whole fruit increase with

[2] Vegetables and fruits were selected for the model based on commonly redeemed varieties. The cost per cup-equivalent was determined based on Economic Research Service price data. See Appendix R for details.

this change. The change in cost per food package ranges from +$0.29 to +$15.29 because of variance in the total cost of the increased CVV in the revised packages. The effects on the overall average per-participant food cost are narrower, ranging from +$0.03 to +$0.50.

Alternatives to the revised packages compared to the current packages Increasing the value of the CVV further in the revised package may compensate for the reduced amounts of vitamin C from juice (a lower-priority nutrient for some women) and result in increased levels of several other micronutrients, including magnesium, potassium, copper, thiamin, niacin, vitamin B6, folate, and choline. As was the case for the previous tests applied to the increased CVV, the HEI–2010 score for total vegetables increased for food package IV-B (for children). Total fruit scores did not decrease beyond the 8 percent threshold with the tests for reductions in juice. The change in cost for these tests ranges from +$0.77 to +$17.29 per food package, and from +$0.22 to +$0.57 per-participant overall.

Evaluation A cost-neutral shift from juice to the CVV increases the level of fiber and whole fruit, but decreases the amount of vitamin C and total fruit in the food packages. A further increase in the CVV may compensate for reduced vitamin C from juice and increase the level of other nutrients as well as increase total vegetables, total fruit, and whole fruit. Although the costs per food package for both the revised packages and additional tests vary widely, the effects on the overall average per-participant food costs are smaller because the largest increases in the CVV are for a package that represents approximately 3 percent of participants (fully breastfeeding women).

The Addition of Fish to Food Packages or Changes in Amounts of Fish

Fish is included in all revised food packages for children and women. This is a new food for several of the food packages because fish is currently only included in food package VII (for fully breastfeeding women). Therefore, several sensitivity tests were developed to evaluate the effect of including fish, as well as the effect of potential increases or decreases in redemption from the rate assumed for the revised packages (see Table 8-6).

Revised packages compared to the current packages Providing 10 ounces of fish every 3 months in the rotation did not result in changes to essential nutrients above the threshold of 8 percent, based on the redemption rate applied. A key nutrient in allowed fish, omega-3 fatty acids, was not evaluated because there is only an adequate intake (AI) for alpha-linolenic acid, the precursor to synthesis of eicosapentaenoic acid (EPA) and docosahexaenoic acid (DHA), and readily available data on fish composition

TABLE 8-5 Impact of Changes to Juice and the CVV Combined on Nutrient and Food Group Food Package Profiles and on the HEI–2010 Scores Relative to the Current Food Packages for Children Ages 2 to Less Than 5 Years (IV-B), Pregnant Women (V-A), and Fully Breastfeeding Women (VII)[a]

Food Package	Adjustments (Amount and Redemption Rate)[b]	Nutrients	Food Group(s)[c]	HEI Score[d]	Package Per-Participant Cost	WIC Average Per-Participant Cost	Appendix S Table Reference
IV-B	Revised: –64 oz, 78%; +$4 CVV	(+) fiber (–) vitamin C	(+) total vegetables, whole fruit (–) total fruit	(+) total vegetable score[e]	+$0.87	+$0.32	S-14
	Test 1: –64 oz 75%; +$4 CVV	(+) fiber (–) vitamin C	(+) total vegetables, whole fruit (–) total fruit	(+) total vegetable score[e]	+$0.77	+$0.28	S-14
	Test 2: –128 oz, +$18 CVV	(+) fiber, copper, vitamin B6, choline, (–) vitamin C	(+) total vegetables, whole fruit (–) total fruit	(+) total vegetable score[e]	+$2.91	+$0.32	S-14
V-A	Revised: –80 oz, +$4 CVV	(+) fiber (–) vitamin C	(+) total vegetables, whole fruit (–) total fruit	NA	+$0.29	+$0.03	S-15

	Test 1: −144 oz, +$10 CVV	(+) fiber, copper, choline (−) vitamin C	(+) total vegetables, whole fruit (−) total fruit	NA	+$2.29	+$0.22	S-15
VII	Revised: −80 oz, +$24 CVV	(+) fiber, magnesium, potassium, copper, vitamin C, thiamin, niacin, vitamin B6, folate, choline	(+) total vegetables, total fruit, whole fruit	NA	+$15.29	+$0.50	S-16
	Test 1: −144 oz, +$41 CVV	(+) fiber, magnesium, potassium, copper, vitamin C, thiamin, niacin, vitamin B6, folate, choline, vitamin A	(+) total vegetables, total fruit, whole fruit	NA	+$17.29	+$0.57	S-16

NOTES: (+) = increased amount (an increased amount for saturated fat, added sugars, and sodium is undesirable); (−) = decreased amount (a decreased amount for saturated fat, added sugars, and sodium is desirable); CVV = cash value voucher; HEI = Healthy Eating Index–2010; NA = unable to calculate change in HEI score for any but food package IV-B. Changes to nutrients and vegetables/fruits are based on the committee's assumptions applied about participant preferences for specific varieties of vegetables and fruits. Nutrient and food group composition of the food packages were based on the assumptions outlined in Appendix R.

[a] Notations for nutrients and food groups in the table represent changes of 8% or greater. Not all nutrients or food groups listed were identified in Chapter 5 as a priority for the target population subgroup.

[b] The adjustment is in reference to the current food package amounts.

[c] Food group noted corresponds to the appropriate food group or subgroup from the *Dietary Guidelines for Americans*.

[d] The committee created a tool to estimate the HEI for children ages 2 to less than 5 years considering the revised package change or test. To do this, the difference between the redeemed amounts of the HEI components for the current food package and the redeemed amounts of the HEI components for the test food package were added to the median intake estimated using NHANES 2011–2012.

[e] No shifts in fruit scores were observed because the HEI scores for total and whole fruit are at the maximum level based on median intake.

TABLE 8-6 Impact of Changes to Fish Redemption on Nutrient and Food Group Food Package Profiles and on the HEI–2010 Scores Relative to the Current Food Packages for Children Ages 2 to Less Than 5 Years (IV-B), Pregnant Women (V-A), and Fully Breastfeeding Women (VII)[a]

Food Package	Adjustments (Amount and Redemption Rate)[b]	Nutrients	Food Groups[c]	HEI Score[d]	Package Per-Participant Cost	WIC Average Per-Participant Cost	Appendix S Table Reference
IV-B	Revised: +10 oz every 3 months, 68%	—[e]	(+) total protein, seafood	(+) seafood and plant protein score	+$0.46	+$0.16	S-17
	Test 1: +10 oz every 3 months, 59%	—[e]	(+) total protein, seafood	(+) seafood and plant protein score	+$0.40	+$0.14	S-17
	Test 2: +10 oz every 3 months, 79%	—[e]	(+) total protein, seafood	(+) seafood and plant protein score	+$0.53	+$0.19	S-17
V-A	Revised: +10 oz every 3 months, 68%	—[e]	(+) total protein, seafood	NA	+$0.46	+$0.04	S-18
	Test 1: +10 oz every 3 months, 59%	—[e]	(+) seafood	NA	+$0.40	+$0.04	S-18
	Test 2: +10 oz every 3 months, 79%	(+) selenium[e]	(+) total protein, seafood	NA	+$0.53	+$0.05	S-18

VII	Revised: –10 oz per month, 68%	(–) selenium, niacin[e]	(–) total protein, seafood	NA	–$1.47	–$0.05	S-19
	Test 1: –10 oz per month, 59%	(–) selenium, niacin[e]	(–) total protein, seafood	NA	–$1.83	–$0.06	S-19
	Test 2: –10 oz per month, 79%	—[e]	(–) total protein, seafood	NA	–$1.02	–$0.04	S-19

NOTES: — = indicates that no changes were in the range of more than approximately ± 8%; (+) = increased amount (an increased amount for saturated fat, added sugars, and sodium is undesirable); (–) = decreased amount (a decreased amount for saturated fat, added sugars, and sodium is desirable); HEI = Healthy Eating Index–2010; NA = unable to calculate change in HEI score for any but food package IV-B. Nutrient and food group composition of the food packages were based on the assumptions outlined in Appendix R.

[a] Notations for nutrients and food groups in the table represent changes of 8% or greater. Not all nutrients or food groups listed were identified in Chapter 5 as a priority for the target population subgroup.

[b] The adjustment is in reference to the current food package amounts.

[c] Food group noted corresponds to the appropriate food group or subgroup from the *Dietary Guidelines for Americans*. For current food packages in which no fish is provided, the seafood food group is noted as increasing.

[d] The committee created a tool to estimate the HEI for children ages 2 to less than 5 years considering the revised package change or test. To do this, the difference between the redeemed amounts of the HEI components for the current food package and the redeemed amounts of the HEI components for the test food package were added to the median intake estimated using NHANES 2011–2012.

[e] Authoritative guidance recommends inclusion of fish in the diet as a source of omega-3 fatty acids. However, the quantity provided could not be assessed because omega-3 fatty acids are not included in the USDA Standard Reference Database for nutrient composition of foods.

are limited. Fish also provides niacin, the quantities of which decrease in the revised food package VII (in which the quantity of fish provided was reduced). As intended, provision of fish (a higher-priority food group for all WIC participants) adds the seafood food group to the food packages where it was previously not included. The addition of fish to food packages IV-B (for children) and V-A (for pregnant women) increases the package cost by $0.46. The average per-participant food cost is increased from $0.04 to $0.16. The reduction in fish in food package VII saves $1.47 for that package, and $0.05 for the average package.

Alternatives to the revised packages compared to the current packages For the food packages evaluated, the redemption rate for fish was both increased and decreased. At a higher rate of redemption (79 percent), the amount of selenium provided becomes more apparent. The HEI–2010 scores for seafood and plant protein increased for all tests conducted on food package IV-B. Increasing the redemption rate of fish in food packages IV-B and V-A increases the package costs by $0.53, but cost savings remain in food package VII because of the reduction from the current food package amount. For these tests, the change in the average per-participant food cost ranges from –$0.06 to +$0.19.

Evaluation Inasmuch as the amounts of fish added to some food packages are small (3 ounces per month in some cases), a large effect on nutrients provided by the food package does not occur. However, inclusion of fish allows the food packages to provide the seafood food group, and omega-3 fatty acids, the amount of which could not be estimated. The cost of adding fish per food package and for the average per-participant food package are relatively high considering the small amounts added to food packages IV-B and V-A.

Rotating Peanut Butter, Legumes, and Fish

In some of the revised food packages, peanut butter, legumes, and fish are rotated over a 3-month period. Sensitivity tests were developed to evaluate the possible effect on nutrients, food groups, and redemption (in the case that the rotation resulted in confusion for participants about which food is issued in a particular month) because this is a new concept (apart from the current choice of peanut butter or legumes in some packages). The rotations were also evaluated without fish to determine the effect of its inclusion or exclusion from the rotation on nutrients and food groups (see Table 8-7).

Revised packages compared to the current packages Changing to a rotation of peanut butter and legumes, and adding fish to food package IV-B (for children) did not change nutrient levels more than ±8 percent. For food package V-A (for pregnant women), this rotation reduced fiber (a higher-priority nutrient for all WIC participants), magnesium, copper, and niacin (lower priorities for some women) in the package, but it also reduced added sugars and saturated fat (higher-priority "nutrients to limit" for most WIC participants). Inclusion of fish expanded the food package coverage of the DGA food groups to include seafood (a higher-priority food group for all WIC participants). The rotation also resulted in a reduction in provision of total vegetables, specifically the vegetables subgroup of beans, and nuts, seeds, and soy. The rotation in the revised food packages changes the per package cost between –$0.64 and +$0.11. The effect on the per-participant average food cost ranges from –$0.06 and +$0.04.

Alternatives to the revised packages compared to the current packages Removing fish from the food package rotation did not result in any changes above the 8 percent threshold for nutrients in food package IV-B. The HEI–2010 scores, however, decreased by more than 8 percent for greens and beans in the revised package and for the additional tests, but the overall HEI–2010 score changed by less than 8 percent. Increasing redemption of legumes from 53 percent (the assumption in the revised packages) to 69 percent did not affect level of fiber and achieved a cost savings. The cost change incurred from the additional tests ranged from –$1.09 to +$0.37. The average per-participant cost ranged from –$0.13 to +$0.13.

Evaluation The rotation of peanut butter, legumes, and fish in the revised food packages potentially reduces the level of fiber, magnesium, copper, and niacin, but it also reduces the amount of saturated fat and added sugars in the food packages. Inclusion of fish in the rotation achieved the addition of the DGA seafood food group to the packages where it was previously not included. For food package IV-B, although the HEI–2010 scores for greens and beans and seafood and plant proteins decreases, the overall change in HEI–2010 scores does not exceed the 8 percent threshold. The rotation results in a net savings because of the reduction of the amounts of peanut butter and legumes, despite the cost of adding fish.

Jarred Infant Food Vegetables and Fruits

Food package II is provided to all infants (fully formula-fed, partially breastfed, or fully breastfed) ages 6 to less than 12 months. Quantities of jarred infant food vegetables and fruits are reduced in the revised food package II for fully breastfeeding infants. In addition, a CVV substitution for the jarred infant food vegetables and fruits is allowed for all infants who receive this package. Given these changes, tests were developed for

TABLE 8-7 Impact of Changes to Amounts and Redemption in the Peanut Butter/Legumes/Fish Rotation on Nutrient and Food Group Food Package Profiles and on the HEI–2010 Scores Relative to the Current Food Packages for Children Ages 2 to Less Than 5 Years (IV-B) and Pregnant Women (V-A)[a]

Food Package	Adjustments (Amount and Redemption Rate)[b]	Nutrients	Food Group(s)[c]	HEI Score[d]	Package Per-Participant Cost	WIC Average Per-Participant Cost	Appendix S Table Reference
IV-B	Revised: –2.7 oz legumes/mo, 53%; –3 oz peanut butter/mo; +3.3 oz fish/mo	—	(+) seafood (–) total vegetables; beans; nuts, seeds, and soy	(–) greens and beans score	+$0.11	+$0.04	S-20
	Test 1: –2.7 oz legumes/mo, 53%; –3 oz peanut butter/mo; no fish	—	(–) total vegetables; beans; total protein; nuts, seeds, and soy	(–) greens and beans score; seafood and plant proteins score	–$0.34	–$0.13	S-20
	Test 2: –2.7 oz legumes/mo, 38%; –3 oz peanut butter/mo; +3.3 oz fish/mo	(–) copper	(+) seafood (–) total vegetables; beans; nuts, seeds, and soy	(–) greens and beans score	–$0.13	–$0.05	S-20
	Test 3: –2.7 oz legumes/mo, 69%; –3 oz peanut butter/mo; +3.3 oz fish/mo	—	(+) seafood (–) beans; total protein; nuts, seeds, and soy	(–) greens and beans score	+$0.37	+$0.13	S-20
V-A	Revised: –5.3 oz legumes/mo, 53%; –12 oz peanut butter/mo; +3.3 oz fish/mo	(–) fiber, magnesium, copper, niacin, added sugars, saturated fat	(+) seafood (–) total vegetables; beans; total protein; nuts, seeds, and soy	NA	–$0.64	–$0.06	S-21

Test 1: –5.3 oz legumes/mo, 53%; –12 oz peanut butter/mo; no fish	(–) fiber, magnesium, copper, niacin, saturated fat, added sugars	(–) total vegetables, beans, total protein, nuts, seeds, and soy	NA	–$1.09	–$0.10	S-21
Test 2: –5.3 oz legumes/mo, 38%; –12 oz peanut butter/mo; +3.3 oz fish/mo	(–) fiber, magnesium, copper, niacin, saturated fat, added sugars	(+) seafood (–) total vegetables, beans, total protein, nuts, seeds, and soy	NA	–$1.02	–$0.10	S-21
Test 3: –5.3 oz legumes/mo, 69%; –12 oz peanut butter/mo; +3.3 oz fish/mo	(–) copper, saturated fat	(+) seafood (–) beans, total protein, nuts, seeds, and soy	NA	–$0.25	–$0.02	S-21

NOTES: — = indicates that no changes were in the range of more than approximately ± 8%; (+) = increased amount (an increased amount for saturated fat, added sugars, and sodium is undesirable); (–) = decreased amount (a decreased amount for saturated fat, added sugars, and sodium is desirable); HEI = Healthy Eating Index–2010; NA = unable to calculate change in HEI score for any but food package IV-B. Nutrient and food group composition of the food packages were based on the assumptions outlined in Appendix R.

[a] Notations for nutrients and food groups in the table represent changes of 8% or greater. Not all nutrients or food groups listed were identified in Chapter 5 as a priority for the target population subgroup.

[b] The adjustment is in reference to the current food package amounts. Redemption rates are only noted if changed in the series of tests.

[c] Food group noted corresponds to the appropriate food group or subgroup from the *Dietary Guidelines for Americans*. For current food packages in which no fish is provided, the seafood food group is noted as increasing.

[d] The committee created a tool to estimate the HEI for children ages 2 to less than 5 years considering the revised package change or test. To do this, the difference between the redeemed amounts of the HEI components for the current food package and the redeemed amounts of the HEI components for the test food package were added to the median intake estimated using NHANES 2011–2012.

the revised food package II (weighting the feeding modes by participation) and the substitution option. No nutrient changes greater or less than 8 percent were observed for the revised food package. Similarly, a test of a 50 percent substitution of the jarred foods with a CVV did not result in changes beyond the 8 percent threshold. The 50 percent CVV substitution decreased the package cost by $0.31 and decreased the average per-participant package cost by $0.04 (see Appendix S, Table S-22).

Shifts in Participation from Formula-Feeding to Partially Breastfeeding

In the revised food packages, a 5 percent shift in participants from a formula-feeding to partially breastfeeding dyad was incorporated. The overall change in the weighted average per-participant cost from the current set of packages increases less than 1 percent, including or excluding formula rebates (see Table 8-8). Shifting 8 percent of participants from formula to partially breastfeeding resulted in a change of the same magnitude, but at a cost-savings. Costs initially increased with the 5 percent shift in participants because postpartum women stay on the program after 6 months if they are partially breastfeeding. As a greater number of participants shift to partial breastfeeding, there is a cost savings, primarily because infant formula is expensive and less of it is provided.[3]

SUMMARY

In this chapter, results of the sensitivity analyses are presented and discussed. The sensitivity tests were applied to food packages IV-B, V-A, and VII, and assessed the degree to which changes to the quantities of foods and other assumptions applied in the committee's food package model affect nutrients, food groups, and costs. The analyses conducted evaluated both major changes to the current food packages to create the revised food packages, as well as additional tests that altered quantities of food amounts in the packages and the assumptions applied to create the revised food packages. To summarize the effects for the various assumptions tested, the committee applied an 8 percent threshold as a potentially meaningful change. However, the degree to which the change observed can be considered meaningful is a function of the specific nutrient or food group, the target population group or subgroup, and the outcome of interest, as prioritized by USDA-FNS. The tables provided in Appendix S can serve as a detailed reference to support future regulatory decisions. The committee's overall findings from this analysis are summarized below in Table 8-9.

[3] See Appendix U for a description of the methodology applied for assessing shifts in participation.

TABLE 8-8 Impact of Shifting Participation from Formula-Feeding to Partially Breastfeeding on Cost

Food Package	Current Participation		Revised: Shift 5% of FF to FF/BF		Test 1: Shift 8% of FF to FF/BF	
	Cost Without Rebates ($)	Cost with Rebates ($)	Cost Without Rebates ($)	Cost with Rebates ($)	Cost Without Rebates ($)	Cost with Rebates ($)
I (0 to <6 mo, FF, BF, FF/BF)	123.00	43.57	120.04	42.52	118.26	41.89
II (6 to <12 mo, FF, BF, FF/BF)	115.37	51.37	113.28	50.63	112.02	50.19
Average food package (I–VII)	53.45	37.28	52.98	37.34	52.68	37.24
Average change from current			–0.46	+0.06	–0.77	–0.03
Average change from current (%)			–0.87	+0.16	–1.44	–0.09

NOTES: BF = breastfed; FF = fully formula-fed; FF/BF = partially breastfed; FP = food package.

TABLE 8-9 Sensitivity Testing of Changes and Assumptions in the Revised Food Packages: Overall Findings and Conclusions

Aspect of the Revised Food Packages Tested in the Sensitivity Analysis	Finding(s) and Conclusion(s)
Overall magnitude of changes observed	In most cases, the change to nutrient amounts in the revised package is less than 8% of the amount in the current package. Exceptions are cases in which larger reductions in milk or larger increases in the CVV are made. For food groups, larger proportional changes are observed, primarily due to reductions in legumes and peanut butter, and the increase of the CVV. In parallel, the estimated HEI–2010 sub-scores for children receiving food package IV-B generally change 8% or more from the current HEI–2010 score in the direction of the food group change. However, the overall HEI–2010 score changes less than 1%.
Changes in substitutions within food categories	The nutrients provided and the costs of the food packages depend on participants' selection among the options offered such as their selection of dairy substitution options.
Shift in funds from juice to the CVV	Shifting funds from juice to the CVV increases fiber in the food packages by at least 8%, but also decreases potassium and vitamin C by at least 8% unless additional funds are added to the CVV. The nutrients provided through redemption of the CVV ultimately depend on the participants' selection of specific vegetables and fruits.
Change to all whole grain-rich breakfast cereals	If cereals in the revised food package are redeemed at the current rate (instead of at a reduced rate), the change to whole grain-rich cereals increases provision of several micronutrients and whole grains in comparison to the current food package; however, the cost of the whole grains cereals is higher.
Addition or reduction of fish	Fish is a relatively expensive component of the food packages and changes in amounts affect the package costs. The inclusion of fish increases the contribution of the food packages to the seafood food group. Fish also provides omega-3 fatty acids, but the lack of a DRI and readily accessible composition data limited the committee's ability to conduct a quantitative assessment.
Effects on overall program costs for food	The effects on overall program costs for food (measured through the average food cost per person) depend on the proportion of participants represented by the changed food package. Of the packages evaluated, changes to food package IV-B (for children ages 2 to less than 5 years) have the largest proportional effect on overall program costs.

NOTES: CVV = cash value voucher; DRI = Dietary Reference Intake; HEI–2010 = Healthy Eating Index–2010.

REFERENCES

Fung, E. B., L. D. Ritchie, B. H. Walker, G. Gildengorin, and P. B. Crawford. 2010. Randomized, controlled trial to examine the impact of providing yogurt to women enrolled in WIC. *Journal of Nutrition Education and Behavior* 42(3 Suppl):S22–S29.

USDA/ARS (U.S. Department of Agriculture/Agricultural Research Service). 2014. *Food Patterns Equivalents Database 2011-12: Methodology and user guide*. http://www.ars.usda.gov/SP2UserFiles/Place/80400530/pdf/fped/FPED_1112.pdf (accessed December 20, 2016).

USDA/ARS. 2016. USDA National Nutrient Database for Standard Reference, Release 28. Beltsville, MD: USDA/ARS. https://ndb.nal.usda.gov/ndb (accessed September 14, 2016).

USDA/HHS (U.S. Department of Agriculture/U.S. Department of Health and Human Services). 2016. *Dietary Guidelines for Americans 2015–2020*. Washington, DC: U.S. Government Printing Office. https://health.gov/dietaryguidelines/2015 (accessed August 29, 2016).

9

How the Revised Food Packages Meet the Criteria Specified

This chapter illustrates the committee's approach to revising the food packages in alignment with the criteria that were first described in Chapter 1 (see Box 9-1). Each criterion is presented and discussed in sequence to show how the proposed food package revisions align with the criterion. Several of the proposed food package revisions align with more than one criterion. Consistent with the study task, for each criterion, revisions were made in consideration of the 2015–2020 *Dietary Guidelines for Americans* (DGA) food groups and subgroups. Throughout the chapter, alignment of the food package revisions with the criteria is evaluated in reference to redeemed amounts (not provided amounts) to reflect the effect of the food packages on meeting participants' needs more accurately. Table 9-1 summarizes how the food packages were revised to meet the seven criteria.

CRITERION 1

Criterion 1 states: "The packages provide a balanced supplement to the diets of women and children."

To meet this criterion, the committee reduced food group or subgroup quantities that met or exceeded 100 percent of recommended food group or subgroup intakes. At the same time, it increased food group or subgroup quantities that were either missing or present below an amount that was considered supplemental (and for which intakes were below recommended levels). Together, these two actions reapportioned the food groups and subgroups offered in a way that achieves a more balanced food package. Preferences and cost were also factors in determining the final amounts of

BOX 9-1

Criteria for Inclusion of Foods in the WIC Food Packages

1. The packages provide a balanced supplement to the diets of women and children.
2. The packages contribute to reduction of the prevalence of inadequate nutrient intakes and of excessive nutrient intakes.
3. The packages contribute to an overall dietary pattern that is consistent with the *Dietary Guidelines for Americans* for individuals 2 years of age and older.
4. The packages contribute to an overall diet that is consistent with established dietary recommendations for infants and children less than 2 years of age, including encouragement of and support for breastfeeding.
5. The foods in the packages are available in forms and amounts suitable for low-income persons who may have limited transportation options, storage, and cooking facilities.
6. The foods in the packages are readily acceptable, commonly consumed, widely available, take into account cultural eating patterns and food preferences, and provide incentives for families to participate in the WIC program.
7. The foods in the packages do not create an undue burden on state agencies or vendors.

foods in the revised packages. To illustrate the concepts of "balanced" and "supplemental," Figure 9-1 compares the currently offered food groups and subgroups, as redeemed, to the amounts of food groups and subgroups in the revised package, as redeemed, for food package IV-B (children ages 2 to less than 5 years). Food package IV-B is used as an example throughout this chapter, as was done in Chapter 8.[1] As shown in Figure 9-1, the proportions of food groups or subgroups provided at above-supplemental levels are reduced while the proportions provided at levels below-supplemental are increased. A comparison of all current and revised food packages as the

[1] As noted in Chapter 8, only food package IV-B is used for assessment of the effects of the revised package on intake. In this chapter, the assessments include the nutrient gap analysis, the food group gap analysis, and the change in Healthy Eating Index–2010 (HEI–2010). Reasons for using only food package IV-B include (1) the *Dietary Guidelines for Americans* (DGA) food patterns apply only to individuals 2 years of age and older and therefore are not applicable to younger children and infants; (2) the National Health and Nutrition Examination Survey (NHANES) subgroup size for children of these ages yielded more robust intake data due to being much larger compared to other subgroups of women and children; (3) because of small sample sizes, intake data for women were available only for NHANES 2005–2012 combined, which did not allow assessment of the intakes based on the current package; and (4) children make up more than 35 percent of the WIC-participating population, so this analysis represents the estimated effect of the food packages on a large proportion of participants.

proportion of DGA food groups and subgroups is presented in Appendix T, Figures T-1 through T-5.

As a result of the constraint to remain cost neutral, the committee was unable to meet criterion 1 fully. Adding servings of some food groups, particularly of vegetables and fruits, seafood, and whole grain cereals, is expensive relative to the cost of servings from the other food groups or subgroups that were replaced. Inasmuch as each food group contains unique and important nutrients, rebalancing of food groups to align with the DGA necessarily increases some nutrients while decreasing others.

CRITERION 2

Criterion 2 states: "The packages contribute to reduction of the prevalence of inadequate nutrient intakes and of excessive nutrient intakes."

Nutrient Levels in the Current, Compared to the Revised Food Packages, as Redeemed

The committee's analyses show that the proposed revisions to the food packages provide a better balance of the availability of most of the priority nutrients (see Appendix T). For example, Table T-11b in Appendix T illustrates that, in the current food package IV-B, the proportion of the Estimated Average Requirement (EAR) provided ranges from 63 to 199 percent. In the revised food package IV-B, the proportion of the EAR provided ranges from 57 to 191 percent.[2] The level of the higher-priority nutrient potassium increases (as redeemed), and the levels of saturated fat and sodium are reduced in the revised food package IV-B (as redeemed) compared to the current food package IV-B.

Changes to the Prevalence of Nutrient Inadequacy are Anticipated to Be Minimal

The gap analysis presented in Table 9-2 illustrates that revisions to close nutrient gaps for priority nutrients identified for food package IV-B are likely to be too minimal to affect nutrient adequacy. In general, the magnitude of nutrient availability from food group adjustments was limited by the need to remain cost neutral. This allowed the committee to predict similar small increments in nutrient adequacy across other population subgroups. More precise predictions of nutrient adequacy related to the food package revisions would require information on consumption of Special

[2] Exclusive of vitamins E and B_{12}.

TABLE 9-1 Overview of How the Revised Food Packages Meet the Criteria

DGA Food Group and Recommended Food Package Change	Criteria						
	1. Balanced Supplement to the Diet	2. Reduce Inadequate or Excessive Nutrient Intakes	3. Diet Aligned with DGA	4. Diet Aligned with Guidance for Children <2 y	5. Availability of Suitable Forms and Amounts Suitable for Low-Income Persons	6. Acceptability, Availability, and Cultural Suitability	7. Pose No Undue State Agency or Vendor Burden
Total fruits							
Increase CVV	✓	✓	✓	✓	✓	✓	
Reduce fruit juice	✓		✓	✓		✓	
Reduce jarred infant food fruits	✓						
Substitute CVV for juice or jarred infant fruits			✓	✓		✓	✓
Total vegetables							
Increase CVV	✓	✓	✓	✓		✓	
Reduce legumes	✓		✓				
Offer canned beans		✓			✓	✓	
Vendors stock three varieties							✓
Reduce jarred infant food vegetables	✓						
Substitute CVV for jarred infant foods				✓		✓	

Offer a canned, frozen, or dried form (vegetable or fruit)					✓	✓	
Allow legumes to substitute for eggs						✓	
Total dairy							
Reduce amount (except in FP VI)	✓						
Increase substitution options	✓	✓				✓	
Offer a range of yogurt amounts							✓
Retain only low-fat or fat-free forms for 2 y or older			✓				
Remove "dangling quart"*							✓
Whole grains							
Require whole grain-rich breakfast cereals	✓	✓	✓				✓
Retain RTE breakfast cereal form		✓					
Offer additional whole grain forms		✓				✓	
Offer range of sizes for whole wheat bread and grains		✓				✓	✓
Reduce infant cereal	✓			✓			

continued

TABLE 9-1 Continued

DGA Food Group and Recommended Food Package Change	Criteria						
	1. Balanced Supplement to the Diet	2. Reduce Inadequate or Excessive Nutrient Intakes	3. Diet Aligned with DGA	4. Diet Aligned with Guidance for Children <2 y	5. Availability of Suitable Forms and Amounts Suitable for Low-Income Persons	6. Acceptability, Availability, and Cultural Suitability	7. Pose No Undue State Agency or Vendor Burden
Total protein							
Offer seafood	✓	✓	✓	✓	✓		
Reduce peanut butter	✓		✓			✓	
Reduce jarred infant food meat	✓			✓			
Substitute fish for jarred infant food meat		✓		✓		✓	
Calories for other uses							
Reduce total sugars limit in yogurt	✓	✓	✓	✓			✓
Limit added sugars in milk alternatives	✓	✓	✓	✓			✓
Reduce saturated fat by reducing dairy	✓	✓	✓				

NOTES: CVV = cash value voucher; DGA = *Dietary Guidelines for Americans*; FP = food package; RTE = ready-to-eat.
* The term "dangling quart" refers to the quart of milk that remains in some food packages when cheese is substituted for milk.

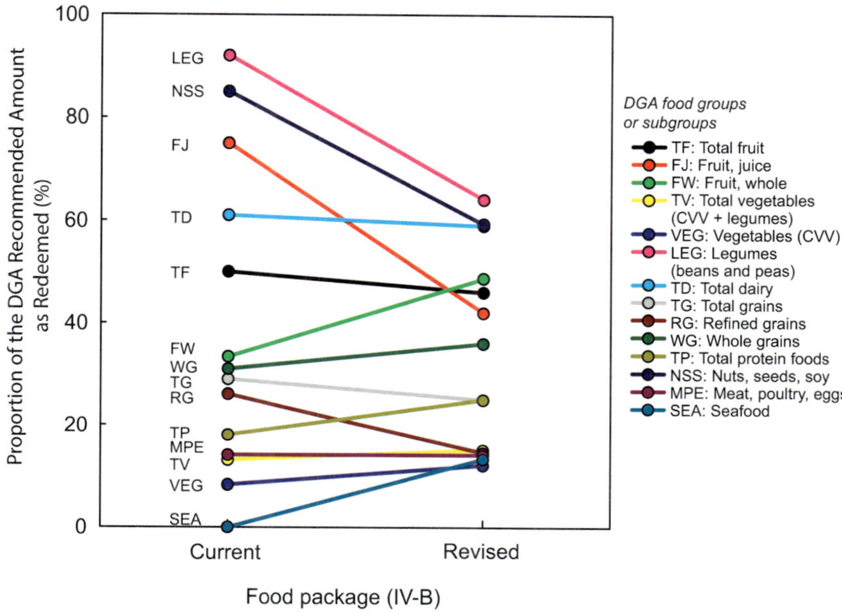

FIGURE 9-1 Proportion of the *Dietary Guidelines for Americans* (DGA) food groups and subgroups provided in the current and revised food package IV-B as redeemed.
NOTE: The methodology for calculating redemption rates is detailed in Appendix R.

Supplemental Nutrition Program for Women, Infants, and Children (WIC) foods.[3]

Fifty Percent of the Estimated Average Requirement (EAR) or Adequate Intake (AI) Provided for Most Priority Nutrients

Overall, each food package provides at least 50 percent of the EAR/Adequate Intake (AI) for *most* priority nutrients. Some priority nutrients (as described in Chapter 5) were retained in the revised packages at levels below 50 percent of the EAR or AI, including potassium and fiber (high priority across WIC participant subgroups), choline (high priority, pregnant women), vitamin D (low priority, pregnant women), and copper (low priority, postpartum women). Potassium, vitamin D, vitamin E, and choline are four nutrients for which adequacy goals are not met in almost all DGA

[3] Owing to lack of detail, the Nutrient-Based Diet Quality index was not a useful tool for evaluation of nutrient adequacy given the revised packages.

TABLE 9-2 Effects of the Food Package Revisions on Priority Nutrient Intakes: Gap Analysis for Food Package IV-B Based on Redemption*

Priority Nutrients[a]	AI or Upper Limit	Median Nutrient Intake	Current Redeemed Amounts[b]	Revised Redeemed Amounts[b]	Current Daily Gap[c]	Revised Daily Gap[d]	Change in Gap[e]	Evaluation of the Change in the Gap[f]
Nutrients to Increase								
Potassium (mg)	3,800	2,071	927	940	1,729	1,716	–13	Small narrowing
Fiber (g)	25	12	4.3	4.0	13	13	+0.3	Small widening
Nutrients to Reduce[g]		95th Percentile of Intake						
Sodium[h] (mg)	1,900	2,995	412	367	1,095	1,051	–44	Small narrowing
Saturated fat (g)	14	18	4.5	3.9	15	14	–0.6	Small narrowing
Added sugars (g)	33	60	4.3	4.6	59	59	+0.4	Small widening

NOTES: Redemption rates for each WIC food category were primarily based on information provided to the committee. The methodology applied to calculate redemption is described in Appendix R. AI = Adequate Intake. *Some values in this table are corrected from the original prepublication.

[a] Priority nutrients were determined using the committee's decision tree, as described in Chapter 5.

[b] Application of redemption rates and assumptions applied to develop the food package nutrient profiles are described in Appendix R.

[c] See Appendix L for details on calculation of the gap.

[d] Based on the difference between redeemed amounts of the current and revised food packages.

[e] A negative value for change in gap is favorable, indicating that participants in the subgroup are moved closer to the recommended intake when the food package is consumed as redeemed.

[f] A small narrowing or widening in the gap was defined as less than 10 percent of the AI, Tolerable Upper Intake Level (UL), or other upper limit.

[g] For nutrients to reduce, the following limits were applied: sodium, the UL; saturated fat, 10 percent of the calculated Estimated Energy Requirement (EER) for the subgroup (33 g); added sugars, 10 percent of the calculated EER for the subgroup (14 g).

[h] The gap analysis for sodium was based on the UL for children ages 4 to 8 years. Using the UL of 1,500 for children ages 1 to 3 years also results in a small narrowing.

food patterns (USDA/HHS, 2016), which indicates that there are some limitations to meeting recommended intakes for these specific nutrients. The same challenges were apparent in the revised food packages. Details of the nutrient composition of the current compared to the revised food packages are provided in Appendix T.

Changes in Sodium, Saturated Fat, and Added Sugars

The revised food packages provide less sodium and saturated fat. Reductions in the amounts of dairy foods were the primary drivers of reducing saturated fat and sodium in all revised food packages (see Appendix T). However, added sugars increase in some packages because of the additional yogurt substitution option.[4] Evidence reviewed in the DGA indicates that added sugars in some foods (yogurt is a provided example) can promote consumption of nutrient-dense foods (USDA/HHS, 2016). Thus, additional yogurt was included as a means of promoting intakes of dairy consumption, which was found to be below recommended amounts across WIC population subgroups.

CRITERION 3

Criterion 3 states: "The package contributes to an overall dietary pattern that is consistent with the *Dietary Guidelines for Americans* for individuals 2 years of age and older."

The committee met criterion 3 by rebalancing the WIC package food groups and subgroups consistent with its definition of supplemental. As illustrated in Figure 9-1, this process reduced the food groups and subgroups offered at levels greater than that required to meet recommended intakes and increased amounts of food groups and subgroups offered at lower levels. The revised food packages are better aligned with the DGA because:

- *Fruit is shifted from juice to whole fruit.* Although total fruit offered varies depending on the food package, overall, the revisions decrease juice and increase whole fruit in all food packages. These changes align with the DGA, which recommend greater consumption of whole fruit in proportion to fruit juice.

---

[4] The food package nutrient profiles were created assuming 70 percent flavored yogurt containing 30 g total sugars per serving, and 30 percent plain yogurt. Participants may choose a flavored yogurt that contains less than 30 g total sugars, if available on state food lists. Details of the assumptions applied can be found in Appendix R.

- *Grains are shifted from refined to whole grains.* The proposed revisions increase the proportion of whole grains compared to refined grains in all food packages, consistent with the recommendations of the DGA.
- *Fish is available in all WIC food packages.* The revised food packages provide fish to all WIC participants,[5] no longer only to exclusively breastfeeding women.
- *Total sodium is reduced.* Appendix T, Tables T-6a through T-11b illustrate that sodium is reduced in all of the food packages, primarily due to the reductions in dairy.
- *Contributions to "calories for other uses (COU)" are reduced.* Overall, the contribution of the food packages to the total daily limits for COU are reduced or remained relatively stable (see Table 9-3).
- *Estimates indicate that food group intakes are either unchanged or change slightly.* Estimating the effects on intake of food groups is highly dependent on knowing the distribution of both redemption and consumption of WIC foods relative to the food package issued. As noted elsewhere in the report, this information was not uniformly available to the committee. Thus, to generate a rough estimate of effects of the revised packages on intake of food groups, the committee conducted a second "gap analysis" to assess the effect of changes in food groups or subgroups provided in food package IV-B on the gap (i.e., the difference between the food group or subgroup intake at the median [50th percentile]). The results of this analysis are presented in Table 9-4.

As shown in Table 9-4, most of the food package changes are expected to either not affect intake or to reduce the gap in food group or subgroup intake. For dairy and nuts, seeds, and soy, however, the gap is increased. This should be interpreted with attention to the fact that these foods are provided in the current food package in amounts that are nearly, or exceed, 100 percent of that recommended. For this food subgroup, the amount in the revised food package IV-B still exceeds 100 percent of recommended amounts owing to container size limitations.

The Healthy Eating Index–2010 Score May Improve

Estimates indicate that the Healthy Eating Index–2010 (HEI–2010) score may improve slightly. The committee estimated the effects of the revised food package against the HEI–2010 for food package IV-B (see

[5] Excluding young infants and older formula-fed or partially breastfed infants.

TABLE 9-3 Comparison of COUs Based on Redemption in the Current and Revised Food Packages for Children and Women*

Food Package and Kcal Pattern Applied	Proportion of the Total Daily Limit (%)[a]		
	Current	Revised	Difference
V-A: Women, pregnant (based on a 2,600-kcal pattern)	18	13	–5
V-B: Women, partially breastfeeding (based on a 2,600-kcal pattern)	18	13	–5
VI: Women, postpartum (based on a 2,300-kcal pattern)	15	14	–2
VII: Women, fully breastfeeding (based on a 2,600-kcal pattern)	22	15	–6
IV: Children ages 2 to <5 years (based on a 1,300-kcal pattern)	55	52	–3

NOTES: COU = calories for other uses, defined in the 2015–2020 *Dietary Guidelines for Americans* (DGA) as the combined calories from saturated fats (solid fats), added sugars, refined added starches, and alcohol; kcal levels patterns were selected based on the calculated estimated energy requirements for WIC participants, using NHANES 2011–2012 (children) or 2005–2012 (women). The methodology applied to develop the food package nutrient profiles and to calculate redemption is described in Appendix R. *Some values in this table are corrected from the original prepublication version.

[a] To calculate this value, the COU that are allotted to each kcal level as noted in the DGA food patterns were assumed. The values represent the proportion of those kcals that are contributed by the food packages.

SOURCES: USDA/ARS, 2005–2012; USDA/ARS, 2016; USDA/HHS, 2016

Table 9-5).[6] The difference in redeemed amounts of the food groups corresponding to HEI–2010 components between the current and revised food package was calculated, making the assumption that the median intake of participants would increase or decrease by this difference. The new intake values were then used to calculate the HEI–2010 score for the revised food packages. As shown in Table 9-5, the revised food package IV-B is predicted to increase several HEI–2010 subscores (e.g., total vegetables, whole grains, and total protein foods, refined grains, and sodium with increases of at least 0.1 points), while decreasing others (e.g., greens and beans, dairy, seafood, and plant proteins with decreases of at least 0.1 points). The scores for components to consume in moderation (refined grains, sodium, and empty calories) were increased or unchanged. Overall, the total HEI–2010 score

[6] This spreadsheet method was validated by comparing the HEI–2010 value calculated using Excel and intake data to the value calculated using the method described in Appendix J and reported in Chapter 4. The value calculated using the Excel spreadsheet method is 66.26, slightly higher that the value presented in Chapter 4 of 65.02. The committee therefore concluded that the spreadsheet method was adequate for generating a rough estimate of the effects of the revised food package IV-B on the HEI–2010.

TABLE 9-4 Estimated Effect of the Revised Food Packages on DGA Food Group and Subgroup Intakes Based on Redemption: Children Ages 2 to Less Than 5 Years, Food Package IV-B

USDA Food Pattern Group	DGA Recommendation	Median Food Group Intake	Current Redeemed Amounts	Revised Redeemed Amounts	Current Daily Gap	Revised Daily Gap	Change in Gap[c]	Evaluation of Change in Gap[d]
Total fruit	1.25	1.4	0.63	0.57	0	0	NA	No effect
Fruit, whole (CVV)[a]	0.63	0.71	0.25	0.37	0	0	NA	No effect
Total vegetables	1.50	0.6	0.19	0.22	0.89	0.86	–0.04	Small narrowing
Vegetables (CVV)[b]	1.50	0.6	0.12	0.18	0.89	0.84	–0.06	Small narrowing
Legumes (beans and peas)	0.07	0.05	0.06	0.04	0.02	0.04	+0.02	Moderate widening
Total dairy	2.50	1.9	1.51	1.48	0.56	0.59	+0.03	Small widening
Total grains	4.50	4.7	1.29	1.13	0	0	NA	No effect
Whole grains	2.25	0.6	0.70	0.81	1.67	1.56	–0.11	Small narrowing
Total protein foods	3.50	2.9	0.62	0.86	0.57	0.34	–0.23	Small narrowing
Nuts, seeds, and soy	0.36	0.2	0.31	0.21	0.16	0.25	+0.09	Moderate widening
Meat, poultry, eggs	2.36	2.5	0.32	0.32	0	0	NA	No effect
Seafood	0.57	0.1	0.00	0.08	0.47	0.39	–0.08	Moderate narrowing

NOTES: CVV = cash value voucher; DGA = *Dietary Guidelines for Americans*; NA = not applicable. The 2015–2020 DGA do not include recommendations for intake of fruit juice or refined grains; therefore these food subgroups were not considered in this analysis. The methodology applied to estimate redemption is described in Appendix R.

[a] Includes estimated intake from whole fruit purchased with the CVV.

[b] Includes estimated intake from legumes and vegetables purchased with the CVV.

[c] A reduction in the gap indicates a change that moves food group intakes closer to the DGA recommended amounts.

[d] The evaluation categorizes a change in the gap of less than 10 percent of recommended amounts as "small," and categorizes a change of less than 50 percent of recommended amounts as "moderate." A narrowing of the gap (i.e., a negative value) indicates an improvement in dietary intake.

is improved, increasing by approximately 1 point, a positive change of approximately 1.4 percent. This small increase may be important because WIC participants generally have poor diets.

The revised food package changes align with select DGA recommendations in other ways as well, as summarized in Table 9-6. Recommendations related to physical activity or alcohol consumption were not considered relevant to this review.

CRITERION 4

Criterion 4 states: "The packages contribute to an overall diet that is consistent with established dietary recommendations for infants and children less than 2 years of age, including encouragement of and support for breastfeeding."

The dietary recommendations for infants and children less than 2 years of age that were considered by the committee are summarized in Chapter 3, Table 3-10. The recommendations cover breastfeeding, formula feeding, complementary feeding, and the promotion of healthy eating habits.

Table 9-7 presents a side-by-side comparison of how the revised food packages align with these recommendations. The revised food packages account for the nutritional needs of exclusively breastfed, partially breastfed, and formula-fed infants in the first few months of life, the developmental and nutritional needs during the first 2 years of life, the promotion of healthy eating patterns, and the safety of foods consumed.

In addition to the comparisons in Table 9-7, the revised food packages are designed to provide incentives for breastfeeding of any intensity with 3 strategies: (1) further increasing the value of the exclusive breastfeeding package by increasing the CVV, (2) increasing the value of the packages for partially breastfeeding women by increasing the CVV and allowing more fish compared to the postpartum package, and by (3) increasing the flexibility of the food packages in the first month so that women may be issued the amount of formula needed based on a professional assessment, instead of having only the choices of no formula, nine cans of formula, or, in states where it is offered, one can of formula.

CRITERION 5

Criterion 5 states: "The foods in the packages are available in forms and amounts suitable for low-income persons who may have limited transportation options, storage, and cooking facilities."

The 2009 food package revisions included the addition of several options for tailoring food packages to meet participant needs related to transportation and limited storage and/or cooking facilities. The revised

TABLE 9-5 Estimated Effect of the Revised Food Packages on the Healthy Eating Index–2010 of Children Ages 2 to Less Than 5 Years: Food Package IV-B Based on Redemption

HEI–2010 Component	Serving-Equivalents per Day[a] Median Food Group Intake	Serving-Equivalents per Day[a] Change in Food Group Intake	Current Food Group Density[b]	New Food Group Density[b]	HEI–2010 Max Score[c]	Density for Min Score	Density for Max Score	Estimated Current Food Group Score	Estimated New Food Group Score
Adequacy									
Total fruit	1.4	–0.05	0.91	0.88	5.00	0.00	0.80	5.00	5.00
Fruit, whole	0.7	0.11	0.47	0.55	5.00	0.00	0.40	5.00	5.00
Total vegetables	0.6	0.05	0.41	0.44	5.00	0.00	1.10	1.84	1.98
Greens and beans[d]	0.1	–0.01	0.04	0.04	5.00	0.00	0.20	1.10	0.92
Whole grains	0.6	0.11	0.39	0.46	10.00	0.00	1.50	2.59	3.06
Total dairy	1.9	–0.03	1.29	1.27	10.00	0.00	1.30	9.95	9.79
Total protein foods	2.9	0.19	1.95	2.08	5.00	0.00	2.50	3.90	4.16
Seafood and plant proteins	0.3	–0.06	0.20	0.16	5.00	0.00	0.80	1.25	1.00
Fatty acids (ratio to SFA)[e]	34.7	–1.26	1.95	1.90	10.00	<1.2	>2.5	5.79	5.41

Moderation									
Refined grains	3.9	−0.26	2.61	2.44	10.00	>4.30	<1.80	6.76	7.45
Sodium	2,182	−44.9	1,455	1,425	10.00	>2000	<1,100	6.06	6.39
Empty calories (kcal)[f]	354	−0.20	23.60	23.59	20.00	>50	<19	17.0	17.0
Total HEI–2010								66.26	67.21
% Change									1.4

NOTES: HEI–2010 = Healthy Eating Index–2010; SFA = saturated fatty acid. It was assumed that changes in the food groups offered in the WIC packages, as redeemed, will alter the median intake of the recipients by the same amount (either increase or decrease). The methodology applied to estimate redemption is described in Appendix R.

[a] Fatty acids are expressed in g; sodium is expressed in mg; empty calories are expressed in kcal.

[b] Food group density expressed per 1,000 kcal; intake of 1,500 kcal per day was assumed for this example, based on the median reported energy intake for this subgroup. Because the energy in the current and revised food packages differ by only 8 kcal as redeemed, 1,500 kcals is used for all density calculations.

[c] The minimum score for each HEI–2010 component is always zero.

[d] No change in greens intake is assumed, because intake of these vegetables was seldom reported, and is unlikely to increase substantially even with an increased value of the CVV. The intake of legumes is included in the greens and beans component because protein foods were close to recommended intakes.

[e] Because the monounsaturated fatty acid (MUFA) and polyunsaturated fatty acid (PUFA) content of the food packages was not determined, MUFA + PUFA as estimated and total fat minus saturated fat. Although this calculation will overestimate MUFA + PUFA, it should have little effect on the magnitude of the change in the ratio.

[f] Although the HEI–2010 typically applies solid fats in the calculation of empty calories, saturated fat was used for this calculation because data for the solid fat composition of foods in the food packages was not available.

TABLE 9-6 Consistency of the Revised Food Packages with Selected Recommendations from the 2015–2020 *Dietary Guidelines for Americans* for Individuals Ages 2 Years and Older (Criterion 3)

Recommendation from the DGA	How the Revised Food Packages Contribute to an Overall Dietary Pattern That Is Consistent with the DGA
To meet nutrient needs within calorie limits, choose a variety of nutrient-dense foods across and within all food groups in recommended amounts	• Emphasize nutrient-dense foods such as seafood, vegetables and fruits, whole grains, dairy • Allow additional dairy and whole grains options to improve acceptability • Reduce contribution to COU • Reduce contribution to the proportional limit for COU for food packages V-A, V-B, VI, VII, and IV-B, as redeemed • Allow additional yogurt substitution option, which provides some additional added sugars, but may increase dairy intake
Consume a variety of vegetables from all of the subgroups	• Increase CVV, which allows participants to redeem more/wider variety of vegetables • Require a frozen, canned, or dried option for vegetables, which may improve the variety available to participants across seasons
Intake of fruit should be at least 50 percent whole fruit and not more than 50 percent 100% fruit juice	• Increase ratio of whole fruit to juice
At least half of grains should be whole grains	• Add more whole grain alternatives and expand the allowable size for whole grains from 16 to 24 oz to encourage redemption • Require 100% whole wheat bread • Require cereal (cooked and ready-to-eat) to meet "whole grain-rich" criteria • Increase ratio of whole grains to refined grains
Consume fat-free or low-fat dairy products	• Retain nonfat or low-fat milk for participants aged 2 years and older (current policy is unchanged)*
Consume less than 10% of energy from saturated fats	• Reduce dairy, which reduces saturated fat
Consume less than 10% of energy from added sugars	• Reduce total sugars limits specifications for yogurt • Propose total sugars limit for soy beverages • Retained total sugars limit for cereals
Stay within the limits for "calories for other uses" for specific food-pattern energy levels	• Revised packages V-A, V-B and VII fall within the limits of COUs relative to the energy content of the food packages and the appropriate food pattern

TABLE 9-6 Continued

Recommendation from the DGA	How the Revised Food Packages Contribute to an Overall Dietary Pattern That Is Consistent with the DGA
Limit sodium intake to less than 2,300 mg per day for individuals ages 14 years and older, less than 1,900 for children age 4 years, and less than 1,500 for children ages 1 to 3 years	• Reduce sodium in all packages by reducing dairy
The general population should consume 8 oz of seafood a week that are high in EPA/DHA. Pregnant and breastfeeding women should consume 8 to 12 oz of seafood a week from choices that are high in EPA/DHA and lower in methyl mercury	• Add currently authorized canned fish options high in omega-3 fatty acids and low in mercury to additional packages
Women should consume between 320 and 520 μg DFE per day, depending on life stage	• Increase CVV and added options for fortified corn masa flour • Encourage states to authorize tortillas made with fortified corn masa flour when available

NOTES: CVV = cash value voucher; DFE = dietary folate equivalents; DGA = *Dietary Guidelines for Americans*; EPA/DHA = eicosapentaenoic acid/docosapentaenoic acid; COU = calories for other uses.

* Low-fat cheese may be offered by states, but is not required. Low-fat cheese may be less available across WIC-approved vendors and if not commonly carried, it is likely to be offered at a higher price.

food packages retain these options, and include additional changes that allow for further flexibility in meeting the needs of participants with limited transportation. Table 9-8 summarizes how the WIC food packages (including current policies and recommended changes) address criterion 5.

CRITERION 6

Criterion 6 states: "The foods in the packages are readily acceptable, commonly consumed, widely available, take into the account cultural eating patterns and food preferences, and provide incentives for families to participate in the WIC program."

The 2009 food package changes also included several additional options to improve alignment with cultural eating patterns and food preferences, as reviewed in Chapter 3. In particular, the increase of the CVV with very few restrictions on choice provides participants with the flexibility to choose

TABLE 9-7 Consistency of the Revised Food Packages with Selected Dietary Recommendations for Infants and Children Less Than 2 Years of Age (Criterion 4)

Recommendation[a]	How the Revised Food Packages Meet the Recommendation
Breastfeeding	
All infants should be exclusively breastfed for about 6 months, followed by continued breastfeeding as complementary foods are introduced, with continuation of breastfeeding for 1 year or longer as mutually desired by mother and infant.[b]	• Increase the CVV from $11 to $35 to enhance the value of the fully breastfeeding package
To improve the intake of omega-3 long-chain fatty acids by breastfed infants, it is recommended that their mothers consume 1–2 servings of "ocean-going" fish per week to achieve a maternal intake of 200–300 mg of omega-3 long-chain fatty acids.[c]	• Provide 10 oz of fish per month in food package V-B • Provide 20 oz of fish per month in food package VII
Formula Feeding	
For infants who are not breastfeeding, iron-fortified infant formula is the recommended alternative for feeding the baby during the first year of life.	• Provide only iron-fortified infant formula throughout the first year after birth (current policy is unchanged)[d]
Therapeutic (noncontract) formula should be made available through physician prescription for specific medical conditions.	• Provide therapeutic (noncontract) formula to infants with a doctor's prescription (current policy is unchanged)
Complementary Feeding	
Complementary foods should be gradually introduced to infants at approximately 6 months of life.	• Provide only infant formula in food packages for infants under 6 months of age (current policy unchanged)
Complementary foods rich in iron and zinc (fortified cereals and meats) should be introduced to exclusively breastfed infants at about 6 months of age depending on developmental readiness. Recommended amounts are 2 servings per day of cereal (2 tablespoons/serving) or 1 to 2 oz of meat per day.	• Provide iron-fortified infant cereals to all infants and infant food meats to fully breastfed infants starting at 6 months of age • Reduce amounts to align better with AAP (2014) recommendations
Introduce single-ingredient new foods, one at a time, observing for adverse reactions or intolerance.	• Provide complementary foods in the food package for older infants (current policy is unchanged)

TABLE 9-7 Continued

Recommendation[a]	How the Revised Food Packages Meet the Recommendation
Avoid cow's milk until age 1 year. Whole milk may be provided at age 1 year. During the second year of life, low-fat milk may be considered if weight gain is appropriate, if weight gain is excessive, or family history is positive for obesity, dyslipidemia, or cardiovascular disease. Recommended total daily milk intake is 16 to 24 oz. Intakes above 25 oz/day may contribute to iron deficiency.	• Do not provide cow's milk to infants (current policy is unchanged) • Provide whole milk to children ages 1 to less than 2 years (current policy is unchanged)
Introduce a variety of foods. By 7 to 8 months, infants should be consuming foods from all food groups. Provide foods of varying textures (e.g., pureed, blended, mashed, finely chopped, and soft lumps). Gradually increase table foods. Avoid mixed textures, such as broth with vegetables.	• Include jarred infant food vegetables and fruits to support introduction of a variety of foods • Allow caretakers to select a variety of vegetables and fruits, and prepare with varying textures using a CVV in place of jarred infant food vegetables and fruits
Promoting Healthy Eating Patterns	
Allow lower fat milks for children age 1 year and older for whom obesity or overweight is a concern.	• Issue, at state agency option, fat-reduced milks to children under 2 years of age for whom overweight or obesity is a concern, as determined by individual nutrition assessment and consultation with the child's health care provider (current policy is unchanged)
Total daily juice intake should be limited to 4 to 6 oz per day from 1 to 6 years of age. Encourage whole fruit intake over juice.	• Reduce juice amounts for children to provide a supplemental amount of the recommended limit
Avoid added sugar and added salt.	• Limit the amount of added sugars and salt (sodium) in foods (current policy is unchanged) • Introduce new total sugars limits for yogurt and soy beverages. Retain total sugars limit for RTE cereals
Repeat exposure to new foods and flavors may be required to optimize acceptance. Early exposure may promote the selection of a varied diet later in life.	• Provide a CVV option for all infants ages 6 to less than 12 months in place of jarred infant food vegetables and fruits, which expands the variety of possible flavors and textures to which infants may be exposed • Retain all of the foods currently provided in the food packages, adjusting amounts to obtain improved balance across food groups

continued

TABLE 9-7 Continued

NOTES: AAP = American Academy of Pediatrics; CVV = cash value voucher; RTE = ready-to-eat. Guidance related to supplementation is not addressed in this table as it falls outside of the constraints of the food packages.

[a] References for each recommendation are presented in Table 3-10.

[b] There is some controversy regarding whether exclusive breastfeeding meets energy requirements of infants at 6 months of age in developed countries (Fewtrell et al., 2007). Fewtrell et al. (2007, p. 637S) states, "A reasonable interpretation of the available scientific data is that there are currently insufficient grounds to confidently recommend an optimal duration of exclusive breastfeeding of 6 as opposed to 4–6 months for infants in developed countries."

[c] Concern regarding the possible risk from intake of excessive mercury or other contaminants is offset by the neurobehavioral benefits of an adequate DHA intake and can be minimized by avoiding the intake of predatory fish (e.g., pike, marlin, mackerel, tilefish, swordfish) (AAP, 2014).

[d] "Current policy is unchanged" indicates, both in this table and in Tables 9-8 and 9-9, that the current food package(s) is already aligned with a specific recommendation and that no changes were proposed.

SOURCES: As indicated in Chapter 3, Table 3-10, of this report.

vegetables and fruits that meet cultural needs (Sucher et al., 2017). Redemption data indicate that the CVV is among the most well-redeemed components of the food packages (see Chapter 2, Table 2-14). The revised food packages increase the value of the CVV further, to the maximum extent possible, while balancing other nutrient and food group priorities and maintaining cost neutrality. Additionally, changes were made that consider participants' personal preferences and cultural needs and/or to incorporate container sizes that are more commonly available (see Table 9-9).

CRITERION 7

Criterion 7 states: "The foods in the packages do not create an undue burden on state agencies or vendors."

For each proposed change to the food packages, the committee considered the effects on program administration across state and local WIC agencies and vendors. These considerations were informed by public comments from stakeholder groups and the committee members' observations during their WIC shopping experiences. Table 9-10 summarizes the major issues that were considered and how the proposed changes address these concerns.

SUMMARY

As was done in the previous WIC report (IOM, 2006), the committee's proposed revisions to the WIC food packages are based on a set of criteria. As elaborated in this chapter, the revised food packages meet these criteria

TABLE 9-8 How the Revised Food Packages Can Be Tailored for Suitability for Individuals with Limited Resources (Criterion 5)

Suitability Requirements of Criterion 5	How the Revised Food Packages Correspond with the Suitability Requirements of Criterion 5
Food forms and amounts available are convenient to participants' transportation options	• Allow dried, powdered, or concentrated forms of a number of foods, including dried fruit, powdered milk, and concentrated juice (current policy is unchanged) • Permit 30 to 32 oz of yogurt to allow authorization of smaller (5 oz) containers • Include some small packages (e.g., 5 oz cans of fish) in the cost evaluation, which eases transportation and storage
Food forms and amounts available for different storage options	• Allow forms of foods that do not require refrigeration and that are less perishable (current policy is unchanged) • Include some small sizes (e.g. 5 oz cans of fish) in cost evaluation, allowing consumption of the full container at one time • Allow fruits, vegetables, and legumes in a form (fresh, canned, frozen, dried) suitable for various storage conditions (current policy is unchanged) • Require at least one form of canned, frozen, or dried fruit and one form of canned, frozen, or dried vegetable, which may be in nonperishable forms
Food forms and amounts available for diverse cooking facilities	• Allow for ready-to-feed infant formulas, full-strength juices, and jarred infant foods (current policy is unchanged) • Allow whole grain selections to include ready-to-eat items (e.g., bread), quick-cooking choices (e.g., parboiled brown rice), and slow-cooking grains (e.g., regular-cooking brown rice) (current policy is unchanged) • Require at least one form of canned, frozen, or dried fruit and one form of canned, frozen, or dried vegetable • Require provision of legumes in dried and canned forms

as closely as possible. However, because of specified cost constraints, meeting the criteria required making trade-offs among food groups and subgroups, as well as considering allowable substitutions within food groups. Generally, the proposed revisions improve the balance of nutrients and food groups provided with respect to the current Dietary Reference Intake and DGA, they are consistent with authoritative dietary guidance for individuals less than 2 years of age, and they increase choice by including additional substitution options and a higher CVV. In addition, women have more flexibility to breastfeed to the extent possible in the first month.

Revising the WIC food packages to satisfy alignment with the DGA may not by itself optimize nutrient adequacy; such optimization also requires that participants actually redeem and consume the foods in the packages. In addition, the likelihood of a change in intakes of nutrients or recommended

TABLE 9-9 How the Revised Food Packages Were Tailored to Be Readily Acceptable (Criterion 6)

Suitability Requirements for Criterion 6	How the Revised Food Packages Correspond with the Suitability Requirements of Criterion 6
Commonly consumed foods	• Modify foods and options based on identification of more or less preferred foods using redemption data • Allow fish as a substitution for a portion of infant food meat based on redemption and other data indicating that jarred infant food meat is not commonly redeemed or consumed
Widely available foods	• Retain current WIC foods that are widely available • Change some allowable sizes to better reflect availability in the marketplace (e.g. ranges are allowed for grains [16 to 24 oz] and for yogurt [30 to 32 oz]) • Require states to offer one canned, frozen, or dried form of fruit and one canned, frozen, or dried form of vegetable which may improve the availability of a variety of vegetables and fruits across seasons • Set limit on total sugars in yogurt and soy beverages and retain limit for whole grain cereal options. Market research reviewed by the committee indicate that yogurts containing 30 g of total sugars or less and the number of whole grain cereals are likely to be widely available to meet participant preferences
Culturally suitable foods and foods and preferred foods	• Include additional options for grains to align with cultural eating patterns • Increase CVV and option to substitute a CVV for fruit juice and/or jarred infant food vegetables and fruits provides participants with increased flexibility • Retain yogurt, tofu, and soy beverage as culturally suitable options (current policy is unchanged) • Add a yogurt substitution option to suit individuals who prefer this product over fluid milk • Add soy-based cheese and soy-based yogurt substitute options • Allow participants following a vegan diet to select legumes in place of eggs
Foods that provide incentive for participation in the WIC program	• Enhance the food packages for fully and partially breastfeeding women • Increase the value of the CVV in all food packages; mandate for canned, frozen, or dried options may increase the purchasing power of the CVV; additional options to substitute a CVV for juice and jarred infant food vegetables and fruits provide additional flexibility • Add canned fish to nearly all food packages

NOTES: CVV = cash value voucher.

TABLE 9-10 How the Revised Food Packages Address Selected Concerns for Impact on WIC Agencies and Vendors (Criterion 7)

Concerns About Potential Administrative Burden for WIC Staff and Retail Vendors	How the Revised Food Packages Address the Concern
WIC state agencies	
The restriction to one can of infant formula in the first month does not allow the CPA/lactation trained staff to assign a food package based on the nutritional needs of the infant.	• Allow an amount of infant formula up to that suitable for a partially breastfed infant in the first month
Allowing only fresh vegetables and fruits to be purchased with the infant CVV is not compatible with some state EBT systems.	• Allow the purchase of frozen or canned vegetables and fruits with any CVV
WIC local agencies	
With nutrition education that follows the DGA, staff instruct participants to limit intake of juice in favor of whole fruit; this is in conflict with the provision of juice in the food packages.	• Reduce amounts of juice; offer participant option to substitute a CVV for juice
The FNS Infant Nutrition and Feeding Guide indicates that around 9 months of age most infants are developmentally ready to consume foods of increased texture and consistency.	• Allow a CVV in place of jarred infant food vegetables and fruits
Additional culturally-suitable options are needed.	• See "culturally suitable foods" in Table 9-7
Vendors[a]	
Concern that 16 oz size of bread and 16 oz whole wheat pasta are difficult to obtain.	• Expand the range of grains to 16 to 24 oz to accommodate more commonly available bread and grain sizes
Vegetable juices are not available in 48 oz sizes.	• Provide 64 oz of juice in all packages
Substitution options result in the issuance of less available sizes (e.g. the "dangling quart"[b] of milk).	• Substitution options for milk that no longer result in a "dangling quart"

NOTES: CPA = competent professional authority; CVV = cash value voucher; DGA = *Dietary Guidelines for Americans*; EBT = electronic benefit transfer; FNS = USDA's Food and Nutrition Service.

[a] The committee did not receive many comments from vendors; however, several comments submitted by other stakeholders relate to vendor administrative burden.

[b] In the current food packages, when participants choose a particular set of milk substitutions, a quart of milk may remain. This quart size is generally less available and may also be more expensive.

food groups based on the revised compared to the current food packages depends on both the nutrient or food group (or food subgroup) and also the food package being considered. In some cases, the expected change may be large relative to current consumption (when current consumption is especially low) and, in other cases, it may be modest at best. Overall, the revised packages are not different enough from the current packages to change the likely effect of the food packages on participants' health. It is noteworthy that if participants were to use the CVV to consume a higher proportion of vegetables (relative to fruits) than anticipated in the committee's modeling, this could create a substantial increase in both their fiber intake and their intake of several food groups and subgroups (see Appendix T, Tables T-11 and T-12).

Expanding the container size ranges for some foods relieves the vendor burden to stock uncommon sizes and increases the likelihood of increasing the availability of these foods to participants. Inasmuch as these changes build on the food package changes implemented in 2009, the committee anticipates that administration of these revisions will be less burdensome than those recommended in 2006.

REFERENCES

AAP (American Academy of Pediatrics). 2014. *Pediatric nutrition*. 7th ed. Edited by R. E. Kleinman and F. R. Greer. Elk Grove Village, IL: American Academy of Pediatrics.

Fewtrell, M. S., J. B. Morgan, C. Duggan, G. Gunnlaugsson, P. L. Hibberd, A. Lucas, and R. E. Kleinman. 2007. Optimal duration of exclusive breastfeeding: What is the evidence to support current recommendations? *American Journal of Clinical Nutrition* 85(2):635S–638S.

IOM (Institute of Medicine). 2006. *WIC food packages: Time for a change*. Washington, DC: The National Academies Press.

Sucher, K., P. G. Kittler, and M. Nelms. 2017. *Food and culture*. 7th ed. Boston, MA: Cengage Learning.

USDA/ARS (U.S. Department of Agriculture/Agricultural Research Service). 2005–2012. *What we eat in America, NHANES 2005–2012*. http://www.cdc.gov/nchs/nhanes/wweia.htm (accessed December 15, 2016).

USDA/ARS. 2016. *USDA National Nutrient Database for Standard Reference, release 28*. http://www.ars.usda.gov/ba/bhnrc/ndl (accessed September 14, 2016).

USDA/HHS (U.S. Department of Agriculture/U.S. Department of Health and Human Services). 2016. 2015–2020 *Dietary Guidelines for Americans*. https://health.gov/dietaryguidelines/2015 (accessed August 29, 2016).

10

The Regulatory Impact Analysis (Abridged)

This chapter presents an abridged regulatory impact analysis (RIA) for the proposed revisions to the Special Supplemental Nutrition Program for Women, Infants, and Children (WIC) food packages. The preceding chapters have explained the nature and need for the food package changes, have provided background on the WIC program, and have described the food package changes proposed and the rationale for each. For brevity, such discussions have been omitted from this chapter and the cost-estimate methodology provided herein is a broad overview. Expanded versions of these sections are provided in the complete RIA (see Appendix U).

An overview of the types of estimates in this RIA is presented in Box 10-1. Throughout this chapter, the committee compares the projected costs of the revised set of food packages (assuming all recommendations are fully implemented) to the projected costs of the status quo, namely the current set of food packages. Estimated costs are based on forecasted program participation levels, estimated redemption of each food package item, and inflated prices of each food package item. Unless otherwise noted, cost differences describe how much more the revised food packages would save or cost across the program, compared to the current food packages.

KEY CONSIDERATIONS

Assumptions underlie this analysis. Some—such as how program participation and prices are projected to change through fiscal year (FY) 2022—pertain to one specific component of the analysis and are described in detail in Appendix U. Other assumptions affect the interpretation of the estimated

BOX 10-1

Overview of the Types of Estimates Presented in This Regulatory Impact Analysis

Current Food Costs
- Costs to the WIC program if the current food package regulations are left intact.

Revised Food Costs
- Costs to the WIC program if all proposed revisions are fully implemented.

Total Food Costs
- The sum of food costs from fiscal year (FY) 2018 through FY2022.

Cost Differences
- Current food costs subtracted from the revised food costs
  - Negative values (–) indicate that the revised food packages costs less than the current food packages.
  - Positive values (+) indicate that the revised food packages costs more than the current food packages.

Total Cost Differences (Total Cost Savings, Total Cost Increases)
- The sum of the cost differences.
- Describe how much more the revised food packages will cost or save compared to the current food packages or another food package scenario.

Unadjusted
- Assumes all state agencies fully implement the revisions as of April 1, 2018.

Phased-In
- Assumes one-third of participants will be served by an agency that implements the revised food packages on April 1, 2018. The remaining state agencies are assumed to implement the food package revisions on October 1, 2019.

costs and cost differences. Three such broad considerations are the representativeness of the available data, timing of implementation, and food package nomenclature.

Representativeness of the Available Data

A number of factors affect the total food costs to the WIC program, including interstate variation in food prices, caseload composition, and cost-containment practices (USDA/ERS, 2005). Accurate estimates of total food costs, therefore, should be based on data that capture this variability. To project the cost effects associated with specific changes to the food packages, data should provide insight into how each individual food item within each specific food package contributes to the total food costs. At the present, this level of granularity does not exist in data sources representative of the entire WIC program.

The committee estimated total food costs and cost differences by integrating the various sources of WIC-specific data.[1] Despite the fact that several of the data sources came from a limited number of state agencies, this analysis necessarily assumes that the data are representative of the WIC-participating population at large because no other data were available to the committee. The committee recognizes, however, that its cost estimates are not identical to costs derived from the U.S. Department of Agriculture's Food and Nutrition Service (USDA-FNS) administrative data. For FY2015, the committee estimated the per-participant food cost to be $37.09[2] per month, based on assumptions about prices per unit, substitutions of allowable options, and redemption of each food package item. USDA-FNS, however, reported the FY2015 per-participant food costs to be $43.37 per month. The committee was unable to discern what component(s) of its analysis led to this difference, because some of the data available to the committee were de-identified and the majority of the data represented only a small portion of states and territories. The estimates presented in this RIA should be interpreted in context of these limitations.

Timing of Implementation

The magnitude of the cost effects and stability of the projections in this analysis are largely defined by the time frame evaluated. The committee assumes that the earliest implementation of the revised food packages could occur would be April 1, 2018, approximately 15 months after the release of this consensus report. Food-cost estimates for both the current and revised food packages are projected through FY2022. This RIA, therefore, encompasses a 54-month period.[3]

---

[1] WIC data sources used in this analysis include the participation data from the *WIC Participant and Program Characteristics 2014: Food Package Report* (USDA/FNS, 2016a), national participation levels presented on the USDA-FNS website (USDA/FNS, 2016b), redemption data from six de-identified state agencies provided to the committee by USDA-FNS (see Appendix U for additional details), redemption data provided to the committee from six individual state agencies, and a 2014 report detailing redemption in three states as they transitioned to electronic benefit transfer (EBT) food benefit issuance method (USDA/ERS, 2014).

[2] A per-participant cost of $37.27 per month was presented previously in this report. This higher estimate reflects the $1 increase in women's cash value voucher, which was implemented in FY2016 (from $10 to $11). The committee used this monthly per participant cost to assess the cost neutrality of the revised food packages, because it reflects current regulations. The $37.09 estimate, in contrast, reflects the regulations that existed in FY2015.

[3] The fiscal year starts October 1. April 1, 2018, is halfway through FY2018.

The committee assumes that, within each state agency, all proposed food package changes will be fully implemented at one time but that, across the WIC program, state agencies may begin offering the revised food packages at different times. As such, two sets of cost projections were generated: unadjusted and phased in. Unadjusted estimates assume that all agencies fully implement the revised food packages on April 1, 2018. Phased-in estimates, in contrast, account for states implementing the revised food packages at different times. The phased-in scenario assumes that states with electronic benefit transfer (EBT) systems operational as of the August 2016 EBT Detail Status Report (USDA/FNS, 2016c) would be early implementers of the proposed food package changes (i.e., those implementing the changes on April 1, 2018).[4] The remaining state agencies would have up to 18 additional months to implement the proposed food package changes (i.e., implemented by October 1, 2019). As evidenced by the final implementation dates from the previous food package revision (USDA/FNS, 2012), most state agencies instituted changes on the regulatory deadline, rather than before or after. This analysis assumes the same will occur for these proposed revisions. Accordingly, the phased-in cost differences between the current food packages and proposed revised food packages are 33.3 percent of the unadjusted cost differences for FY2018 (6 months) and FY2019 (12 months), and 100 percent of the unadjusted differences thereafter. The dates and rates of implementation used in this RIA are not intended to be prescriptive or to be the committee's recommended timeline for implementation, but rather they are the committee's informed assumptions necessary for this analysis.

Food Package Nomenclature

The WIC food packages are specific to the age, life stage, physiological state, and, if applicable, breastfeeding status of the participant. Several of the broad food package categories (both current and revised) are actually composed of two or more specific food package types. Both the quantity of foods and the food items prescribed in each specific food package can differ within a broad food package category, and therefore have cost implications.

As Table 10-1 highlights, the proposed revisions largely leave the

[4] This estimate was calculated by identifying agencies that have implemented EBT statewide as of August 2016 (USDA/FNS, 2016c) and determining what proportion of participants are served by those agencies from total participation administrative data (USDA/FNS, 2016b). For FY2015, EBT states serve 34.3 percent of WIC participants. Given this, the assumption for the phased-in estimate is that one-third of participants would be served by an "early implementer" state agency. This assumption only affects the phased-in estimates, not the unadjusted estimates.

current structure of the food packages unchanged. There are, however, three important considerations:

1. Food package V is currently a single food package prescribed to both pregnant women and partially (mostly) breastfeeding women, up to 1 year postpartum. Under the proposed revisions, it would be split into two distinct food packages, V-A for pregnant women and V-B for partially (mostly) breastfeeding women.
2. Revised food package I-BF/FF-A (partially [mostly] breastfed infant, age 0 to less than 1 month) is retained as its own food package in this analysis, as the committee expects that recipients of this food package would continue to be prescribed only small quantities of infant formula. Upon implementation of the proposed revisions, however, it may be decided to consolidate this food package with food package I-BF/FF-B (partially [mostly] breastfed infant, age 1 to less than 4 months), because both would have the same maximum prescription ("up to") amount for infant formula.
3. Food package "N/A" is listed as a food package because it is included in an assumption about how participation is expected to change with the revised food packages. Women who are minimally breastfeeding and with infants more than 6 months of age that receive more formula than is allowed for a partially breastfeeding infant do not receive a food benefit (referred to herein as "food package N/A"), but are still eligible to continue to receive breastfeeding support, nutrition education, health and social services referrals, and other program benefits (USDA/FNS, 2013). These program participants do not contribute to the total food costs of the program.

SUMMARY OF PROPOSED CHANGES

The food package revisions recommended in this report reflect the consensus of an expert committee and account for the nutritional intake, health status, and cultural needs of the program participant population, while simultaneously considering the efficiency and efficacy of program operations and administration. The proposed changes to the food packages affect a broad range of individuals and entities associated with the WIC program, including, but not limited to, USDA-FNS; the 90 agencies that administer WIC and their associated staff; authorized vendors; food producers, manufacturers, and distributors; and program participants. As summarized in Table 10-2, the committee considered the effect of each key food package revision on these stakeholder groups.

TABLE 10-1 Current and Revised Food Packages and Corresponding Participant Categories

Food Package	Abbreviation of Specific Food Package	Applicable Version of the Food Packages	Participant Category
I	I-BF-A	Current, revised	Fully breastfed infants, ages 0 to less than 4 months
	I-BF-B	Current, revised	Fully breastfed infants, ages 4 to less than 6 months
	I-BF/FF-A	Current, revised[a]	Partially (mostly) breastfed infants,[b] ages 0 to less than 1 month
	I-BF/FF-B	Current, revised	Partially (mostly) breastfed infants,[b] ages 1 to less than 4 months
	I-BF/FF-C	Current, revised	Partially (mostly) breastfed infants,[b] ages 4 to less than 6 months
	I-FF-A	Current, revised	Fully formula-fed infants, ages 0 to less than 4 months
	I-FF-B	Current, revised	Fully formula-fed infants, ages 4 to less than 6 months
II	II-BF	Current, revised	Fully breastfed infants, ages 6 to less than 12 months
	II-BF/FF	Current, revised	Partially breastfed infants, ages 6 to less than 12 months
	II-FF	Current, revised	Fully formula-fed infants, ages 6 to less than 12 months
III	III[c]	Current, revised	Infants, children, and women with a qualifying condition[d]
IV	IV-A	Current, revised	Children, ages 1 to less than 2 years
	IV-B	Current, revised	Children, ages 2 to less than 5 years
V	V	Current	Pregnant women Partially (mostly) breastfeeding women,[b] up to 1 year postpartum
V-A	V-A	Revised	Pregnant women

V-B	V-B	Revised	Partially (mostly) breastfeeding women,[b] up to 1 year postpartum
VI	VI	Current, revised	Nonbreastfeeding postpartum women, up to 6 months postpartum Partially (minimally) breastfeeding women,[e] up to 6 months postpartum
VII	VII	Current, revised	Fully breastfeeding women, up to 1 year postpartum
N/A	N/A	Current, revised	Partially (minimally) breastfeeding women, more than 6 months postpartum[e]

[a] Despite revised food packages I-BF/FF-A and I-BF/FF-B having the same maximum ("up to") amount for infant formula, the two food packages remain separate in this analysis. The committee supports issuance of infant formula to food package I-FF/BF-A recipients only on a case-by-case basis after a breastfeeding assessment. Accordingly, the committee assumes the average quantity of infant formula prescribed in food package I-BF/FF-A to be less than the average amount prescribed to I-BF/FF-B recipients. Food package I-BF/FF-A may not ultimately be operationalized as separate from food package I-BF/FF-B for partially (mostly) breastfed infants, ages 1 month to less than 4 months.

[b] The parenthetical "mostly" is determined by the amount of formula provided to the infant through the WIC program. Women and their infants are classified as partially (mostly) breastfeeding if the infant's formula prescription does not exceed the monthly maximum allowance for the age-specific BF/FF food packages.

[c] Food package III recipients are prescribed food packages appropriate to their age and physiological state. There are specific food packages for women, infants, and children within food package III that correspond to specific food packages I, II, IV, V, VI, and VII.

[d] Participants prescribed food package III have one or more medically documented qualifying conditions. Recipients are eligible to receive WIC formula (i.e., infant formula, exempt infant formula, and WIC-eligible nutritionals) and supplementary foods.

[e] The parenthetical "minimally" is determined by the amount of formula provided to the infant through the WIC program. Women and infants are classified as partially (minimally) breastfeeding if the infant's formula prescription exceeds the monthly maximum allowance for the age-specific BF/FF food packages but does not exceed the full amount allowed in the age-specific fully formula-fed food packages. Women who are minimally breastfeeding less than 6 months postpartum receive food package VI, along with breastfeeding support. Women who are minimally breastfeeding and with infants more than 6 months of age that receive more formula than is allowed for a partially breastfeeding infant do not receive a food benefit. These women, however, are eligible to continue to receive other benefits through WIC, such as breastfeeding support, nutrition education, and health and social services referrals (USDA/FNS, 2013). This group of participants is included in one of the committee's assumption regarding the revised food package cost estimates, and is therefore included in the above table.

TABLE 10-2 Summary of Key WIC Food Package Revisions

Current Rules, Proposed Revisions, and Projected Net Cost Differences[a]	Effect of the Proposed Revision			
	USDA/Federal Government	State/Local Agencies	Vendors/Industry	WIC Participants
Current rule: State agencies have the option to prescribe breastfed infants up to 104 fl oz of infant formula (not more than one can of powdered infant formula) during the first 30 days of life, on a case-by-case basis. *Proposed revision:* Breastfed infants can be prescribed up to 364 fl oz of infant formula during the first 30 days of life, on a case-by-case basis after a breastfeeding assessment by a competent professional authority, and remain categorically classified as a partially breastfed infant. (*Net cost effect: savings*)	The cost of food package I-BF/FF-A itself may slightly increase, depending on how frequently competent professional authorities identify need for issuance of formula beyond 104 fl oz. The anticipated shift in fully formula fed dyads toward the partial (mostly) breastfeeding food packages is expected to largely offset additional costs of the infant formula.	At the staff and clinic level, the proposed revision is expected to provide greater flexibility in tailoring the partially (mostly) breastfed infant's food package and create opportunities to support partial breastfeeding in dyads who would otherwise be considered fully formula-fed. Management Information Systems will need to be updated. State and local agencies will encounter a short-term burden of retraining staff.	The effect on vendors or industry is anticipated to be minimal. The anticipated shift in fully formula-fed dyads to the partial (mostly) breastfeeding food packages may slightly reduce the amount of infant formula purchased by WIC participants with their food benefit.	The revision is intended to prevent women and infants from being categorized as postpartum (nonbreastfeeding or minimally breastfeeding) and fully formula fed, respectively, in the first month or soon thereafter. The proposed revision is intended to provide security for women who may try to breastfeed in the immediate postpartum period but are not yet certain they can succeed.
Current rule: The maximum monthly allowance of formula	The cost effect of the proposed revision will depend on the extent to	At the staff and clinic level, the proposed revision is expected to	The effect on the vendors will depend on the amount of infant formula	Participants would still have access to the quantities of infant

should not be used as the standard for issuance unless the mother is not breastfeeding the infant at all. *Proposed revision:* The quantity of infant formula prescribed to infants should be tailored based on needs. All maximum monthly allowances for infant formula should be considered "up to" amounts. (*Net cost effect: minimal*)	which infant formula tailoring occurs. If minimal tailoring occurs, the cost effects would be minimal. If it is fully executed, the proposed revision would result in a cost savings.	provide greater flexibility in tailoring the amount of formula provided to infants. Management Information Systems will need to be updated. State and local agencies will encounter a short-term burden of retraining staff.	tailoring that occurs. If minimal tailoring occurs, the effect on infant formula sales would be minimal. Full execution is likely to result in a decrease of infant formula sales to WIC participants using their food benefit.	formula currently being offered by WIC. The proposed revision, however, would help participants receive the amount of infant formula needed to meet their infants' needs.
Current rule: All food package II recipients are prescribed 24 oz of infant cereal per month *Proposed revision:* Food package II-BF recipients are prescribed 16 oz of infant cereal per month; II-FF and II-BF/FF recipients are prescribed 8 oz per month (*Net cost effect: savings*)	The proposed revision would reduce the cost of food package II. This reduction helps offset costs elsewhere in the food packages.	Administrative burden is expected to be minimal. State agencies currently authorize 8 oz infant cereal containers; some state agencies also authorize 16 oz containers. Management Information Systems will need to be updated. State and local agencies will encounter a short-term burden of retraining staff and communicating the change to participants when the revisions are initially implemented.	The proposed revision may result in reduced infant cereal sales to WIC participants. It is not anticipated to affect stocking requirements.	Although infants will receive less infant cereal under the revised food package, the amount provided is more consistent with current complementary feeding recommendations.

continued

TABLE 10-2 Continued

Current Rules, Proposed Revisions, and Projected Net Cost Differences[a]	Effect of the Proposed Revision			
	USDA/Federal Government	State/Local Agencies	Vendors/Industry	WIC Participants
Current rule: Food package II-BF recipients are prescribed 256 oz of jarred infant food vegetables and fruits per month. All other food package II recipients receive 128 oz of jarred infant food vegetables and fruits. Up to 16 oz of jarred infant food fruits can be substituted with fresh bananas, 1 banana per 4 oz jar. *Proposed revision:* All infants receiving food package II are prescribed 128 oz of jarred infant food vegetables and fruits. A CVV can be prescribed for partial substitution ($10 for 64 oz jarred infant food vegetables and fruits) or complete substitution ($20 for the 128 oz). The CVV can be used to purchased	Despite the decrease in jarred infant vegetable and fruit issuance to fully breastfed infants, the option for CVV substitution are expected to lead to an increase in redemption, thereby increasing costs to the program.	Administrative burden is expected to be minimal. Management Information Systems will need to be updated, but overall it will improve Management Information Systems efficiency by authorizing the same vegetable and fruit varieties for all CVVs. State and local agencies will encounter a short-term burden of retraining staff and communicating the change to participants when the revisions are initially implemented. State and local agencies will also face an administrative burden developing educational messages and materials related to selecting and preparing vegetables and fruits appropriate for complementary feeding.	The proposed revision may result in slight reductions in jarred infant food vegetable and fruit sales to WIC participants, but it may increase fresh, frozen, and/or canned vegetables and fruits via the CVV. This is not anticipated to affect stocking requirements.	The proposed revision is intended to provide fully breastfed infants with a supplemental quantity of infant food vegetables and fruits, in the absence of definitive guidance on recommended intake. The CVV substitution option provides participants the opportunity to prepare their own infant food vegetables and fruits, which can be used to better meet diverse cultural needs, personal preferences, and the infant's developmental stage. Participants may be able to buy more servings of vegetables or fruit using the CVV compared to the jarred varieties.

vegetables and fruits in all forms authorized by the state agency (i.e., fresh, frozen, canned) except dried. (*Net cost effect: increase*)				
Current rule: Food package II-BF recipients are prescribed 77.5 oz of infant food meat per month. *Proposed revision*: Food package II-BF recipients are prescribed 40 oz of infant food meat per month. Ten oz of canned fish can be substituted for 4 jars (10 oz) of infant food meat per month. (*Net cost effect: savings*)	Because redemption of infant food meat is low, reducing the amount prescribed is expected to result in slight cost savings. The option for substitution of canned fish may slightly increase redemption in this category. Given that canned fish is currently less expensive per oz than jarred infant food meat, increase in redemption may be offset by the slightly lower price.	Implementation of the proposed revision will require training WIC staff and participants of the change and new substitution option. Management Information Systems will need to be updated.	The revision may reduce the amount of infant food meat purchased by WIC participants. The substitution option may slightly increase the amount of canned fish purchased by WIC participants.	The proposed revision addresses participants' feedback about the quantity and preference in the infant food meat category, while still providing key nutrients to fully breastfed infants. The substitution option provides participants with greater flexibility in this food category.
Current rule: Food package III is reserved for participants who have one or more qualifying conditions that	Clarifies that WIC formula is not an absolute requirement of food package III. The cost effects of the proposed	Administrative burden increases in the short term. Management Information Systems will need to be updated.	No impact.	Some participants receiving food package III may be prescribed a package that is more appropriate for their needs.

continued

TABLE 10-2 Continued

Current Rules, Proposed Revisions, and Projected Net Cost Differences[a]	Effect of the Proposed Revision			
	USDA/Federal Government	State/Local Agencies	Vendors/Industry	WIC Participants
require an exempt infant formula or WIC-eligible nutritional (formerly WIC-eligible medical food) to supplement their nutrition needs, as determined by the participant's health care professional. *Proposed revision:* Participants with a qualifying condition in which a WIC formula is not medically necessary are still eligible to receive appropriate supplementary foods through food package III. (*Net cost effect: minimal*)	revision will be minimal, as the number of applicable participants is expected to be extremely small.			
Current rule: Children are prescribed 128 fl oz of juice per month; pregnant, partially (mostly) breastfeeding, and fully breastfeeding	The reduction in juice prescribed would reduce the costs of the food packages. This reduction helps offset costs elsewhere in the food packages.	Implementation of the proposed revision will require training WIC staff and participants of the change and new substitution option.	Less juice would be purchased with the WIC food benefits. The minimum stocking requirements for juice would be simplified, as	The proposed revision provides a supplemental amount of juice, which can help participants meet their daily fruit intake goals. The CVV

women are prescribed 144 fl oz of juice per month; postpartum and partially (minimally) breastfeeding women are prescribed 96 fl oz of juice per month. *Proposed revision:* Children, pregnant women, partially (mostly) breastfeeding women, and fully breastfeeding women are prescribed 64 fl oz of juice per month. Recipients may opt to substitute a $3 CVV for the 64 fl oz of juice. Postpartum and partially (minimally) breastfeeding women no longer receive juice. (*Net cost effect: savings*)		Management Information Systems will need to be updated.	all participants prescribed juice would receive 64 fl oz (or frozen equivalent).	substitution option allows participants greater flexibility to tailor their food package for personal preferences. The reduction and eliminations (food package VI) of juice from the food packages also allowed for larger CVVs across all food packages provided to children and women.
Current rule: Food package IV and VI recipients are prescribed 16 qt of milk per month. Food package V recipients are prescribed 22 qt of milk per month. Food package VII recipients are	The proposed revisions would reduce the costs of the food packages. This reduction helps offset costs elsewhere in the food packages.	The administrative burden is expected to be short term, as the revision changes quantities, rather than adding new items. It will require training WIC staff and participants of the changes and revised	The total amount of milk purchased by WIC participants with their food benefit is expected to decrease. The revised quantities and substitution options eliminate participants' need for	The proposed revisions provide supplemental quantities of milk across the food packages. The substitution structure eliminates the possibility of a dangling quart and may be more compatible

continued

TABLE 10-2 Continued

Current Rules, Proposed Revisions, and Projected Net Cost Differences[a]	Effect of the Proposed Revision			
	USDA/Federal Government	State/Local Agencies	Vendors/Industry	WIC Participants
prescribed 24 qt of milk per month. Three qt of milk can be substituted for 1 lb of cheese, with the maximum amount of cheese being 1 lb for food packages IV, V, and VI and 2 lb for food package VII. Food package VII recipients are also prescribed 1 lb of cheese as a separate food package category. At state agency option, 1 qt of yogurt may be substituted for 1 qt of milk for women and children in food packages III–VII. No more than 1 qt of yogurt is authorized per participant. No more than a total of 4 qt of milk may be substituted for a combination of cheese, yogurt or tofu for children and women in food packages IV–VI. No		substitution options. Management Information Systems will need to be updated.	milk in a quart-sized container. More yogurt may be purchased by WIC participants under the revised substitution options, as 1 and 2 qt substitution options are allowed. The state agency option of a range of yogurt container sizes (30 to 32 oz) may also lead to increased redemption. Stocking requirements are not expected to substantially expand or change.	with cultural needs or preferences.

more than a total of 6 qt of milk may be substituted for a combination of cheese, yogurt or tofu for women in food package VII.

Proposed revision:
Food package IV-A recipients are prescribed 12 qt of milk per month. Food package IV-B recipients are prescribed 14 qt of milk per month. All women are prescribed 16 qt of milk per month. Cheese is no longer offered as a separate food package item. Children and women can substitute up to 4 qt of milk per month, choosing either to substitute 2 qt of yogurt for 2 qt for milk or to substitute 1 lb of cheese and 1 qt of yogurt for 4 qt of milk. Fully breastfeeding women can choose from a third substitution option of 2 lb of cheese for 6 qt of milk.

continued

TABLE 10-2 Continued

Current Rules, Proposed Revisions, and Projected Net Cost Differences[a]	Effect of the Proposed Revision			
	USDA/Federal Government	State/Local Agencies	Vendors/Industry	WIC Participants
Only one substitution option can be selected per month. At the discretion of the state agency, yogurt may be prescribed as a range of 30 to 32 oz, to accommodate different container sizes available on the market. (*Net cost effect: savings*)				
Current rule: Food packages V and VII recipients are prescribed 1 lb of whole wheat bread or other authorized options. Food package IV recipients are prescribed 2 lb of whole wheat bread or other authorized options. Authorized whole grain options include brown rice, bulgur, oats, whole grain barley, tortillas, and macaroni (pasta).	The proposed revisions are expected to decrease food package costs. The expanded list of whole grain options is available at the discretion of state agencies, within cost-containment parameters.	The expanded list of whole grain options that states can authorize is intended to better meet the cultural and personal preferences of the participants they serve, within cost containment parameters. The expansion of whole grain sizes will require the Management Information Systems to be updated. WIC staff, vendors, and	The range of whole wheat bread sizes may lead to the elimination of the 16 oz bread size in the market, which was principally created for the WIC population. The proposed revision is likely to lead to stocking requirements that better reflect widely available sizes. Vendors will need to train personnel to identify WIC-eligible breads and grains.	WIC participants will benefit by allowing whole wheat breads that are readily available in the market. The expanded state options for substitutions may allow options that better meet diverse cultural needs and personal preferences.

Proposed revision: Food packages IV, V, and VII recipients are prescribed one 16 to 24 oz 100% whole wheat bread or other authorized whole grain option. Allowable whole grain options include brown rice, bulgur, oats, whole grain barley, tortillas, macaroni (pasta), corn masa flour (non-whole grain), cornmeal, teff, and buckwheat. (*Net cost effect: savings*)		participants will need to be trained on new sizes and options.		
Current rule: Food package VII recipients are prescribed 30 oz of canned fish per month. May be packed in water or oil. Pack may include bones or skin. May be regular or lower in sodium content. At the state agency's option, added sauces and flavorings are allowable.	Addition of fish across the food packages will increase food packages costs. The additional costs are offset by other changes across food packages.	Implementing the proposed change will increase the short-term administrative burden. Management Information Systems will need to be revised. WIC staff, vendors, and participants will need to be trained on new quantities and rotation pattern for food packages IV, V-A, and VI.	The proposed revision is expected to increase the amount of water-packed canned fish purchased by WIC participants with their food benefit. The revision may increase minimum stocking requirements for small vendors. Vendors will need to train personnel to identify authorized canned fish products.	Provision of water-packed canned fish provides a high nutrient-density source of nonperishable seafood, and better aligns the food packages with DGA recommendations.

continued

TABLE 10-2 Continued

Current Rules, Proposed Revisions, and Projected Net Cost Differences[a]	Effect of the Proposed Revision			
	USDA/Federal Government	State/Local Agencies	Vendors/Industry	WIC Participants
Proposed revision: Food packages IV, V-A, and VI recipients are prescribed 10 oz of fish once every 3 months. Food package V-B recipients are prescribed 10 oz of fish every month and food package VII recipients are prescribed 20 oz per month. May be packed in water, but may not be packed in oil. All other specifications remain the same. (*Net cost effect: increase*)		The burden is expected to be relatively minor, as all food packages would be authorized the same canned fish.		
Current rule: Food packages IV and VI recipients have the option of being prescribed 1 lb dried legumes (or 64 oz of canned legumes) or 16 to 18 oz of peanut butter per month. Food	Reduction of the amount of legumes and peanut butter prescribed in food packages IV through VII will result in a cost savings.	States and local agencies will need to educate participants about the legume and peanut butter rotation patterns for children and women. States that do not currently authorize	Sales of legumes and peanut butter to WIC participants using their food instrument will decrease. Market effect is expected to be minimal.	This change brings children's and women's food packages in better alignment with the concept of supplemental and the recommendations of the DGA. Cost savings help offset costs of

packages V and VII are prescribed 1 lb legumes (or 64 oz of canned legumes) and 16 to 18 oz of peanut butter per month. *Proposed revision:* Food package IV recipients receive peanut butter, legumes, and canned fish in rotation over 3 months. All women receive legumes and peanut butter once each in a quarter. Both canned and dried legumes must be allowed by all state agencies. (*Net cost effect: savings*)		canned legumes will incur a short-term administrative burden of expanding to include the canned option. Management Information Systems will need to be revised.		revisions throughout the food packages.
Current rule: Children are prescribed an $8 CVV per month. Women are prescribed an $11 CVV per month. *Proposed revision:* The monthly CVVs for food packages IV, V-A, V-B, VI, and VII are $12,	Increasing the CVV across the food packages will increase food package costs. The additional costs are offset by other changes across food packages.	The infrastructure already exists to provide the CVV through the program, which greatly reduces the administrative burden associated with the proposed changes. Management Information Systems will need to be	Sales of vegetables and fruits will increase through WIC participants using their food benefit. Minimum stocking requirements will slightly increase for vendors that meet the current federal minimum stocking	Increasing the CVV expands the amount of vegetables and fruits participants are able to buy with their food instrument. Provision of a dollar amount, allows participants flexibility and choice to meet cultural

continued

TABLE 10-2 Continued

Current Rules, Proposed Revisions, and Projected Net Cost Differences[a]	Effect of the Proposed Revision			
	USDA/Federal Government	State/Local Agencies	Vendors/Industry	WIC Participants
$15, $25, $15, and $35, respectively. (*Net cost effect: increase*)		updated. States and local agencies will need to develop ways to communicate the change in the short term, and encourage use of the CVV for vegetables, to align use with the DGA.	requirement vegetables. Vendors in states that currently only allow fresh fruits may experience additional stocking requirements, as frozen, canned, and/or dried options are authorized.	needs and personal preferences. Larger CVV values in food packages V-B and VII are intended as incentives to partial (mostly) and full breastfeeding.

NOTES: BF = breastfeeding; CVV = cash value voucher; DGA = *Dietary Guidelines for Americans*; fl oz = fluid ounce(s); lb = pound(s); oz = ounce(s).

[a] The projected net cost differences described in this table are contingent on the committee's assumptions, which are detailed in the "Cost" section of this chapter and in Appendix U. The magnitude and even the direction of some of the cost differences can change with different assumptions that would still be considered reasonable. The cost effects of various different assumptions are evaluated in the "Uncertainties" section of this chapter and in Appendix U.

COST

Proposed Revisions to the Benefit

Unadjusted Estimates of Food Costs and Total Cost Differences

Table 10-3 presents unadjusted food cost estimates for the current and revised food packages. The total unadjusted food costs from FY2018 through FY2022 are estimated to be $17.7 billion (averaging $3.93 billion per year) for the current food packages and $17.4 billion (averaging $3.87 billion per year) for the revised food packages. Over the course of FY2018 through FY2022, the proposed revisions are projected to lead to a total unadjusted cost savings of $263 million, compared to the current food packages.

Phased-in Cost Differences

Table 10-4 presents the phased-in cost differences between the current and revised food packages, from FY2018 through FY2022. Assuming phased-in implementation across the WIC program inherently decreases the projected total cost savings because, overall, the revised food packages result in a long-term cost savings. The total phased-in cost savings for FY2018 through FY2022 are approximately $42 million less than the total unadjusted cost savings ($220.4 million versus $262.8 million). The estimated cost differences not only reflect changes to the type and quantity of items in the specific food packages, but also the proportion of participants who are prescribed each food package. The cost savings in food package I in FY2021 and FY2022, for example, is driven by the anticipated 5 percent shift of mother–infant dyads from fully formula-fed to the partially (mostly) breastfeeding categories, as a result of the incentives included in the revised food packages (see the "Participation" subsection in the section titled "Cost Estimate Methodology" for additional details about this assumption).

Sources of Cost Differences

Cost Difference of Each Food Package Item

To determine the source(s) of the projected cost savings of the revised food package, the committee evaluated the total costs of each food package item category within the current and revised food packages. The total costs of each of the food items presented in Table 10-5 include assumptions about substitutions and allowable options within each category and assumptions about changes in redemption rates (see "Cost Estimate Methodology" for

TABLE 10-3 Estimated Unadjusted Food Costs of the Current and Proposed Food Packages, FY2018 Through FY2022

Food Package Version	Food Package	Unadjusted Food Costs ($, millions)					
		FY2018[a]	FY2019	FY2020	FY2021[b]	FY2022	Total, FY2018 Through FY2022
Current	I	213.5	441.3	451.0	461.8	472.9	2,040.6
	II	300.3	620.5	634.2	649.4	665.0	2,869.4
	III[c]	45.2	93.4	95.3	97.5	99.7	431.2
	IV-A	277.7	571.7	582.1	593.7	605.5	2,630.7
	IV-B	616.5	1,268.9	1,291.9	1,317.4	1,343.6	5,838.3
	V	202.4	416.3	423.5	431.6	448.1	1,922.0
	VI	128.2	263.5	267.8	272.7	284.0	1,216.3
	VII	76.9	158.3	161.2	164.5	170.2	731.1
Total food costs		1,860.7	3,833.9	3,907.1	3,988.7	4,089.2	17,679.6
Revised	I	213.5	441.3	451.0	450.7	461.5	2,018.1
	II	297.5	614.7	628.3	634.0	649.2	2,823.7
	III[c]	45.4	93.7	95.7	97.8	100.0	432.6
	IV-A	264.8	544.5	553.7	563.9	574.3	2,501.2
	IV-B	602.2	1,237.9	1,258.7	1,281.9	1,305.6	5,686.4
	V-A	166.0	340.9	346.3	352.3	358.4	1,563.9
	V-B	35.4	72.4	73.4	97.6	99.1	377.9
	VI	129.0	264.5	268.4	259.0	263.2	1,184.1
	VII	87.6	179.4	184.0	186.5	191.3	828.8
Total food costs		1,841.4	3,789.5	3,859.4	3,923.7	4,002.7	17,416.7
Total unadjusted cost differences[d]		*–19.2*	*–44.4*	*–47.7*	*–65.0*	*–86.6*	*–262.8*

NOTES: Unadjusted costs and cost differences assume full implementation of the proposed revisions in all state agencies as of April 1, 2018. Column and row totals may not be exact owing to independent rounding.

[a] This analysis assumes the earliest date of implementation of the proposed changes would be April 1, 2018. Accordingly all estimates for FY2018 only encompass a 6-month period.

[b] This analysis assumes the proposed revisions will incentivize partially (mostly) breastfeeding food packages for the dyads. The cost estimates for the revised food package anticipates a 5 percent shift of fully formula-fed dyads to the partially (mostly) breastfed participant categories in the year after full implementation of the food package revisions under the phased-in implementation assumption. Difference in food package costs in FY2021 and FY2022 are due, in part, to this anticipated shift in participants.

[c] Estimated costs for food package III only include standard issuance food package items, and does not account for exempt infant formula or WIC-eligible nutritionals.

[d] Calculated by subtracting the current food package costs from the revised food package costs. Negative values (–) indicate that the revised food packages result in cost savings compared to the current food packages. Positive values (+) indicate that the revised food packages result in cost increases compared to the current food packages.

TABLE 10-4 Estimated Phased-in Cost Differences of the Proposed Revised Food Packages Compared to the Current Food Packages, FY2018 Through FY2022

Food Package	Phased-in Cost Differences of the Revised Food Packages Compared to Current Food Packages ($, millions)[a]					
	FY2018[b,c]	FY2019[c]	FY2020	FY2021[d]	FY2022[d]	Total, FY2018 Through FY2022
I	0.0	0.0	0.0	−11.1	−11.4	−22.5
II	−0.9	−1.9	−5.9	−15.4	−15.8	−40.0
III[e]	+0.1	+0.1	+0.3	+0.3	+0.3	+1.1
IV-A	−4.3	−9.1	−28.4	−29.8	−31.2	−102.8
IV-B	−4.8	−10.3	−33.1	−35.6	−38.0	−121.8
V-A[f]	−2.1	−4.6	−14.7	−15.6	−23.5	−60.5
V-B[f]	+1.8	+3.6	+10.8	+33.9	+32.9	+83.0
VI	+0.2	+0.3	+0.5	−13.6	−20.8	−33.4
VII	+3.6	+7.0	+22.8	+22.0	+21.1	+76.5
Total phased-in cost differences	*−6.4*	*−14.8*	*−47.7*	*−65.0*	*−86.6*	*−220.4*

NOTES: Phased-in estimates assume full implementation of the proposed revisions in state agencies serving one-third of all WIC participants as of April 1, 2018. All other state agencies are assumed to implement the proposed revisions as of FY2020. FY = fiscal year.

[a] Cost differences were calculated by subtracting the estimated food costs for the current food packages from the estimated food costs for the revised food packages. Negative values (−) indicate that the revised food packages result in cost savings compared to the current food packages. Positive values (+) indicate that the revised food packages result in cost increases compared to the current food packages. Column and row totals may not be exact owing to independent rounding.

[b] This analysis assumes the earliest date of implementation of the proposed changes would be April 1, 2018. Accordingly all estimates for FY2018 only encompass 6 months.

[c] Phased-in cost differences in FY2018 and FY2019 are 33.3 percent of the unadjusted cost differences.

[d] This analysis assumes the proposed revisions will incentivize partially (mostly) breastfeeding food packages for the dyads. Accordingly, the cost estimates for the revised food package anticipates a 5 percent shift of fully formula-fed dyads to the partially (mostly) breastfed participant categories in the year after full implementation of the food package revisions. The participant shift is assumed to take place in FY2021. The shift is expected to be sustained, but to not recur in FY2022. The difference in food package costs for both FY2021 and FY2022 is due, in part, to the participant shift assumptions.

[e] Estimates for food package III only include standard issuance food package items for both the current and revised food packages. Costs and cost differences do not account for exempt infant formula or WIC-eligible nutritionals.

continued

TABLE 10-4 Continued

[f] Currently, food package V is issued to both pregnant and partially (mostly) breastfeeding women. To arrive at cost differences, the proportion of food package V recipients categorized as pregnant and partially (mostly) breastfeeding were applied to the estimated costs of food package V for the current food packages to create estimates that could be compared to revised food package V-A and V-B, respectively.

additional details). Across the food package items, the total cost savings are larger than the total added costs, which results in estimated total cost savings of the revised food packages compared to the current food packages. Two major sources of cost differences between the current and revised food packages are juice and the cash value voucher (CVV). In the current food packages, all women and children are prescribed juice. The reduction of total juice in the revised food packages results in a total phased-in cost savings of approximately $627 million over the course of FY2018 through FY2022 compared to the current food packages. In contrast, increasing the value of the CVV for all women and children in the revised food package leads to an estimated total phased-in cost increase of approximately $780 million over the course of FY2018 through FY2022.

Major Cost Differences of Food Package Items Within Each Food Package

To explore the sources of the cost differences further, the committee evaluated the total phased-in cost differences of each food package item within each food package. Table 10-6 presents each food package item revision that resulted in a total phased-in cost difference of at least $25 million in cost saving or cost increases from FY2018 through FY2022 compared to the total cost of the corresponding item in the current food packages. The major total cost differences summarized in the table not only reflect the specific revisions to the items and the quantity prescribed, but also the distribution of participants across the different food packages. Inasmuch as food package IV-B comprises the largest participant group (approximately 36 percent of food package recipients), relatively small changes lead to more substantial cost differences. For example, the CVV in the revised food package IV-B would increase by $3 per month compared to the current food package,[5] leading to an estimated $246-million increase in estimated total

[5] Participants do not receive adjustments in the CVV until the inflated value crosses a $1 increment. The CVV for food package IV is currently $8 per month. By 2018, it is expected to cross the next $1 increment and be adjusted to $9 per month. The proposed revisions would increase the CVV for children to $12 per month.

TABLE 10-5 Phased-in Total Food Cost and Cost Differences (FY2018 Through FY2022) Between the Current and Revised Food Packages by Food Package Item Category, in Descending Order of Additional Costs

Food Package Item[a]	Total Phased-in Food Costs, FY2018 Through FY2022 ($, millions)[b] Current Food Packages	Revised Food Packages	Total Phased-in Cost Difference, FY2018 Through FY2022 ($, millions)[c]
Cash value voucher	1,886.9	2,666.4	+779.5
Canned fish	51.9	165.5	+113.5
Jarred infant vegetables and fruits	578	659.4	+81.4
Eggs	513.5	513.6	+0.2[d]
Infant food meat	52.1	32.6	–19.4
Breakfast cereal	1,321.8	1,300.0	–21.7
Infant formula, postrebate	3,321.2	3,279.8	–41.5[d]
Cheese[e]	45.9	0	–45.9
Infant cereal	142.6	64.4	–78.1
Milk	3,747.7	3,662.2	–85.5
Legumes and peanut butter	410.4	286.9	–123.6
Whole wheat bread	559.5	406.9	–152.6
Juice	1,251.6	625.0	–626.6

NOTES: Phased-in estimates assume full implementation of the proposed revisions in state agencies serving one-third of all WIC participants as of April 1, 2018. All other state agencies are assumed to implement the proposed revisions as of FY2020. FY = fiscal year.

[a] Broadly describes the food package item category. Cost differences include assumptions about substitutions and selection of allowable options within each category.

[b] Calculated by summing the food cost of each specific food package item from FY2018 through FY2022. To account for the phased-in implementation, the food costs for FY2018 and FY2019 are one-third the estimated unadjusted food costs. Phased-in and unadjusted food costs are identical for FY2020 through FY2022. The estimated phased-in total food costs reflect assumptions about redemption, substitutions, prices, and program participation.

[c] Cost differences were calculated by subtracting the estimated phased-in food costs for the current food packages from the estimated food costs for the revised food packages. Negative values (–) indicate that the revised food packages result in cost savings compared to the current food packages. Positive values (+) indicate that the revised food packages result in cost increases compared to the current food packages. Row totals may not be exact owing to independent rounding.

[d] This analysis assumes the proposed revisions will incentivize partially (mostly) breastfeeding food packages for the mother–infant dyads. Accordingly, the cost estimates for the revised food package anticipates a 5 percent shift of fully formula fed dyads to the partially (mostly) breastfed participant categories in the year after full implementation of the food package revisions. The participant shift is assumed to take place in FY2021. The shift is expected to be sustained, but to not recur in FY2022. The projected cost difference is attributed solely to this shift, rather than revisions to the food item in the food package.

TABLE 10-5 Continued

[e] Describes the total food cost and cost difference of cheese as a separate food package category for food package VII. The costs associated with cheese as a substitution option for fluid milk is incorporated into the estimates for the milk category.

phased-in costs compared to the current food package. In contrast, the CVV for fully breastfeeding women (food package VII)—who comprise approximately 3 percent of food package recipients—would increase by $24 per month in the revised food packages, and would only lead to an estimated $200 million increase in estimated phased-in costs.

Cost Differences of Food Package Items Over Time

The preceding sections evaluate the cost implications of each food package item, summed across all projected years. As presented in Table 10-7, the phased-in costs differences during FY2018 through FY2022 reflect the assumptions of the analysis. Cost differences in FY2018 and FY2019 are markedly lower than in subsequent years, for example, because they reflect the phased-in implementation of the revised food package. The values for these 2 years are one-third of the unadjusted value. The cost differences for FY2018 are even less, because the values only encompass a 6-month period.

Some of the variations in cost differences over time result from assumptions about participation. In FY2021 and FY2022, infant formula is projected to cost less and eggs are projected to cost slightly more in the revised food packages compared to the current food packages. The analysis does not assume changes in quantities or the rate of redemption between the current and revised food packages for either food package item. Instead, the cost differences result from the 5-percent shift in fully formula fed mother–infant dyads to partially (mostly) breastfeeding dyads that the committee projects to take place in FY2020 for the revised food packages. The slight increase in egg costs in the revised food packages is attributed to the women shifting from being classified as partially (minimally) breastfeeding at more than 6 months postpartum (i.e., receiving food package N/A) to partially (mostly) breastfeeding (i.e., receiving the revised food package V-B). Partially (mostly) breastfeeding women may receive food package benefits for up to 1 year postpartum.

Most of the projected variations in cost differences over time are the result of a complex interplay among several factors. The CVV serves as a prime example. The proposed revisions add value to the CVV across all food packages for women and children. In FY2020 and FY2022, the CVV for women in the revised food package VII is projected to be adjusted for inflation by $1, increasing to $36 and $37 per month, respectively.

TABLE 10-6 Revisions to Food Package Items That Lead to Major Total Phased-in Cost Differences from FY2018 Through FY2022, by Food Package

Food Package	Food Package Revision	Total Phased-in Cost Difference, FY2018 Through FY2022 ($, millions)[a]
I	• No revision leading to a major cost difference[b]	—
II	• Infant vegetable and fruit redemption is projected to increase with the addition of the CVV substitution option	+69
	• Infant cereal is reduced	–71
III	• No revision leading to a major cost difference[c]	—
IV-A	• CVV is increased	+107
	• Canned fish is added to the food package	+27
	• Milk[d] is reduced	–45
	• Whole wheat bread[e] is reduced	–52
	• Juice is reduced	–116
IV-B	• CVV is increased	+246
	• Canned fish is added to the food package	+62
	• Legumes and peanut butter are reduced	–47
	• Whole wheat bread[e] is reduced	–119
	• Juice is reduced	–264
V-A	• CVV is increased	+129
	• Milk[d] is reduced	–29
	• Legumes and peanut butter are reduced	–37
	• Juice is reduced	–84
V-B	• CVV is increased	+26
VI	• CVV is increased	+65
	• Juice is reduced	–109
VII	• CVV is increased	+200
	• Cheese[f] is eliminated as its own food package item	–46

NOTES: The committee defined a major total cost difference as a revision within a specific food package resulting in a total phased-in cost difference of at least $25 million over the course of FY2018 through FY2022. The major total cost differences not only reflect the specific revisions to the items and the quantity prescribed, but also the distribution of participants across the different food packages. Food packages that represent a smaller proportion of WIC participants generally have fewer major cost differences. Not all savings and costs are reflected in the table. CVV = cash value voucher; FY = fiscal year.

continued

TABLE 10-6 Continued

[a] Phased-in estimates assume full implementation of the proposed revisions in state agencies serving one-third of all WIC participants as of April 1, 2018. All other state agencies are assumed to implement the proposed revisions as of FY2020. Cost differences were calculated by subtracting the estimated cost for the current food package item from the estimated costs corresponding to the food item in the revised food package. Negative values (–) indicate that the revised food packages result in cost savings compared to the current food packages. Positive values (+) indicate that the revised food packages result in cost increases compared to the current food packages.

[b] This analysis assumes the incentives in the proposed revisions will result in a 5 percent shift of fully formula fed mother–infant dyads to the partially (mostly) breastfed participant categories in the year after full implementation of the food package revisions across the entire WIC program under the phased-in assumption. The total amount of formula prescribed in the revised food packages I and II is expected to decrease because of this shift in participants. For food package I, the total cost difference for FY2018 through FY2022 is expected to result in $22.5 million in savings.

[c] Because food package III recipients comprise a small proportion of food package recipients, all food package revisions resulted in total phased-in cost differences of less than $25 million over the course of FY2018 through FY2022.

[d] The estimated cost differences for milk includes assumptions about the proportion of participants purchasing fluid milk (e.g., whole milk, 2%), milk alternatives (e.g., lactose-free milk, soy-based beverage), and substitutions (e.g., cheese, yogurt).

[e] The estimated cost difference for whole wheat bread includes assumptions about the proportion of participants purchasing options available under the current food packages and proposed revisions (e.g., corn tortillas, instant oatmeal).

[f] The proposed revisions removes cheese as a separate food package category prescribed to food package VII participants. Cheese remains a substitution option for milk across all children's and women's food packages.

Similarly, an inflation adjustment of $1 is projected for the revised food package V-B (for partially [mostly] breastfeeding women), increasing the CVV to $26 per month. Also during FY2021, the committee anticipates a 5 percent shift of fully formula fed dyads to partially (mostly) breastfed dyads, which would shift a portion of postpartum women to the larger CVV in the revised food package V-B (compared to the revised food package VI CVV). These adjustments and assumptions in the revised food packages do not have a dramatic effect on total cost differences because participants in food packages VII and V-B are only a small proportion of the total WIC-participating population. In FY2022, however, the trajectory of the cost difference for the CVV changes, decreasing from +$230 million in FY2021 to +$215 million in FY2022. This is the result of a $1 inflation adjustment that is projected to affect all food packages for women in the current food packages. Although the revised CVV values result in positive cost differences (i.e., cost increases) compared to the CVV values in the current food packages for each fiscal year assessed, the difference across the years is not consistent. Assumptions regarding the CVV are described

TABLE 10-7 Phased-in Cost Differences Between the Current and Revised Food Packages by Food Package Item Category, by Fiscal Year (FY)

	Phased-in Cost Differences of the Revised Food Packages Compared to Current Food Packages ($, millions)[b]				
Food Package Item[a]	FY2018[c,d]	FY2019[d]	FY2020	FY2021	FY2022
Cash value voucher	+36.5	+73.9	+224.1	+229.7	+215.2
Canned fish	+5.0	+10.3	+31.6	+32.9	+33.7
Jarred infant vegetables and fruits	+3.6	+7.5	+22.9	+23.4	+24
Eggs	0	0	0	+0.1	+0.1
Infant food meat	–0.9	–1.8	–5.5	–5.6	–5.7
Breakfast cereal	–1.0	–2.0	–6.2	–6.2	–6.3
Infant formula, postrebate	0	0	0	–20.5	–21.0
Cheese[e]	–2.0	–4.2	–12.9	–13.2	–13.5
Infant cereal	–3.5	–7.2	–22.0	–22.5	–23.0
Milk	–3.9	–8.1	–24.7	–24.1	–24.7
Legumes and peanut butter	–5.5	–11.3	–34.8	–35.6	–36.4
Whole wheat bread	–6.8	–14.1	–43.4	–43.6	–44.6
Juice	-27.9	-57.7	-176.9	-179.9	-184.2

NOTES: Phased-in estimates assume full implementation of the proposed revisions in state agencies serving one-third of all WIC participants as of April 1, 2018. All other state agencies are assumed to implement the proposed revisions as of FY2020. FY = fiscal year.

[a] Broadly describes the food package item category. Cost differences include assumptions about substitutions and selection of allowable options within each category.

[b] Cost differences were calculated by subtracting the estimated phased-in food cost for each item in the current food packages from the estimated food costs of the corresponding item in the revised food packages. Negative values (–) indicate that the revised food packages result in cost savings compared to the current food packages. Positive values (+) indicate that the revised food packages result in cost increases compared to the current food packages.

[c] This analysis assumes the earliest date of implementation of the proposed changes would be April 1, 2018. Accordingly all estimates for FY2018 only encompass a 6-month period.

[d] Phased-in cost differences in FY2018 and FY2019 are 33.3 percent of the unadjusted cost differences.

[e] Describes the cost difference of cheese as a separate food package category for food package VII. The costs associated with cheese as a substitution option for fluid milk is incorporated into the estimates for the milk category.

in the "Cost Effect Methodology" section that follows and in Appendix U. Alternative assumptions and their effects on total cost differences are tested in the "Uncertainty" section later in this chapter.

Cost-Estimate Methodology

This analysis projects costs of each food package in the current and revised sets of food packages through FY2022. The committee estimated the monthly costs of a food package by multiplying the projected number of recipients of the package, the average proportion of each food package item projected to be redeemed, and the estimated prices of each item in the food package and then summing these values within the food package. This process was repeated for each specific food package. Monthly costs were multiplied by 12 to arrive at annual estimates for each fiscal year in the analysis (FY2018[6] through FY2022). The sections that follow provide a brief overview of how the committee projected participation, redemption, and prices. Details of the methodology are presented in Appendix U.

Participation

The committee used two data sources to estimate program participation, as described previously in Chapter 7. The 2014 *Food Package Report* (USDA/FNS, 2016a) was used to determine the distribution of participants across the specific food packages. To estimate the average numbers of participants that are issued each specific food package in a month, the distributions in the *Food Package Report* were applied to the administrative data posted on FNS's website[7] (USDA/FNS, 2016d). The participation estimates the committee derived from these data sources served as the basis for both the current and revised food package cost estimates that were used for the cost analysis presented in Chapter 7 and this chapter. The complete regulatory impact analysis (see Appendix U) includes a detailed explanation of how participation for each food package was determined.

Estimating participation for FY2018 through FY2022 To forecast participation through FY2022, the committee extrapolated the FY2015 WIC participation levels based on the relationship between WIC participation and the general economy (unemployment rates and the forecast of the civilian labor force). During and following the economic recession

[6] FY2018 in this analysis only encompasses 6 months. As such, monthly estimates were multiplied by 6 rather than 12.

[7] Administrative data includes all state agencies, Indian Tribal Organizations, and territories.

of 2008–2009, WIC participation grew. As that recession waned, WIC participation declined. With the general economy forecasted to improve moderately and then stabilize, the committee expects that WIC participation levels will decrease initially, then increase slightly and stabilize. The committee forecasts WIC participation to decline by 2.2 percent between FY2015 and FY2018. From FY2018 to FY2022, the committee forecasts WIC participation to increase by 1.5 percent. As a result, the committee forecasts that the FY2022 participation levels will be 0.7 percent lower than the FY2015 levels.

Anticipating a shift in fully formula fed mother–infant dyads under the proposed revisions Participation projections are identical between the current and proposed revised food packages, with one exception. As described in Chapter 7 (and in more detail in Appendix U), the committee incorporated a 5 percent shift of participants from the fully formula-feeding to the partially breastfeeding dyad. The committee anticipates that the 5 percent shift will take place after all the revisions have been implemented in all states and will be sustained over time. Accordingly, the shift has been incorporated in FY2021 participation estimates, which corresponds to the year after full implementation under the phased-in assumption.

Redemption

As described in Chapter 7, USDA-FNS provided the committee with 12 months (August 2013 through July 2014) of price and redemption data from a convenience sample of six WIC state agencies, representing five of the seven regions of the country (hereafter referred to as the FNS redemption dataset). Additional details related to this data source, and the methods applied to calculate redemption rates for the current and revised food packages using this and other sources are presented in Chapter 7 and further detailed in Appendix R. The calculated redemption rates for each food package item served as the quantity multipliers used in the estimation of total food package costs.

Prices

Prices for each food package item were primarily estimated from the FNS redemption dataset, supplemented by data from the 2014 Information Resources, Inc. (IRI) Consumer Network Database as described in Chapter 7 and in Appendix U. Chapter 7 and Appendix U also describe the development of composite prices for certain WIC food categories and the inflation of prices to the base of FY2015.

Projecting prices after FY2015 For years after FY2015, prices for items that are prescribed as a fixed quantity (e.g., 16 quarts of milk) were inflated using the Congressional Budget Office's March 2015 Baseline Thrifty Food Plan estimates (CBO, 2015). The inflation assumptions are presented in Table 10-8.

Inflating the cash value voucher The CVV does not inflate the same way as items prescribed as a fixed quantity. Instead, its inflation depends on an annual average of the Consumer Price Index (CPI) for fresh fruits and vegetables (7 C.F.R. § 246.16). Under the current rule, the average CPI for fresh fruits and vegetables from April 2006 through March 2007 is assigned to FY2008 and considered the baseline CPI. Each subsequent year follows the same pattern (e.g., FY2009 value is the average CPI from April 2007 through March 2008). To inflate the CVV, the average CPI for the fiscal year being considered is divided by the baseline CPI value and multiplied by the base values of each CVV ($8 for children, $10 for women). Participants only receive an increase in value when the inflated CVV crosses a $1 increment. This inflation adjustment recently occurred in the food packages for women, with the $10 CVV increased to $11 beginning in FY2016. Provision of the CVV in dollar increments, rather than prescribing the exact inflated value, is easier from an administrative perspective, as adjustments only have to be made periodically. It also decreases participant burden, as the benefit is provided in a round number and a consistent value

TABLE 10-8 Inflation Assumption for Food Package Items Prescribed as a Fixed Quantity, FY2016–FY2022

Year	Thrifty Food Plan (inflation rate)[a]
FY2016[b]	1.026
FY2017[b]	1.020
FY2018	1.020
FY2019	1.021
FY2020	1.021
FY2021	1.023
FY2022	1.023

NOTES: The base year of this analysis is FY2015. FY = fiscal year.

[a] The percent change is relative to the fiscal year preceding it. Prices for FY2016, for example, were projected to be 2.6 percent higher than in FY2015.

[b] Year not included in the cost estimates presented in this regulatory impact analysis, but was necessary to arrive at price estimates for FY2018 through FY2022.

SOURCE: CBO, 2015.

month-to-month. This inflation approach was used for estimating the costs of the current food packages in this analysis.

Under the proposed revisions, all women and children receive a CVV of higher value. Had the committee kept FY2008 as the baseline CPI value under the proposed revisions, in FY2018 the $12, $15, $25, and $35 CVVs would already have been inflated to $13, $17, $28, and $39, respectively, because of the inflation that has taken place in the decade between FY2008 and FY2018. Accordingly, the CVV under the proposed revision required a new inflation baseline, which was assumed to be the first year of implementation (FY2018).

The CPI values used in the inflation of the CVV encompass the 6 to 18 months prior to the fiscal year they describe. Accordingly, actual CPI values were used through FY2017 of this analysis. The committee could not identify forecasts for the retail price of fresh vegetables and fruits that extended to FY2022. A forecast for 2017 projected a 1 to 2 percent relative change in price from FY2016 (USDA/ERS, 2016). Therefore, a relative change in average CPI of 1.5 percent was used for FY2018 through FY2022. The cost effect of using alternate baseline years for the CPI inflation values for the revised food packages are tested in the "Uncertainties" section.

UNCERTAINTIES

The estimated costs of the current food packages and proposed revised food packages are sensitive to key assumptions made in the preceding sections. The cost implications of several of these assumptions are tested below. The uncertainty scenarios specifically evaluate changing one or multiple assumptions about the revised food package and evaluating the cost effects. The "primary analysis" refers to the assumptions, food costs, and cost differences presented in the preceding sections of this chapter. "Base assumption" refers to the specific assumption(s) used in the primary analysis.

For each uncertainty scenario tested, the phased-in cost differences are presented. The phased-in cost differences presented for each assumption scenario (i.e., base assumption, each uncertainty scenario) indicate the cost effect as it compares to the current food packages. Negative values (–) indicate that the specific scenario costs less than the current food packages, whereas a positive value (+) indicates that the specific scenario costs more than the current food packages. The cost differences between the base assumption and each uncertainty scenario are also presented. These describe how much the base assumption costs or saves, compared to the tested uncertainty scenario. For these differences, a negative value (–) indicates that the base assumption used in the primary analysis costs less than the uncertainty scenario; a positive value (+) indicates that the base assumption costs more than the uncertainty scenario. This section presents select uncertainties tested by the committee. A broader range of uncertainties is explored in the complete RIA (see Appendix U).

The cost differences presented in this section must be considered in context of estimated overall food costs of the current and revised food packages. Over the course of FY2018 through FY2022, the food packages in this analysis are projected to cost approximately $17 billion, averaging to approximately $3.9 billion per year, both under the current and revised food packages.

Assumptions About the CVV

The CVVs are estimated to cost approximately $780 million more in the revised food packages compared to the CVVs in the current food packages. The proposed revisions allow for a CVV to be a substitution option for juice and jarred infant food vegetables and fruits. Given the CVV's increased prominence in the revised food packages, it is essential to evaluate different aspects of the assumptions underlying the primary cost analysis.

Different CVV Redemption Projections Under the Proposed Revisions

In the primary analysis, CVV redemption was estimated to be 77.2 percent in the current food packages and 75.0 percent in the revised food packages (rationale presented in Appendix U). The cost implications of two alternative redemption scenarios are presented in Table 10-9. Scenario 1 shows that increasing the redemption assumption to 85 percent for the revised food packages would result in the estimated $220.4 million savings projected in the primary analysis becoming $135.1 million in additional costs compared to the current food packages ($355.5 million in additional costs compared to the base assumption). Similarly, scenario 2 shows that lower redemption of the revised CVV (65 percent redemption) results in an additional $355.5 million savings from FY2018 through FY2022, compared to the base assumptions in the primary analysis. This lower redemption assumption for the CVVs in the revised food packages results in a total cost savings of approximately $580 million over the course of FY2018 through FY2022, compared to the current food packages.

Different CPI Base Year for the Revised Food Packages

In the revised food packages, FY2018 serves as the base year to which subsequent years are compared for CVV inflation. Table 10-10 explores the cost differences associated with different CPI base years for the revised food packages. In scenario 1, changing the base year to inflate the revised

TABLE 10-9 Projected Phased-in Cost Difference of WIC Food Package Revisions, Increase or Decrease in Redemption Assumption of Cash Value Voucher

Scenario	CVV Assumption, Percent Redeemed	Phased-in Cost Differences of the Revised Food Packages Compared to Current Food Packages ($, millions)[a]					
		FY2018	FY2019	FY2020	FY2021	FY2022	Total Cost Difference, FY2018 Through FY2022
Base assumption[b]	75	-6.4	-14.8	-47.7	-65.0	-86.6	-220.4
Uncertainty scenario 1[b]	85	+10.2	+18.8	+53.4	+37.0	+15.8	+135.1
Cost difference of base assumption compared to uncertainty scenario 1[c]		**-16.6**	**-33.6**	**-101.1**	**-101.9**	**-102.3**	**-355.5**
Base assumption[b]	75	-6.4	-14.8	-47.7	-65.0	-86.6	-220.4
Uncertainty scenario 2[b]	65	-23.0	-48.4	-148.8	-166.9	-188.9	-575.9
Cost difference of base assumption compared to uncertainty scenario 2[c]		**+16.6**	**+33.6**	**+101.1**	**+101.9**	**+102.3**	**+355.5**

NOTES: This table shows the phased-in cost difference between the revised and current food packages, along with the cost differences between different redemption assumptions for the revised CVV (85 and 65 percent redemption) and the current food packages. The primary analysis of the regulatory impact analysis assumes 75 percent redemption of the revised CVVs. All other assumptions in the primary analysis remain constant. Column and row totals may not be exact owing to independent rounding. CVV = cash value voucher; FY = fiscal year.

[a] Phased-in estimates assume full implementation of the proposed revisions in state agencies serving one-third of all WIC participants as of April 1, 2018. All other state agencies are assumed to implement the proposed revisions as of FY2020.

[b] Describes the increases or savings of the base assumption or uncertainty scenario ("assumption scenario") compared to the current food packages. Negative values (–) indicate that the assumption scenario costs less than the current food packages. Positive values (+) indicate that the assumption scenario costs more than the current food packages.

[c] Describes the increases or savings of the base assumption compared to the uncertainty scenario. Negative values (–) indicate that the base assumption costs less than the uncertainty assumption. Positive values (+) indicate that the base assumption costs more than the uncertainty scenario.

TABLE 10-10 Projected Phased-in Cost Difference of WIC Food Package Revisions, Changing the Base Comparison Year for CVV Inflation

Scenario	Base Year for CVV Inflation in the Revised Food Packages	Phased-in Cost Differences of the Revised Food Packages Compared to Current Food Packages ($, millions)[a]					
		FY2018	FY2019	FY2020	FY2021	FY2022	Total Cost Difference, FY2018 Through FY2022
Base assumption[b]	FY2018	−6.4	−14.8	−47.7	−65.0	−86.6	−220.4
Uncertainty scenario 1[b]	FY2015	−5.8	−13.6	−31.1	−8.6	−32.4	−91.6
Cost difference of base assumption compared to uncertainty scenario 1[c]		**−0.6**	**−1.2**	**−16.6**	**−56.4**	**−54.1**	**−128.8**
Base assumption[b]	FY2018	−6.4	−14.8	−47.7	−65.0	−86.6	−220.4
Uncertainty scenario 2[b]	FY2016	−6.4	−14.0	−46.5	−62.6	−72.3	−201.8
Cost difference of base assumption compared to uncertainty scenario 2[c]		**0.0**	**−0.8**	**−1.2**	**−2.3**	**−14.3**	**−18.6**
Base assumption[b]	FY2018	−6.4	−14.8	−47.7	−65.0	−86.6	−220.4
Uncertainty scenario 3[b]	FY2017	−6.4	−14.0	−46.5	−62.6	−73.8	−203.4
Cost difference of base assumption compared to uncertainty scenario 3[c]		**0.0**	**−0.8**	**−1.2**	**−2.3**	**−12.8**	**−17.1**

NOTES: This table shows the phased-in cost difference between the revised and current food packages, along with the cost differences between different base years for CVV inflation and the current food packages. The primary analysis of the RIA assumes that the base year of the CVV inflation is FY2018. All other assumptions in the primary analysis remain constant. Column and row totals may not be exact owing to independent rounding. CVV = cash value voucher; FY = fiscal year.

[a] Phased-in estimates assume full implementation of the proposed revisions in state agencies serving one-third of all WIC participants as of April 1, 2018. All other state agencies are assumed to implement the proposed revisions as of FY2020.

[b] Describes the increases or savings of the base assumption or uncertainty scenario ("assumption scenario") compared to the current food packages. Negative values (−) indicate that the assumption scenario costs less than the current food packages. Positive values (+) indicate that the assumption scenario costs more than the current food packages.

[c] Describes the increases or savings of the base assumption compared to the uncertainty scenario. Negative values (−) indicate that the base assumption costs less than the uncertainty assumption. Positive values (+) indicate that the base assumption costs more than the uncertainty scenario.

CVV to FY2015 would cost an additional $128 million over the FY2018 through FY2022, compared to using FY2018 as the base year. Both scenarios 2 and 3 demonstrate that there are relatively small costs effects of selecting either FY2016 or FY2017 as the base year for CVV inflation in the revised food packages.

Assumptions About Use of "Up to" Amounts

The primary analysis assumes that infant formula prescription practices will not change between the current and revised food packages. Table 10-11 projects the cost effects of different formula prescription practices for the revised food packages. In scenario 1, prescribing all infants in food package I-BF/FF-A the maximum "up to" amount of infant formula would result in approximately $20 million in additional costs in the revised food packages over the course of FY2018 through FY2022, compared to the base assumption used in the primary analysis. The revised food packages would still be projected to cost approximately $201 million less than the current food packages, over the course of FY2018 through FY2022. In contrast, if the average amount of infant formula prescribed across all food packages was 95 percent of the maximum "up to" amount for each food package (scenario 2), the total cost savings of the revised food packages would increase by $145 million over the course of the FY2018 through FY2022, compared to the base assumption used in the primary analysis. This would result in an estimated $366 million in total savings compared to the current food packages.

Assumptions About Shifts in Fully Formula-Fed Dyads

A key assumption of the primary analysis is that, under the proposed revisions, 5 percent of fully formula fed mother–infant dyads will shift to corresponding fully (mostly) breastfeeding food packages. The committee considered the 5 percent shift conservative, given evidence that the 2009 food package, which allowed women to choose between formula-feeding or fully breastfeeding in the infant's first month of life, resulted in an approximately 7 to 11 percent shift of dyads from breastfeeding to formula-feeding (USDA/FNS, 2011).

Table 10-12 presents the cost effect of this assumption. The cost differences only affect FY2021 and FY2022, because the base assumption is that the shift would occur 1 year after full implementation in all state agencies under the phased-in implementation assumption. Assuming no shift in participants in the revised food packages (scenario 1) would cost approximately $25 million more over the course of FY2018 through FY2022, compared to the assumption of a 5 percent shift. A 3 percent shift of

TABLE 10-11 Projected Phased-in Cost Difference of WIC Food Package Revisions, Changing the Maximum Amount of Formula in Food Packages I and II

Scenario	Maximum Formula Assumption, Amount Change	Phased-in Cost Differences of the Revised Food Packages Compared to Current Rule ($, millions)[a]					
		FY2018	FY2019	FY2020	FY2021	FY2022	Total Cost Difference, FY2018 Through FY2022
Base assumption[c]	Identical to current food package[b]	–6.4	–14.8	–47.7	–65.0	–86.6	–220.4
Uncertainty scenario 1[c]	All I-BF/FF-A recipients prescribed maximum "up to" amount	–5.6	–13.1	–42.6	–58.8	–80.3	–200.5
Cost difference of base assumption compared to uncertainty scenario 1[d]		**–0.8**	**–1.6**	**–5.1**	**–6.1**	**–6.3**	**–19.9**
Base assumption[c]	Identical to current food package[b]	–6.4	–14.8	–47.7	–65.0	–86.6	–220.4
Uncertainty scenario 2[c]	95 percent of maximum "up to" amounts	–13.0	–28.5	–89.6	–105.9	–128.5	–365.5
Cost difference of base assumption compared to uncertainty scenario 2[d]		**+6.6**	**+13.7**	**+41.9**	**+41.0**	**+41.9**	**+145.1**

NOTES: This table shows the phased-in cost difference between the proposed revisions and the current rule, along with the cost differences of different assumptions regarding the maximum amount of formula in food packages I and II. All other assumptions in the primary analysis remain constant. Column and row totals may not be exact owing to independent rounding. FY = fiscal year.

[a] Phased-in estimates assume full implementation of the proposed revisions in state agencies serving one-third of all WIC participants as of April 1, 2018. All other state agencies are assumed to implement the proposed revisions as of FY2020.

[b] Base assumptions for maximum formula under the proposed revisions are as follows: I-BF/FF-A (104 fluid ounces), I-BF/FF-B (424 fluid ounces), I-BF/FF-C (510 fluid ounces), I -FF-A (861 fluid ounces), I -FF-B (948 fluid ounces), II-BF/FF (371 fluid ounces), II-FF (683 fluid ounces). The formula amounts are the weighted average of the monthly maximum allowances across the different forms of infant formula. The base assumption is that the quantity of formula prescribed will remain unchanged.

[c] Describes the increases or savings of the base assumption or uncertainty scenario ("assumption scenario") compared to the current food packages. Negative values (–) indicate that the assumption scenario costs less than the current food packages. Positive values (+) indicate that the assumption scenario costs more than the current food packages.

[d] Describes the increases or savings of the base assumption compared to the uncertainty scenario. Negative values (–) indicate that the base assumption costs less (provides more savings) than the uncertainty assumption. Positive values (+) indicate that the base assumption costs more than the uncertainty scenario.

TABLE 10-12 Projected Phased-in Cost Difference of WIC Food Package Revisions, Changing Assumptions About Percent of Fully Formula-Fed Dyads Shift to Partially (mostly) Breastfed Food Packages

Scenario	Dyadic Shift Assumption, Percent of Fully Formula Fed Projected to Shift[a]	Phased-in Cost Differences of the Revised Food Packages Compared to Current Food Packages ($, millions)[b]					
		FY2018	FY2019	FY2020	FY2021	FY2022	Total Cost Difference, FY2018 Through FY2022
Base assumption[c]	5	–6.4	–14.8	–47.7	–65.0	–86.6	–220.4
Uncertainty scenario 1[c]	0	–6.4	–14.8	–47.7	–52.8	–74.0	–195.7
Cost difference of base assumption compared to uncertainty scenario 1[d]		0.0	0.0	0.0	**–12.1**	**–12.5**	**–24.7**
Base assumption[c]	5	–6.4	–14.8	–47.7	–65.0	–86.6	–220.4
Uncertainty scenario 2[c]	3	–6.4	–14.8	–47.7	–60.1	–81.5	–210.6
Cost difference of base assumption compared to uncertainty scenario 2[d]		0.0	0.0	0.0	**–4.9**	**–5.0**	**–9.9**
Base assumption[c]	5	–6.4	–14.8	–47.7	–65.0	–86.6	–220.4
Uncertainty scenario 3[c]	8	–6.4	–14.8	–47.7	–72.2	–94.1	–235.2
Cost difference of base assumption compared to uncertainty scenario 3[d]		0.0	0.0	0.0	**+7.3**	**+-7.5**	**+14.8**
Base assumption[c]	5	–6.4	–14.8	–47.7	–65.0	–86.6	–220.4
Uncertainty scenario 4[c]	5 (only dyads <6 months postpartum)[d]	–6.4	–14.8	–47.7	–57.5	–78.9	–205.30
Cost difference of base assumption compared to uncertainty scenario 4[d]		0.0	0.0	0.0	**–7.5**	**–7.7**	**–15.1**

NOTES: This table shows the phased-in cost difference between the revised and current food packages, along with the cost differences of different assumptions regarding the percent of fully formula-fed mother–infant dyads shifting to partially (mostly) breastfeeding food packages. All other assumptions in the primary analysis remain constant. Column and row totals may not be exact owing to independent rounding. FY = fiscal year.

[a] The shift describes the percent of participants prescribed food package I-FF-A, I-FF-B, II-FF, VI, and N/A shifting to corresponding partially (mostly) breastfeeding food packages. Approximately 21 and 79 percent of participants shifting from food package I-FF-A were assigned to food packages I-BF/FF-A and I-BF/FF-B, respectively. All women shifting from being classified as more than 6 months postpartum (i.e., food package N/A) were assigned to food package V-B. The shift is projected to occur in the year after full implementation of the proposed revisions (FY2021). The effect on participation is expected to be sustained but additional shifts are not projected in subsequent years.

[b] Phased-in estimates assume full implementation of the proposed revisions in state agencies serving one-third of all WIC participants as of April 1, 2018. All other state agencies are assumed to implement the proposed revisions as of FY2020.

[c] Describes the increases or savings of the base assumption or uncertainty scenario ("assumption scenario") compared to the current food packages. Negative values (–) indicate that the assumption scenario costs less than the current food packages. Positive values (+) indicate that the assumption scenario costs more than the current food packages.

[d] Describes the increases or savings of the base assumption compared to the uncertainty scenario. Negative values (–) indicate that the base assumption costs less (provides more savings) than the uncertainty assumption. Positive values (+) indicate that the base assumption costs more than the uncertainty scenario.

participants would decrease estimated total cost savings by $9.9 million (Scenario 2), whereas an 8 percent shift would increase estimated total cost savings by $14.8 million (Scenario 3), compared to the base assumption in the primary analysis. If the shift only occurs for infants less than 6 months old and women less than 6 months postpartum, the estimated total cost savings of the revised food packages would decrease by $15.1 million over the course of FY2018 through FY2022, compared to the base assumption.

ALTERNATIVES

The committee considered several alternatives to current food package items and amounts that were ultimately rejected. Some of these alternatives and the committee's rationale for not including them in the revised food packages are outlined in the sections that follow. As with the uncertainty scenarios, the "primary analysis" refers to the set of base assumptions that led to a total phased-in cost savings of $220 million for the revised food packages compared to the current food packages, over the course of FY2018 through FY2022.

For each alternative tested, the phased-in cost differences are presented. They indicate the cost effect as it relates to the current food packages. Negative values (–) indicate that the specific scenario costs less than the current food packages, whereas a positive value (+) indicates that the specific scenario costs more than the current food packages. The cost difference between the base assumption and the alternative are also presented. These describe how much the base assumption costs or saves, compared to the tested alternative. For these differences, a negative value (–) indicates the base assumption used in the primary analysis costs less than the alternative; a positive value (+) indicates the base assumption costs more than the alternative. This section presents select alternatives tested by the committee. Additional alternatives are explored in the complete RIA (see Appendix U).

More Canned Fish

To support the *Dietary Guidelines for Americans* (DGA) recommendation to increase seafood intake, the committee proposes adding canned fish to all children's and women's food packages and offering it as a substitution option for jarred infant-food meat. To maintain cost neutrality and create incentives for partially (mostly) and fully breastfeeding women, different quantities and rotation patterns were created for canned fish. The amount prescribed in food packages IV-A, IV-B, V-A, and VI are relatively low compared to the DGA recommended intake. Table 10-13 shows the cost effects of prescribing additional canned fish to these food packages. Increasing the prescribed amount to 20 ounces every 3 months for

TABLE 10-13 Projected Phased-in Cost Difference of WIC Food Package Revisions, Prescribing Additional Fish to Food Packages IV-A, IV-B, V-A, and VI

		Phased-in Cost Differences of the Revised Food Packages Compared to Current Food Packages ($, millions)[a]					
Scenario	Quantity of Fish Prescribed to Food Packages IV-A, IV-B, V-A, and VI	FY2018	FY2019	FY2020	FY2021	FY2022	Total Cost Difference, FY2018 Through FY2022
Base assumption[b]	10 oz once every 3 months	−6.4	−14.8	−47.7	−65.0	−86.6	−220.4
Alternative 1[b]	20 oz once every 3 months	−1.0	−3.6	−13.4	−30.0	−50.8	−98.8
Cost difference of base assumption compared to alternative 1[c]		**−5.4**	**−11.2**	**−34.3**	**−35.0**	**−35.8**	**−121.6**
Base assumption[b]	10 oz once every 3 months	−6.4	−14.8	−47.7	−65.0	−86.6	−220.4
Alternative 2[b]	10 oz per month	4.4	7.6	20.9	4.9	−15.0	22.8
Cost difference of base assumption compared to alternative 2[c]		**−10.8**	**−22.4**	**−68.6**	**−69.9**	**−71.6**	**−243.2**

NOTES: This table shows the phased-in cost difference between the revised and current food packages, along with the cost differences of alternative quantities of canned fish prescribed to participants receiving food packages IV-A, IV-B, V-A, and VI. All other assumptions in the primary analysis remain constant. Column and row totals may not be exact owing to independent rounding. FY = fiscal year.

[a] Phased-in estimates assume full implementation of the proposed revisions in state agencies serving one-third of all WIC participants as of April 1, 2018. All other state agencies are assumed to implement the proposed revisions as of FY2020.

[b] Describes the increases or savings of the base assumption or alternative compared to the current food packages. Negative values (−) indicate that the base assumption or alternative costs less than the current food packages. Positive values (+) indicate that the base assumption or alternative costs more than the current food packages.

[c] Describes the increases or savings of the base assumption compared to the alternative. Negative values (−) indicate that the base assumption costs less (provides more savings) than the uncertainty assumption. Positive values (+) indicate that the base assumption costs more than the uncertainty scenario.

these food packages (alternative 1) costs approximately $122 million more than the base assumption. Alternative 1 would be considered cost neutral from FY2018 through FY2022, as the total food package costs would be approximately $99 million less than the projected costs for the current food packages (from FY2018 through FY2022). However, the parameter of cost neutrality the committee was operating under was +/–$0.10 per-participant cost per month, based on FY2015 prices. When 20 ounces of canned fish every 3 months is used in this pricing scenario, the revised food packages would cost $0.37 more per-participant per month than the current food packages. Alternative 2 shows that 10 ounces per month in the food packages would cost approximately $23 million more than the current food packages.

MARKET ANALYSIS

The food package revisions will result in changes in the quantities and types of foods that WIC participants buy with their WIC food benefit. Although the market effects of the changes are difficult to quantify accurately, the committee expects them to be minor.

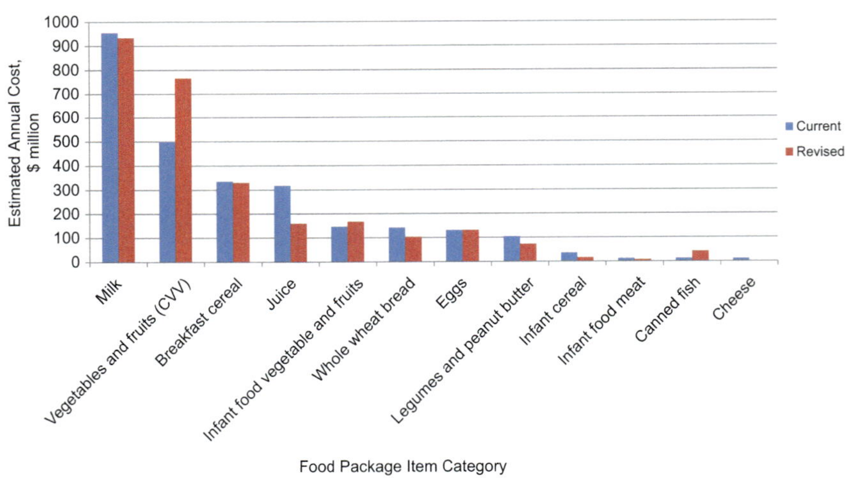

FIGURE 10-1 Estimated annual cost of food package item categories, current and revised food packages, FY2015.
NOTES: The food package item categories encompass substitutions and allowable options. Estimates for the revised food packages includes the 5 percent participant shift from the fully formula-feeding mother–infant dyads to partially (mostly) breastfeeding food packages. Vegetables and fruits (CVV) estimates for the current food packages use $11 for all women's food packages. CVV = cash value voucher.

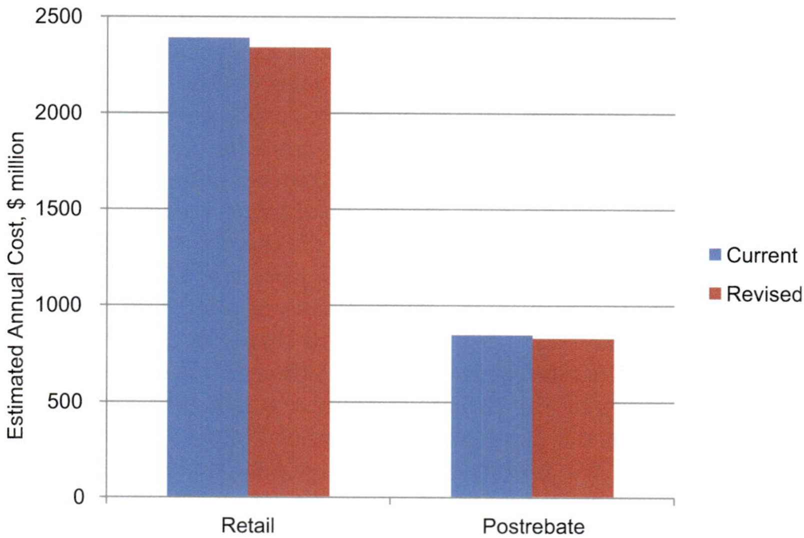

FIGURE 10-2 Estimated annual cost of infant formula, current and revised food packages, FY2015.
NOTES: Estimates for the revised food packages includes the 5 percent participant shift from the fully formula-feeding mother–infant dyads to partially (mostly) breastfeeding food packages.

Based on the assumptions in the primary analysis, the committee estimated the total value of WIC sales for each food item using the quantities in the current and revised food packages for FY2015.[8] Figure 10-1 shows the estimated sales for each category prescribed in the current food package side-by-side with estimates for the revised package. Each food item represents the food-item category, which encompasses assumptions about substitutions and allowable options within that category (e.g., yogurt and cheese substitution are included in the milk category). Estimated sales of infant formula using retail prices are presented in Figure 10-2.

Changes in total sales are estimated to be relatively small for most food categories, with the possible exception of juice, vegetables and fruits, and

[8] To reflect current regulations, women's CVV in this portion of the analysis is $11 for the current food package. The committee acknowledges that this inflation-based increase in CVV was not effective until FY2016. Using a $10 CVV for women in this portion of the analysis would result in the estimated annual cost of fruits and vegetables to be approximately $483 million for the current food package.

milk. However, WIC sales of each of these categories are a small portion of the total retail market. The committee did not have access to data that would permit it to estimate the total retail sales of WIC food categories. Instead, the analysis is based on the committee's assessment of likely market effects using aggregate retail data available from the RIA conducted for the Interim Rule (USDA/FNS, 2007). The estimates presented in that RIA are summarized in Table 10-14. WIC sales of juice were estimated to be 2 percent of the total retail juice market in the interim rule. WIC sales of vegetables and fruits were estimated to be 2.7 percent of the retail vegetable and fruit market. In the Interim Rule RIA, sales of milk were estimated to be 4.4 percent of the retail milk market, and cheese sales were estimated to be 2 percent of the retail cheese market. Although it is difficult to gauge accurately how sales of any individual product within that composite will be affected, data for the dairy products examined in the Interim Rule suggest that effects of the proposed revisions will be small. The categories estimated to experience the largest changes in sales under the revised packages represent small shares of their respective total retail markets, and the committee expects minimal market impacts as a consequence of the revision to the food package.

TABLE 10-14 Estimated Percent of the Market Attributed to WIC Sales, as Presented in the Interim Rule Regulatory Impact Analysis

	Estimated WIC Percent of the Market of the Interim Rule Food Packages Calendar Year 2005	
WIC Food Item	Assuming No Substitutions	Assuming Full Substitution
Formula	65.5	56.3
Beans	8.9	9.5
Peanut Butter	4.8	4.8
Milk	4.5	4.4
Adult Cereal	4.1	4.1
Juice	2.0	2.0
Vegetables and Fruits	2.7	2.7
Eggs	2.3	2.3
Cheese	2.0	2.0
Bread	0.5	0.6
Canned Fish	0.6	0.6

SOURCE: USDA/FNS, 2007.

SUMMARY

The proposed revisions to the WIC food packages are anticipated to have largely beneficial effects across a wide range of stakeholders, including the USDA-FNS, state and local WIC agencies, vendors, industry, and program participants. The committee estimates that the revised food packages save approximately $220 million program-wide over the course of FY2018 through FY2022, compared to the current food packages. Revisions to juice in the food packages are projected to lead to substantial cost savings, allowing for other changes in the food packages, such as increasing the value of the CVV. The projected cost effects of the revised food packages, compared to the current food packages, are contingent on the assumptions made in the analysis. Many of the key assumptions the committee tested maintained or increased the costs savings of the revised food packages. The committee expects the market effects of the revised food packages to be relatively minimal.

REFERENCES

CBO (Congressional Budget Office). 2015. *Supplemental Nutrition Assistance Program—CBO's March 2015 baseline*. https://www.cbo.gov/sites/default/files/51312-2015-03-SNAP.pdf (accessed October 3, 2016).

USDA/ERS (U.S. Department of Agriculture/Economic Research Service). 2005. *Interstate variation in WIC food package costs: The role of food prices, caseload composition, and cost-containment practices*. Washington, DC: USDA/ERS. http://ageconsearch.umn.edu/bitstream/33811/1/fa050041.pdf?origin=publication_detail (accessed October 3, 2016).

USDA/ERS. 2014. *Transition to EBT in WIC: Review of impact and examination of participant redemption patterns: Final report*. Washington, DC: Altarum Institute. http://altarum.org/sites/default/files/uploaded-publication-files/Altarum_Transition%20to%20WIC%20EBT_Final%20Report_071614.pdf (accessed March 2, 2016).

USDA/ERS. 2016. *Food price outlook—Consumer Price Index, changes in food price indexes, 2014 through 2017*. Washington, DC: USDA/ERS. http://www.ers.usda.gov/data-products/food-price-outlook.aspx (accessed October 3, 2016).

USDA/FNS (U.S. Department of Agriculture/Food and Nutrition Service). 2007. Special Supplemental Nutrition Program for Women, Infants and Children (WIC): Revisions in the WIC food packages; interim rule, 7 C.F.R. § 246.

USDA/FNS. 2011. *Evaluation of the birth month breastfeeding changes to the WIC food packages*. Alexandria, VA: USDA/FNS. http://www.fns.usda.gov/sites/default/files/BirthMonth.pdf (accessed March 9, 2016).

USDA/FNS. 2012. *Special Supplemental Nutrition Program for Women, Infants, and Children (WIC) erroneous payments to vendors: Annual estimates for FY2011*. Alexandria, VA: USDA/FNS. http://www.fns.usda.gov/sites/default/files/WICErroneousPayment_2011.pdf (accessed October 3, 2016).

USDA/FNS. 2013. *Breastfeeding promotion in WIC: Current federal requirements*. Alexandria, VA: USDA/FNS. http://www.fns.usda.gov/wic/breastfeeding-promotion-wic-current-federal-requirements (accessed October 3, 2016).

USDA/FNS. 2016a. *WIC participant and program characteristics 2014: Food package report.* Alexandria, VA: USDA/FNS. http://www.fns.usda.gov/wic-participant-and-program-characteristics-2014-food-package-report (accessed August 30, 2016).

USDA/FNS. 2016b. *WIC program, state-level participation.* http://www.fns.usda.gov/pd/wic-program Alexandria, VA: USDA/FNS. (accessed October 3, 2016).

USDA/FNS. 2016c. *August 2016 EBT detail status report*. Alexandria, VA: USDA/FNS. http://www.fns.usda.gov/sites/default/files/wic/August2016EBTDetailStatusReport.pdf (accessed October 3, 2016).

USDA/FNS. 2016d. *Monthly data—state level participation by category and program costs.* Alexandria, VA: USDA/FNS. http://www.fns.usda.gov/pd/wic-program (accessed October 3, 2016).

11

Recommendations for Implementation and Research

As part of the study task, the U.S. Department of Agriculture's Food and Nutrition Service (USDA-FNS) asked the committee to develop recommendations to maximize effective implementation of the revised food packages and for research on improved methodological approaches, data collection, and analyses designed to document effects of the recommended food package revisions. This chapter begins with recommendations for implementation, followed by research recommendations. In each section, recommendations are placed in order of priority. Additionally, the committee outlines its suggestions for modifications to the packages should available funds exceed or fall short of the cost-neutral level. The chapter concludes with a brief review of multilevel approaches to improve intake of foods in the Special Supplemental Nutrition Program for Women, Infants, and Children (WIC) food packages, and some final remarks.

RECOMMENDATIONS FOR IMPLEMENTATION OF THE REVISED FOOD PACKAGES

The Complexities of Implementation

As noted in Chapter 2, administration of the WIC food packages involves stakeholders at many levels: federal, state, local, participant, clinic, vendor, and food manufacturer. At each level, a series of factors ease or pose barriers to redemption of WIC foods by program participants. This was apparent to the committee in their WIC site visits and shopping experiences, from the review of literature conducted in phase I (NASEM, 2016), and from information presented at several workshops and public comment sessions organized for this study. Box 11-1 provides a summary of challenges that affect participant redemption of WIC foods. Once electronic benefit transfer (EBT) systems have been implemented nationwide and adaptation to these systems is complete, some of the barriers noted may be reduced in magnitude or may no longer be present.

BOX 11-1

Challenges That Affect Participant Redemption of WIC Foods

State level
- Authorizing widely available food options
- Maintaining a Universal Product Code (UPC) list
- Keeping apprised of market developments
- Identifying and authorizing vendors conveniently located for participant access
- Keeping apprised of and addressing vendor challenges

Participant level
- Accessing WIC-vendors
- Identifying WIC-approved foods
- Translating the cash value voucher (CVV) into a quantity of vegetables and fruits; keeping track of the CVV balance
- Checking out with ease
- Understanding the electronic benefit transfer (EBT) system and maintaining a list of nonredeemed foods

Clinic level
- Assisting WIC participants in identifying local WIC vendors, particularly when authorized vendors change
- Adapting to the EBT system
- Training staff

- Vendor level
- Adapting to the EBT system
- Keeping required WIC products in stock
- Updating UPC coding of WIC-approved products
- Training staff
- Providing refrigeration at small stores
- Maintaining inventory of WIC-approved foods while maintaining a viable business

Manufacturer level
- Meeting WIC food specifications for composition and sizes

SOURCES: Evidence derived from the literature review (see the phase I report, NASEM, 2016), also informed by the committee site visits and workshop presentations and discussion, July 29, 2016 (see Appendix D).

Key Recommendations Related to Implementation

The committee was charged to optimize implementation of the revised food packages by considering how to maximize the cost-effectiveness and efficiency of program administration. To achieve this goal, the committee offers the following recommendations:

11-1. The U.S. Department of Agriculture's Food and Nutrition Service (USDA-FNS) should develop the tools and strategies needed to assist state agencies, local agencies, and vendors to inform participants about and support them to make the best use of the expanded options of the revised food packages.

Rationale: The revised food packages include a variety of new options. Given the complexities of implementation listed in Box 11-1, it is essential that USDA-FNS strategically support states, agencies, clinics, and vendors to minimize barriers to WIC food redemption. Tools and strategies may include the development or support of Web-based materials and/or smart phone applications ("apps") that assist participants and vendors in maximizing redemption at the point of purchase. USDA-FNS could also lead dissemination of these tools and strategies among states and regions. Content that demonstrates the expanded options for vegetables and fruits, fish, dairy, and whole grains may enhance the shopping experience for WIC participants. Given that the revised packages may require vendors to offer more options, collaboration with vendors and food manufacturers to address challenges with stocking of WIC foods is essential to enhance participants' ability to locate and redeem these foods. Finally, with expansion of the cash value voucher (CVV), particularly for breastfeeding women, it will be important for USDA-FNS to encourage states that are not yet using the EBT system to issue paper CVVs in amounts that encourage full redemption (e.g., increments of $5 to $10).

11-2. USDA-FNS should maximize the extent to which the revised food packages motivate the choice to initiate and continue breastfeeding among all racial and ethnic groups by enhancing and stabilizing the funding available (independent of the food packages) for peer counseling and other lactation support staff at WIC sites.

Rationale: The committee's vision for WIC in the future is that all women receive adequate counseling and support prenatally through the first month postpartum and that the issuance of formula is individually tailored (not routinely issued) to meet the unique needs of every mother–infant dyad in the first 30 days after the infant's birth. After 30 days, food packages would continue to be designed to support each participant's level of breastfeeding.

The committee recognizes that that there are substantial societal barriers to breastfeeding that are outside of USDA's control. Improvements to the food packages for breastfeeding women are insufficient to support breastfeeding by themselves. Evidence indicates that enhanced breastfeeding support (e.g., the WIC Loving Support© program) is essential for improving breastfeeding outcomes among WIC participants (see the phase I report [NASEM, 2016] for a complete literature review). This support includes having WIC staff work closely with pregnant women and mothers as they make early feeding decisions, particularly during the third trimester of pregnancy through the first month postpartum. To meet demand, breastfeeding support programs need to be funded adequately and consistently from year to year.

Additional Considerations for Implementation

In its evaluation of the food packages, the committee reviewed the current federal implementation guidance to states. Several aspects of this guidance were considered particularly important to retain and/or enhance as part of the food package revisions. These are:

- **Continue to encourage state agencies to authorize as many food options as feasible within the limits of cost-containment, stocking requirements, and the redemption patterns of WIC participants.** *Rationale:* WIC participants appreciate choice in meeting their nutritional needs and accommodating their cultural and personal food preferences. The additional choices being offered in the revised packages also promote redemption of the WIC benefit. Examples of these additional choices include multiple forms of whole grains in addition to whole wheat bread and allowing a range of container sizes for yogurt (i.e., 30–32 ounces to accommodate purchase of multiple 5-ounce containers).
- **Continue to encourage state agencies to include lower-sodium options (where available) on state WIC food lists.** *Rationale:* The 2015-2020 *Dietary Guidelines for Americans* (DGA) recommend that individuals limit their sodium intake. As a result, added sodium is not permitted in the specifications for some WIC food categories (e.g., frozen vegetables and fruits). In other food categories (e.g., canned vegetables), lower-sodium products are now widely available but are not always included in state food lists. Including them in such lists would allow WIC participants access to these lower-sodium choices.

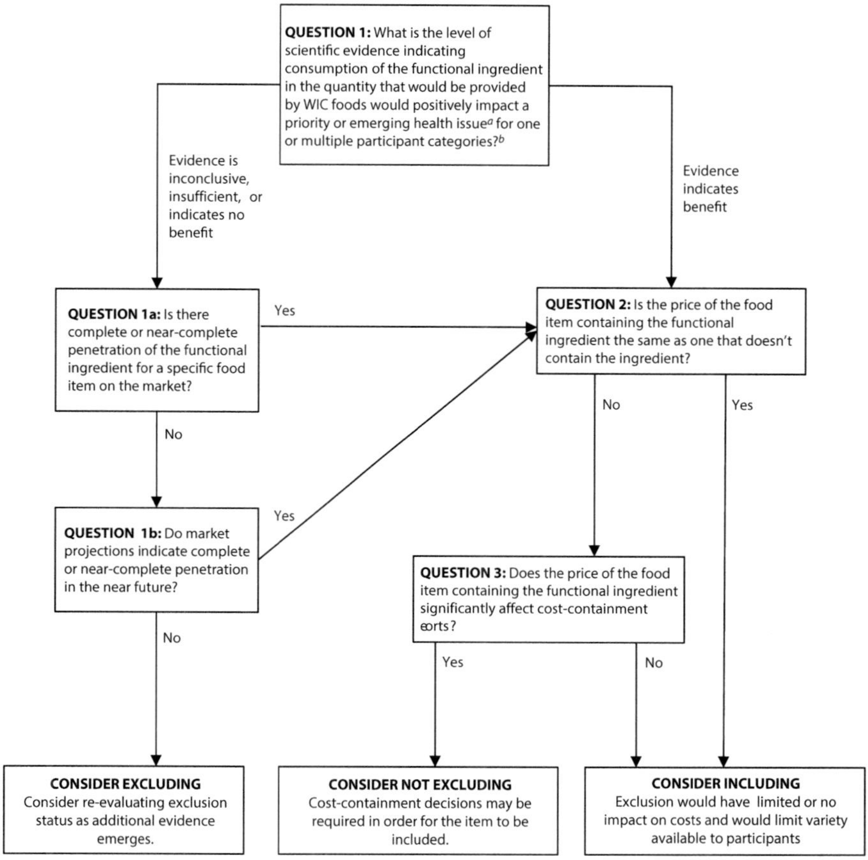

FIGURE 11-1 Proposed U.S. Department of Agriculture's Food and Nutrition Service (USDA-FNS) decision tree for evaluating inclusion of foods and infant formulas containing functional ingredients.
NOTES: This schematic assumes that the safety of infant formulas, foods, and ingredients permitted therein are assured by the U.S. Food and Drug Administration's (FDA's) regulatory processes. Each individual food item or formula should undergo the full evaluation presented.

[a] A priority or emerging health issue as indicated in the phase I Review of WIC Food Packages report (NASEM, 2016), or based on other evidence collected by USDA-FNS specific to the WIC-eligible population.

[b] The assessment of scientific evidence is conducted by a review of (1) statements or assessments of authoritative bodies such as the American Academy of Pediatrics, the Academy of Nutrition and Dietetics, or others deemed appropriate by USDA-FNS; (2) evaluation of Cochrane reviews; (3) evaluation of systematic reviews that follow a generally accepted and transparent procedure, and (4) other sources deemed appropriate by USDA-FNS.

- **Initiate discussions with national and state Medicaid programs to address barriers to ensuring they are the payer of the full cost of all exempt infant formulas and medical foods issued to WIC participants nationally.**
  Rationale: The purpose and scope of WIC does not include providing care to medically fragile infants (7 C.F.R. § 246.1); therefore, Medicaid is the appropriate primary payer (see WIC Policy Memorandum #2015-07). Enhanced collaboration between USDA-FNS and Medicaid at the national and state levels could reduce the complexity of the reimbursement process and remove WIC as the payer.
- **Evaluate inclusion of foods and infant formulas containing functional ingredients using the decision tree developed by the committee.**
  Rationale: The committee was tasked to consider the current science on functional ingredients[1] added to foods for infants, children, and adults (see the phase I report, NASEM [2016]) to determine how USDA-FNS might approach the inclusion of foods containing these ingredients in the WIC food packages. For this report, the committee outlined an approach that could be applied by USDA-FNS, and, potentially, state agencies, to determine whether foods or formula with these ingredients should be included in food packages (see Figure 11-1).

RESEARCH AND DATA COLLECTION RECOMMENDATIONS FOR EVALUATION OF THE WIC FOOD PACKAGES

Consistent with its task, the committee developed a prioritized list of recommendations for research and data collection. The majority of the research gaps identified also align with the research areas identified in the 2010 workshop, Planning a WIC Research Agenda (IOM, 2011), which indicates that many of the same data needs persist. Three high-priority research gaps were:

1. How the food packages affect participants' diet quality, food security, program satisfaction, and participation in WIC in combination with other nutrition assistance programs;

[1] At the time this report was written, the FDA had not established a definition for functional foods or ingredients. Functional ingredients are permitted in foods if evidence indicates the ingredients are safe at estimated national levels of consumption, but efficacy of these ingredients is not evaluated or regulated by the FDA. Broadly, functional foods and ingredients are thought to provide a "health benefit beyond basic nutrition," and may be beneficial to long-term health (Crowe and Francis, 2013).

2. The effect of program support and the food packages on the choice to initiate and continue breastfeeding; and
3. How choices regarding the purchase of vegetables and fruits can be optimized through the enhanced CVV.

Coordination of future WIC research timelines to allow completion by 2024 would ensure availability for the next review of WIC food packages. The specific recommendations that align with these priorities follow.

11-3. USDA-FNS should fund research to evaluate the effects of the recommended revisions to the WIC food packages on participant satisfaction, participation in the program, redemption of WIC foods, and participants' diets and health.

11-3a. USDA-FNS should collect WIC state agency policies on an annual basis and establish a national database of electronic benefit transfer (EBT) expenditures by program participants.

11-3b. USDA-FNS and the U.S. Department of Health and Human Services should collaborate to achieve expansion of nationally representative collection of data on the dietary intakes for pregnant, breastfeeding, and postpartum women and breastfed infants in the National Health and Nutrition Examination Survey. USDA-FNS should request that the data on breastfeeding women include an indicator on the intensity of breastfeeding (i.e., exclusive or partial).

Rationale: Although results from regional and state studies provided the committee with important evidence about the effects of the 2009 food package changes, no nationally representative study evaluated how the new food packages affected participant satisfaction, participation in the program, and use of the new WIC foods.[2,3] In addition, only limited information was

---

[2] To understand the effect of policy changes on participant purchasing patterns and/or nutrition and health outcomes, a study that applies the difference-in-difference approach, which is common in economics and health information research, to the timing of the policy changes is needed. For example, the U.S. Department of Agriculture created a Supplemental Nutrition Assistance Program (SNAP) Policy Database that includes information on the timing of policy changes and how they affect outcomes. Availability of these data has resulted in informative research about SNAP policies and how they affect outcomes. To understand the effects of the WIC program, it is also important to know when non-participants become participants, and vice-versa, particularly for children.

[3] Near the close of the committee's deliberations, Oh et al. (2016), which is a nationally representative study of whole grain purchases by WIC participants, was published.

available on how participants from different racial, ethnic, and cultural groups selected and used foods in the revised packages.

The EBT system, scheduled for implementation in all states by the year 2020, provides a unique opportunity to collect participant- and state-level data on redemption of issued foods (USDA/ERS, 2014). Under the direction of USDA-FNS, these individual-level data could be collected, anonymized,[4] and analyzed (or, importantly, left disaggregated and made publicly available) to provide, for example, information about regional and national purchasing patterns, price variations, and how purchasing patterns and price variation interact with state-level regulations about cost containment. To determine whether the food package is meeting the needs of participants, it is essential to link the food redeemed to the specific food package. It is also essential that the timing of implementation nationally is clearly documented. Given that it may only be possible to collect these data in states using EBT, data collected before food package revisions are implemented would ensure that a strong baseline is established. Annual collection of state-level policies, paired with the creation of a national EBT database, would help USDA-FNS and other researchers examine the effect of variations in food package policies on redemption of WIC foods and participation in the program. These data could also be added to other online datasets as part of the current open-data initiative (TWH, 2016) to allow access to information collected via the EBT system.[5]

The committee lacked information on how foods in the WIC packages are used in the context of participants' overall diets, in conjunction with participation in other programs, such as the Supplemental Nutrition Assistance Program (SNAP), and in combination with foods purchased with participants' own funds. Such data would inform how the WIC food packages can be designed to optimize the overall diet and complement other food resources. The recently released Food Acquisition and Purchase Survey (FoodAPS) dataset holds the potential for evaluating food acquisition and purchase in addition to household participation in multiple programs. Although there are limitations in the currently available data,[6] subsequent rounds of this survey could modify data collection to better address these issues, in addition to having data on low-income nonparticipants.

Research questions that could complement the various data sources mentioned here, applied in studies that use causal techniques, include:

[4] Data for this purpose would be stripped of all personally identifying information.

[5] Data that are not open-access could be made available by allowing researchers to apply for restricted access to anonymized data in a setting where confidentiality can be protected, following the model of the Federal Statistical System Research Data Centers.

[6] The Food Acquisition and Purchase Survey dataset is limited in terms of verifying WIC participation with administrative data and in linking specific food items acquired and purchased to the use of WIC benefits.

- How do changes to the WIC food packages affect purchasing patterns and redemption of WIC foods?
- How do food purchasing patterns change with WIC participation compared to purchases made in the absence of WIC benefits?
- Do the revised food packages increase participants' satisfaction and improve participation in the program?
- What is the effect of the revised food packages on participants' diets, as measured by Healthy Eating Index–2010 (HEI–2010) score?
- What is the effect of WIC participation on household food security?
- Is there an effect of WIC participation on participant maternal and neonatal health outcomes?

11-4. USDA-FNS should fund data collection and analysis of that data toward optimizing support for breastfeeding and increasing the proportion of WIC participants who choose to initiate and continue breastfeeding, and tailoring food package options to best meet the needs and goals of the breastfeeding dyad. USDA-FNS should examine how breastfeeding outcome data are captured in WIC Management Information Systems and work toward a set of universal breastfeeding indicators that can be captured across systems.

Rationale: Achievement of the committee's vision for further improvements in breastfeeding support through the WIC program requires a targeted research initiative. The proposed revisions to the food packages are intended to support a woman's choice to breastfeed by increasing the quantity and variety of foods available to the breastfeeding mother during the infant's first 6 months. The objective is to increase proximal incentives (closer in time) as well as the distal incentive (further in time) of extended food benefits already being provided in the current packages from 6 to 12 months. The "up to" amounts for formula in the revised packages are intended to allow staff to calibrate formula amounts that meet the needs of each dyad. It is not expected that the food package alone will be sufficient incentive to breastfeed because a woman's decision to breastfeed is influenced by numerous complex factors.

Continued improvements in the coverage and quality of breastfeeding counseling available to WIC participants are necessary to achieve national breastfeeding goals. Adequate support by state and local agencies is important to determine the level of breastfeeding support provided through nutrition services administration funds as well as through peer-counseling funding and other sources. Piloting of various approaches to formula distribution by state and local WIC agencies, particularly in the first 30 days postpartum, would provide a strong evidence base to determine whether providing breastfeeding counseling in conjunction with customizing infant formula helps women to achieve their breastfeeding goals. Behavioral economics research may help elucidate how breastfeeding can be promoted through further revisions to the food packages and/or increased investments in sound breastfeeding protection, promotion, and support efforts.

Specific research questions could include

- From birth to age 1 year, what are the patterns of breastfeeding exhibited by mother–infant dyads on WIC? How well are these patterns aligned with the food packages issued? How is breastfeeding affected by the food package change?
- Paired with support, how does tailoring the food package to provide an amount of formula that supports the needs of the dyad in the first 30 days affect the duration and intensity of breastfeeding?
- What incentives motivate WIC participants to choose to breastfeed as well as to continue to breastfeed beyond 4 to 6 weeks postpartum? Did the package changes affect these outcomes?
- Outside of the food package for mother–infant dyads, what level and type of support (peer counseling, lactation consultation, etc., for what duration/periodicity) is optimal to promote and support breastfeeding?

To investigate these research questions, it will be necessary to collect and evaluate state-level data on the efficacy of various breastfeeding promotion and support practices and policies, including the number of peer counselors available at local agency sites, the ratio of peer counselors to women participants, the state agency formula issuance policy, and demographic characteristics (including race and ethnicity) of WIC participants at the state level. These data could be collected on a routine basis (e.g., once annually), linked to participant outcome data, and disseminated to researchers. If possible, it would be ideal to test different approaches for the promotion of breastfeeding through randomized controlled trials. USDA-FNS could provide funding (and waivers if needed) to allow states to explore how varying policies and resources affect breastfeeding initiation, exclusive breastfeeding duration, and overall duration. This evidence could help ensure that cost-effective approaches are used.[7]

11-5. USDA-FNS should fund research to assess how inclusion of the cash value voucher as a component of WIC food packages affects: food package redemption rates; participant choice of

[7] In alignment with 7 C.F.R. § 246.26, all participant or applicant information would remain confidential.

vegetable and fruit varieties; overall diet quality; and vendor stocking practices.

Rationale: There is a lack of comprehensive national data on WIC food package redemption rates; participant choice of vegetable and fruit varieties; overall diet quality; and vendor stocking practices. EBT redemption data should be used to the fullest extent to capture data on use of the CVV to elucidate redemption rates and vegetable and fruit choices made with the revised CVV. For the next WIC program review, it is also important to understand the extent to which the recommended increased CVV assists WIC participants in meeting their nutritional goals.

Future evaluations of the WIC food packages would also benefit from information on vendor stocking practices for vegetables and fruits as an outcome of increasing the CVV. It would be valuable to understand the feasibility of stocking the new WIC food options as well as the effects of vendor stocking practices on participant purchasing patterns.

Specific research questions could include

- What are the CVV redemption rates, and what factors (CVV amount, region in the United States, participant characteristics, etc.) are associated with higher and lower rates of redemption?
- What do participants purchase with the CVV, and how do participants apportion their purchases of vegetables and fruits, including the variety of vegetables and fruits and selection of vegetables versus fruits?
- Does the revised CVV assist participants to consume a nutritionally adequate diet and meet the recommendations for consumption of vegetables and fruits of the DGA?
- What are the changes in the availability of vegetables and fruits at WIC authorized vendors and in vendor stocking practices before and after changes in the CVV amount? Do vendors increase the diversity of their vegetable and fruit offerings? Do vendors change their WIC authorization status in response to the package changes? How does vendor size relate to stocking requirements and participant options?

11-6. USDA-FNS should fund research to evaluate the feasibility of adjusting the value of the cash value voucher (CVV) in high-cost states and territories (Alaska, Guam, Hawaii, and the U.S. Virgin Islands).

Rationale: Higher amounts of WIC program funds are allotted per-participant to states and territories with a high cost of living, including Alaska, Guam,

Hawaii, and the U.S. Virgin Islands. The average food package costs in these areas are 21, 18, 81, and 82 percent higher, respectively, than the average for all U.S. states and territories (USDA/FNS, 2016a). For most foods in the WIC package, participants receive a specific quantity of the WIC-approved food, an amount that does not vary with the price of the food. However, as a cash benefit, the amount of food available to the participant through the CVV reflects the regional price difference and thus, it is likely that fewer vegetables and fruits can be purchased with the CVV in those high-cost areas. For example, the U.S. Department of Agriculture's Economic Research Service (USDA-ERS) (2011) reported that commonly purchased vegetables and fruits may cost up to 70 percent more in the most expensive markets, compared to the least expensive markets. Therefore, the available benefit varies at the participant level if participants nationwide receive a flat purchase value with the CVV. In the proposed revised food packages, the CVV makes up a larger proportion of the food package benefit than the current packages; thus vegetable and fruit intake may be influenced to a greater degree by geographic variations in their price.

A first step to address the inequity in high-cost areas is to adjust the CVV using the SNAP cost adjustments assigned to these four high-cost regions (see USDA/FNS, 2016b).[8] If adjusted in this manner, on average, the CVV would be 49 percent higher (unweighted; 60 percent when weighted by the state population) for WIC participants in these areas. Inasmuch as WIC participants in these areas make up 1 percent of the total WIC population (USDA/FNS, 2016a), the effect on overall program costs will be minor. A second step would be to consider adjustments that account for higher costs of vegetables and fruits in additional states.

PRIORITIES FOR FUNDING OUTSIDE COST-NEUTRALITY

USDA-FNS asked that the committee identify changes to the food packages that should be made if funding for the WIC food packages is either 10 percent higher or 10 percent lower than cost neutrality. The committee's priority in case of additional funding is enhancement of food package IV (for children).

11-7. The committee recommends that in the case that USDA-FNS has funding above cost neutrality, the value of the CVV should be increased for all children on the program.

---

[8] An alternative for Alaska and Hawaii is to use an adjustment factor based on the Thrifty Food Plan food cost estimates for these two states (USDA/CNPP, 2016).

Rationale: A CVV of $23 (approximately 10 percent above cost-neutral) would allow children adhering to a 1,300-kcal food pattern to meet half of their recommendations for consumption of vegetables and fruits. Retention of children in the WIC program is a concern. Inasmuch as this food package represents approximately 53 percent of all food packages issued, changes to food package IV have a significant effect on overall program costs for food. As a result, the degree to which the committee could enhance this food package within cost-neutral constraints was severely limited, and any changes in this food package likewise limited the degree to which other food packages could be enhanced. The reasons for the decline in WIC participation at 1 year of age and beyond are unknown and likely multifaceted. In the absence of additional information, one strategy to improve child retention may be to enhance food package IV for children ages 1 to less than 5 years.

11-8. The committee recommends that in the case that USDA-FNS has funding below cost neutrality, provision of juice should be further reduced or eliminated across food packages.

Rationale: Elimination of juice would reduce the food package costs by approximately 4 percent. Both the DGA and authoritative guidance for children less than 2 years of age indicate that fruit juice is a less preferred way to meet fruit intake recommendations, compared to whole fruit. Moreover, these sources suggest upper limits for juice intake rather than recommended amounts. The nutrients in juice are also present in many other foods, specifically, whole vegetables and fruits, dairy foods, legumes, and ready-to-eat breakfast cereals.

Should further reductions be needed, the committee recommends targeting the following foods in priority order:

1. Eliminate peanut butter from the food packages. Because of the availability and price of smaller container sizes, it is difficult to provide a supplemental quantity of peanut butter. This is a relatively inexpensive food with a long shelf-life. WIC dollars may be better allocated to foods that provide nutrients more critical to the WIC population than those provided by peanut butter.
2. Further reduce the amount of milk in food package IV-B to 12 quarts. Milk in the proposed revised food package IV-B, although reduced, still provides 75 percent of the recommended dairy intake. Inadequate calcium intake in children of this age group was found to be less than 5 percent.
3. Reduce the quantity of fish that has been added to the revised food packages. Participant acceptability of fish in the revised food

packages is not known. An alternate option would be to add fish only to food packages for women and then assess participant acceptability before revising the food packages for children.

MULTILEVEL APPROACHES TO IMPROVING CONSUMPTION OF WIC FOODS

Nutrition Education

WIC is the only federal nutrition assistance program that *requires* nutrition education as part of its core services. There is some evidence to suggest that the WIC program is a key resource for nutrition education within the WIC-participating population (Hromi-Fiedler et al., 2016; USDA/FNS, 2016a). Effective nutrition education and counseling are essential to encourage WIC participants to consume the foods provided in the food packages. Nutrition education is also a means of encouraging overall healthy dietary behaviors among the WIC population. There is growing recognition that individual and group-based direct education efforts alone are less effective than when they are implemented in the context of multilevel interventions and in connection with the broader community and public health approaches (IOM, 2012). Therefore, it is important to provide effective opportunities for WIC participants to increase their knowledge and skills related to food purchasing, storage, handling, and preparation.

A review of best practices of nutrition education strategies for low-income audiences indicated that effective nutrition education should be theory driven and evidence based; target multiple levels (individual, family, organization, community, and policy); consider the goals, learning styles, culture, and literacy level of participating audiences; and include experiential activities and incentives to reinforce behaviors (Baker et al., 2014). Additionally, models and approaches should allow sites and educators to offer nutrition education strategies in the appropriate frequency and duration to produce behavior change but also with enough flexibility to tailor strategies across contexts and settings (Baker et al., 2014). For example, there is some evidence that the use of hands-on cooking instruction with low-income families is associated with improved dietary behaviors (Hersch et al., 2014; Reicks et al., 2014; Eisenberg and Burgess, 2015). Moreover, recent studies have shown that innovative approaches currently being implemented in WIC, such as Internet-based and participant-centered education, show great promise (Au et al., 2016a,b). USDA-FNS recently released a report describing delivery of nutrition education within WIC, phase I of a three-phase study (USDA/FNS, 2016c). Phase II of the study tests the effect of nutrition education in six pilot regions and phase III is to design a national study. The results will represent the first national study of the efficacy of WIC nutrition education and will be useful in the subsequent review of WIC food packages.

Collaboration between WIC and other USDA programs, such as SNAP-Education and the Expanded Food and Nutrition Education Program as well as other community stakeholders, is a way to provide additional experiences for hands-on nutrition education (USDA/FNS, 2016c) for program participants, as well as increase the availability and affordability of healthy food options through policy, system, and environmental change initiatives, and promote effective use of the CVV within the shopping experience. Use of funds allocated to these programs for nutrition education could be made more effective by coordinating messaging across programs.

In Chapter 4, the committee describes its findings on the high intakes of sodium, saturated fat, and added sugars among WIC participants. Many vegetables and fruits are commonly served with added sodium, saturated fat, or added sugars. Additionally, more participants may have access to canned vegetables as a result of the recommended requirement that states now offer a canned, frozen, or dried form and provide an option to purchase canned legumes. Thus, it is important to include in nutrition education some science-based guidance on how to limit the addition of sodium, saturated fat, and added sugars to foods so that the foods consumed by WIC participants align with the DGA.

Optimizing Redemption and Consumption of WIC Foods

To increase the availability of vegetables and fruits to WIC participants, the committee increased the value of the CVV in the revised food packages by \$4 to \$24. This decision was prompted by evidence that vegetable intakes were particularly low across participant subgroups (see Chapter 4), and evidence that the CVV is more often used to obtain fruits than vegetables. One strategy to encourage participants to select more vegetables with their CVV is "nudging," for example, intentionally naming vegetables first (e.g. "the vegetable and fruit voucher") or suggesting to participants that they should use the CVV as a "vegetable voucher" first and then buy fruits if funds are still left.

Behavioral Approaches Beyond Nutrition Education

A number of studies have cited the shopping experience as a key barrier to selecting and redeeming vouchers or electronic benefits for WIC foods (Woelfel et al., 2004; Bertmann et al., 2014). As discussed in Chapter 5, emerging evidence indicates that behavioral economics approaches could potentially provide additional strategies to overcome this and other barriers to consumption of foods provided in the food packages. Behavioral science draws from principles in economics, marketing, and psychology to influence decision making processes that guide behavior. USDA has maintained a strong focus on the use of behavioral economics approaches to improve dietary quality among individuals and families participating in federal food and nutrition assistance programs (USDA/ERS, 2007). In particular, approaches to reducing cognitive load (the amount of information that must be processed at one time) have been demonstrated to improve individual food-choice behavior (USDA/ERS, 2007; USDA/FNS, 2014). A number of other behavioral economics studies of potential relevance to WIC participants are currently under way, funded through the Behavioral Economics Research Center at Duke University (Ammerman, 2016; BECR, 2016). Outcomes of this and future work may yield additional practical and applicable strategies for improving WIC participant redemption and intake of foods provided in the food packages.

CONSIDERATIONS FOR THE NEXT REVIEW

The committee evaluated a number of potential revisions to the food packages that ultimately were rejected. The committee's key ideas are shown in Appendix Q. In many cases, revisiting these ideas at the time of the next review of the WIC food packages may be helpful as a result of changes in the landscape of food availability, nutritional needs, and participant preferences. Among the potential revisions considered, support for breastfeeding emerged as a priority concern and therefore is discussed below.

Infant Nutrition Needs in the First 6 Months of Life

In contrast to other components of the WIC food packages that were reduced to conform to the committee's definition of "supplemental," the provision of infant formula was retained at its current level of approximately 100 percent of infant needs from birth to 6 months. The committee was concerned that reducing the amount of infant formula currently provided would impose a cost burden on families served by the program. Additionally, the committee found no suitable alternatives for these participants. Moreover, the committee found that, until breastfeeding was fully and universally supported by the program, it would remain aspirational for many WIC participants.

Thus, the committee retained the recommendations of the prior committee (IOM, 2006), which revised the amount of formula provided to infants. However, the committee believes that the provision of formula by WIC should be reconsidered at the time of the next review. Revisions to Dietary Reference Intakes may have occurred by then as well as changes to the composition of infant formulas used in the program. As noted elsewhere in the report, infant formula is procured by WIC through a competitive bidding process with few bidders. The formulas available to WIC participants closely track options available to nonparticipants. Changes to these products have been frequent in recent years, as have increases in prices to the consumer (see section above on functional ingredients). As a result, a future committee could face a different infant formula market, one that could influence the ability of the WIC program to meet an infant's full need for formula.

The fact that WIC currently meets nearly 100 percent of young infants' needs for infant formula as well as the perceived value of that formula may influence women's choices to breastfeed (Haughton et al., 2010; Jensen and Labbok, 2011; Varela Ruiz et al., 2011; Hedberg, 2013). The committee received comments suggesting that reducing the perceived value of the infant packages by reducing the amount of formula provided would result in a shift in women's breastfeeding choices. In the absence of pilot studies demonstrating that this would be the outcome from such a change, paired with uncertainty that the infrastructure currently exists to ensure that all women have the support needed to breastfeed, the committee considered it important to ensure that all needs of young infants continue to be met. In accordance with the recommendation in this report that protection, promotion, and support of breastfeeding should be evaluated and fully supported, it may be warranted for USDA-FNS to consider reducing the amount of formula provided to infants once there is sufficient evidence to do so, and there is adequate support in place for WIC participants who choose breastfeeding. The Center for Nutrition Policy and Promotion Nutrition Evidence Library work under way to support the 2020 DGA (USDA, 2016) is likely to yield information pertinent to further refinement of the infant packages.

CONCLUDING REMARKS

Although the committee completed its task, much work remains. Three major issues emerged as priorities for future consideration: support for breastfeeding, encouraging consumption of vegetables, and availability and use of WIC data.

Historically, the WIC program has given priority to exclusive breastfeeding by optimizing the food package for women who exclusively breastfeed. This committee continued that practice. However, given the barriers to breastfeeding faced by low-income women in the United States, it is possible that WIC may be reaching nearly all those who are willing and able to breastfeed exclusively. To promote and encourage any breastfeeding, the committee also chose to enhance the food package for partially breastfeeding women and allow issuance of this package in the first month postpartum. As stated above, the committee's vision is that all women should receive adequate counseling and support for breastfeeding prenatally through the first month postpartum. This is especially the case for women who find exclusive breastfeeding incompatible with other constraints in their lives, but are nonetheless interested in breastfeeding and can be successful with partial breastfeeding. WIC can enhance its stated commitment to breastfeeding (USDA/FNS, 2016d) by reaching and supporting these women. However, achieving the committee's vision will require the expansion and full coordination of the several WIC resources that promote and support breastfeeding. The committee strongly encourages USDA-FNS to meet this challenge.

Although the committee was able to respond to its primary task by increasing the variety and balance of foods in the WIC food packages, providing some priority nutrients in adequate amounts (i.e., potassium, vitamin D, and choline) is limited even in the DGA food patterns. In addition, finding ways to encourage redemption of vegetables with the CVV remained a challenge. This is because of WIC participants' preference for fruits. Participants who receive the largest increase in the CVV in the revised food packages should be able to satisfy their preference for fruits and begin to purchase more vegetables. However, to increase vegetable redemption, the CVV may have to be substantially increased for all participants and accompanied by appropriate nutrition education and perhaps further incentives as well. In a cost-neutral environment, this may require reductions in the amount of other high-cost items such as dairy products and infant formula, which are provided in amounts at the high end of "supplemental" in the recommended revised packages. To assist USDA-FNS in identifying ways to accomplish this goal, the committee's recommendations include specific ideas for data collection and analyses.

This committee had access to a limited amount of data on redemption and also the distribution of redemption of WIC foods. This information was crucial for understanding how participants use the program, but more such data as well as many other kinds of data that would have assisted the committee were unavailable, so the committee has provided recommendations to address these data needs for future decision making. Moreover, the committee views it as essential that WIC identify ways to increase the availability of program data so interested researchers can contribute their expertise to determine which aspects of the program work and how and which aspects are cost effective and scalable.

The committee's strategy for revisions included several noteworthy innovations that are anticipated to lead to improvements to the WIC food packages. Highlights of these innovations include development of the concept of "supplemental" and its use as a criterion for the revision of the food packages (the concept of supplemental is discussed in Chapter 6); use of data on redemption and the distribution of redemption to inform estimates of actual use of the food packages (an explanation of how redemption data were used is provided in Chapter 7); and consideration of the dyadic nature of infant feeding related to the contents of the food packages (the committee's consideration of the mother–infant dyad is discussed in Chapters 6 and 7). These innovations permitted the committee to make important revisions to the food packages within the constraint of cost neutrality. In particular, the committee was able to balance the food packages to increase the variety of foods included, increase participants' choices within food categories, and develop a more thoughtful and comprehensive approach to the use of the packages to support breastfeeding of all durations and intensities. To be fully effective, the committee's recommended revisions to the food package should be accompanied by the recommendations for implementation presented in this chapter. As the committee's experience indicated, it is necessary for USDA-FNS to invest in data collection and research that can inform the next revision of these packages. These revisions to the food packages, when accompanied by their successful implementation, should improve both the attractiveness of the program to participants and success in meeting the WIC program's goals to promote and support breastfeeding and to safeguard the health of low-income women, infants, and children through the provision of foods that provide key nutrients.

REFERENCES

Ammerman, A. 2016. Buying wisely and well: Managing WIC food costs while improving the WIC customer's shopping experience. *BECR Center at Duke-UNC*. https://becr.sanford.duke.edu/wp-content/uploads/2016/05/BECR-WIC-Research-Brief.pdf (accessed October 3, 2016).

Au, L. E., S. Whaley, K. Gurzo, M. Meza, and L. D. Ritchie. 2016a. If you build it they will come: Satisfaction of WIC participants with online and traditional in-person nutrition education. *Journal of Nutrition Education and Behavior* 48(5):336–342.

Au, L. E., S. Whaley, N. J. Rosen, M. Meza, and L. D. Ritchie. 2016b. Online and in-person nutrition education improves breakfast knowledge, attitudes, and behaviors: A randomized trial of participants in the Special Supplemental Nutrition Program for Women, Infants, and Children. *Journal of the Academy of Nutrition and Dietetics* 116(3):490–500.

Baker, S. A., C. MacKinnon, A. Ammerman, G. Hanula, B. Lohse, M. Scott, E. Serrano, E. Tucker, and M. Wardlaw. 2014. *Best practices in nutrition education for low-income audiences*. Colorado State University. https://snaped.fns.usda.gov/snap/CSUBestPractices.pdf (accessed September 30, 2016).

BECR (Duke-UNC USDA Center for Behavioral Economics and Healthy Food Choice Research). 2016. *Funded 2015 WIC white papers*. https://becr.sanford.duke.edu/funding/wic (accessed August 30, 2016).

Bertmann, F. M., C. Barroso, P. Ohri-Vachaspati, J. S. Hampl, K. Sell, and C. M. Wharton. 2014. Women, infants, and children cash value voucher (CVV) use in Arizona: A qualitative exploration of barriers and strategies related to fruit and vegetable purchases. *Journal of Nutrition Education and Behavior* 46(3 Suppl):S53–S58.

Crowe, K. M., and C. Francis. 2013. Position of the Academy of Nutrition and Dietetics: Functional foods. *Journal of the Academy of Nutrition and Dietetics* 113(8):1096–1103.

Eisenberg, D. M., and J. D. Burgess. 2015. Nutrition education in an era of global obesity and diabetes: Thinking outside the box. *Academic Medicine* 90(7):854–860.

Haughton, J., D. Gregorio, and R. Pérez-Escamilla. 2010. Factors associated with breastfeeding duration among Connecticut Special Supplemental Nutrition Program for Women, Infants, and Children (WIC) participants. *Journal of Human Lactation* 26(3): 266–273.

Hedberg, I. C. 2013. Barriers to breastfeeding in the WIC population. *MCN The American Journal of Maternal/Child Nursing* 38(4):244–249.

Hersch, D., L. Perdue, T. Ambroz, and J. L. Boucher. 2014. The impact of cooking classes on food-related preferences, attitudes, and behaviors of school-aged children: A systematic review of the evidence, 2003–2014. *Preventing Chronic Disease* 11:E193.

Hromi-Fiedler, A., D. Chapman, S. Segura-Pérez, G. Damio, P. Clark, J. Martinez, and R. Pérez-Escamilla. 2016. Barriers and facilitators to improve fruit and vegetable intake among WIC-eligible pregnant Latinas: An application of the health action process approach framework. *Journal of Nutrition Education and Behavior* 48(7):468–477.

IOM (Institute of Medicine). 2006. *WIC food packages: Time for a change*. Washington, DC: The National Academies Press.

IOM. 2011. *Planning a WIC research agenda: Workshop summary*. Washington, DC: The National Academies Press.

IOM. 2012. *Accelerating progress in obesity prevention: Solving the weight of the nation.* Washington, DC: The National Academies Press.

Jensen, E., and M. Labbok. 2011. Unintended consequences of the WIC formula rebate program on infant feeding outcomes: Will the new food packages be enough? *Breastfeeding Medicine* 6(3):145–149.

NASEM (National Academies of Sciences, Engineering, and Medicine). 2016. *Review of WIC food packages: Proposed framework for revisions: Interim report*. Washington, DC: The National Academies Press. doi: 10.17226/21832.

Oh, M., H. Jensen, and I. Rahkovsky. 2016. Did revisions to the WIC program affect household expenditures on whole grains? *Applied Economic Perspectives and Policy* 38(4):578-598. doi: 10.1093/aepp/ppw020.

Reicks, M., A. C. Trofholz, J. S. Stang, and M. N. Laska. 2014. Impact of cooking and home food preparation interventions among adults: Outcomes and implications for future programs. *Journal of Nutrition Education and Behavior* 46(4):259–276.

TWH (The White House). 2016. *Open government initiative*. https://www.whitehouse.gov/open (accessed September 30, 2016).

USDA (U.S. Department of Agriculture). 2016. *USDA-HHS Dietary Guidance Development Project for Pregnancy & Birth to 24 Months (P/B-24)*. http://www.nel.gov/birth-to-24-overview (accessed October 24, 2016).

USDA/CNPP (U.S. Department of Agriculture/Center for Nutrition Policy and Promotion). 2016. *USDA food plans: Cost of food*. https://www.cnpp.usda.gov/USDAFoodPlans CostofFood (accessed September 30, 2016).

USDA/ERS (U.S. Department of Agriculture/Economic Research Service). 2007. *Could behavioral economics help improve diet quality for nutrition assistance program participants?* http://ben.cornell.edu/pdfs/USDA-BeEcon.pdf (accessed December 9, 2016).

USDA/ERS. 2011. *The WIC fruit and vegetable cash voucher: Does regional price variation affect buying power?* https://www.ers.usda.gov/webdocs/publications/eib75/7452_eib75.pdf (accessed December 2, 2016).

USDA/ERS. 2014. *Cost containment in the WIC program: Vendor peer groups and reimbursement rates*. https://www.ers.usda.gov/webdocs/publications/err171/48701_err171_summary.pdf (accessed December 2, 2016).

USDA/FNS (U.S. Department of Agriculture/Food and Nutrition Service). 2014. *Evaluation of the healthy incentives pilot (HIP): Final report*. http://www.fns.usda.gov/sites/default/files/HIP-Final.pdf (accessed December 9, 2016).

USDA/FNS. 2015. *WIC policy memorandum #2015-7 to WIC state agency directors: Medicaid primary payer for exempt infant formulas and medical foods*.

USDA/FNS, 2016a. *WIC program data*. http://www.fns.usda.gov/pd/wic-program (accessed November 7, 2016).

USDA/FNS. 2016b. *FY 2016 maximum allotment amounts for Alaska, Hawaii, Guam and U.S. Virgin islands*. http://www.fns.usda.gov/sites/default/files/snap/FY16-Allotments-AKHIGUVI-1.pdf (accessed September 30, 2016).

USDA/FNS. 2016c. *WIC nutrition education study, phase I report*. http://www.fns.usda.gov/wic-nutrition-education-study-phase-I-report (accessed November 7, 2016).

USDA/FNS. 2016d. *Breastfeeding policy and guidance*. http://www.fns.usda.gov/sites/default/files/wic/WIC-Breastfeeding-Policy-and-Guidance.pdf (accessed November 4, 2016).

Varela Ruiz, M., H. Arroyo, R. R. Davila Torres, M. I. Matos Vera, and V. E. Reyes Ortiz. 2011. Qualitative study on WIC program strategies to promote breastfeeding practices in Puerto Rico: What do nutritionist/dietician's think? *Maternal and Child Health Journal* 15(4):520–526.

Woelfel, M. L., R. Abusabha, R. Pruzek, H. Stratton, S. G. Chen, and L. S. Edmunds. 2004. Barriers to the use of WIC services. *Journal of the American Dietetic Association* 104(5):736–743.

Appendix A

Acronyms and Abbreviations

αTOC	α-tocopherol
μg	microgram or micrograms
AAP	American Academy of Pediatrics
ACC	American College of Cardiology
ADA	American Diabetes Association
AHA	American Heart Association
AHRQ	Agency for Healthcare Research and Quality
AI	Adequate Intake
AMDR	acceptable macronutrient distribution range
AND	Academy of Nutrition and Dietetics
ARA	arachidonic acid
ARS	Agricultural Research Service, U.S. Department of Agriculture
BF	breastfeeding/breastfed
BLS	U.S. Bureau of Labor Statistics
BLUP	best linear unbiased predictor
BMI	body mass index
c	cup or cups
CACFP	Child and Adult Care Food Program
CCRP	California Cancer Research Program
CDC	U.S. Centers for Disease Control and Prevention
CDHS	California Department of Health Services

C.F.R.	Code of Federal Regulations
CG	comparison group
CNPP	Center for Nutrition Policy and Promotion, U.S. Department of Agriculture
COU	calorie for other uses
CPI	Consumer Price Index
CPS	Current Population Survey
CVD	cardiovascular disease
CVV	cash value voucher
d	day or days
DASH	Dietary Approaches to Stop Hypertension
DE	design effect
DFE	dietary folate equivalent
DGA	*Dietary Guidelines for Americans*
DGAC	Dietary Guidelines Advisory Committee
DGV	dark green vegetables
DHA	docosahexaenoic acid
DRI	Dietary Reference Intake
EAR	Estimated Average Requirement
EBT	electronic benefit transfer
ECLS-B	Early Childhood Longitudinal Study-Birth Cohort
EER	Estimated Energy Requirement
EFNEP	Expanded Food and Nutrition Education Program
EPA	eicosapentaenoic acid
EPA	U.S. Environmental Protection Agency
eq	equivalent
ERS	Economic Research Service, U.S. Department of Agriculture
FAFH	food away from home
FAH	food at home
FDA	U.S. Food and Drug Administration
FE	fixed effect
FF	formula fed
FITS	Feeding Infants and Toddlers Study
fl oz	fluid ounce or ounces
FNB	full nutrition benefit
FNS	Food and Nutrition Service, U.S. Department of Agriculture
FoodAPS	National Household Food Acquisition and Purchasing Survey

FP	food package
FPED	Food Patterns Equivalent Database
FPID	Food Patterns Ingredients Database
FY	fiscal year
g	gram or grams
GAO	U.S. Government Accountability Office
GDM	gestational diabetes mellitus
GI	glycemic index
HBW	high birth weight
HCP	health care provider
HEI	Healthy Eating Index
HHS	U.S. Department of Health and Human Services
HMD	Health and Medicine Division, The National Academies of Sciences, Engineering, and Medicine
IFPS II	Infant Feeding Practices Study II
IOM	Institute of Medicine
IRI	Information Resources, Inc.
ISU	Iowa State University
ITO	Indian Tribal Organization
IU	international unit
IV	instrumental variable
kcal	kilocalorie or kilocalories
kg	kilogram or kilograms
KQ	key question
lb	pound or pounds
LBW	low birth weight
LGA	large-for-gestational age
LVL	local vendor liaison
mg	milligram or milligrams
MIS	Management Information System
MMA	maximum monthly allowance
mo	month or months
MUFA	monounsaturated fatty acid
MULO	Total Multi-Outlet
N	sample size
NA	not applicable

NASS	National Agricultural Statistical Service, U.S. Department of Agriculture
NATFAN	National Food and Nutrition Survey
NBDQ	Nutrient-Based Diet Quality
NCGS	non-celiac gluten sensitivity
NCI	National Cancer Institute, U.S. Department of Health and Human Services
NDB	National Nutrient Database for Standard Reference
NHANES	National Health and Nutrition Examination Survey
NHIS	National Health Interview Survey
NIH	National Institutes of Health
NIS	National Immunization Survey
NPNL	nonpregnant, nonlactating
NR	no recommendation or not redeemed
NSA	nutrition services and administrative
NSLP	National School Lunch Program
NSWP	National Survey of WIC Participants
NUPC	national Universal Product Code database
nutr	nutrients
oz	ounce or ounces
P	pregnant
PC	peer counselor
PC-SIDE	PC Software for Intake Distribution Estimation
PedNSS	Pediatric Nutrition Surveillance System
PIH	pregnancy-induced hypertension
PIM	perceived insufficient milk
PIR	poverty-to-income ratio
PNSS	Pregnancy Nutrition Surveillance System
PP	postpartum
PRAMS	Pregnancy Risk Assessment Monitoring System
PUFA	polyunsaturated fatty acid
qt	quart or quarts
RACC	reference amount customarily consumed
RAE	retinol activity equivalent
RD	regression discontinuity
RDA	Recommended Dietary Allowance
Red-Or	red and orange vegetables
RIA	regulatory impact analysis
RTE	ready-to-eat

RTF	ready-to-feed
RWJF	Robert Wood Johnson Foundation
SAS	Statistical Analysis System
SE	standard error
SFA	saturated fatty acid
SGA	small-for-gestational age
SNAP	Supplemental Nutrition Assistance Program
SNAP-Ed	Supplemental Nutrition Assistance Program-Education
SPADE	Statistical Program for Age-adjusted Dietary Assessment
SSI	Supplemental Security Income
TANF	Temporary Assistance for Needy Families
tbsp	tablespoon or tablespoons
tsp	teaspoon or teaspoons
UI	unemployment insurance
UL	Tolerable Upper Intake Level
UPC	Universal Product Code
USDA	U.S. Department of Agriculture
USDA-CNP	U.S. Department of Agriculture, Food and Nutrition Service, Child Nutrition Programs
USDA-FNS	U.S. Department of Agriculture, Food and Nutrition Service
veg/fr	vegetables and fruits
WG	whole grain or whole grain-rich
WHO	World Health Organization
WIC	Special Supplemental Nutrition Program for Women, Infants, and Children
WIC-AI	WIC availability index
wk	week or weeks
WP	white potatoes
WWEIA	What We Eat in America (NHANES)
y	year or years

Appendix B

Glossary

Acceptable macronutrient distribution range (AMDR)	Range of macronutrient intake that is associated with reduced risk of chronic disease, while providing recommended intakes of other essential nutrients
Added sugars	Sugars that are added to foods or beverages when they are processed or prepared, not naturally occurring in foods
Adequate Intake (AI)	The recommended average daily intake level based on observed or experimentally determined estimates of nutrient intake of groups of apparently healthy people that are assumed to be adequate; used when an Estimated Average Requirement (EAR) cannot be determined
Administrative burden	Includes adding unreasonably to staff time and effort, requiring additional systems that are not already in place, or requiring any program modifications that would be disproportionate to the benefit of the change
Anemia	Condition that occurs when the body does not have enough red blood cells or when the red blood cells do not function properly

Baby-Friendly Hospital Initiative	Global program launched by the World Health Organization and the United Nations Children's Fund in 1991 to encourage and recognize hospitals and birthing centers that offer an optimal level of care for infant feeding and mother/baby bonding
Bioavailability	Accessibility of a nutrient to participate in unspecified metabolic and/or physiologic processes
Buckwheat	A proposed WIC whole grain alternative, technically not a grain or related to wheat, derived from the seed of the buckwheat plant
Calories for other uses (COU)	The 2015–2020 *Dietary Guidelines for Americans* defines "calories for other uses" as calories from added sugars and saturated fat, along with calories from added refined starch, as well as additional calories from the recommended food groups, and alcohol
Cash value voucher (CVV)	A monthly voucher in the WIC food package (currently $11 for women and $8 for children) that allows for the purchase of a variety of vegetables and fruits
Celiac disease	An autoimmune disorder that can occur in genetically predisposed people where the ingestion of gluten leads to damage in the small intestine
Competent Professional Authority (WIC Program)	An individual authorized to determine nutritional risks and prescribe supplemental foods. Physicians, registered dietitians, registered nurses and nutritionists are all examples of Competent Professional Authorities
Complementary foods	Foods other than breast milk or infant formula introduced to an infant to provide nutrients
Corn masa flour	A very soft flour made from finely ground hominy or dried corn kernels that have been cooked and soaked in limewater
Cornmeal	Dried corn kernels ground less finely than those in corn masa flour

Cost-neutrality	Refers to the condition that the weighted average per-participant cost of the revised set of food packages falls within 10 cents of the weighted average per-participant cost of the current set of food packages. Under this constraint, the effects of each food package on cost depend on the number of participants represented by that package
Culturally suitable	Foods should align with food preferences and feeding practices based on an individual's ethnic identity and religion
DASH eating plan	The Dietary Approaches to Stop Hypertension (DASH) eating plan is a dietary pattern shown to prevent and control hypertension emphasizing vegetables and fruits, whole grains, and lean meats, while limiting sodium and sugar
Dietary Guidelines for Americans (DGA)	A report published every 5 years by the U.S. Department of Agriculture containing nutritional and dietary information and guidelines for the general public, required by P.L. 101-445, 7 U.S.C. 5341 to be based on the preponderance of current scientific and medical knowledge
Docosahexaenoic acid (DHA)	An omega-3 fatty acid found in cold-water, fatty fish
Dyad	Mother–infant pair in WIC program
Electronic benefit transfer (EBT)	An electronic system that allows a recipient to authorize transfer of their government benefits from a federal account to a retailer account to pay for products received
Estimated Average Requirement (EAR)	A nutrient intake value that is estimated to meet the requirement of half the healthy individuals in a population
Estimated Energy Requirement (EER)	The average dietary energy intake that is predicted to maintain energy balance in a healthy adult of a defined age, gender, weight, height, and level of physical activity consistent with good health

Federal poverty guidelines	Guidelines used by the U.S. government to determine financial eligibility for certain federal programs, issued each year in the *Federal Register* by the U.S. Department of Health and Human Services (HHS)
Final Rule	7 C.F.R. § 246 in the *Federal Register* updated on March 4, 2014, to reflect revisions to the WIC food packages proposed in the 2006 Institute of Medicine report *WIC Food Packages: Time for a Change*
Food allergy	An adverse health effect arising from a specific immune response that occurs reproducibly on exposure to a given food
Food composition data	Calorie and nutrient content of foods
Food insecurity	Limited or uncertain availability of nutritionally adequate and safe foods or limited or uncertain ability to acquire acceptable foods in socially acceptable ways
Food package	A specific set of foods prescribed to each WIC participant on a monthly basis. There are currently seven food packages (eight in the revised set), assigned by age and physiological state (pregnant; breastfeeding; or postpartum, nonbreastfeeding)
Food security	The World Food Summit of 1996 defined food security as existing "when all people at all times have access to sufficient, safe, nutritious food to maintain a healthy and active life"
Full-redemption	All foods prescribed in WIC package were purchased in the quantities available using monthly benefits
Fully breastfed	"Exclusive breastfeeding" is defined by the World Health Organization as giving no other food or drink—not even water—except breast milk. It does, however, allow the infant to receive oral rehydration salts (ORSs), drops, and syrups (vitamins, minerals, and medicines)

Functional ingredient	Nutrient or non-nutrient component added to foods that may provide a health benefit beyond basic nutrition and is considered safe at estimated national levels of consumption
Gestational diabetes	Type of diabetes that is first seen in a pregnant woman who did not have diabetes before she was pregnant
Gestational weight gain	Amount of weight gained during pregnancy
Gluten	Proteins found in wheat, rye, barley, and triticale
Halal	When used in relation to food products, halal refers to any foods that are allowed to be eaten according to Islamic Sharia law. Foods that are not considered halal include pork and its byproducts, alcohol, and animals not slaughtered properly according to Islamic law
Healthy Eating Index–2010 (HEI–2010)	A measure of diet quality that assesses conformance to the *Dietary Guidelines for Americans*
Healthy People 2020	A set of goals and objectives released by the U.S. Department of Health and Human Services with 10-year targets designed to guide national health promotion and disease prevention efforts to improve the health of all people in the United States
Heme iron	Easily absorbed form of dietary iron that comes primarily from meat
Hydrolyzed protein	Protein that has been broken down into its component amino acids
Hypoglycemia	A condition characterized by an abnormally low level of blood sugar (glucose)
Income-to-poverty ratio	Measurement of the depth of poverty as determined by how close a family's or individual's income is to their poverty threshold. Families and individuals with an income-to-poverty ratio of less than 100 percent are identified as being in poverty. An income-to-poverty ratio of 50 percent indicates a family or person is living with in deep poverty

Indian Tribal Organization	Any tribe, band, nation, or other organized group or community, including any Alaska Native village, regional corporation, or village corporation that is recognized by the Secretary of the Interior as eligible for the special programs and services provided by the United States to Indians because of their status as Indians
ISU method	Method developed at Iowa State University (ISU) to estimate the distributions of usual intake of nutrients, foods consumed almost daily, and other dietary components
Jarred infant food meat	Any variety of commercial infant food meat or poultry meeting WIC specifications. Texture may range from pureed through diced
Kosher	When used in relation to food products, kosher means that the item in question meets the dietary requirements of Jewish law. Restrictions include those pertaining to types of animals that can be eaten, the process by which they are slaughtered, and the separation of meat and milk
Lactose intolerance	An inability to digest lactose, which causes symptoms such as bloating, diarrhea, and gas after eating or drinking milk or milk products
Legumes	Any type of mature dry beans, peas, or lentils in dry-packaged or canned forms
Loving Support©	The U.S. Department of Agriculture's (USDA's) national breastfeeding promotion and support campaign (Loving Support Makes Breastfeeding Work©) that provides education, training and outreach materials for staff of the Special Supplemental Nutrition Program for Women, Infants, and Children (WIC). Resources are also available for women and their families and friends and health care providers and community partners
Macronutrient	Dietary components that constitute the bulk of the diet and supply energy and many essential nutrients, including carbohydrates, proteins (including essential amino acids), and fats (including essential fatty acids)

Management Information System (MIS)	A computerized database of information organized and programmed in such a way that it produces regular reports on operations for management in an organization
Maximum monthly allowance (MMA)	The maximum amount of a specific food a participant is allowed in WIC food packages
Micronutrient	Dietary component required by the body in small amounts that are vital to development, disease prevention, and well-being. Micronutrients are not produced in the body and must be derived from the diet
Micropolitan area	Urban areas in the United States that are centered on an urban cluster with a population at least 10,000 but less than 50,000
Nonceliac gluten sensitivity (NCGS)	A form of gluten intolerance that neither meets the diagnostic criteria for celiac disease nor those for wheat allergy
Nonredemption	No foods prescribed in WIC package were purchased using monthly benefits
Nutrient-Based Diet Quality (NBDQ) Index	An index developed for this report to measure of the adequacy of nutrient intake and diet quality in the WIC population based on the mean probability of adequacy for the nine shortfall nutrients, calculated for each individual, as compared to Dietary Reference Intake (DRI) values
Nutrients of public health concern	According to the 2015 Dietary Guidelines Advisory Committee, within the larger category of shortfall nutrients (nutrients inadequately consumed by the U.S. population), nutrients of public health concern are of particular importance because their underconsumption has been linked to adverse health outcomes
Omega-3 fatty acid	An unsaturated fatty acid occurring chiefly in fish oils, reported to benefit cardiovascular health
Partial-redemption	Some amount of foods prescribed in WIC package was purchased with some benefit remaining at the end of the month

Partially breastfed	The World Health Organization's definition of partial breastfeeding is "giving a baby some breastfeeds, and some artificial feeds, either milk or cereal, or other food"
Patient Protection and Affordable Care Act	Comprehensive health insurance reforms enacted to improve access, affordability, and quality of health care for Americans
PC Software for Intake Distribution Estimation (PC-SIDE)	Software for intake distribution estimation developed at Iowa State University
Phased-in cost estimates	Cost estimates for food packages for the 5-year period fiscal year (FY) 2018–FY2022 calculated to account for states implementing the revised food packages at different times
Postpartum women	Women up to 6 months after giving birth, as defined by the *Federal Register*
Preeclampsia	Pregnancy-induced hypertension that occurs after the 20th week (late second or third trimester) of pregnancy
Pregnancy-induced hypertension	A pregnancy complication characterized by high blood pressure, swelling due to fluid retention, and protein in the urine
Rebate	The amount of money refunded under cost containment procedures to any state agency from the manufacturer of the particular food product as the result of the purchase of the supplemental food with a voucher or other purchase instrument by a participant in each state agency's program
Redeemed foods	Foods actually purchased by WIC participants, compared to foods prescribed to WIC participants
Redemption rates	Percentage of prescribed foods issued that are obtained by the participant at the WIC vendor. Rates used in this report were derived through various methods, including consideration of three types of redemption practices: full redemption, partial redemption, and nonredemption

Regression discontinuity	A study design that compares people who are just below an eligibility threshold with those who are just above it, which provides internally valid estimates of eligibility on outcomes—provided that these individuals cannot manipulate their presence below or above the threshold. This design requires using the measure of income that is used by the program rather than survey data
Regulatory impact analysis	A systemic approach to critically assessing the positive and negative effects of proposed and existing regulations and nonregulatory alternatives, from a cost perspective
Revised food packages	Proposed revisions to WIC food packages
Selection bias	A distortion of the measured effect resulting from procedures used to select subjects such that the relation between exposure and disease is different for those who participate and those who would be eligible but do not participate
Sensitivity analysis	Study of how the uncertainty in the output of a model can be attributed to different sources of uncertainty in the model inputs
Shortfall nutrients	Nutrients identified by the Dietary Guidelines Advisory Committee as underconsumed by the U.S. population relative to Dietary Reference Intake (DRI) recommendations
Split tender	Participants may pay the difference out of pocket if their fruit and vegetable purchase exceeds the amount on the cash value voucher
State agency	State agencies administering the WIC program
Statistical Program for Age-adjusted Dietary Assessment (SPADE)	Statistical method for estimating usual dietary intake distributions

Substitutions — Foods that may be selected in place of the prescribed WIC foods in a food category of the WIC food packages. Substitutions for a food in the WIC food categories "must be nutritionally equivalent or superior to the food it is intended to replace"

Supplemental (the concept of) — A committee-developed concept that was used as a target for the food package revisions. It refers to the amounts of nutrients and food groups that the WIC packages that would provide a moderate proportion of an individual's requirement for a particular nutrient or food group. The supplementation target (i.e., proportion of requirement or recommended amount) may differ depending on the nutrient requirement or recommended amount of a food group, the degree to which foods appropriate for the food package and available in the marketplace499 can supply these recommended amounts, and the degree to which cultural food patterns or food preferences can be met

Supplemental food — "Those foods containing nutrients determined by nutritional research to be lacking in the diets of pregnant, breastfeeding, and postpartum women, infants, and children, and foods that promote the health of the population served by the WIC Program as indicated by relevant nutrition science, public health concerns, and cultural eating patterns, as prescribed by the Secretary" (P.L. 95-627 § 17)

Teff — A fine, whole grain—about the size of a poppy seed—that comes in a variety of colors, from white and red to dark brown. Grown predominantly in Ethiopia and Eritrea

Temporary Assistance for Needy Families (TANF) — Federal program that provides grant funds to states and territories to provide financial assistance and related support services to pregnant women and families with one or more dependent children. State-administered programs may include childcare assistance, job preparation, and work assistance

Tolerable Upper Level Intake (UL)	The highest average daily nutrient intake level that is likely to pose no risk of adverse health effects to almost all individuals in the general population
Type 2 diabetes	Chronic condition that affects the metabolism of glucose caused by the body's ineffective use of insulin
Unadjusted estimates	Cost estimates for food packages for the 5-year period FY2018–FY2022 based on the assumption that all WIC agencies implement all changes on April 1, 2018
Universal Product Code (UPC)	A unique 12-digit number assigned to retail goods that identifies both the product and the vendor that sells the product
USDA or DGA food pattern	Food patterns grouped by kilocalorie levels developed by the U.S. Department of Agriculture to help individuals carry out *Dietary Guidelines for Americans* recommendations
Vegan diet	A diet that excludes all animal foods and products
Vegetarian diet	A diet that does not include animal flesh foods (i.e., meat, seafood), but does include other animal products (e.g., eggs, milk, cheese, yogurt)
Vendor (or WIC vendor)	Authorized WIC retailer where participants may redeem WIC foods that are obtained using WIC benefits
Whole grain-rich	Foods that contain at least 50 percent whole grains with the remaining grains enriched, or foods that contain 100 percent whole grains
Whole grains	Whole grains or foods made from them contain all the essential parts and naturally-occurring nutrients of the entire grain seed (bran, germ, and endosperm) in their original proportions

Appendix C

WIC Food Package Regulation

TABLE C-1 Comparison of IOM 2006 Recommendations and USDA and State Implementation Specific to Meeting Dietary Guidance

2006 IOM Report		USDA Action	
Major Proposed Changes	Specific Recommendation	Federal Regulation[a]	State Option
Include fruits and vegetables for all individuals ages 6 months and older	Provide a CVV for fruit and vegetable purchases, \$8 for children and \$10 for women; allow fresh and processed; allow jarred infant vegetables and fruits to infants ages 6 to 12 months. One lb of fresh bananas may replace 8 oz of infant food	Provide a CVV of \$8 for children; \$10 for women; vegetables and fruits may be fresh or processed with no added sugars or fats; vendors must stock at least 2 fruits and 2 vegetables; jarred vegetables and fruits for infants ages 6 to 12 months, may substitute ½ of jars with a CVV for infants ages 9 to 11 months	States must allow fresh and may allow processed; may restrict packaging[b]; may allow farmer's markets to accept vouchers; for infants ages 9 to 11 months, substitution of a portion of jarred infant food vegetables and fruits with a CVV (\$8 for fully BF; \$4 for others) by individual assessment; states may allow the substitution of bananas for infant food as specified in the IOM (2006) report
Include more whole grain products	Allow only whole grain breakfast cereals[c] Allow whole grain bread with other possible whole grain substitutions	At least ½ of all breakfast cereal on each state agency's authorized food list must have whole grain as the primary ingredient by weight *and* meet labeling requirements for making a health claim as a "whole grain food with moderate fat content"	States may select authorized cereals

		Allow whole grain bread, brown rice, bulgur, oats, whole-grain barley, soft corn or whole wheat tortillas, and whole wheat macaroni (pasta) products	States may select authorized breads and substitutions
Reduce amounts of saturated fat for participants ages 2 years and older (thereby reducing cholesterol and total fat provided)	Reduce amounts of milk	Reduce amounts of milk	No option to increase milk amounts
	Permit whole milk for children ages 1 to 2 years; for others milk must be 2% milkfat or less	Permit whole milk between ages 1 and 2 years only; for others milk must be nonfat or 1% only	States may issue fat-reduced milks to infants 1 year of age if weight is a concern
	Reduce quantity of cheese	Reduce cheese and limit substitution rate	No option to increase substitution of cheese for milk
	Reduce quantity of eggs[d]	Reduce quantity of eggs	No option for eggs
Provide more flexibility for WIC state agencies and more variety and choice for WIC participants	In grain category, allow soft corn or whole wheat tortillas, brown rice, oats, bulgur, and barley, as bread substitutes; allow soy beverage, tofu, and yogurt as milk substitutes; allow canned beans; allow tuna, salmon, sardines, and mackerel	Whole grain tortillas (corn or wheat), brown rice, oats, bulgur, barley, and whole wheat macaroni (pasta) products may be substituted for bread; tofu may be substituted for milk; 1 qt yogurt may be substituted for 1qt milk; dried or canned beans; tuna, salmon, sardines, and mackerel permitted as fish options	States must provide bread, milk, dry or canned beans, and at least 2 fish options; additional substitutions at state option States may offer various substitutions in the whole grains category

continued

TABLE C-1 Continued

2006 IOM Report		USDA Action	
Major Proposed Changes	Specific Recommendation	Federal Regulation[a]	State Option
Promote and support breastfeeding, especially full breastfeeding	Provide a $10 CVV for all women	Provide a $10 CVV for all women	No option to change the CVV amount
	Reduce formula to partially breastfed infants	No routine issuance of formula to partially breastfed infants	States may tailor amounts of formula up to the maximum allowance
	Infant formula not provided in the first month to breastfeeding infants	Infant formula may be provided to breastfed infants in the first month, but this should not be standardized	No routine issuance in the first month to breastfeeding mothers, or may provide 1 can of powdered infant formula in the first month
	Fully breastfed infants receive jarred infant food meats in addition to greater amounts of jarred infant food vegetables and fruits	Individual needs should be assessed and the food quantities issued accordingly	Assess individual needs to tailor packages
	Additional quantities of milk, eggs, and cheese; also fish, for fully breastfeeding mothers	Additional quantities of milk, eggs, and cheese; also fish, for fully breastfeeding mothers	No option
Address developmental needs of infants and young children	Slightly increase formula amounts for fully formula-fed infants ages 4 to 5 months	Fully formula fed infants ages 4 to 5 months received a slightly increased amount of infant formula	No option

	Reduce formula amounts for infants ages 6 to 11 months; infant foods provided only at 6 months of age or older (and exclusion of juice)	Reduced maximum amounts of formula; no infant foods provided from 0 to less than 6 months of age	No option
	Jarred infant food and fresh bananas for infants	From 9 months to less than 1 year, half of jarred foods may be substituted with fresh vegetables and fruits[e]; for infants ages 6 months to less than 1 year, fresh bananas may be substituted for a limited amount of jarred infant food fruit	State option to allow the infant fruit and vegetable substitutions
Address obesity concerns	Slightly decrease total food energy provided by the packages after age 4 months (except for fully breastfed infants) including reduced milk, cheese, eggs, and juice	Milk, cheese, eggs, and juice quantities were reduced overall	No option
	Limit sugars in jarred infant food, processed vegetables and fruits, breakfast cereals and whole grains	Limits placed on added or total sugars content of jarred infant foods, processed vegetables and fruit, breakfast cereals, and yogurt	States may further reduce total sugars limits

NOTES: BF = breastfeeding or breastfed; CVV = cash value voucher; lb = pound; oz = ounce; qt = quart or quarts.

[a] Federal regulation information is from the Final Rule issued March 4, 2014. See the documentation for the minimum requirements and specifications for foods including sugar limits and Standards of Identity.

[b] States may not selectively choose the vegetable and fruit varieties allowable, but may restrict packaging type and packaging sizes. Types may be restricted if vendor or participant confusion is anticipated.

[c] At least 51 percent of the grain in the product was required to be whole grain.

[d] The primary reason for reducing the quantity of eggs was to maintain cost-neutrality; fat and cholesterol reduction was a secondary result.

[e] Partially breastfed or fully formula-fed infants may receive a $4 CVV plus 64 ounces of infant food vegetables and fruits; fully breastfed infants may receive an $8 CVV plus 128 ounces of infant food vegetables and fruits.

SOURCES: IOM, 2006; USDA/FNS, 2014a.

TABLE C-2 Timeline for Implementation of the Most Recent WIC Food Package Changes

Deadline for Implementation	Action of State Agencies	Source
1992	FP VII was created to encourage breastfeeding, added two new items: carrots and canned tuna, along with increased amounts of juice, cheese, legumes and peanut butter for women who exclusively breastfeed their infants	WIC Program: Background, Trends, and Economic Issues (USDA/ERS, 2015)
October 1, 2009	New WIC food packages effective February 4, 2008 (CVV for vegetables and fruits, added whole grains, reduced amount of juice, milk, cheese and eggs, allowed greater substitution of foods), must be implemented by August 5, 2009, according to the Interim Rule, later changed to October 1, 2009, to align with the federal fiscal year	WIC Interim Rule (USDA/FNS, 2007); WIC Program: Background, Trends, and Economic Issues (USDA/ERS, 2015)
June 2, 2014	CVV must increase for children from $6 to $8	WIC Final Rule (USDA/FNS, 2014a)
October 1, 2014	State agencies may issue authorized soy-based beverages or tofu to children who receive FP IV based on the determination of a competent professional authority	WIC Final Rule (USDA/FNS, 2014a)
October 1, 2014	States must require only low-fat (1%) or nonfat milks for children over age 2 and women in FP IV through VII	WIC Policy Memorandum 2014-6 (USDA/FNS, 2014b)
April 1, 2015	Split tender CVV must be implemented	WIC Final Rule (USDA/FNS, 2014a)
April 1, 2015*	States may authorize yogurt for children and women in FP III through VII	WIC Final Rule (USDA/FNS, 2014a)
July 1, 2015	States are required to include white potatoes to be eligible for purchase with CVV 15 days after the date of enactment (December 31, 2014), all implementations including education and new product lists completed by July 1, 2015	WIC Policy Memorandum 2015-3 (USDA/FNS, 2015a)
October 1, 2015	CVV for women must increase from $10 to $11	WIC Policy Memorandum 2015-4 (USDA/FNS, 2015b)

NOTES: CVV = cash value voucher; FP = food package.
*Effective date.

CHRONOLOGY OF STATUTES PERTAINING TO THE DEFINITION OF WIC SUPPLEMENTAL FOODS

September 26, 1972: Public Law No. 92-433. The term "supplemental foods" is defined in the original WIC statute, Child Nutrition Act, as amended.

> § 17(f)(3): "Supplemental foods" shall mean those foods containing nutrients known to be lacking in the diets of populations at nutritional risks and, in particular, those foods and food products containing high-quality protein, iron, calcium, vitamin A, and vitamin C. Such term may also include (at the discretion of the Secretary) any food product commercially formulated preparation specifically designed for infants.

July 11, 1973: In what appears to be the first WIC rule (*Federal Register* p. 18447):

> § 246.2(v): "Supplemental food" means any food authorized to be made available under the WIC program.

October 7, 1975: Public Law No. 94-105. Child Nutrition Act §17(f)(3) is amended to include a new, final sentence:

> The contents of the food package shall be made available in such a manner as to provide flexibility, taking into account medical and nutritional objectives and cultural eating patterns.

January 12, 1976: Interim "Revision, Reorganization, and Republication" (*Federal Register* p. 1743) reads:

> § 246.2(t): "Supplemental foods" means the foods authorized by FNS in this part to be made available under the WIC program.

January 9, 1979: Proposed Rule, to comply with section 3 of Public Law No. 95-627 § 3 (beginning *Federal Register* p. 2114) deletes the definition of supplemental foods (no explanation is provided for this change):

> § 246.2 (no "letter" designation): "Supplemental foods" [Reserved]

July 27, 1979: Final Rule, to comply with Public Law No. 95-627 § 3 (beginning *Federal Register* p. 44422):

> § 246.2 (no "letter" designation): "Supplemental foods" [Reserved].

July 8, 1983: Proposed Rule (beginning on *Federal Register* p. 31502) issued to "reduce the regulatory burden on State and local agencies." It states:

> A definition of "supplemental foods" was reserved in the 1979 regulations because of the pending issuance of the proposed food package Regulations. A definition consistent with the legislative definition and past regulatory definitions is proposed in this rulemaking.
>
> § 246.2 (no "letter" designation): "Supplemental foods" means those foods containing nutrients determined to be beneficial for pregnant, breastfeeding, and postpartum women, infants and children, as prescribed by the Secretary in section 246.10.

November 10, 1989: Public Law No. 101-147. Child Nutrition and WIC Reauthorization Act of 1989 continues the statutory emphasis on providing nutrients for which WIC participants are most vulnerable to deficiencies and adds concern regarding nutrient density and how to effectively provide the priority nutrients.

June 30, 2004: Public Law No. 108-265. Child Nutrition and WIC Reauthorization Act of 2004 continues the statutory emphasis on nutrients that are lacking. It also adds language about foods to the definition, still at (b)(14), and adds material to (f)(11) without altering the sentences inserted in 1978. The new (b)(14) reads:

> (b)(14): "Supplemental foods" means those foods containing nutrients determined by nutritional research to be lacking in the diets of pregnant, breastfeeding, and postpartum women, infants, and children, and those foods that promote the health of the population served by the program authorized by this section, as indicated by relevant nutrition science, public health concerns, and cultural eating patterns, as prescribed by the Secretary. State agencies may, with the approval of the Secretary, substitute different foods providing the nutritional equivalent of foods prescribed by the Secretary, to allow for different cultural eating patterns.

Child Nutrition Act § 17, includes the following relevant provisions in a paragraph primarily addressing state operations:

> "(f)(11) SUPPLEMENTAL FOODS—
>
> (A) IN GENERAL—The Secretary shall prescribe by regulation the supplemental foods to be made available in the program under this section.
>
> (B) APPROPRIATE CONTENT—To the degree possible, the Secretary shall assure that the fat, sugar, and salt content of the prescribed foods is appropriate."

REFERENCES

IOM (Institute of Medicine). 2006. *WIC food packages: Time for a change*. Washington, DC: The National Academies Press.

USDA/ERS (U.S. Department of Agriculture/Economic Research Service). 2015. The WIC program: Background, trends, and economic issues, 2015 edition. Washington, DC: USDA/ERS. http://www.ers.usda.gov/media/1760725/eib134.pdf (accessed April 13, 2016).

USDA/FNS (U.S. Department of Agriculture/Food and Nutrition Service). 2007. Special Supplemental Nutrition Program for Women, Infants and Children (WIC): Revisions in the WIC food packages; interim rule, 7 C.F.R. § 246.

USDA/FNS. 2014a. Special Supplemental Nutrition Program for Women, Infants and Children (WIC): Revisions in the WIC food packages; final rule, 7 C.F.R. § 246.

USDA/FNS. 2014b. WIC policy memorandum #2014-6: Final WIC food package rule: Implementation of low-fat (1 percent) and nonfat milks provision. Alexandria, VA: USDA/FNS.

USDA/FNS. 2015a. WIC policy memorandum #2015-3 to WIC state agency directors: Eligibility of white potatoes for purchase with the cash-value voucher. Alexandria, VA: USDA/FNS.

USDA/FNS. 2015b. WIC policy memorandum #2015-4 to WIC state agency directors: Increase in the cash value voucher for pregnant, postpartum, and breastfeeding women. Alexandria, VA: USDA/FNS.

Appendix D

Details of the Committee's Information-Gathering Strategies

WORKSHOP AGENDAS

Examining Evidence on a Role for White Potatoes in WIC Food Packages
Committee to Review WIC Food Packages
October 14, 2014

8:30 am Registration

Introduction and Opening Remarks

9:00 Welcome
Kathleen Rasmussen, Chair, Committee to Review WIC Food Packages

9:10 Opening Remarks
Jay Hirschman, USDA's Food and Nutrition Service

Session 1: Trends in Market Availability and Consumption of White Potatoes

Moderated by Mary Kay Fox, Mathematica Policy Research

9:20 Trends in the Production and Pricing of White Potatoes
Jennifer Bond, USDA's Economic Research Service

9:40 Potato Consumption Trends: Data from the Economic Research Service
Joanne Guthrie, USDA's Economic Research Service
Elizabeth Frazao, USDA's Economic Research Service

10:00 WIC Voucher Purchase Patterns for Fresh Fruits and Vegetables
Stacy Gleason, Altarum Institute

10:20 Panel Discussion with Speakers

Session 2: Products, Processing, and Composition of White Potatoes
Moderated by Rachel Johnson, University of Vermont

10:50 White Potato Products and Processing—Healthy Options
Maureen Storey, Alliance for Potato Research and Education

11:10 Nutrient Content and Bioavailability of White Potatoes
Connie Weaver, Purdue University

11:30 Carbohydrates, Fiber, and Resistant Starch in White Potatoes—Links to Health Outcomes
Joann Slavin, University of Minnesota

11:50 Panel Discussion with Speakers

12:15 pm Lunch

1:00 Public Comments

4:00 Adjourn

Phase I Data-Gathering Workshop
Methods and Approaches to the Assessment of WIC Food Packages
Committee to Review WIC Food Packages
March 12, 2015

8:00 am Registration

Introduction and Opening Remarks

8:30 Welcome
Kathleen Rasmussen, Chair, Committee to Review WIC Food Packages

8:35 Opening Remarks
Jay Hirschman, USDA's Food and Nutrition Service

Session 1: DGAC 2015 and Assessing Food and Nutrient Intakes of the WIC Population
Moderated by Patsy Brannon

8:45 Key Findings from the 2015 Dietary Guidelines Advisory Committee (DGAC) Report with Potential Relevance to the Review of WIC Food Packages
Alice H. Lichtenstein, Tufts University

9:05 USDA Food Patterns Update from the DGAC 2015 Report
Trish Britten, USDA's Center for Nutrition Policy and Promotion

9:25 Proposed Revision of Dietary Reference Intakes for Energy in Preschool-Age Children
Nancy Butte, Baylor College of Medicine

9:45 Dietary Guidance Development Project for Children Birth to 24 Months and Pregnant Women
Joanne Spahn, USDA's Center for Nutrition Policy and Promotion

10:05 Panel Discussion with Speakers

10:25 Break

Session 2: Breastfeeding, Formula Feeding, and Complementary Feeding
Moderated by Susan Baker

10:45 The Impact of the 2009 Food Package Revisions on Breastfeeding in the WIC Population—Lessons Learned
Parke Wilde, Tufts University

11:05 Key Breastfeeding Needs and the Role of WIC Food Packages in Supporting Breastfeeding
Rafael Pérez-Escamilla, Yale University

11:25 Transitioning to Foods
Virginia Stallings, Children's Hospital of Philadelphia

11:45 Panel Discussion with Speakers

12:05 pm Lunch

Session 3: Barriers and Incentives for WIC Participants
Moderated by Shannon Whaley

1:00 Administrative and Participant Experience
Geraldine Henchy, Food Research & Action Center

1:15 Rewards-Based Incentive Programs on Fruit and Vegetable Purchases
Etienne (Tina) Phipps, Einstein Healthcare Network

1:30 Barriers and Incentives from a State Perspective
Stan Bien, Michigan WIC Program

1:45 Panel Discussion with Speakers

Session 4: Characterizing the WIC Population: Health Status and Cultural Food Preferences
Moderated by Tamera Hatfield

2:00 Characterization of Nutrition and Health of Low-Income Populations and Changes Over Time
Jackson Sekhobo, New York State Department of Health

2:20 Food Preferences of Racial/Ethnic Groups Represented in the WIC Population
Lucia Kaiser, University of California, Davis

2:40 Considerations for Medically Fragile Participants
Virginia Stallings, Children's Hospital of Philadelphia

3:00 Panel Discussion with Speakers

3:15 Break

Session 5: The WIC Food Package: Economic and Regulatory Considerations
Moderated by Marianne Bitler

3:30 The Store Environment
Annemarie Kuhns, USDA's Economic Research Service

3:50 Impact of the Infant Formula Market on WIC
Victor Oliveira, USDA's Economic Research Service

4:10 Vendor Response to the 2009 Food Package Revisions
Tatiana Andreyeva, University of Connecticut

4:30 Regulatory Impact Analyses
Edward Harper, USDA's Food and Nutrition Service

4:50 Panel Discussion with Speakers

5:15 Adjourn

Methods and Approaches to the Assessment of WIC Food Packages
Committee to Review WIC Food Packages: Public Comment Session
March 13, 2015

8:30 am Registration

Introduction and Opening Remarks

9:00 Welcome
Kathleen Rasmussen, Chair, Committee to Review WIC Food Packages

Public Comments

9:15 Public Comments

Phase II Data Gathering Workshop
Informing WIC Food Package Recommendations: State, Vendor, and Manufacturer Considerations
Committee to Review WIC Food Packages
March 31, 2016

8:00 am Registration

Introduction and Opening Remarks

8:30 Welcome
Kathleen Rasmussen, Chair, Committee to Review WIC Food Packages

8:40 Opening Remarks
Ronna Bach, Special Nutrition Program Director for the Western Region
Melissa Abelev, Assistant Deputy Administrator, Office of Policy Support

Session 1: Food and Nutrient Intake of WIC Participants
Moderated by Mary Kay Fox

9:25 The 2015 *Dietary Guidelines for Americans*: Overview of Key Changes from 2010 and Relevance to the WIC Population
TusaRebecca Schap, USDA's Center for Nutrition Policy and Promotion

10:00 NHANES: Data Collection Strategy and Future Directions
Kirsten Herrick, U.S. Centers for Disease Control and Prevention

10:35 Break

10:50 Eating Behavior in Young Children
Susan L. Johnson, University of Colorado

11:25 PANEL: Culturally Appropriate Food Options
Janet Jackson Charles, Washington State WIC Director
Delores James, University of Florida
Christina McGeough, Institute for Family Health
Joseph Sharkey, Texas A&M University

12:30 pm Lunch

1:30 The Family Food Economy: The Role of WIC in Meeting Needs
Craig Gundersen, University of Illinois at Urbana-Champaign

Session 2: Implementation and Administration of the Food Packages
Moderated by Shannon Whaley

2:10 PANEL: Program Administration and Vendor Management in WIC
Mary Blocksidge, Massachusetts Vendor Manager
Janet Jackson Charles, Washington State WIC Director
Janet Moran, Wyoming WIC Director
Lindsay Rodgers, Texas WIC Director
Debi Tipton, Project Director, Chickasaw Nation WIC

3:30 Break

Moderated by David Davis

3:45 PANEL: Vendor and Manufacturer Perspectives
Cary Frye, International Dairy Foods Association
Tammy Seitel, General Mills
Clyde Steele, MOM's Fresh Foods
Jeff Stilgenbauer, Kroger

4:45 Break

Moderated by Shannon Whaley and David Davis

5:00 PANEL: WIC Staff and Vendor/Manufacturer Cross-Talk

5:30 Adjourn

Public Comments Session
April 1, 2016

8:00 am Registration

Introduction and Opening Remarks

8:30 Welcome
Kathleen Rasmussen, Chair, Committee to Review WIC Food Packages

8:40 Public Comments

Phase II
Review of WIC Food Packages: Final Data Gathering Session
Optimizing Implementation
June 29, 2016

8:00 am Registration

Introduction and Opening Remarks

8:30 Welcome
Kathleen Rasmussen, Chair, Committee to Review WIC Food Packages

8:40 Opening Remarks
Danielle Berman, USDA's Food and Nutrition Service, Review of Nutrition Education Efforts within WIC

Primary Session
Moderator: Shannon Whaley, Vice-Chair, Committee to Review WIC Food Packages

9:20 Does Nutrition Education Produce Behavior Change?
Jamie Dollahite, Cornell University

9:55 Understanding WIC Fruits and Vegetables Redemption in Virginia
Chuanyi Tang, Old Dominion University
Harry Zhang, Old Dominion University by WebEx

10:30 Break

11:00 Understanding the WIC Shopping Experience
Elizabeth Racine, University of North Carolina at Charlotte

11:35 Federal and State Stocking Regulations Affecting Small WIC Vendors
Jennifer Pelletier, Minnesota Department of Health

12:10 pm Understanding Small Vendor Stocking Challenges and Distribution Systems
Deb Bentzel, The Food Trust
Candace Young, The Food Trust

12:45 Adjourn and Lunch

Public Comments Session

1:00 Registration

Introduction and Opening Remarks

2:00 Welcome
Kathleen Rasmussen, Chair, Committee to Review WIC Food Packages

2:10 Public Comments

EVIDENCE REVIEW STRATEGY

A comprehensive literature review[1] was conducted in phase I to gather evidence to support the final recommendations (see NASEM, 2016, Appendix I). The search was run again in phase II to capture relevant publications released since the phase I interim report. The first step to design the search strategy in phase I was development of a draft of key research questions based on the statement of task, the literature review questions developed for the letter report (IOM, 2015), and other topics outlined by the U.S. Department of Agriculture's Food and Nutrition Service (USDA-FNS) for committee consideration (see Table D-1). In collaboration with National Academies of Sciences, Engineering, and Medicine's Health and Medicine Division staff and committee consultants, committee members refined the key questions, as well as the literature search strategy, study eligibility criteria, and the synthesis of search results, using an iterative process.

Literature Search Strategy

Updated literature searches were conducted to capture relevant studies published after the search end date of the phase I interim report. Electronic literature searches of studies indexed in MEDLINE, PubMed, Agricola, CINAHL (Cumulative Index to Nursing and Allied Health Literature), ERIC (Educational Resources Information Center), PsychINFO, Scopus (including Embase), EconLit, Ageline, GPO Monthly Catalogue, HealthStar, ProQuest Social Science Journals, and ProQuest Dissertation & Thesis Full Text were conducted. First, a broad search was conducted to identify all studies including WIC programs or WIC populations without restrictions to any outcome or study design. Searches were conducted using the National Library of Medicine's Medical Subject Headings (MeSH) keyword nomenclature. All relevant studies with human subjects that were published in the English language from 2005 onward were identified. Duplicate citations across databases were removed before screening. Separate search strategies were developed to identify studies conducted among low-income populations living in the United States. The MEDLINE database was searched using a combination of search terms relating to Medicaid, poverty, and low income, plus search terms relating to firstly, culture or race/ethnicity and diet or feeding behavior or, secondly, food access or accessibility, food environment, food costs, store, and vendor. Furthermore, another MEDLINE search strategy was developed for identifying interventional breastfeeding studies conducted among low-income populations living in

[1] Time and resources were inadequate to carry out a full systematic review. Specifically, the last two steps of a systematic review process were not completed: (1) risk of bias evaluation, and (2) evidence synthesis (which includes evaluation of the strength of the evidence).

TABLE D-1 Evidence Review Key Questions and Study Eligibility Criteria

Key Question (KQ)	Study Eligibility Criteria
1. Nutritional status of WIC Populations	
1a. Are there differences in the status of nutrients of concern, dietary quality, or dietary patterns comparing WIC participants with nonparticipants? 1b. Are there differences in the status of nutrients of concern, dietary quality, or dietary patterns that are associated with the 2009 WIC food package revisions among WIC populations? 1c. Are 2009 WIC food package revisions associated with differences in food package redemption rates? 1d. Are there geographical differences in the status of nutrients of concern, dietary quality, or dietary patterns in the WIC populations?	**Populations of interest:** WIC participants **Exposures of interest:** For KQ 1a, WIC participants versus any definition of nonparticipants For KQ 1b, any definition of pre- and post-2009 WIC food package revisions For KQ 1c, food package redemption rates (WIC benefits redeemed) For KQ 1d, different geographical area (e.g., urban versus rural) **Outcomes of interest:** Intake or biomarker levels of the nutrients of concern, including at least one of the following: vitamin D, vitamin C, iron, folate, potassium, calcium, and dietary fiber WIC food intake levels, and fruits and vegetables or whole grain intake levels Any dietary pattern/index Any measure of diet quality **Study designs of interest:** Any
2. Health status of WIC populations	
2a. What is the prevalence of health outcomes among WIC participants? 2b. Are there differences in health outcomes comparing WIC participants with nonparticipants? 2c. Are there differences in health outcomes that are associated with the 2009 WIC food package revisions among WIC populations? 2d. What is the relationship between the status of nutrients of concern, dietary quality or dietary patterns and health outcomes in the WIC populations?	**Populations of interest:** WIC participants **Exposures of interest:** For KQ 2b, WIC participants versus any definition of nonparticipants For KQ 2c, any definition of pre- and post-2009 WIC food package revisions For KQ 2d, nutrients of concern includes at least one of the following: vitamin D, vitamin C, iron, folate, potassium, calcium, and dietary fiber; any measure of dietary pattern/index or diet quality **Health outcomes of interest:** Child overweight and obesity Maternal/postpartum overweight and obesity Maternal BMI Gestational weight gain Postpartum weight retention Diabetes control Growth outcomes: failure to thrive (rare), underweight, stunting Cognitive development

continued

TABLE D-1 Continued

Key Question (KQ)	Study Eligibility Criteria
	Visual acuity Anemia Iron status Folate status Pregnancy outcomes: birth weight, preterm birth, infant mortality, neural tube defect **Study designs of interest:** Any (except for KQ 2a, see exclusion criteria below) **Exclusion criteria for KQ 2a & 2b:** Case-control study and intervention studies (any design) Not analyses of population-based datasets at the national or state level (such as NHANES, PRAMS, PNSS, or the WIC Minimum Data Set)
3. Breastfeeding promotion and incentivizing	
3a. Is participation in WIC associated with breastfeeding initiation, longer duration, and exclusivity (compared with non-WIC participants)? 3b. What are the factors associated with breastfeeding initiation, duration, and exclusivity among WIC participants? 3c. What are the associations between breastfeeding and [health outcomes] among WIC participants? 3d. What are the effects of breastfeeding promotion on breastfeeding initiation, duration, and exclusivity among WIC participants and among WIC-eligible or low-income populations?* 3e. Are there differences in breastfeeding initiation, duration, or exclusivity that are associated with the 2009 WIC food package revisions among WIC populations?	**Population of interest:** WIC participants For KQ 3d, WIC participants, and WIC-eligible or low-income populations **Exposures of interest:** For KQ 3c, exposures of interest are breastfeeding initiation, duration, or exclusivity For KQ 3e, any definition of pre- and post-2009 WIC food package revisions **Outcomes of interest:** Breastfeeding initiation, duration, and exclusivity Any barriers to breastfeeding For KQ 3c, outcomes of interest are described in "Health outcomes of interest" above under KQ 2. **Study designs of interest:** Any (except for KQ 3d, see below) For KQ 3d, include only interventional studies or programmatic studies with active intervention to promote breastfeeding

TABLE D-1 Continued

Key Question (KQ)	Study Eligibility Criteria
4. The role of WIC food packages in preventing food insecurity	
4a. Is food insecurity associated with WIC participation? 4b. What are the associations between food insecurity and [health outcomes] of WIC populations? 4c. Are there differences in food insecurity that are associated with the 2009 WIC food package revisions among WIC households?	**Population of interest:** WIC participants **Exposures of interest:** For KQ 4a, WIC participants versus any definition of nonparticipants For KQ 4b, exposures of interest are any measure of food insecurity/security, and outcomes of interest are described in "Health outcomes of interest" under KQ 2 For KQ 4c, any definition of pre- and post-2009 WIC food package revisions **Outcomes of interest:** For KQ 4a, any measure of food insecurity/security **Study designs of interest:** Any
5. Racial or ethnic differences in infant/child feeding practices and food intake patterns	
5a. Among caregivers of WIC participants, nonparticipants, or low-income infants or children, are there racial or ethnic differences in their practices or beliefs regarding infant/child feeding and food intake patterns? 5b. Among WIC participants, nonparticipants, or low-income women, are there racial or ethnic differences in their personal food intake patterns, eating practices, or beliefs?	**Population of interest:** For KQ 5a, caregivers of WIC participants, non-participants or low-income infants or children For KQ 5b, WIC participants, nonparticipants or low-income women **Exposures of interest:** Different racial or ethnic groups **Outcomes of interest:** Assessment of diet quality in WIC participants or low-income women and/or children comparing race/ethnicities or focusing on one race/ethnicity Breastfeeding behaviors, perceptions, intentions, cultural factors, and experiences in WIC participants or low-income women comparing race/ethnicities or focusing on one race/ethnicity Parental feeding practices, beliefs, and behaviors comparing race/ethnicities or focusing on one race/ethnicity Diet and overweight/obesity comparing race/ethnicities or focusing on one race/ethnicity Food purchasing and preparation among different race/ethnicities or focusing on one race/ethnicity Ethnic differences in home food environment among WIC or low-income families Perceptions of eating healthy among low-income mothers and children **Exclusion criteria:** Not relevant to low-income mothers and children Not in the United States Not related to food and nutrition

continued

TABLE D-1 Continued

Key Question (KQ)	Study Eligibility Criteria
6. Market availability of current WIC foods	
6a. What are the availability, costs, or purchase patterns of WIC foods among WIC vendors or vendors in low-income neighborhoods nationwide? 6b. What is the accessibility of WIC participants (or low-income individuals) to WIC foods? 6c. What are the determinants of store choice for WIC participants (or low-income consumers)? 6d. Were there changes in WIC food purchase patterns or availability associated with the 2009 WIC food package changes?	**Inclusion criteria:** Economics of food choices and availability in low-income neighborhoods Retail food environment and healthy food availability in low-income neighborhoods Geographic, racial, ethnic, and socioeconomic disparities in the availability of food stores among low-income women Fruit and vegetable availability and selection Regional food price variations in low-income neighborhoods **Exclusion criteria:** Not relevant to low-income mothers and children Not in the United States Not related to food and nutrition
7. Administrative feasibility and efficiency for vendors	
7a. Are there differences in sales or other concerns that are associated with the 2009 WIC food package revisions among WIC-authorized vendors?	**Inclusion criteria:** Qualitative interviews of WIC vendor store owners or employees Any study comparing sales between pre- and post-2009 WIC food package revisions among WIC vendors
8. Barriers and incentives for WIC participants, potential participants, and their families	
8a. What are the barriers and incentives to WIC program participation or acceptance of WIC food packages?	**Inclusion criteria:** Any relevant data related to barriers and incentives to WIC program participation or acceptance of WIC food packages

NOTES: BMI = body mass index; KQ = key question; NHANES = National Health and Nutrition Examination Survey; PNSS = Pregnancy Nutrition Surveillance System; PRAMS = Pregnancy Risk Assessment Monitoring System.

*A supplemental search on Medline was conducted to identify interventional studies of breastfeeding promotion or support in low-income populations for this key question.

the United States using the combinations of the low-income search with additional MeSH terms for culture and continental population groups and a broad search for breastfeeding, infant nutrition, and human milk. The search strategies are described in Table D-2.

Study Selection

Abstrackr software (abstrackr.cebm.brown.edu), Endnote, and Microsoft Excel were used to manage the search outputs, screening, and data abstraction. After a training session to ensure understanding of the inclusion and exclusion criteria, title/abstract screening was conducted in duplicate using a screening form that listed the inclusion and exclusion criteria and allowed selection of reasons for exclusion. A third reviewer reconciled the discrepant title/abstract selections. Full-text articles of all accepted title/abstracts were then retrieved and screened by one reviewer based on the study eligibility criteria. Second-level screening of full text articles was conducted by two reviewers and differences reconciled by a third reviewer. The literature search and study selection are summarized in Table D-2 and Figure D-1.

Identification of Relevant Reports

In addition to the literature search described above, relevant IOM reports and government reports related to the task, also published since 2005, were identified and evaluated. The U.S. Department of Agriculture's Economic Research Service (USDA-ERS), USDA-FNS, and Agricultural Research Service (USDA-ARS) websites were searched for reports relevant to WIC and other topics identified as relevant by the key questions.

Additional Literature Searches

In phases I and II, additional literature searches were conducted to address specific chapter topics, for example, to identify information to support a review of relevant nutrition-related health risks, to understand food allergies, and other food intolerances, and to understand the health effects of fruit juice or high-fat dairy as examples.

COMMITTEE WIC SITE VISITS AND SHOPPING EXPERIENCE

USDA-FNS asked that the majority of committee members visit a WIC site and experience shopping as a WIC participant prior to development of the phase II report. Between March and June 2015, committee members visited a total of 14 WIC sites and vendors either in their home state, another state, or both. The visits were organized to ensure geographic and cultural diversity, a balance of sites issuing paper vouchers versus using electronic benefit transfer (EBT), committee member availability, site staff availability, and activity at the site (e.g., days of greater participant flow and provision of group education). A list of sites visited by city and state is presented in Table D-3.

TABLE D-2 Medline Search Strategy to Identify Relevant Literature

Search No.	Search Terms
	WIC search
1	"Women, Infants, and Children".af. [af=all fields]
2	WIC.af.
3	"Special Supplemental Nutrition Program".af.
4	1 or 2 or 3
5	limit 4 to (english language and yr="2005-Current")
	Supplemental low-income search for KQ 5 and KQ 6
1	exp Medicaid or exp Poverty [exp=search for requested subject heading and terms related to subject heading]
2	("low income" or "low-income").mp. [mp=search title, abstract, original title, name of substance word, subject heading word, protocol supplementary concept, rare disease supplementary concept, unique identifier]
3	1 or 2
4	United States.cp. [cp=country of publication]
5	3 and 4
6	exp Food
7	(access or accessibility).mp.
8	exp Environment or environment.mp.
9	costs.mp. or exp "Costs and Cost Analysis"
10	"purchase pattern".tw. [tw = search title, abstract, MeSH headings, other terms, chemical names, secondary source identifier, person name as subject]
11	store.mp.
12	vendor.mp.
13	or/7-12
14	6 and 13
15	5 and 14
16	exp Diet
17	exp Breast Feeding/ or exp Bottle Feeding/ or exp Feeding Behavior
18	16 or 17
19	exp Culture
20	exp Continental Population Groups
21	ethnicity.mp.
22	or/19-21
23	18 and 22

TABLE D-2 Continued

Search No.	Search Terms
24	5 and 23
25	15 or 24
	Supplemental breastfeeding intervention search for KQ 3e
1	infant nutrition.mp. or exp Milk, Human/
2	human milk.mp.
3	(human adj2 milk).tw.
4	breast milk.mp.
5	breastmilk.mp.
6	breast feeding.mp.
7	breastfeeding.mp.
8	breastfeed$.mp.
9	breast fed.mp.
10	breastfed.mp.
11	(breast adj2 fed).tw.
12	exp lactation/
13	(lactating or lactation).mp.
14	or/1-13
15	limit 14 to english language
16	follow-up studies/
17	(follow-up or followup).tw.
18	exp Case-Control Studies/
19	(case adj20 control).tw.
20	exp Longitudinal studies/
21	longitudinal.tw.
22	exp Cohort Studies/
23	cohort.tw.
24	(random$ or rct).tw.
25	exp randomized controlled trials/
26	exp random allocation/
27	exp double-blind method/
28	exp single-blind method/
29	randomized controlled trial.pt.
30	clinical trial.pt.

continued

TABLE D-2 Continued

Search No.	Search Terms
31	controlled clinical trials/
32	(clin$ adj trial$).tw.
33	((singl$ or doubl$ or trebl$ or tripl$) adj (blind$ or mask$)).tw. (82507)
34	exp PLACEBOS/
35	placebo$.tw.
36	exp Research Design/
37	exp Evaluation Studies/
38	exp Prospective Studies/
39	exp Comparative Study/
40	or/16-39
41	15 and 40
42	limit 41 to (addresses or bibliography or biography or case reports or congresses or consensus development conference or consensus development conference, NIH or dictionary or directory or editorial or festschrift or government publications or interview or lectures or legal cases or legislation or letter or news or newspaper article or overall or patient education handout or periodical index)
43	limit 41 to comment and (letter or editorial).pt.
44	41 not (42 or 43)
45	limit 44 to humans
46	exp Medicaid/ or exp Poverty/
47	("low income" or "low-income").mp.
48	46 or 47
49	United States.cp.
50	48 and 49
51	45 and 50
52	limit 51 to yr="2005 -Current"
53	exp Culture/
54	exp Continental Population Groups/
55	ethnicity.mp.
56	or/53-55
57	45 and 56
58	United States.cp.
59	57 and 58
60	limit 59 to yr="2005 -Current"
61	52 or 60

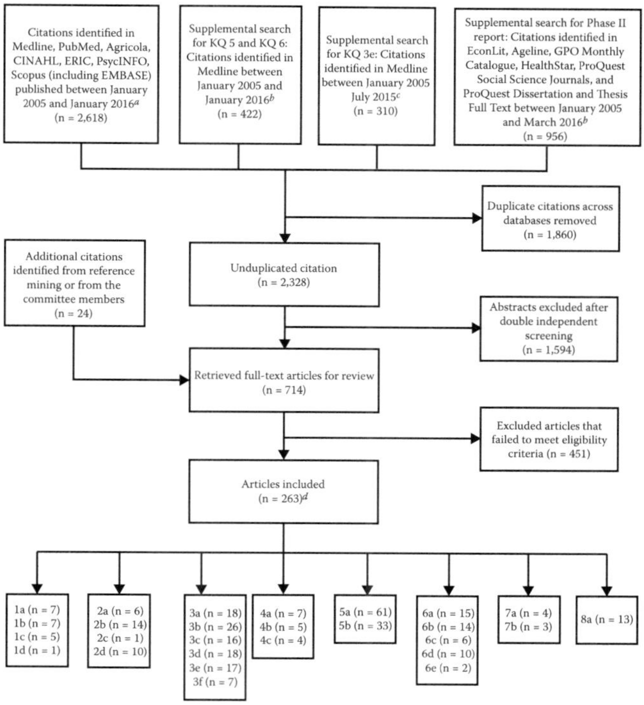

FIGURE D-1 Literature search and study selection flow.
NOTES: CINAHL = Cumulative Index to Nursing and Allied Health Literature; ERIC = Education Resources Information Center; GPO = Government Publishing Office; KQ = key question.

[a] Search strategy was designed for identifying all studies conducted in WIC programs or WIC populations without restriction to any outcome or study design (referred to as "WIC search" herein).

[b] For KQ 5 and KQ 6, a separate search strategy was developed for identifying studies conducted among low-income populations living in the United States using a combination of MeSH or search terms for Medicaid, poverty, and low income (referred to as *low-income search* herein). The low-income search was then combined with search terms relating to culture or race/ethnicity and diet or feeding behavior (KQ5), as well as terms relating to food access or accessibility, food environment, food costs, store, and vendor (KQ6).

[c] A supplemental search of Medline was developed for identifying breastfeeding interventional studies conducted among low-income populations living in the United States using a combination of the low-income search with additional MeSH terms for Culture and Continental Population Groups and a broad search for breastfeeding, infant nutrition, and breast milk (KQ 3e).

[d] Sum of the total number of articles across all KQs is greater than the total number of articles included because one article can provide data relevant to more than one KQ.

TABLE D-3 WIC Sites Visited by the Committee to Review WIC Food Packages

State	City
Connecticut	Hartford
Illinois	Chicago
Iowa	Ames
Kentucky	Newport
Massachusetts	Sommerville
Michigan	Detroit
Nevada	Las Vegas
New York	Kenmore
Oklahoma	Chickasaw Nation
Texas	McAllen
Vermont	Burlington
Virginia	Alexandria
West Virginia	Charleston
Wyoming	Cheyenne

The committee members adhered to the following agenda during site visits:

- Become familiar with the flow of clinic operations and intake.
- If possible, observe a WIC enrollment from start to finish. Alternatively, observe a WIC certification appointment from start to finish.
- If occurring at the time of the visit, observe a group education class.
- If occurring at the time of the visit, observe a prenatal and/or breastfeeding class.
- Observe the orientation to WIC foods and use the voucher/EBT card.
- If a breastfeeding Peer Counselor is available, learn about delivery of such services at that site.
- Obtain an EBT card or voucher to complete the shopping experience.
- Visit a local WIC-authorized vendor to locate and purchase WIC foods.

Committee members prepared written reports and shared their experiences during a closed session. The most outstanding comment from committee members was the variability across WIC sites in several programmatic aspects, as summarized in Box D-1. As described elsewhere in this report,

BOX D-1

Committee Site Visits: Key Perceptions

A key take-away for committee members was that states vary widely in their structure and program implementation. The U.S. Department of Agriculture's Food and Nutrition Service (USDA-FNS) offers states a variety of implementation options. A summary of the points of variability is provided here with examples.

Program Component	*Variations*
Services offered in conjunction with WIC	Medical, dental, sexually-transmitted disease testing, immunization check, voter registration; other sites offer exclusively WIC-based services
Clinic flow	Depends on the size of the staff; the process may be handled largely by one or a different staff person for each stage
Breastfeeding support	Breastfeeding support offered via peer counseling or collocated breastfeeding clinic paid for by WIC funds varies. Some sites have International Board-Certified Lactation Consultants (IBCLCs) on staff. Time spent talking to prenatal participants about breastfeeding plans varies. Provision of materials and supplies (including pumps, educational pamphlets, and incentives to breastfeed) varies
Education	Group classes, one-on-one instruction, and/or online instruction. Detail of food guides vary (with or without photos, multiple languages)
Vendors	WIC-only vendors, WIC-authorized grocery and corner stores, home delivery (Vermont only)
State food options	Forms of produce permitted for purchase with the cash value voucher vary widely, with some states offering fresh only. States vary in the number of options and brands of WIC foods as well as in the availability of state-approved foods at each vendor. Choices may sometimes be made at the store or, alternatively, must be made before the food package is issued
Cost-containment practices	These include "least expensive brand" policies and offering of regular-sodium or regular-fat only options

continued

BOX D-1 Continued

In-store labeling	All WIC foods labeled, specific foods labeled, or no WIC foods labeled
Checkout process	With the exception of one state, the electronic benefit transfer (EBT) process is faster and less noticeable to other shoppers than the paper voucher process; the ease of the transaction depends on staffing and staff knowledge, food labeling, consumer knowledge, accuracy of store databases, and other factors

Other notes:

Participant racial and ethnic diversity is wide overall, but varies by state. The staff is typically attuned to the needs of participants in their region, providing education accordingly. Mechanisms were usually in place to serve clients in multiple languages. There was positive feedback from users of mobile-based applications when available in the state.

WIC foods that were difficult to find on more than one occasion include the 16-ounce loaf of bread or whole wheat pasta and yogurt with the required sugar limits.

difficulties finding a 1-pound loaf of whole wheat bread were noted. Similarly, in states where whole wheat pasta is permitted for purchase, finding a product meeting the 1-pound specification was difficult. Check-out efficiency, although not quantifiable, appeared to be qualitatively improved with the EBT instrument.

Some WIC personnel with whom the committee met on site visits expressed concern about the 18-ounce container of peanut butter, because not all peanut butter vendors offer this size. They and also public commenters expressed concern that manufacturers frequently change package sizes. These changes can affect availability to participants when WIC state agencies define the allowable package sizes to contain costs, which may not align with package size revisions. WIC participants are an important customer base, and it benefits manufacturers to be cognizant of WIC rules, particularly considering potential variation across states.

PUBLIC COMMENTS

A summary of the major public comment themes received over the course of the study is presented in Table D-4.

TABLE D-4 Summary of Public Comments Submitted for Review by the Committee to Review WIC Food Packages

Proposed Modification	Rationale Provided
CVV:	
Mandate that states offer both fresh and some form of processed fruit and vegetable in the CVV	There is no nutritional loss in other forms Would reduce confusion for participants with family members whose CVV does allow the purchase of other forms Longer shelf life Offering all forms of fruits and vegetables improves self-efficiency and correlates with greater consumption Offering all forms of fruits and vegetables maximizes the CVV benefit
Increase the CVV and reduce the juice benefit	The DGA support nutrient dense foods in their whole form. Excess juice consumption is a risk factor for increased calorie consumption and tooth decay
Milk:	
Allow purchase of 2% or whole milk	Literature shows no difference between 1% and 2% milk in childhood weight gain. Some WIC participants will only drink nonfat or low-fat milk if they add chocolate syrup to it
Reduce the amount of milk and increase the CVV amounts of cheese/yogurt	WIC gives too much milk. If more than one family member on WIC, gallons of milk would not fit standard refrigerator. Allowing whole and 2% milk while reducing the amount of milk would save money and still provide the enough of the dairy recommendation for a supplemental program
Allow almond, rice, or coconut milk to accommodate allergies	Some participants have both milk and soy allergies
Whole grains:	
Offer more whole grain options (e.g., whole grain pasta, rolls)	Increase flexibility
Consider adding "ancient grains": spelt, kamut, quinoa, farro, teff, amaranth, chia, sorghum, freekeh, and millet	Provide a greater variety of gluten-free alternatives
Increase whole grain bread sizes to 24–26 oz per month	Difficult to find certain sizes; would likely be cost neutral as stores charge the same for 16 oz versus 26 oz loaves
Include enriched pasta. Permit flexibility of whole grain pasta package sizes up to 16 oz	Increase flexibility

continued

TABLE D-4 Continued

Proposed Modification	Rationale Provided
Canned fish:	
Offer pregnant women canned seafood	The DGA recommend more seafood. Women are under-consuming seafood. Canned fish are a convenient, versatile, and nutritious form of protein
Add canned wild Alaskan salmon	Comments regarding nutritional value and supporting local economy in Alaska
Offer tuna as an option for children	Pediatricians recommend introducing solid foods, including seafood into a children's diet around 4–6 months. Survey data show that only 10% of children meet the recommendation for seafood intake
Cereal:	
Increase options for hot cereals (e.g. single packages)	Participants would like more options
Allow only high fiber and low sugar cereal	Cereals with a high glycemic load can have a large impact on blood glucose levels throughout the day. High fiber cereals can help prevent chronic diseases
Reduce options or amounts of breakfast cereals	WIC should not be encouraging consumption of processed foods like ready-to-eat cereals
Yogurt:	
Allow all fat levels of yogurt for all participants	Concerns that the restriction for only whole milk yogurt for 1-year-olds is challenging at the retail levels (limited yogurt availability in some stores; yogurt not labeled as whole milk)
Reduce the allowed sugar content of yogurt to align with the DGA. Consider reducing to 30 grams of sugar per 8 oz of yogurt	Specification of <40 grams of total sugar is too generous given that many popular yogurts contain lower levels. Manufacturers are working to lower sugar contents. CACFP recently adopted a level of 23 grams of sugar per 6 oz of yogurt
Increase the amount of yogurt allowed as a substitute for milk	Many families would prefer to have more yogurt to reduce the amount of excess milk they receive. Yogurt is a preferred food
Consider flexibility in yogurt package sizes to allow 30 to 32 oz combined	The majority of yogurts on the market are smaller container sizes. Smaller sizes are more likely to be on sale. Yogurts may be mixed to meet a 30 to 32 oz requirement

TABLE D-4 Continued

Proposed Modification	Rationale Provided
Cheese:	
Allow cheese for pregnant and postpartum women	Cheese can be tolerated better than milk for those who are lactose intolerant
Allow additional cheese as a substitute for milk	Over the past 4 decades, consumption patterns of fluid milk have fallen while cheese and yogurt consumption have shown increased acceptance in the American diet
Peanut Butter/Legumes:	
Make canned beans an option	Offering canned beans in addition to dry maximizes likelihood of consumption and participant satisfaction. Canned beans outsell bagged dry beans 11 to 1. Preparation time should be taken into consideration for dried beans
Decrease amount of peanut butter, consider limiting additives allowed for peanut butters including hydrogenated oils and sweeteners added as "seasoning," allow natural nut butters	Packages have too much peanut butter. Many participants have peanut allergy
Eggs:	
Increase egg allowance	Eggs are an important protein source for toddlers and pregnant moms
Allow more eggs in place of beans/peanut butter; allow more beans/peanut butter in place of eggs	Cholesterol is important for central nervous system development Accommodate participant preferences
Juice:	
Increase CVV and remove or reduce juice	Participants ask for more fruits and vegetables in place of juice
Allow partial or full replacement of the juice benefit with CVV	The DGA support nutrient dense foods in their whole form to optimize nutrient content. Juice increases risk of tooth decay Mixed message of recommending that clients reduce juice intake and then issuing benefits for large quantities of juice Request by recipients to reduce juice
Infant foods:	
Allow states to issue infant CVV in addition to jarred infant fruits and vegetables to offer additional forms of fruits/vegetables	Would reduce confusion among participants and allows more shelf stable fruits/vegetables for families in rural areas

continued

TABLE D-4 Continued

Proposed Modification	Rationale Provided
Reduce infant food meats for fully breastfed infants. Consider replacing with beans or raw ground meats	Staff report that the majority of families do not redeem infant meats. They are seen as unpalatable Families can make their own baby foods
Flexibility for infants ages 6–12 months to use fresh fruits and vegetables instead of jarred foods	Excessive amounts of baby foods increase risk of abuse by moms selling foods for cash
Reduce the amount of baby foods to exclusively breastfed infants	Infant cereal and infant fruits and vegetables provided by WIC are inappropriate texture for this age group. Infant cereal is under-redeemed and WIC participants request adult cereal for their growing infant to transition to finger feeding
Consider additional complementary foods for infants ages 9–11 months as they are transitioning to soft table foods such as regular breakfast cereal	Many infants at this age are well transitioned to table foods and reject jarred infant food. May also incentivize parents to recertify their child at the end of the first year
Allow 11-month-old infants to opt for the child food package	
Special diets and other:	
Expand substitutions for food allergies and vegetarians Offer vegan substitutions in the eggs/fish categories	Currently no vegan WIC substitutions for egg and fish categories. DGA recommend increased consumption of plant foods. Vegetarians might be at risk for protein, iron, B12, zinc, calcium, and vitamin D deficiencies
Continue to allow organic foods and Farmers Market Nutrition Program benefits Expand organic food options at the state level	Organic foods are perceived by many participants to be of improved safety or nutritional quality compared to conventionally produced foods
Administration:	
Consider a flexible range of package sizes that allow practical and cost-effective implementation	16-oz size of bread and 16-oz whole wheat pasta are difficult to obtain, vegetable juices not available in 48 oz sizes
Consider practical application of recommendations	Often difficult for staff to explain allowable items and difficult for participants to find items at store
Incentivize breastfeeding by increasing the dollar amount of CVV for fully breastfeeding women above postpartum, pregnant, and partially breastfeeding	The food package is a powerful vehicle for supporting breastfeeding in WIC. Since the original implementation of the interim rule, the amount of CVV in other food packages for women has also increased, diluting the value of the incentive for fully breastfeeding women

TABLE D-4 Continued

Proposed Modification	Rationale Provided
Allow states to convert food dollars equal to the amount spent on a fully formula fed infant to administrative funds for breastfeeding education.	This would be consistent with CACFP rule that allows participants to receive reimbursement when mother directly breastfeeds her infant and receives no additional food component
Simplify method for determining infant formula quantities/add flexibility to minimum and maximum ranges	The current method makes it difficult for programs to accommodate frequent industry changes to package sizes
Provide CVVs instead of specific foods for all food groups	Simplify shopping experience, eliminate need for cost containment (participants will be elastic consumers), reduce vendor fraud
Revisit cost containment of formula	Rebate model is unsustainable and some argue it violates the World Health Organization code
Do not place the 67 kcal per 100 mL minimum energy requirement on standard infant formula but allow for the regulatory range of 63 to 71 kcal per 100 mL	Increasing prevalence of childhood obesity. The best estimates for the energy content of breastmilk is in a somewhat lower range than earlier studies, between 62–63 and 65–71 kcal per mL. Current recommendation is at odds with AAP and European guidelines
Redefine "fully breastfed"	Definition of "fully breastfed" is not helpful
Ensure implementation dates allow for adequate planning, food list printing, local staff and vendor training, and data system updates. Staggering of implementation dates is undesirable for coordinating these components.	Effectively administer the WIC program, ensure integrity, and facilitate efficiency
Fully utilize the overage allowance for "cost neutral"	Maximize opportunities to supplement nutrition while remaining within parameters of cost neutrality

NOTES: AAP = American Academy of Pediatrics; CACFP = Child and Adult Care Food Program; CVV = cash value voucher; DGA = *Dietary Guidelines for Americans*; oz = ounce or ounces. This table summarizes only the public comments relevant to the task or very commonly submitted and is not inclusive of all submitted comments. All public comments are accessible through the National Academies Public Access File (Email: paro@nas.edu).

REFERENCES

IOM (Institute of Medicine). 2015. *Review of WIC food packages: An evaluation of white potatoes in the cash value voucher: Letter report*. Washington, DC: The National Academies Press.

NASEM (National Academies of Sciences, Engineering, and Medicine). 2016. *Review of WIC food packages: Proposed framework for revisions: Interim report*. Washington, DC: The National Academies Press. doi: 10.17226/21832.

Appendix E

USDA-Funded Studies of the 2009 Food Package Changes

TABLE E-1 USDA-Funded Studies Evaluating Outcomes of the 2009 WIC Food Package Revisions

Reference	Funding Source	Study Design and Objective	Population	General Findings
Andreyeva and Luedicke, 2013: Federal food package revisions: Effects on purchases of whole-grain products	USDA	Pre-post design using scanner data to assess how the revisions affected purchases of bread and rice among WIC-participating households in Connecticut and Massachusetts	2,137 WIC-participating households in Connecticut and Massachusetts	2009 revisions significantly increased purchases of whole grain bread and rice among WIC participating families.
Andreyeva and Luedicke, 2014: Incentivizing fruit and vegetable purchases among participants in the Special Supplemental Nutrition Program for Women, Infants, and Children	USDA	Pre-post design using scanner data to examine the impact of the newly implemented CVV on fruit and vegetable purchases	2,137 WIC-participating households in Connecticut and Massachusetts	Fresh and frozen vegetable purchases increased by 17.5% and 27.8% respectively, and fresh fruit purchases increased by 28.6%.
Andreyeva et al., 2011: Changes in access to healthy foods after implementation of the WIC food package revisions	USDA	Evaluate the impact of the WIC food package revisions using multiple determinants of access to healthy food	252 (all) convenience stores and non-chain grocery stores in 5 towns of Connecticut, including 33 WIC-authorized stores and 219 non-WIC stores	Strong evidence that stores responded to the food package revisions by improving the availability and variety of healthy foods in urban and suburban settings, especially in WIC-authorized stores

Andreyeva et al., 2012: Positive influence of the revised Special Supplemental Nutrition Program for Women, Infants, and Children food packages on access to healthy foods	USDA	Pre-post design using a standardized store inventory instrument to evaluate the impact of the revisions using multiple determinants of access to healthy food	252 (all) convenience stores and nonchain grocery stores in five towns of Connecticut, including 33 WIC-authorized stores and 219 non-WIC stores	Access to healthy foods improved using a composite score measure mostly due to increased availability and variety of whole grain products in urban and suburban settings, especially in WIC-authorized stores.
Andreyeva et al., 2013: Effects of reduced juice allowances in food packages for the Women, Infants, and Children Program	USDA	Pre-post design using scanner data to describe changes in purchases of 100% juice and other beverages among WIC participants after the revisions	2,137 WIC-participating households in Connecticut and Massachusetts	Purchases of 100% juice among WIC households declined by 25%. Little compensation occurred from non-WIC funds for juice or other beverages.
Andreyeva et al., 2014: The positive effects of the revised milk and cheese allowances in the Special Supplemental Nutrition Program for Women, Infants, and Children	USDA	Pre-post design using scanner data to examine the effect of the revisions on milk and cheese, and saturated fat intakes	515 WIC households in Connecticut and Massachusetts	Whole-milk share declined in WIC milk purchases with no change in non-WIC purchases. Total milk volume fell by 14.2%, whole milk by half, and WIC-eligible cheese by 37.2%. Saturated fat from milk and cheese declined by 85 g/month per household in Connecticut and 107 g/month per household in Massachusetts.

continued

TABLE E-1 Continued

Reference	Funding Source	Study Design and Objective	Population	General Findings
Gleason and Pooler, 2011: The effects of changes in WIC food packages on redemptions: Final report	USDA	Multimethod, cross-sectional exploratory study to assess participant satisfaction with the revisions by monitoring redemptions before and 6, 12, or 18 months after the 2009 food package changes	WIC participants in Wisconsin: 126,850 prior to the food package change and 116,956 after the food package change	Overall positive response to the food package changes. Decreases were noted in redemptions that differed among racial and ethnic subpopulations. Use of the CVV among racial and ethnic subpopulations were also disproportionate.
Herman et al., 2006: Choices made by low-income women provided with an economic supplement for fresh fruit and vegetable purchase	CCRP, CDHS, USDA, NIH, ASNS	Nonequivalent control-group design to investigate whether supplemental financial support specifically for purchase of fresh fruits and vegetables (bimonthly vouchers at the level of $10/wk for 6 months) would result in high uptake of the supplement, and what the individuals would choose to purchase	602 women enrolled at 3 WIC sites in Los Angeles, California	Wide variety of items purchased at supermarket and farmers' market sites. The 10 most frequently mentioned items: oranges, apples, bananas, peaches, grapes, tomatoes, carrots, lettuce, broccoli, and potatoes. Farmers' market potatoes: 9.1% of total fruit and vegetable items reported. Supermarket potatoes: 10.4% of total fruit and vegetable items reported.

IOM, 2011: Planning a WIC research agenda—workshop summary	USDA	Workshop to guide planning for the use of significant WIC research dollars	Considered the WIC target population	Defined research priorities in the areas of birth outcomes, obesity, breastfeeding, food security, nutritional status, and nutrition education, as well as cost, benefits, and effectiveness of the program.
Joyce and Reeder, 2015: Changes in breastfeeding among WIC participants following implementation of the new food package	USDA/ ERS	Linear regression of national survey data to analyze changes in breastfeeding among WIC participants before and after the new food package	PRAMS in 19 states 2004–2010, PedNSS in 16 states 2007–2010, NIS from 50 states and DC 2004–2010	Data showed steady upward trends in ever-breastfed infants on WIC but not statistically different from trends in breastfeeding among non-WIC low-income.
Kim et al., 2013: Mothers prefer fresh fruits and vegetables over jarred infant fruits and vegetables in the new Special Supplemental Nutrition Program for Women, Infants, and Children food package	USDA	Repeated cross-sectional survey to examine WIC participant use and satisfaction with jarred infant foods, preference for CVVs versus jarred infant foods, and variations among ethnic groups	2,996 participants who received WIC in California in 2010 and California WIC redemption data	Participants reported high satisfaction with the CVV and jarred infant foods with significant variations across ethnic groups. About two-thirds of participants preferred CVV over jarred infant foods. Redemption rates for jarred foods declined with increasing age of infant across all ethnic groups.
Kreider et al., 2016: Identifying the effects of WIC on food insecurity among infants and children	USDA	NHANES analysis to examine the effects of WIC on the nutritional well-being and food security of infants and young children	4,614 low-income infants and children less than 5 from 1999–2008 NHANES	WIC was estimated to reduce the prevalence of child food insecurity by at least 3.6 percentage points (20%).

continued

TABLE E-1 Continued

Reference	Funding Source	Study Design and Objective	Population	General Findings
May et al., 2015: Special Supplemental Nutrition Program for Women, Infants, and Children (WIC) Infant and Toddler Feeding Practices Study 2 (ITFPS-2): Intention to Breastfeed	USDA	Pre-post telephone survey to examine the effects of WIC on attitudes around breastfeeding; comparing data from 1995 to 2013	A nationally representative sample of 2,649 women either pregnant or having a child under 3 months of age	Overall increase in perceptions of the positive benefits of breastfeeding; overall decrease in the number of women with specific perceived barriers to breastfeeding; increase in number of women reporting that breastfeeding is painful, and no one else can feed the infant.
O'Malley et al., 2014: Use of a new availability index to evaluate the effect of policy changes to the Special Supplemental Nutrition Program for Women, Infants, and Children (WIC) on the food environment in New Orleans	CDC, USDA	Assess changes before and after revisions using a new index developed to monitor the retail environment's adoption of these new food supply requirements (WIC-AI)	139 and 128 supermarkets, medium and small WIC stores, and non-WIC food stores in New Orleans, LA, were surveyed before and after 2009 package changes, respectively	Median WIC-AI score increased in medium and small stores. In small stores, this increase was mostly attributed to increased availability of cereals and grains, juices and fruit, and infant fruits and vegetables.
Ritchie et al., 2014: Satisfaction of California WIC participants with food package changes	USDA	Cross-sectional telephone interviews to assess California WIC participant satisfaction with the revisions, compare based on language preference and timing of WIC enrollment	2,996 WIC participants in California in 2010	Most (91.3%) were satisfied with checks for new WIC foods (fruits/vegetables, whole grains, and lower-fat milk), and 82.7% were satisfied with amounts of foods reduced in the new packages in WIC before the revisions.

				(milk, cheese, eggs, juice). A higher percentage of Spanish speakers than English speakers reported satisfaction. A higher percentage of newer enrollees reported satisfaction compared to those participating
Rose et al., 2014: The influence of the WIC food package changes on the retail food environment in New Orleans	CDC, USDA	Pre-post comparison group design with repeat in-store observations to examine the effect of the revisions on the availability of healthy foods in small stores	102 small stores in New Orleans were visited in 2009 and 91% of these revisited in 2010 (27 WIC and 66 non-WIC)	WIC stores were more likely to improve the availability of lower-fat milks than non-WIC stores and more likely to improve the availability of whole grains. WIC stores showed a relative increase in varieties of fresh fruits and shelf life of vegetables.
USDA/FNS, 2011: Evaluation of the birth month breastfeeding changes to the WIC food packages	USDA	Pre-post study to examine changes in breastfeeding initiation, duration, or intensity that occurred following issuance of the 2007 Interim Rule, detailing the food package revisions	17 randomly sampled local WIC agencies, data collected shortly before and shortly after implementation of the Interim Rule	Notable differences in package assignments were observed, including decreases in the partial breastfeeding package, and increases in the full breastfeeding and full formula packages; infants receiving no formula in the first month increased; the proportion receiving the maximum allowance of formula also increased. No differences were observed in breastfeeding rates or intensity; a slight increase in duration was observed.

continued

TABLE E-1 Continued

Reference	Funding Source	Study Design and Objective	Population	General Findings
USDA/FNS, 2012: Effects of the Special Supplemental Nutrition Program for Women, Infants, and Children (WIC): A review of recent research	USDA	Comprehensive literature review on WIC program impacts between 2002 and 2010 (published research) and 1999 to 2010 ("gray" literature). Report is intended as an update of the review published by USDA/ERS in 2004	Peer-reviewed studies focusing on WIC published between 2002 and 2010 or unpublished studies completed between 1999 and 2010	Prenatal WIC participation is consistently positively associated with gestational age and mean birth weight and negatively associated with incidence of low and very low birth weight when not adjusted for gestational age. There is no clear evidence of an association between WIC and adequate weight gain during pregnancy.
USDA/FNS, 2013: WIC food cost report, fiscal year 2010	USDA	Estimate the average monthly food costs for each WIC participant subgroup and total dollars spent on 17 major categories of WIC-eligible foods in 2010; data are compared to 2005	National estimates for participation and national average retail prices for each WIC food category were used to generate cost estimates for each food package	The average monthly food cost with rebates in 2010 was $41.44. Costs increased 11% compared to 2005, below the Consumer Price Index for food at home. The relative cost of the infant food package increased.
USDA/FNS, 2015: WIC food packages policy options II	USDA	Examine state agency responses to policy options in the Final Rule, determine differences in food options and cost containment measures across state agencies, observe changes in WIC food lists before and	86 state agencies representing 99.98% of all WIC participants	WIC participants were offered more options after the implementation of the revisions. WIC participants have access to foods consistent with recommendations made by the *Dietary Guidelines*

		after implementation of the revisions		*for Americans* and by the American Academy of Pediatrics. State agencies employ a variety of cost containment strategies while increasing options for participants.
USDA/FNS, 2016: WIC participant and program characteristics 2014: Food package report	USDA	A supplement to the WIC participant and program characteristics (PC) report, this report provides an overview of the foods prescribed to participants, including a description of the changes in prescription amounts due to the revisions	PC 2014 dataset of participant data submitted by 90 state agencies, approaching 100% of all WIC participants	Between 2008 and 2012, prescriptions of infant formula dropped by 2.3 to 2.4% for younger and middle infants and 4.1% for older infants.
Whaley et al., 2012: Revised WIC food package improves diets of WIC families	USDA	Pre-post cross-sectional telephone surveys to explore the impact of the revisions on WIC participant consumption of fruit, vegetables, whole grain food, and lower-fat milk	3,004 California WIC participants in 2009; 2,996 in 2010	Whole grain consumption increased by 17.3 percentage points. Whole milk consumption by caregivers and children who usually consumed whole milk decreased by 15.7 and 19.7% respectively. Lower-fat milk consumption increased accordingly. Small but significant increases in consumption of vegetables and fruits were observed.

continued

TABLE E-1 Continued

Reference	Funding Source	Study Design and Objective	Population	General Findings
Wilde et al., 2012: Food-package assignments and breastfeeding initiation before and after a change in the Special Supplemental Nutrition Program for Women, Infants, and Children	USDA	Measure changes pre-post WIC package changes in WIC food-package assignments, WIC infant formula amounts, and breastfeeding initiation	National random sample of 17 local WIC agencies. Administrative records for 206,092 dyads with an infant age 0–5 months in the sampled WIC agencies	After the revisions, fewer mothers received the partial breastfeeding package. More mothers received the full breastfeeding package and the full formula package.
Zenk et al., 2012: Fruit and vegetable availability and selection: Federal food package revisions, 2009	USDA, RWJF	Quasi-experimental design with two pre-policy and one post-policy observation to examine availability and selection of commonly consumed and culturally specific vegetables and fruits at authorized WIC vendors before and after the revisions	Data from WIC vendors in 7 northern Illinois counties from 2008 to 2010 (n = 329, 346, and 364 in 2008, 2009, and 2010, respectively)	Availability and selection of overall fresh vegetables and fruits and availability of African-American culturally specific fresh vegetables and fruits improved after the policy change. Modest improvements in overall availability of canned low-sodium vegetables and frozen vegetables and fruits were observed.
Zenk et al., 2014: Impact of the revised Special Supplemental Nutrition Program for Women, Infants, and Children (WIC) food package policy on fruit and vegetable prices	USDA, RWJF, NIH	Quasi-experimental design with two pre-policy and one post-policy observation to observe changes in fruit and vegetable prices pre-post WIC policy changes	Data from WIC vendors in 7 northern Illinois counties from 2008 to 2010	Revisions contributed to modest reductions in fruit and vegetable prices. WIC participants' purchasing power can differ depending on type of WIC vendor and neighborhood.

NOTES: ASNS = American Society of Nutrition Sciences; CCRP = California Cancer Research Program; CDC = Centers for Disease Control and Prevention; CDHS = California Department of Health Services; CVV = cash value voucher; ERS = USDA's Economic Research Service; NHANES = National Health and Nutrition Examination Survey; NIH = National Institutes of Health; NIS = National Immunization Survey; PedNSS = Pediatric Nutrition Surveillance System; PRAMS = Pregnancy Risk Assessment Monitoring System; RWJF = Robert Wood Johnson Foundation; USDA = U. S. Department of Agriculture; WIC-AI = WIC availability index.

REFERENCES

Andreyeva, T., and J. Luedicke. 2013. Federal food package revisions: Effects on purchases of whole-grain products. *American Journal of Preventive Medicine* 45(4):422–429.

Andreyeva, T., and J. Luedicke. 2014. Incentivizing fruit and vegetable purchases among participants in the Special Supplemental Nutrition Program for Women, Infants, and Children. *Public Health Nutrition* 18(1):33–41.

Andreyeva, T., J. Luedicke, A. E. Middleton, M. W. Long, and M. B. Schwartz. 2011. Changes in access to healthy foods after implementation of the WIC food package revisions. Washington, DC: USDA/ERS.

Andreyeva, T., J. Luedicke, A. E. Middleton, M. W. Long, and M. B. Schwartz. 2012. Positive influence of the revised Special Supplemental Nutrition Program for Women, Infants, and Children food packages on access to healthy foods. *Journal of the Academy of Nutrition and Dietetics* 112(6):850–858.

Andreyeva, T., J. Luedicke, A. S. Tripp, and K. E. Henderson. 2013. Effects of reduced juice allowances in food packages for the Women, Infants, and Children Program. *Pediatrics* 131(5):919–927.

Andreyeva, T., J. Luedicke, K. E. Henderson, and M. B. Schwartz. 2014. The positive effects of the revised milk and cheese allowances in the Special Supplemental Nutrition Program for Women, Infants, and Children. *Journal of the Academy of Nutrition and Dietetics* 114(4):622–630.

Gleason, S., and J. Pooler. 2011. *The effects of changes in WIC food packages on redemptions: Final report*. Altarum Institute. http://naldc.nal.usda.gov/download/50613/PDF (accessed March 2, 2016).

Herman, D. R., G. G. Harrison, and E. Jenks. 2006. Choices made by low-income women provided with an economic supplement for fresh fruit and vegetable purchase. *Journal of the American Dietetic Association* 106(5):740–744.

IOM (Institute of Medicine). 2011. *Planning a WIC research agenda: Workshop summary*. Washington, DC: The National Academies Press.

Joyce, T., and J. Reeder. 2015. Changes in breastfeeding among WIC participants following implementation of the new food package. *Maternal and Child Health Journal* 19(4):868–876.

Kim, L. P., S. E. Whaley, P. H. Gradziel, N. J. Crocker, L. D. Ritchie, and G. G. Harrison. 2013. Mothers prefer fresh fruits and vegetables over jarred baby fruits and vegetables in the new Special Supplemental Nutrition Program for Women, Infants, and Children food package. *Journal of Nutrition Education and Behavior* 45(6):723–727.

Kreider, B., J. V. Pepper, and M. Roy. 2016. Identifying the effects of WIC on food insecurity among infants and children. *Southern Economic Journal* 82(4):1106–1122.

May, L., C. Borger, S. McNutt, G. Harrison, N. Weinfield, C. MacAllum, and J. Montaquila. 2015. *WIC ITFPS-2 infant report: Intention to breastfeed*. Rockville, MD: Westat http://www.fns.usda.gov/sites/default/files/ops/WICITFPS2-Prenatal.pdf (accessed June 1, 2016).

O'Malley, K., B. G. Luckett, L. F. Dunaway, J. N. Bodor, and D. Rose. 2014. Use of a new availability index to evaluate the effect of policy changes to the Special Supplemental Nutrition Program for Women, Infants, and Children (WIC) on the food environment in New Orleans. *Public Health Nutrition* 18(1):25–32.

Ritchie, L. D., S. E. Whaley, and N. J. Crocker. 2014. Satisfaction of California WIC participants with food package changes. *Journal of Nutrition Education and Behavior* 46(3 Suppl):S71–S78.

Rose, D., K. O'Malley, L. F. Dunaway, and J. N. Bodor. 2014. The influence of the WIC food package changes on the retail food environment in New Orleans. *Journal of Nutrition Education and Behavior* 46(3 Suppl):S38–S44.

USDA/ERS (U.S. Department of Agriculture/Economic Research Service). 2004. *Effects of Food Assistance and Nutrition Programs on Nutrition and Health: Volume 3, Literature Review.* Washington, DC: U.S. Department of Agriculture. https://www.ers.usda.gov/webdocs/publications/fanrr193/30240_fanrr19-3_002.pdf?v=41479 (accessed March 1, 2017).

USDA/FNS (U.S. Department of Agriculture/Food and Nutrition Service). 2011. *Evaluation of the birth month breastfeeding changes to the WIC food packages*: USDA/FNS. http://www.fns.usda.gov/sites/default/files/BirthMonth.pdf (accessed March 9, 2016).

USDA/FNS. 2012. *Effects of the Special Supplemental Nutrition Program for Women, Infants, and Children (WIC): A review of recent research.* Alexandria, VA: USDA/FNS. http://www.fns.usda.gov/sites/default/files/WICMedicaidLitRev.pdf (accessed September 15, 2016).

USDA/FNS. 2013. *Fiscal year 2010: WIC food cost report.* Alexandria, VA: USDA/FNS. http://www.fns.usda.gov/sites/default/files/WICFoodCost2010_0.pdf (accessed December 21, 2016).

USDA/FNS. 2015. *WIC food packages policy options II, final report.* Alexandria, VA: USDA/FNS. http://www.fns.usda.gov/wic-food-package-policy-options-ii (accessed December 21, 2016).

USDA/FNS. 2016. *WIC participant and program characteristics 2014 food package report.* Alexandria, VA: USDA/FNS. http://www.fns.usda.gov/wic-participant-and-program-characteristics-2014-food-package-report (accessed August 30, 2016).

Whaley, S. E., L. D. Ritchie, P. Spector, and J. Gomez. 2012. Revised WIC food package improves diets of WIC families. *Journal of Nutrition Education and Behavior* 44(3):204–209.

Wilde, P., A. Wolf, M. Fernandes, and A. Collins. 2012. Food-package assignments and breastfeeding initiation before and after a change in the Special Supplemental Nutrition Program for Women, Infants, and Children. *American Journal of Clinical Nutrition* 96(3):560–566.

Zenk, S. N., A. Odoms-Young, L. M. Powell, R. T. Campbell, D. Block, N. Chavez, R. C. Krauss, S. Strode, and J. Armbruster. 2012. Fruit and vegetable availability and selection: Federal food package revisions, 2009. *American Journal of Preventive Medicine* 43(4):423–428.

Zenk, S. N., L. M. Powell, A. M. Odoms-Young, R. Krauss, M. L. Fitzgibbon, D. Block, and R. T. Campbell. 2014. Impact of the revised Special Supplemental Nutrition Program for Women, Infants, and Children (WIC) food package policy on fruit and vegetable prices. *Journal of the Academy of Nutrition and Dietetics* 114(2):288–296.

Appendix F

Changes in the WIC Food Packages and Program Participation

To determine whether regulatory changes made to the Special Supplemental Nutrition Program for Women, Infants, and Children (WIC) food packages are associated with coincident changes in program participation, the committee compared the number of WIC participants with data to the number of individuals eligible for program participation at the state level (USDA/FNS, 2015a). The resulting proportion of participants reflects both the program generosity (the income limit for participation in the program) as well as the number of categorically and income-eligible individuals by state and year, with the eligibility calculations including adjustments for income eligibility or eligibility through participation in other programs as well as other adjustments made to the Current Population Survey Annual Social and Economic Supplement data (USDA/FNS, 2015b). The committee plotted these trends and estimated models of these program coverage rates, that is, the number of participants/number eligible by state and year as a function of the share of the year the new package was in effect for, state-fixed effects, and some controls for the state of the economy (the unemployment rate), and, in some specifications, year-fixed effects and program participation rates per-person in the state (participation rates in the Temporary Assistance for Needy Families [TANF] program and the Supplemental Nutrition Assistance Program [SNAP] and participation rates in the regular, extended and emergency Unemployment Compensation program [Bitler and Hoynes, 2016]). The state-fixed effects controlled for time invariant differences in state participation among WIC eligibles, and the year-fixed effects controlled for national-level shocks. The committee included these in the model because there was variation in the exact month of implementation of the 2009 food package change across states, with New York and Delaware implementing in January and many other states not implementing until the regulatory deadline (dates are reported in Appendix F of USDA/FNS, 2012). The models were estimated by both ordinary least squares and weighted least squares methods, with the eligibility totals used as weights to produce population-representative results. The data span the period from 2006 to 2012. The variance/covariance matrices and associated inference allow for arbitrary within-state correlations of the error terms.[1] Note that the eligibility shares were only available for all WIC participants rather than by eligibility category.

Figure 1-3 of the phase I report (NASEM, 2016) shows the time series of the aggregate national program coverage rate components—the national total number of participants by calendar year and the national total number of eligibles by calendar year. There is little evidence that the number of participants in 2009 changes any more than the number of eligible persons. Figure F-1 shows coverage rates (take-up by eligible individuals) for selected states. Again, coverage does not seem to move systematically in 2009. The raw correlation between the annual coverage rate and the share of the year a state had the new package in place is 0.031 (i.e., holding everything else constant, implementing the new package everywhere would be associated with a 3.1 percentage point increase in the coverage rate relative to a pre-2009 rate of 61 percentage points). However, 2009 marks the end of the Great Recession (using the National Bureau of Economic Research ending date); 2009 also marks the peak year for the number of WIC eligibles in the data (see NASEM, 2016, Figure 1-3) suggesting the importance of adjusting these comparisons for the business cycle. Further, associated with the stimulus, there were expansions in the generosity of SNAP benefits (which ended in November 2013), expansions in the Federal Medical Assistance Percentages matching rate for Medicaid expenditures, and a stimulus-associated TANF emergency fund. Since categorically eligible individuals who participate in any of these programs are automatically eligible for WIC, there is possible concern that failing to control for effects of other programs might bias estimates of the effects of the initial rollout of the new food package. The committee therefore estimated a series of regressions with the unemployment rate and unemployment insurance recipiency per capita as well as SNAP and TANF caseloads per capita as controls in addition to state- and year-fixed effects (regression results and controls in Tables F-1 and F-2).

[1] The standard errors are produced using the software package Stata 13.1 and are adjusted for arbitrary correlation of the error terms within state, using a method known as robust clustering. When the independent variable is constant across states or when regression errors are correlated within states, standard errors computed the standard way are inappropriate for hypothesis tests (Rogers, 1993). Robust-clustering corrects standard errors and makes them appropriate for hypothesis testing.

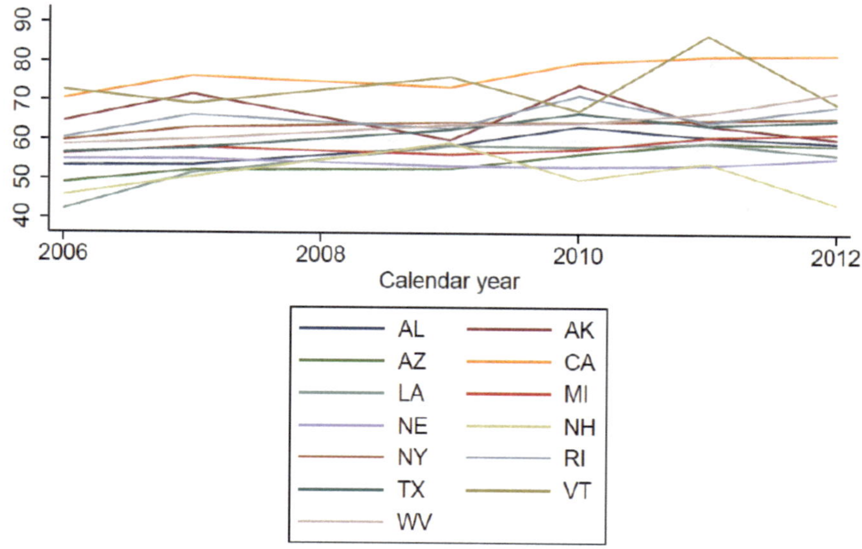

FIGURE F-1 Proportion of individuals participating in WIC of those eligible for WIC by year for selected states.
SOURCES: USDA/FNS, 2011, 2013, 2014, 2015a; Bitler and Hoynes, 2016.

Table F-1 shows the findings controlling for year-fixed effects. However, despite the fact that there is variation across states within 2009 which allows the effect of partial year implementation to be identified in a model with year-fixed effects, another approach might leave out the year-fixed effects. The latter is not the preferred approach because the period before implementation plus most of the period of partial implementation occurred in the middle of the Great Recession. The committee tried to adjust for this with various controls, but prefers the models with year-fixed effects. For comparison, a version without year-fixed effects is also presented (see Table F-2) (thus columns 1 through 3 are the same as in Table F-1).

Once controlling for state-fixed differences and time effects, or alternatively, the unemployment rate, the coefficient on the share of the year for which the new package was in effect falls in magnitude and it is no longer statistically significant. This also holds if we add controls for the monthly average of Aid to Families with Dependent Children/TANF and SNAP caseloads per capita. Table F-2 also illustrates that even without controlling for year-fixed effects, the effect of the implementation of the 2009 food package is small and statistically insignificant. These results suggest no significant difference comparing participation before to participation after implementation of the new food package, with and without the year-fixed

TABLE F-1 Regression Results and Controls, Total WIC Participation per Eligible Individual, 2006–2012

	Regression Number						
	1	2	3	4	5	6	7
Regression Results							
Share of year with new package	0.031[a] (0.007)	0.032[a] (0.008)	0.013 (0.015)	0.014 (0.017)	0.015 (0.018)	0.013 (0.017)	0.013 (0.017)
Unemployment rate				0.787 (0.502)	0.971[a] (0.466)	1.52[a] (0.413)	1.21[a] (0.536)
Regression Controls							
Year-fixed effects	N	N	N	Y	Y	Y	Y
State-fixed effects	N	Y	Y	Y	Y	Y	Y
TANF cases per capita	N	N	N	N	Y	Y	Y
SNAP cases per capita	N	N	N	N	Y	Y	Y
Unemployment insurance recipiency per capita	N	N	N	N	N	Y	Y
Births per capita	N	N	N	N	N	N	Y

NOTES: SNAP = Supplemental Nutrition Assistance Program; TANF = Temporary Assistance for Needy Families. Each column represents a separate regression, and there is one observation per state-year combination. N = 357. The baseline mean for the participation rate is 0.608, and the baseline mean for the unemployment rate is 0.074. The key dependent variable is the state-by-year count of participants in WIC divided by an estimate of the number of WIC eligibles, using a series of reports on WIC-eligible estimation. The key independent variable is the share of each year during which a state had implemented the new food packages taken from USDA/FNS, 2012. The regressions are weighted by the total number of eligibles, and variance-covariance matrices allow for arbitrary autocorrelation within state (implemented using state clustering in Stata version 13.1).

[a] $P < .05$.

SOURCE: USDA/FNS, 2012.

TABLE F-2 Regression Results and Controls, Total WIC Participation per Eligible Individual, 2006–2012, Omitting Year Effects

	Regression Number						
	1	2	3	4	5	6	7
Regression Results							
Share of year with new package	0.031[a] (0.007)	0.032[a] (0.008)	0.013 (0.015)	0.015 (0.011)	0.011 (0.018)	0.008 (0.016)	–0.007 (0.012)
Unemployment rate				0.493[a] (0.166)	0.509[a] (0.149)	1.40[a] (0.411)	0.801[b] (0.474)
Regression Controls							
Year-fixed effects	N	N	N	N	N	N	N
State-fixed effects	N	Y	Y	Y	Y	Y	Y
TANF cases per capita	N	N	N	N	Y	Y	Y
SNAP cases per capita	N	N	N	N	Y	Y	Y
Unemployment insurance recipiency per capita	N	N	N	N	N	Y	Y
Births per capita	N	N	N	N	N	N	Y

NOTES: SNAP = Supplemental Nutrition Assistance Program; TANF = Temporary Assistance for Needy Families. Each column represents a separate regression, and there is one observation per state-year combination. N = 357. The baseline mean for the participation rate is 0.608, and the baseline mean for the unemployment rate is 0.074. The key dependent variable is the state-by-year count of participants in WIC divided by an estimate of the number of WIC eligibles, using a series of reports on WIC-eligible estimation. The key independent variable is the share of each year during which a state had implemented the new food packages taken from USDA/FNS, 2012. The regressions are weighted by the total number of eligibles, and variance-covariance matrices allow for arbitrary autocorrelation within state (implemented using state clustering in Stata version 13.1).

[a] $P < .05$.
[b] $P < .10$.

SOURCE: USDA/FNS, 2012.

effects and other program participation rates. Further, the coefficients on the share of the year the new package was in effect are small in magnitude, with a typical estimate being 0.014 (again, on a pre-2009 baseline mean of 0.61 or 61 percentage points).

REFERENCES

Bitler, M., and H. Hoynes. 2016. The more things change, the more they stay the same? The safety net and poverty in the Great Recession *Journal of Labor Economics* 34(s1):part 2.

NASEM (National Academies of Sciences, Engineering, and Medicine). 2016. *Review of WIC food packages: Proposed framework for revisions: Interim report.* Washington, DC: The National Academies Press. doi: 10.17226/21832.

Rogers, W. H. 1993. Regression standard errors in clustered samples. *Stata Technical Bulletin* 13:19–23. Reprinted in Stata Technical Bulletin Reprints, vol. 3, pp. 88–94. College Station, TX: Stata Press.

USDA/FNS (U.S. Department of Agriculture/Food and Nutrition Service). 2011. *National and state-level estimates of Special Supplemental Nutrition Program for Women, Infants, and Children (WIC) eligibles and program reach, 2000–2009.* Alexandria, VA: USDA/FNS. http://www.fns.usda.gov/sites/default/files/WICEligibles2000-2009Vol1.pdf (accessed August 31, 2016).

USDA/FNS. 2012. *Special Supplemental Nutrition Program for Women, Infants, and Children (WIC) erroneous payments to vendors: Annual estimates for FY 2011.* Alexandria, VA: USDA/FNS. http://www.fns.usda.gov/sites/default/files/WICErroneousPayment_2011.pdf (accessed August 26, 2016).

USDA/FNS. 2013. *National and state-level estimates of Special Supplemental Nutrition Program for Women, Infants, and Children (WIC) eligibles and program reach, 2010.* Alexandria, VA: USDA/FNS. http://www.fns.usda.gov/sites/default/files/WICEligibles2010Vol1.pdf (accessed August 24, 2016).

USDA/FNS. 2014. *National and state-level estimates of the Special Supplemental Nutrition Program for Women, Infants, and Children (WIC) eligibles and program reach, 2011, volume I.* Alexandria, VA: USDA/FNS. http://www.fns.usda.gov/sites/default/files/WICEligibles2011Volume1.pdf (accessed May 22, 2016).

USDA/FNS. 2015a. *National and state-level estimates of the Special Supplemental Nutrition Program for Women, Infants, and Children (WIC) eligibles and program reach, 2012, vol. I.* Alexandria, VA: USDA/FNS. http://www.fns.usda.gov/sites/default/files/ops/WICEligibles2012-Volume1.pdf (accessed August 24, 2016).

USDA/FNS. 2015b. *WIC eligibility requirements.* Alexandria, VA: USDA/FNS. http://www.fns.usda.gov/wic/wic-eligibility-requirements (accessed July 13, 2016).

Appendix G

Barriers to Participation and Redemption

The extent to which the food packages for the Special Supplemental Nutrition Program for Women, Infants, and Children (WIC) can affect food and nutrient intake of the WIC-eligible population is dependent upon the extent to which eligible individuals participate. Factors that affect the decision to participate range from individual level to vendor level to variations in the food environment. Table G-1 summarizes the committee's review of the evidence related to these factors. Table G-2 presents the results of a quasi-experimental study of changes in availability of fruits and vegetables at WIC vendors before and after the 2009 WIC food package changes. The results suggest that benefits yielded by expansion of WIC food options vary by participant ethnicity and vendor type. A detailed discussion of barriers and incentives to participation in WIC can be found in the phase I interim report (NASEM, 2016).

TABLE G-1 Literature Findings on Barriers and Incentives to WIC Participation and Redemption

Article	Barriers	Incentives/Strategies
Bertmann et al., 2014	Negative interactions in stores: annoyance or anger expressed by cashier or other shoppers Confusion over WIC rules: fluctuation in enforcement of redemption rules store to store and week to week Cashiers lack training: participants have to explain the rules Feeling of embarrassment when using CVV	Find strategic choice of times and locations at which to shop Choose particular cashiers Pool CVV (using multiple vouchers at once)
Christie et al., 2006	Long duration of appointment wait time Dissatisfaction with customer service Dissatisfaction with the physical environment	Decrease wait times by extending clinic hours and/or changing clinic flow High level of satisfaction with WIC personnel
Gleason and Pooler, 2011	Underutilization of infant food benefits	Issue a CVV for V/F for caregivers who prefer preparing own infant foods Implement targeted nutrition education to subpopulations with high nonuse of food instruments
Gleason et al., 2011	Maintaining food freshness (small WIC vendors) Availability of products in allowable form (e.g., bread in approved size)	Continue and expand vendor training Continue to engage food suppliers Continue nutrition education of participants Use state WIC data for internal program management, policy making, ongoing monitoring Examine effect of minimum stocking requirements

TABLE G-1 Continued

Article	Barriers	Incentives/Strategies
Gleason et al., 2014	*Participants:* Gaps in knowledge (determining the amount of V/F with CVV) Incorrect information provided by cashier Limited selection of some WIC foods at local vendors and poor quality produce Lack of transportation (e.g., tribe located 30 minutes from a store) *Vendors:* Delivery of spoiled items Difficulty anticipating demand and maintaining adequate supply of some WIC foods Challenges in serving participants who lack knowledge Challenges in communicating with local WIC agency	*Participants:* Use more than one check at a time when transportation is an issue *Vendors:* Adopt practices that will make it easier for participants to shop *WIC Staff:* Use open-ended question and probing to encourage discussion with participants Expand nutrition education opportunities Inform participants of local vendors *Local WIC Directors:* Establish open lines of communication with vendors Increase cross-program collaboration *State WIC Agencies:* Offer additional training opportunities to staff Expand allowable WIC foods to include frozen and canned vegetables Develop a formalized local vendor liaison (LVL) program (CA example: LVL makes visits)
Najjar, 2013	Food package policies (e.g., container size) Negative grocery store experiences and personal misunderstanding and embarrassment	Helpful vendors Vendor and participant understanding about the use of CVV and other WIC benefits
Phillips et al., 2014	Certain individual WIC foods have low rates of full redemption Could not use certain foods (i.e., received too much) Participants or their children disliked the food or did not know how to prepare them	Implement targeted educational efforts to promote full utilization of WIC benefits Tailor nutrition education to include foods that are commonly underused and focus on culturally relevant approaches to incorporating these foods into meals and snacks

continued

TABLE G-1 Continued

Article	Barriers	Incentives/Strategies
USDA/ERS, 2010	Of those exiting WIC at 1 year, transaction costs of participation may be a barrier: program requires too much effort and the benefits are not worth the time (26.2%) or they have scheduling or transportation problems (10%) Program requires too much effort, or scheduling, or transportation problems	
USDA/ERS, 2012	Improved national economic conditions generally reduce participation rates for WIC and other national assistance programs	Poorer economic conditions and unemployment rates tend to improve participation rates when the program is fully funded

NOTES: CA = California; CVV = cash value voucher; V/F = vegetables and fruits; LVL = local vendor liaison.

TABLE G-2 Changes in Fruit and Vegetable Availability and Selection Overall and by Vendor Type, Before Compared to After the 2009 WIC Food Package Changes

	Fresh			Canned			Frozen	
Availability or Selection	Commonly Consumed FV	African-American FV	Latino FV	Vegetables	Low-Sodium Vegetables	Fruits	Vegetables	Fruits
Availability								
Overall change	2.14 (1.31, 3.50)[b]	2.53 (1.31, 5.35)[b]	1.72 (0.84, 3.98)	NE	2.69 (1.17, 6.22)[a]	1.84 (0.91, 3.72)	1.97 (1.05, 3.70)[a]	2.15 (1.06, 4.37)[a]
Change by vendor type								
Large	3.56 (1.22, 10.34)[a]	2.27 (1.31, 5.48)[a]	1.69 (0.94, 5.54)	1.62 (0.81, 3.25)	0.93 (0.25, 3.48)	1.01 (0.41, 2.48)	1.43 (0.91, 2.25)	2.10 (0.86, 5.12)
Small	1.07 (0.51, 2.24)	2.64 (1.09, 6.38)[a]	1.83 (0.65, 5.17)	1.18 (0.47, 2.94)	5.95 (1.74, 20.29)[b]	2.11 (0.95, 4.69)	2.80 (1.13, 6.93)[a]	1.93 (0.68, 5.53)
Pharmacy	NE	1.38 (1.02, 1.88)[a]	1.25 (0.92, 1.69)	NE	0.71 (0.12, 4.18)	1.06 (0.04, 25.53)	1.34 (0.34, 5.24)	2.24 (0.19, 25.74)
Selection								
Overall change	1.67 (1.14, 2.47)[b]	1.14 (1.01, 1.42)	1.17 (1.02, 1.33)	1.22 (1.07, 1.40)[b]	1.13 (0.98, 1.30)	0.96 (0.77, 1.20)	1.09 (0.82, 1.46)	0.92 (0.69, 1.21)
Change by vendor type								
Large	1.67 (1.03, 2.69)[a]	1.13 (1.01, 1.43)	1.22 (1.06, 1.36)[a]	0.84 (0.68, 1.04)	1.05 (0.91, 1.20)	0.88 (0.71, 1.09)	1.02 (0.74, 1.40)	0.93 (0.69, 1.25)
Small	1.71 (1.06, 2.76)[a]	1.17 (0.78, 2.19)	1.05 (0.73, 1.58)	1.32 (0.95, 1.85)	2.01 (1.03, 3.84)[a]	1.05 (0.53, 2.07)	1.34 (0.79, 2.29)	0.80 (0.33, 1.93)
Pharmacy	NE	1.04 (0.93, 1.20)	1.09 (0.95, 1.21)	1.58 (1.31, 1.91)[b]	1.17 (0.18, 7.45)	1.35 (0.06, 30.18)	0.81 (0.32, 2.08)	NE

NOTES: FV = fruits and vegetables; NE = odds ratio not estimated due to lack of variability in outcome by year. Data presented as odds ratio (95% confidence interval). An odds ratio of 1.0 for this contrast indicates that the post-policy change from 2009 to 2010 was greater than the pre-policy change from 2008 to 2009.

[a] $P < .05$.

[b] $P < .01$.

SOURCE: Zenk et al., 2012 (used with permission).

REFERENCES

Bertmann, F. M., C. Barroso, P. Ohri-Vachaspati, J. S. Hampl, K. Sell, and C. M. Wharton. 2014. Women, Infants, and Children cash value voucher (CVV) use in Arizona: A qualitative exploration of barriers and strategies related to fruit and vegetable purchases. *Journal of Nutrition Education and Behavior* 46(3 Suppl):S53-S58.

Christie, C., J. A. Watkins, A. Martin, H. Jackson, J. E. Perkin, and J. Fraser. 2006. Assessment of client satisfaction in six urban WIC clinics. *Florida Public Health Review* 3:35–42.

Gleason, S., and J. Pooler. 2011. *The effects of changes in WIC food packages on redemptions: Final report*. Portland, ME: Altarum Institute. http://naldc.nal.usda.gov/download/50613/PDF (accessed December 21, 2016).

Gleason, S., R. Morgan, L. Bell, and J. Pooler. 2011. *Impact of the revised WIC food package on small WIC vendors: Insight from a four-state evaluation*. Portland, ME: Altarum Institute. http://www.calwic.org/storage/FourStateWICFoodPackageEvaluation-Full_Report-20May11.pdf (accessed December 21, 2016).

Gleason, S., D. McGuire, and R. Morgan. 2014. *Opportunities to enhance American Indian access to the WIC food package: Evidence from three case studies*. Portland, ME: Altarum Institute. http://altarum.org/sites/default/files/uploaded-publication-files/Opportunities%20to%20Enhance%20Am%20Indian%20Access%20to%20the%20WIC%20FP_fmt_04.pdf (accessed December 21, 2016).

Najjar, S. 2013. Barriers to WIC benefits redemption among participants in Washington State. Master's thesis, School of Public Health, University of Washington, Seattle, WA.

NASEM (National Academies of Sciences, Engineering, and Medicine). 2016. *Review of WIC food packages: Proposed framework for revisions: Interim report*. Washington, DC: The National Academies Press. doi: 10.17226/21832.

Phillips, D., L. Bell, R. Morgan, and J. Pooler. 2014. *Transition to EBT in WIC: Review of impact and examination of participant redemption patterns: Final report*. Portland, ME: Altarum Institute. http://altarum.org/sites/default/files/uploaded-publication-files/Altarum_Transition%20to%20WIC%20EBT_Final%20Report_071614.pdf (accessed December 21, 2016).

USDA/ERS (U.S. Department of Agriculture/Economic Research Service). 2010. *WIC participation patterns: An investigation of delayed entry and early exit*. Washington, DC: USDA/ERS. https://www.ers.usda.gov/webdocs/publications/err109/8018_err109.pdf?v=41056 (accessed December 21, 2016).

USDA/ERS. 2012. *How economic conditions affect participation in USDA nutrition assistance programs*. Washington, DC: USDA/ERS. https://www.ers.usda.gov/webdocs/publications/eib100/32191_eib100.pdf (accessed December 21, 2016).

Zenk, S. N., A. Odoms-Young, L. M. Powell, R. T. Campbell, D. Block, N. Chavez, R. C. Krauss, S. Strode, and J. Armbruster. 2012. Fruit and vegetable availability and selection: Federal food package revisions, 2009. *American Journal of Preventive Medicine* 43(4):423-428.

Appendix H

Kosher and Halal Substitution Options

TABLE H-1 Authorization of Kosher and Halal Substitutions

Substitutions Offered for WIC Foods	WIC State Agencies Authorizing Substitutions (%)	Nationwide WIC Participants Covered by the Option (%)*
Kosher	17	34
Kosher and Halal	6	19
No Substitutions	42	27
Not Specified	36	19

NOTES: Results were obtained from a database of WIC food lists for all 90 state agencies as of October 2009, as well as foods that were approved in the period immediately preceding implementation of the Interim Rule. WIC state plans, vendor manuals, and grocery shopping guides were also reviewed. The most recent WIC Food Packages Policy Options Study (USDA/FNS, 2015) did not quantify the number of state agencies allowing Kosher and Halal options nationally. The report indicated that 7 percent of state agencies covering 21.3 percent of WIC participants allowed Kosher milk.

* Percentages represent the number of WIC participants linked to the state agencies offering the option.

SOURCE: USDA/FNS, 2011; with update from personal communication with N. Cole, Mathematica, March 17, 2015.

TABLE H-2 WIC ITFPS-2: Percentage of Mothers Who Have Religious or Lifestyle Beliefs That Influence Feeding, by Belief

Belief	Study Mothers % (SE)
Halal	0.72 (0.30)
Kosher	0.37 (0.16)
Vegetarian	0.37 (0.10)
Vegan	0.09 (0.06)
Other	2.00 (0.25)
Unweighted N*	2,807
Weighted N	442,574

NOTES: Data were collected at month 13 of the study. ITFPS-2 = WIC Infant and Toddler Feeding Practices Study 2; SE = standard error. Two cases indicated multiple responses. One respondent indicated both Vegetarian and Vegan; only Vegan is displayed. Another respondent indicated Kosher and Other; only Kosher is displayed.

* N is the number of mothers who completed interviews at month 13.

SOURCE: Personal communication, K. Castellanos-Brown, USDA-FNS, April 27, 2016.

REFERENCES

USDA/FNS (U.S. Department of Agriculture/Food and Nutrition Service). 2011. WIC food packages policy options study, final report. Alexandria, VA: USDA/FNS. http://www.fns.usda.gov/sites/default/files/WICFoodPackageOptions.pdf (accessed December 21, 2016).

USDA/FNS. 2015. WIC food packages policy options II, final report. Alexandria, VA: USDA/FNS. http://www.fns.usda.gov/wic-food-package-policy-options-ii (accessed December 21, 2016).

Appendix I

Complementary Feeding: Summary of Information Reviewed

To evaluate complementary feeding of infants in this report, the committee relied on food intake data from three large contemporary datasets: (1) Infant Feeding Practices Study II (IFPS II) (Grummer-Strawn et al., 2008), (2) 2008 Feeding Infants and Toddlers Study (FITS 2008) (Deming et al., 2014), and (3) National Health and Nutrition Examination Survey (NHANES) (Grimes et al., 2015). The Special Supplemental Nutrition Program for Women, Infants, and Children (WIC) Infant and Toddler Feeding Practices Study, (WIC ITFPS II) is currently under way, but only limited results were available in time for this report. A summary of the study designs is presented in Table I-1 and key results are outlined in Tables I-2 and I-3.

TABLE I-1 Study Designs and Characteristics of Selected Reports, IFPS II, FITS 2008, and NHANES 2005–2012

	IFPS II[a]	FITS 2008[b]	NHANES, 2005–2012[c]
Design	Longitudinal data collected from the last trimester of pregnancy through infant's first year of life[d]	Cross-sectional evaluation of dietary intake of U.S. children, 0–4 years	Cross-sectional
Data Collection Dates	May 2005–June 2007; 6-year follow-up in 2012[d]	June 2008–January 2009	2005–2012
Recruitment	Pregnant women who were part of a nationally distributed consumer opinion panel	Sample frame came from the New Parent Database and the Consumer Database and the Consumer Database from the Experian, Inc.	Complex, multistage, probability sampling
Eligibility	Women at least 18 years of age Delivered a singleton infant who was at least 35 weeks gestation and weighed at least 5 pounds at birth Both mother and child were free from conditions that could affect feeding	Household had child 0–47 months	Non-institutionalized U.S. population
Sample Size	4,902 qualified in prenatal period 3,033 qualified in neonatal period 1,807 remained by end of study	3,273 infants and children	2,857 children enrolled[e] 2,791 completed the first 24-hour dietary recall 2,740 had reliable dietary recall data 765 infants, 0–5.9 months 854 infants, 6–11.9 months 1,121 toddlers, 12–23.9 months
WIC Participants in Sample	1,112 (36.7%) of enrolled households (mother and/or infant) participated in WIC in the neonatal period 912 (30.1%) of	794 WIC infants and children 117 infants, 0–5.9 months 84 infants, 6–8.9 months 76 infants 9–11.9 months 238 toddlers,	Not identified in this analysis

TABLE I-1 Continued

	IFPS II[a]	FITS 2008[b]	NHANES, 2005–2012[c]
	enrolled households (mother and/or infants) participated in WIC any time from month 1 to 12	12–23.9 months 279 preschoolers, 24–47.9 months	
Data Collection	Mail-based survey Sent monthly approximately 2–7 months postpartum, then approximately every 7 weeks thereafter through 12 months postpartum	Phone-based	Face-to-face interview
Dietary Assessment[f]	Food frequency table of liquids and solids the infant consumed in previous 7 days Quantities consumed not captured	24-hour recall and brief questionnaire Second 24-hour recall performed in a subsample, 7–10 days after first (n = 701)[h] Descriptive findings of unadjusted prevalence are presented for WIC vs. non-WIC participants; analyses used sample weights and groups were compared using t-tests[g]	24-hour proxy-recall[i] Evaluated contributions of foods to energy and nutrient intake

NOTES: FITS = 2008 Feeding Infants and Toddlers Study; IFPS II = Infant Feeding Practices Study II; NHANES = National Health and Nutrition Examination Survey.

[a] Overall study design, Fein et al., 2008; CDC, 2014.

[b] Overall study design, Briefel et al., 2010.

[c] Grimes et al., 2015.

[d] A year 6 follow-up study of children initially assessed in the IFPS II has been conducted, evaluating links between early feeding practices and various health outcomes (Fein et al., 2014).

[e] Number represents sample included in the analysis, not entire NHANES sample.

[f] Information about dietary supplement use was collected in each of the overall study designs, but the three reports on food group intakes did not evaluate supplement use.

[g] Report-specific analysis, Deming et al., 2014.

[h] Two days of dietary intake per sampled child was used to calculate usual nutrient intake distributions, Briefel et al., 2010.

[i] While two 24-hour recalls are part of the NHANES procedures, Grimes et al. (2015) only evaluated intake reported on the first day of recall.

SOURCES: CDC, 2014; Fein et al., 2008, 2014; Grimes et al., 2015.

TABLE I-2 Complementary Food Intake of Infants, Ages 0 to 2 Years, from IFPS II and FITS II

	IFPS II[a]		FITS 2008[b]		
				Percent Consuming on a Given Day	
Food Group	Age in Months	Percent Consuming in the Previous Week	Age in Months	WIC	Non-WIC
Fruit (excluding juice)	3	2.8	0–5.9	8.6[c]	6.4[c]
	6	71.3	6–11.9	69.1	75.6
	9	97.0	12–23.9	62.3	83.6[d]
	12	98.4			
100% Juice	3	5.0	0–5.9	8.2[c]	3.8[c]
	6	33.4	6–11.9	46.1	28.3[e]
	9	62.8	12–23.9	61.9	52.4
	12	76.9			
Vegetables, total	3	1.4	0–5.9	11.2[c]	8.4
	6	73.1	6–11.9	57.7	75.6[e]
	9	97.2	12–23.9	73.5	69.5
	12	98.7			
Grains and grain products, total	3	18.3	0–5.9	26.7	22.7
	6	86.1	6–11.9	91.5[c]	90.3
	9	96.3	12–23.9	99.5[c]	98.4[c]
	12	97.0			
Infant cereal	3	18.2	0–5.9	26.7	21.9
	6	83.7	6–11.9	61.8	66.9
	9	83.4	12–23.9	6.9[c]	11.4
	12	46.6			
Meats and meat substitutes[f]	3	0.7	0–5.9	2.8[c]	0.0[c]
	6	22.0	6–11.9	64.1	53.6
	9	78.4	12–23.9	93.9[c]	94.1
	12	96.6			
Cow's milk, total	3	0.3	0–5.9	0.0	0.0
	6	1.2	6–11.9	13.3	9.4
	9	5.3	12–23.9	86.5	81.0
	12	81.2			
Cow's milk, whole	NR		6–11.9	10.0[c]	7.8
			12–23.9	59.2	64.2
Cow's milk, reduced- or low-fat	NR		6–11.9	2.7[c]	1.1[c]
			12–23.9	31.8	19.7[e]
Cow's milk, nonfat	NR		6–11.9	0.5	0.1[c]
			12–23.9	1.0[c]	1.0
Sweetened beverages	3	1.1	0–5.9	0.0[c]	0.3[c]
	6	3.1	6–11.9	12.3[c]	4.5[c]
	9	6.2	12–23.9	39.6	22.0
	12	14.6			

TABLE I-2 Continued

Food Group	IFPS II[a]		FITS 2008[b]		
	Age in Months	Percent Consuming in the Previous Week	Age in Months	Percent Consuming on a Given Day: WIC	Percent Consuming on a Given Day: Non-WIC
Desserts and candy	3	0.2	0–5.9	1.7[c]	1.1[c]
	6	1.5	6–11.9	22.7	24.8
	9	12.3	12–23.9	63.6	55.5
	12	52.2			

NOTES: NR = not reported.
[a] Grummer-Strawn et al., 2008.
[b] Deming et al., 2014 (data reprinted with permission).
[c] Point estimate imprecise due to small sample size and it being an uncommon or very common response.
[d] Significantly different from WIC group at 0.01 level by t-test.
[e] Significantly different from WIC group at 0.05 level by t-test.
[f] FITS 2008 classified this category as "Meat and other protein sources" and included cheese and yogurt in this category while IFPS II has a separate "Other Dairy" category.
SOURCES: Grummer-Strawn et al., 2008; Deming et al., 2014.

TABLE I-3 Percent of Daily Energy Intake of Complementary Food Groups by Infants Ages 6 to 23.9 Months, NHANES 2005–2012[a]

Food Group	Percent of Daily Energy Intake	
	6–11.9 months	12–23.9 months
Fruit (excluding juice)	2.3	4.8
100% Juice	1.5	5.9
Vegetables	NA[b]	3.2[c]
Grains and grain products		
Mixed dishes—grain-based	2.3	5.5
Bread, rolls, tortillas	1.1	3.8
Crackers	NA	2.4
Ready-to-eat cereal	NA	2.3
Quick breads and bread products	NA	1.6
Cooked cereals	NA	1.4
Meats and meat substitutes		
Poultry	NA	3.6
Cured meats and poultry	NA	2.5
Eggs	NA	2.2
Mixed dishes—meat, poultry, seafood	NA	2.0
Plant-based protein foods	NA	1.6
Dairy		
Cow's milk, all fat levels	3.1	22.4
Cheese	NA	2.6
Yogurt	NA	1.7
Flavored milk	NA	1.3
Desserts, sweetened beverages, and savory snacks		
Sweet bakery products	1.8	4.6
Sweetened beverages	NA	3.1
Savory snacks	NA	2.4
Candy	NA	1.3
Other desserts	NA	1.2

NOTES: NA = data not available.

[a] Intake of human milk and infant formulas not represented in this table.

[b] All NA notations indicate that data were not presented in Grimes et al. (2015), as intake contributed to less than 1 percent of total energy intake.

[c] Sum of "White Potatoes" group and "Vegetables, excluding potatoes" group.

SOURCE: Grimes et al., 2015.

REFERENCES

Briefel, R. R., L. M. Kalb, E. Condon, D. M. Deming, N. A. Clusen, M. K. Fox, L. Harnack, E. Gemmill, M. Stevens, and K. C. Reidy. 2010. The Feeding Infants and Toddlers Study 2008: Study design and methods. *Journal of the American Dietetic Association* 110(12 Suppl):S16–S26.

CDC (Centers for Disease Control and Prevention). 2014. *Infant Feeding Practices Study II and its year six follow-up, chapter 2: Neonatal survey*. http://www.cdc.gov/ifps/pdfs/data/ifps2_tables_ch2.pdf (accessed December 20, 2016).

Deming, D. M., R. R. Briefel, and K. C. Reidy. 2014. Infant feeding practices and food consumption patterns of children participating in WIC. *Journal of Nutrition Education and Behavior* 46(3 Suppl):S29–S37.

Fein, S. B., J. Labiner-Wolfe, K. R. Shealy, R. Li, J. Chen, and L. M. Grummer-Strawn. 2008. Infant Feeding Practices Study II: Study methods. *Pediatrics* 122(Suppl 2):S28–S35.

Fein, S. B., R. Li, J. Chen, K. S. Scanlon, and L. M. Grummer-Strawn. 2014. Methods for the year 6 follow-up study of children in the Infant Feeding Practices Study II. *Pediatrics* 134(Suppl 1):S4–S12.

Grimes, C. A., E. A. Szymlek-Gay, K. J. Campbell, and T. A. Nicklas. 2015. Food sources of total energy and nutrients among U.S. infants and toddlers: National Health and Nutrition Examination Survey 2005–2012. *Nutrients* 7(8):6797–6836.

Grummer-Strawn, L. M., K. S. Scanlon, and S. B. Fein. 2008. Infant feeding and feeding transitions during the first year of life. *Pediatrics* 122(Suppl 2):S36–S42.

Appendix J

Nutrient and Food Intake of WIC Subgroups: Analytical Methods and Results

This appendix presents the methodology and detailed results for the analyses of nutrient and food group intakes and diet quality of the Special Supplemental Nutrition Program for Women, Infants, and Children (WIC) participants and WIC-eligible subgroups using the National Health and Nutrition Examination Survey (NHANES).The WIC subgroup was defined as the subgroup of individuals reporting participation in WIC regardless of income level. Eligible non-WIC was defined as the subgroup of individuals with incomes less than or equal to 185 percent of the federal poverty level who did not report participation in WIC. Results presented in this appendix and summarized in Chapter 4 of this report update the methods and results that were presented in the phase I interim report. The tables presented in this appendix and the corresponding page numbers are listed below. These data, generated by Iowa State University, were checked by the committee members as well as by the staff. Data were also compared to the phase I results and to nationally representative data for reasonability.

TABLES

USING THE DIETARY REFERENCE INTAKES TO ASSESS NUTRIENT ADEQUACY

The committee used the Dietary Reference Intakes (DRIs) (defined in Box J-1 and presented in Tables J-1a through J-1c) to assess nutrient adequacy, which involved examining both inadequate and excessive intakes of nutrients. The methods applied in this report are generally the same as those used in the 2006 Institute of Medicine (IOM) report *WIC Food Packages: Time for a Change* and originally designed by Nusser et al. (1996) and Carriquiry (1999) (see Appendix C of IOM, 2006). Brief descriptions of the approaches are provided here, with modifications noted as appropriate. Nutrients analyzed for this report are listed in Table J-2.

BOX J-1

Dietary Reference Intakes

The Dietary Reference Intakes (DRIs) were developed to serve as standards for nutrient intake and include the following:

Estimated Average Requirement (EAR): The usual daily intake of a nutrient that is expected to meet the requirement of half of healthy individuals in a group defined by age and sex. The requirement is based on a specific indicator of adequacy.

Recommended Dietary Allowance (RDA): The usual daily intake level that is sufficient to meet the nutrient requirements of 97 to 98 percent of healthy individuals in the specified life stage and sex group. If the requirements in a specified group are normally distributed, the RDA is equivalent to the EAR plus two standard deviations.

Adequate Intake (AI): When available evidence is not sufficient to determine the EAR for a nutrient, an AI is set. The AI is the average daily nutrient intake observed in an apparently healthy sex and age group. It is based on experimentally derived intake levels or observations of mean nutrient intakes by a group of apparently healthy people who are maintaining a defined criterion of adequacy. It is not certain where an AI level of intake fits relative to an actual nutrient requirement, as no EAR or RDA have been specified for these nutrients. It is generally believed that the AI would be equal to or exceed the RDA (if one existed).

Acceptable Macronutrient Distribution Range (AMDR): A range of usual intakes for a macronutrient that is associated with reduced risk of chronic disease while providing adequate intakes of essential nutrients. An AMDR is expressed as a percentage of total energy intake.

Tolerable Upper Intake Level (UL): The highest usual daily nutrient intake level that is likely to pose no risk of adverse effects to nearly all healthy individuals in the specified life stage and sex group.

The DRIs were also applied in the previous review of WIC food packages (IOM, 2006). These can be applied to population-level nutrient intake assessments, with the exception of the RDA which is intended for assessment of individuals.

SOURCES: IOM, 2000b, 2002/2005.

Estimating Usual Intake Distributions

Assessing nutrient adequacy involves, first, estimating distributions of usual intake. The Iowa State University (ISU) method proposed by Nusser et al. (1996) and applied in the 2006 IOM report is generally accepted in the nutrition community, and several software packages are now available to generate the mean and variance of usual intake as well as percentiles of intake of the user's choosing. For this report, PC Software for Intake

TABLE J-1a Dietary Reference Intakes Used for Assessing Nutrient Intakes of WIC-Eligible Subgroups

Population Subgroup and Type of DRI	Nutrient								
	Calcium (mg/d)	Copper (μg/d)	Iron (mg/d)	Magnesium (mg/d)	Phosphorus (mg/d)	Selenium (μg/d)	Zinc (mg/d)	Potassium (mg/d)	Sodium (mg/d)
Infants 0–6 mo									
EAR/AI	200*	200*	0.27*	30*	100*	15*	2*	400*	120*
UL	1,000	ND	40	ND	ND	45	4	NA	ND
Infants 6–12 mo									
EAR/AI	260*	220*	6.9	75*	275*	20*	2.5	700*	370*
UL	1,500	ND	40	ND	ND	60	5	NA	ND
Children 1–3 y									
EAR/AI	500	260	3	65	380	17	2.5	3,000*	1,000*
UL	2,500	1,000	40	65	3,000	90	7	NA	1,500
Children 4–8 y									
EAR/AI	800	340	4.1	110	405	23	4	3,800*	1,200*
UL	2,500	3,000	40	110	3,000	150	12	NA	1,900
Females 19–30 y									
EAR/AI	800	700	8.1	255	580	45	6.8	4,700*	1,500*
UL	2,500	10,000	45	350	4,000	400	40	NA	2,300

Females 31–50 y									
EAR/AI	800	700	8.1	265	580	45	6.8	4,700*	1,300*
UL	2,500	10,000	45	350	4,000	400	40	NA	2,300
Pregnancy 19–30 y									
EAR/AI	800	800	22	290	580	49	9.5	4,700*	1,500*
UL	2,500	10,000	45	350	3,500	400	40	NA	2,300
Pregnancy 31–50 y									
EAR/AI	800	800	22	300	580	49	9.5	4,700*	1,500*
UL	2,500	10,000	45	350	3,500	400	40	NA	2,300
Lactation 19–30 y									
EAR/AI	800	1,000	6.5	255	580	59	10.4	5,100*	1,500*
UL	2,500	10,000	45	350	4,000	400	40	NA	2,300
Lactation 31–50 y									
EAR/AI	800	1,000	6.5	265	580	59	10.4	5,100*	1,500*
UL	2,500	10,000	45	350	4,000	400	40	NA	2,300

NOTES: AI = Adequate Intake, used when necessary, followed by an asterisk (*); EAR = Estimated Average Requirement, used when available; NA = not applicable; ND = not determined due to lack of data; UL = Tolerable Upper Intake Level. The UL for magnesium represents intake from pharmacological agents only and does not include intake from food. The AIs for calcium for infants are based on the calcium content of human milk. The UL values for phosphorous and sodium in this table were corrected to mg units from the values in the originally posted prepublication, which were in g units.

SOURCES: Data sources for Table J-1a to J-1c are listed after Table J-1c.

TABLE J-1b Dietary Reference Intakes Used for Assessing Nutrient Intakes of WIC-Eligible Subgroups

Population Subgroup and Type of DRI	Nutrient										
	Vitamin A (μg/d)	Vitamin D (IU/d)	Vitamin E (mg/d)	Vitamin C (mg/d)	Thiamin (mg/d)	Riboflavin (mg/d)	Niacin (mg/d)	Vitamin B6 (mg/d)	Folate (μg DFE/d)	Vitamin B12 (mg/d)	Choline (mg/d)
Infants 0–6 mo											
EAR/AI	400*	400*	4*	40*	0.2*	0.3*	2*	0.1*	65*	0.4*	125*
UL	600	1,000	ND	ND	ND	ND	ND	ND	ND	ND	ND
Infants 6–12 mo											
EAR/AI	500*	400*	5*	50*	0.3*	0.4*	4*	0.3*	80*	0.5*	150*
UL	600	1,500	ND	ND	ND	ND	ND	ND	ND	ND	ND
Children 1–3 y											
EAR/AI	210	400	5	13	0.4	0.4	5	0.4	120	0.7	200*
UL	600	2,500	200	400	ND	ND	10	30	300	ND	1,000
Children 4–8 y											
EAR/AI	275	400	6	22	0.5	0.5	6	0.5	160	1.0	250*
UL	900	3,000	300	650	ND	ND	15	40	400	ND	1,000
Females 19–30 y											
EAR/AI	500	400	12	60	0.9	0.9	11	1.1	320	2.0	425*
UL	3,000	4,000	1,000	2,000	ND	ND	35	100	1,000	ND	3,500

Females 31–50 y											
EAR/AI	500	400	12	60	0.9	0.9	11	1.1	320	2.0	425*
UL	3,000	4,000	1,000	2,000	ND	ND	35	100	1,000	ND	3,500
Pregnancy 19–30 y											
EAR/AI	550	400	12	70	1.2	1.2	14	1.6	520	2.2	450*
UL	3,000	4,000	1,000	2,000	ND	ND	35	100	1,000	ND	3,500
Pregnancy 31–50 y											
EAR/AI	550	400	12	70	1.2	1.2	14	1.6	520	2.2	450*
UL	3,000	4,000	1,000	2,000	ND	ND	35	100	1,000	ND	3,500
Lactation 19–30 y											
EAR/AI	900	400	16	100	1.2	1.3	13	1.7	450	2.4	550*
UL	3,000	4,000	1,000	2,000	ND	ND	35	100	1,000	ND	3,500
Lactation 31–50 y											
EAR/AI	900	400	16	100	1.2	1.3	13	1.7	450	2.4	550*
UL	3,000	4,000	1,000	2,000	ND	ND	35	100	1,000	ND	3,500

NOTES: AI = Adequate Intake, used when necessary, followed by an asterisk (*); EAR = Estimated Average Requirement, used when available; ND = not determined due to lack of data; UL = Tolerable Upper Intake Level.
The UL for vitamin A refers to preformed vitamin A only.
The UL for vitamin E applies to synthetic forms obtained from dietary supplements, and fortified foods, not from vitamin E naturally occurring in foods.
SOURCES: Data sources for Table J-1a to J-1c are listed after Table J-1c.

TABLE J-1c Macronutrient Intake Recommendations for WIC-Eligible Subgroups

	Recommended Intake				
Macronutrient	Infants 0 to Less Than 6 Months	Infants 6 to Less Than 12 Months	Children 1–3 Years	Children and Adolescents 4–18 Years	Adults
Carbohydrate (% of kcal AMDR)[a]	60 g/d	95 g/d	45–65	45–65	45–65
Protein (% of kcal AMDR)	ND	ND	5–20	10–30	10–35
Protein (g/kg/d EAR)[b]	1.52 (AI)	1.0	1.1	0.95	0.88

NOTES: AI = Adequate Intake; AMDR = acceptable macronutrient distribution range; EAR = Estimated Average Requirement. Because the 2015–2020 *Dietary Guidelines for Americans* do not indicate a recommended amount of total fat, intake of this nutrient was not analyzed for this report; ND = not determined.

[a] Units are percent of kcal except where noted.

[b] Values are EAR except where noted.

SOURCES: IOM, 1997, 1998, 2000a, 2001, 2002/2005, 2005, 2011b.

Distribution (PC-SIDE) was used to implement the ISU method (nutrients). To estimate the distribution of dietary components consumed episodically (food groups and subgroups), the Statistical Program for Age-adjusted Dietary Assessment (SPADE), a method similar to the National Cancer Institute method was implemented (Dekkers et al., 2014). These software packages are specifically designed for estimating the usual intake distributions of populations, and are not appropriate for application to individuals (IOM, 2000b).

Assessing the Prevalence of Inadequate Nutrient Intake with EARs

In all of the statistical analyses, intake data were weighted to population values by using survey weights associated with survey participants. Fractional jackknife replicate weights were used to estimate standard errors of estimated percentiles (Fuller, 2009). Usual nutrient intake distributions were estimated using methods that account for the statistical properties of the data (intra-individual variation and reported data that are not normally distributed (Nusser et al., 1996; IOM, 2000b). Beaton (1994) and Carriquiry (1999) suggested that the prevalence of inadequate intakes in the group can be estimated by the proportion of persons in the group whose usual intakes do not reach the Estimated Average Requirement (EAR) for the nutrient. This approach is known as the EAR cut-point method. To estimate the prevalence of inadequacy in a group that includes persons from

TABLE J-2 Nutrients Selected for Intake Analysis

Nutrients Available in WWEIA	Include in Analyses	Rationale for Exclusion in Current Report
Food energy (kcal)	✓	
Protein (g)	✓	
Carbohydrate (g)	✓	
Fat, total (g)		No DGA recommendation
Dietary fiber, total (g)	✓	
Saturated fatty acids, total (g)	✓	
Monounsaturated fatty acids, total (g)		No DRI
Polyunsaturated fatty acids, total (g)		No DRI
Cholesterol (mg)		No DRI or DGA recommendation
Linoleic 18:2 (g)		Used USDA food pattern "oils" as a proxy
Linolenic 18:3 (g)		Used USDA food pattern "oils" as a proxy
EPA 20:5 (g)		No DRI, seafood intake as proxy
DHA 22:6 (g)		No DRI, seafood intake as proxy
Vitamin A as RAE (μg)	✓	
Retinol (μg)	✓	
Vitamin E as alpha-tocopherol (mg)	✓	
Vitamin D (D2 + D3) (μg)	✓	
Vitamin D, 25-Hydroxy (nmol/dL)	✓	Data not available for infants
Vitamin K as phylloquinone (μg)		Inadequacy is extremely rare
Vitamin C (mg)	✓	
Thiamin (mg)	✓	
Riboflavin (mg)	✓	
Niacin (mg)	✓	
Vitamin B6 (mg)	✓	
Folate as DFE (μg)	✓	
Folic acid (μg)	✓	
Vitamin B12 (μg)	✓	
Calcium (mg)	✓	
Iron (mg)	✓	
Magnesium (mg)	✓	
Phosphorus (mg)	✓	
Potassium (mg)	✓	

continued

TABLE J-2 Continued

Nutrients Available in WWEIA	Include in Analyses	Rationale for Exclusion in Current Report
Sodium (mg)	✓	
Zinc (mg)	✓	
Copper (mg)	✓	
Selenium (μg)	✓	
Choline (mg)	✓	

NOTES: DGA = 2015–2020 *Dietary Guidelines for Americans*; DRI = Dietary Reference Intake; USDA = U.S. Department of Agriculture; WWEIA = What We Eat in America.

subgroups that have different EARs, an approach proposed previously is used (IOM, 2000b). This approach consists of rescaling daily intakes for one of the population subgroups so they can be compared to the EAR of the other group (a similar rescaling was used in IOM, 2006). This approach was applied to two of the population subgroups of interest in this work: children ages 2 to less than 5 years (which requires DRIs for ages 1 to 3 years and ages 4 to 8 years), and women ages 19 to 50 years (which requires DRIs for ages 19 to 30 years and ages 31 to 50 years). The EAR cut-point method cannot be used to estimate the prevalence of iron inadequacy for women because requirements are not normally distributed, mostly because of menstrual losses of iron. However, because most of the women in the NHANES analytic sample were pregnant or breastfeeding, and the analytic sample was small, the cut-point method was implemented nonetheless.

Interpretation of intake differs for nutrients with Adequate Intakes (AIs) in that only limited inferences can be made about the prevalence of nutrient inadequacy. If a mean intake level is equal to or exceeds the AI, it is likely that the prevalence of inadequacy is low, but no *conclusion* can be drawn about the prevalence of inadequacy for a mean intake level that falls below the AI (IOM, 2000b). For this reason, in this report, means and usual intake distributions were determined for nutrients with an AI, but the prevalence of inadequacy could only be evaluated as low (the mean was above the AI) or unknown (the mean was below the AI). Because only AIs are available for infants ages 0 to less than 6 months, only this limited evaluation of inadequacy was possible for this age group.

Assessing the Prevalence of Excessive Intakes

Excessive intakes of micronutrients were assessed by comparing estimated usual nutrient intake distributions to the Tolerable Upper Intake

Level (UL) for that nutrient, as described in the 2006 IOM report. Not all nutrients have ULs and, for four nutrients (folate, vitamin E, niacin, and magnesium), the UL is based on intake of supplements, fortificants, or pharmacological agents only (IOM, 1997, 1998, 2000a), not all of which were evaluated for this report. Thus, the prevalence of intakes exceeding the UL was determined only for retinol, vitamin C, vitamin B6, calcium, iron, phosphorous, zinc, copper, selenium, choline, and sodium in this report. Excess zinc intake was not considered of concern for formula-fed infants or children age 1 to less than 2 years because the method used to set the UL resulted in a narrow margin between the Recommended Dietary Allowance (RDA) and the UL (IOM, 2001). For other age groups, there exists no evidence for adverse effects from zinc naturally occurring in food (IOM, 2001), and the committee considers infant formula (and zinc provided therein) to be tightly regulated for safety by the U.S. Food and Drug Administration (FDA). Excess retinol intake was not considered of concern because of a similarly narrow margin between the UL and the RDA (IOM, 2001). Toxicity from excess consumption of retinol rarely occurs without supplemental intake (IOM, 2001). Finally, excess copper and selenium intake in children was not considered of concern because the UL is extrapolated down from adults (IOM, 2001). In addition, adult intakes of up to 12 mg of copper per day from food have not resulted in adverse effects (IOM, 2001).

Assessing the Prevalence of Inadequate and Excessive Consumption of Macronutrients

Acceptable macronutrient distribution ranges (AMDRs) for protein, fat, and carbohydrate intakes are expressed in terms of percent of total calories contributed by these macronutrients. However, for this report, protein intakes were evaluated relative to protein requirements in grams per kilogram of body weight per day (g/kg/d), rather than relative to the AMDR, as this assessment was considered more accurate when evaluating the adequacy of intakes of the WIC populations. Although the proportions of carbohydrate intakes above and below the AMDR were estimated, carbohydrate intakes below the AMDR are not considered of concern given lack of evidence for harm. Because the 2015–2020 *Dietary Guidelines for Americans* (DGA) emphasize saturated and not total fat (USDA/HHS, 2016), intakes of total fat relative to the AMDR were also not evaluated in this report. Added sugars and saturated fat do not have AMDRs, but as indicated in the DGA, the committee applied the guideline of not more than 10 percent of energy from each. Therefore, the upper limit for these nutrients varies depending on the overall kcal level that is appropriate for the individual (USDA/HHS, 2016).

Inadequacy or Excess: The Basis for Concern

The committee was tasked with developing nutrient intake adequacy estimates referenced to the DRIs. On a population level, inadequate or excessive intake of any nutrient is usually considered to be of concern when present in 2.5 percent or more of the population of interest (IOM, 2003). This percent should translate to an equivalent prevalence of impaired function or adverse effect. For example, a 5 percent prevalence of dietary iron inadequacy should translate to a 5 percent prevalence of low iron stores. For this report, a 5 percent threshold was applied (as in IOM, 2011a).This is a slightly relaxed standard, which accounts for some of the uncertainty in setting the EARs, as well as some of the generally accepted errors associated with dietary assessment. The same threshold was applied to proportions of the population with intakes above the UL. For nutrients with an AI, an assessment of adequacy cannot be made. Rather, it can only be stated that the mean usual intakes above the AI imply a low prevalence of inadequacy (IOM, 2000b). To be conservative, mean intakes below the AI were considered potentially indicative of inadequacy in this report. For saturated fat and added sugars, the percent of individuals with intakes exceeding 10 percent of energy were determined (as well as the distribution of intakes in gram amounts).

Special Case: Vitamin D

Evaluation of Vitamin D Adequacy

Both dietary intake and sun exposure contribute to an individual's vitamin D status. It is generally agreed that dietary intake of vitamin D is of limited value in the evaluation of vitamin D adequacy because the relationship between the two is nonlinear (IOM, 2011b). Further, the current U.S. Department of Agriculture (USDA) Food and Nutrient Composition Database does not separate vitamin D from 25-hydroxyvitamin D (25(OH)D) in foods. This results in an underestimate of the bioequivalent vitamin D in foods because 25(OH)D is four to five times more bioequivalent than is the parent form of vitamin D (Cashman, 2012; Cashman et al., 2012).

In contrast, serum 25(OH)D captures both total dietary intake of parent vitamin D and 25(OH)D and sun exposure and has been validated as a biomarker for assessing vitamin D adequacy (IOM, 2011b; Taylor et al., 2013). Data on adults ages 19 to 70 from NHANES 2005–2006 indicate that approximately 71 percent of the U.S. population consumes less than the EAR for dietary vitamin D, but the prevalence of inadequacy assessed by 25(OH)D is only about 19 percent (Taylor et al., 2013).

Vitamin D intake data are presented only for infants ages 0 to less than 12 months in this report because serum 25(OH)D data are not available for this group. Data on serum 25(OH)D were available for individuals ages 1 year and older for NHANES survey years 2005–2006. Current food package content of vitamin D is presented in this report to serve as a reference point for food package changes.

Evaluation of Serum Vitamin D Using NHANES

Estimation of usual serum vitamin D requires two observations. For some individuals only one observation was available. In these cases, the within-person variance in serum 25(OH)D from an earlier NHANES (2001–2002) was applied. By using this external estimate of the within-person variance, the serum 25(OH)D distribution could be adjusted as described in Jahns et al. (2005). Because there is no second day to permit estimation of the within-person variability for children, a value computed for the 2001–2002 NHANES (15 percent) was used to adjust the values. The EAR for serum 25(OH)D is 40 nmol/L for all groups.

Assessing Vitamin D Intake of Individuals Less Than 1 Year of Age

Vitamin D intake data are available for NHANES 2007–2012. Intake data are expressed in μg/d, but the EAR is given in international units (IU). The EAR in IUs was converted to μg by multiplying the amount in IUs by 0.025. For an EAR of 400 IU, the corresponding value in μg is 10.

Estimated Energy Requirements

Some of the analyses in this report used Estimated Energy Requirements (EERs) for the various WIC subgroups. A 2002 IOM committee developed equations to derive EERs that balance total energy expenditure at a level of physical activity consistent with health and support growth rates in children that are compatible with a healthy body size and composition (IOM, 2002/2005). In children, the EER was calculated based on an individual's age, body weight, height, and activity level. For adults, the EER was calculated based on age, gender, body weight, height, and physical activity level. The EER calculations applied in this report assumed a low physical activity level for women and children ages 2 to 5 years. The EER for pregnant and breastfeeding women also includes energy needs associated with the deposition of tissue or the secretion of milk. For pregnant women, the second trimester of pregnancy was assumed to cover all stages of pregnancy. For breastfeeding women, the EER assumed the first 6 months postpartum. Recent research suggested that the IOM (2002/2005) formula may overestimate energy needs for children (Butte et al., 2014), although this finding is yet to be validated broadly. Interpretations of data in this report were considered in light of these recent findings.

Evaluation of Food Group Intakes

Food group intakes can be compared to recommended food patterns for a specific energy level. Food patterns provided as part of the DGA represent a range of energy needs (USDA/HHS, 2016). For women, the food patterns selected were based on the EER (as described above) of WIC-participating subgroups, rounded to the nearest 100 kcal/d. For pregnant and breastfeeding women, this was 2,600 kcal; for postpartum women, this was 2,300 kcal. For women who were income eligible, but not pregnant, breastfeeding, or postpartum, this was 2,200 kcal. For children ages 2 to less than 5 years, the median EER was 1,517 kcals. A food pattern of 1,300 kcal was selected for this age group because (1) 1,500 kcal/d may reflect recent increases in body weights for young children and was considered too high for normal weight children in this age group, particularly in light of efforts to reduce and/or contain the prevalence of childhood obesity; and (2) the 1,300-kcal pattern was applied in both the previous WIC food package review (IOM, 2006) and the Child and Adult Care Food Program (CACFP) report (IOM, 2011a) and should similarly be appropriate for current WIC-participating children of the same ages. Although the 2,300-kcal patterns applied to postpartum women in the current report are somewhat higher than the EERs calculated for the IOM (2006) report (2,163), the patterns selected for this report correspond to the CACFP assumption of 2,400 kcal for women ages 19 to 29 years and 2,300 kcal for women ages 30 to 49 years. The calculated EERs for pregnant and breastfeeding women were approximately 2,600 kcal/d, which corresponds to an additional 300 kcal/d needed by these women relative to nonlactating postpartum women.

Because the food patterns are designed to ensure nutrient intakes that meet almost all of the RDAs, it would be ideal if almost everyone in a population reported usual diets that conformed to the food patterns. However, this goal is almost never achieved, so the committee chose a less restrictive approach in selecting foods group intakes that should be improved: If 50 percent or more of the population fell below the recommended level, then improving intake was considered a priority.

Datasets and Analytical Subgroups

The What We Eat in America Dataset

The primary source of data on food and nutrient intake of the U.S. population is the What We Eat in America (WWEIA) component of NHANES (USDA/ARS, 2005–2012). The WWEIA data used for this report were dietary intake data (foods and nutrients from food sources only, not dietary supplements) collected using the Automated Multiple-Pass Method (AMPM),[1] and demographic information, including age, gender, and physiological status (e.g., pregnant, breastfeeding, or postpartum women [0–1 year after delivery][2]). The only filter applied to create the analytic datasets was the indicator DR1DRSTZ (or DR2DRSTZ for day 2) that identified complete and reliable records. No outliers were removed. By and large, the published NHANES databases have few missing values, in particular for nutrient intake. The population survey weights were applied to all analyses, generating estimated intake values representative of the U.S. population, including by income categories. However, participation in programs such as WIC is not considered in the survey design (USDA/FNS, 2014). In addition, pregnant, breastfeeding, or postpartum women are not oversampled in most survey years (USDA/FNS, 2014), which results in small sample sizes for these physiological states, especially when narrowed to low-income participants.

Food intake data for each survey respondent were translated to USDA food group equivalent values using the Food Patterns Equivalent Database (FPED), a file that identifies the food group and subgroup categories associated with the DGA recommendations (USDA/ARS, 2014). A reasonability check was conducted to compare the output for this report to the nationally representative WWEIA data. Table J-3 presents the FPED component categories that are matched to the main components of the USDA food patterns. Table J-4 presents the definition of the food groups that make up the USDA food patterns, and lists example foods.

Utility of NHANES Datasets in WWEIA for Addressing the Task

The committee was tasked with assessing the nutrient and food group intakes of the WIC-eligible population, as well as low-income women who

---

[1] The AMPM is a computerized method for collecting interviewer-administered 24-hour dietary recalls. In NHANES it is applied in person for the first day and by telephone for the second day of data collection.

[2] Women were selected from NHANES if coded as pregnant, breastfeeding, or if not breastfeeding, coded as 0 to less than 6 months postpartum. Some women reporting WIC participation did not report being pregnant, breastfeeding, or postpartum.

TABLE J-3 Food Groups for Analyses Based on Food Pattern Components in FPID and FPED

Main Components	FPID/FPED Components (2011–2012)
Fruit	Total fruit
Vegetables	Total vegetables
	Dark green vegetables
	Red and orange vegetables
	Starchy vegetables
	Other vegetables
	Beans and peas computed as vegetables
Grains	Total grains
	Whole grains
	Refined grains
Protein foods	Total protein foods
	Meat, poultry, and seafood
	Meat, poultry, and eggs (not seafood)
	Seafood
	Nuts, seeds, soy (nuts and seeds and soybean products)
Dairy	Total dairy (milk, yogurt, cheese, whey)
Oils	Oils
Solid fats	Solid fats
Added sugars	Added sugars

NOTES: FPED = Food Patterns Equivalents Database; FPID = Food Patterns Ingredients Database.
SOURCE: USDA/ARS, 2014.

did not report being pregnant, breastfeeding, or postpartum. USDA's Food and Nutrition Service (USDA/FNS) also requested an evaluation of intakes before and after the 2009 food package changes, and an evaluation of WIC participants separate from eligible non-WIC participants.

USDA-FNS required full implementation of the 2007 (Interim Rule) food package changes by October 2009, and most states implemented the changes at some point between issuance of the 2007 Interim Rule and the October deadline (USDA/FNS, 2012). Given the complications

TABLE J-4 USDA Food Pattern Food Groups, Definitions, and Example Foods*

Food Group	Definition and Unit	Examples of 1 Serving Equivalent
Fruits	Total intact fruits (whole or cut) and fruit juices (c-eq)	1 c raw or cooked fruit; 1 c fruit juice
Vegetables	Total dark green, red and orange, starchy, and other vegetables; excludes legumes (c-eq)	1 c raw or cooked vegetables
Dark green vegetables	Dark green vegetables (c-eq)	1 c raw or cooked dark green vegetables
Red/orange vegetables	Total red and orange vegetables (tomatoes and tomato products + other red and orange vegetables) (c-eq)	1 c raw or cooked red/orange vegetables
Dry beans and peas	Beans and peas (legumes) computed as vegetables (c-eq)	175 g cooked beans; 175 g cooked peas
Starchy vegetables	Total starchy vegetables (white potatoes + other starchy vegetables) (c-eq)	155 g boiled or canned potatoes; 245 g cooked, frozen, or canned pumpkins
Other vegetables	Other vegetables not in the vegetable components listed above (c-eq)	100 g raw cauliflower, 80 g raw eggplant
Grains	Total whole and refined grains (oz-eq)	1/2 c cooked rice, pasta; 1 slice bread
Whole grains	Grains defined as whole grains and contain the entire grain kernel—the bran, germ, and endosperm (oz-eq)	1/2 c cooked whole grain rice, pasta; 1 slice whole grain bread
Protein foods	Total meat, poultry, organ meat, cured meat, seafood, eggs, soy, and nuts and seeds; excludes legumes (oz-eq)	1 egg
Meat, poultry, eggs	Total of meat, poultry, organ meat, and cured meat (oz-eq)	28.35 g cooked, lean meat or poultry
Seafood	Seafood (finfish, shellfish, and other seafood) (oz-eq)	28.35 g cooked fish or shellfish
Nuts, seeds, soy	Peanuts, tree nuts, and seeds; excludes coconut; soy products, excluding calcium fortified soy milk (soymilk) and mature soybeans (oz-eq)	1/2 oz of nuts; 1/2 oz of seeds; 1 tbsp of peanut butter; 1/4 c roasted soybeans
Dairy	Total milk, yogurt, cheese, and whey. For some foods, the total dairy values could be higher than the sum of D_MILK, D_YOGURT, and D_CHEESE because the Miscellaneous Dairy component composed of whey is not included in FPED as a separate variable (c-eq)	1 c milk; 1–2 oz cheese

continued

TABLE J-4 Continued

Food Group	Definition and Unit	Examples of 1 Serving Equivalent
Oils	Fats naturally present in nuts, seeds, and seafood; unhydrogenated vegetable oils, except palm oil, palm kernel oil, and coconut oils; fat present in avocado and olives above the allowable amount; 50% of fat present in stick and tub margarines and margarine spreads (grams)	1.5 g per 100 g in olives and avocados; 100 g per 100 g in vegetable oil; 60 g per 100 g in tub margarine
Solid fats	Fats naturally present in meat, poultry, eggs, and dairy (lard, tallow, and butter); fully or partially hydrogenated oils; shortening; palm, palm kernel and coconut oils; fats naturally present in coconut meat and cocoa butter; and 50% of fat present in stick and tub margarines and margarine spreads (grams)	100 g per 100 g in coconut or palm oil; 81.1 g of 100 g in butter
Added sugars	Foods defined as added sugars: honey, corn syrup, white sugar, brown sugar, fructose (tsp-eq)	1 tsp-eq of added sugars = 4 g of added sugars as honey, corn syrup, etc.

NOTES: c-eq = cup equivalents; oz-eq = ounce equivalents; Tbsp = tablespoon; tsp-eq = tsp equivalents.

* As applied in the 2015–2020 *Dietary Guidelines for Americans.*

SOURCES: USDA/ARS, 2014; USDA/HHS, 2016.

with dividing the NHANES 2009–2010 dataset,[3] the committee estimated prepackage-change intakes using NHANES 2005–2008, and postpackage-change intakes using NHANES 2011–2012, as sample sizes allowed.

The committee evaluated the population sizes to determine which combinations of individuals relevant to the task would allow adequately robust sample sizes. Oversampling of some NHANES population subsets has been discontinued (CDC, 2014), which was a concern for several of the WIC subgroups of interest because small subgroup sizes may result in statistically unreliable population-level estimates. The committee's initial goal was to

[3] NHANES respondents are assigned weights specific to the 2-year datasets. Separation of a 2-year dataset requires recomputation of population weights, which was beyond the scope of this study. It also required knowledge of the location of the participant and the dates of the interviews. Both of these variables are unpublished to preserve privacy of participants.

TABLE J-5 Limitations to the NHANES Datasets Relevant to the Task and Resulting Subgroup Modification

NHANES Dataset Limitation Related to the Task	Modification Implemented
Women ages 14 to 18 years were not identified as participating in WIC in the public use versions of the 2007–2008 and 2009–2010 datasets*	Analyses of these data were limited to women ages 19 to 50 years
NHANES discontinued the oversampling of pregnant women after 2006, which limited the number of pregnant low-income and WIC women surveyed	The survey years 2005–2012 were combined; women were then grouped by physiological state: subgroups of nonparticipating breastfeeding and postpartum women were too small to generate reliable data
No postpartum variable is available in NHANES 2005–2006	For postpartum women, the data span was NHANES 2007–2012
The sample size for eligible non-WIC breastfeeding women across the 2005–2012 survey years was 16	Data for this group were not generated
The sample size for eligible non-WIC postpartum women across the 2005–2012 survey years was 4	Data for this group were not generated
Breastmilk intakes were not quantified for breastfed infants	Only iron and zinc nutrient adequacy were evaluated for infants ages 6 months and older because breastmilk is not a major source of these nutrients
Vitamin D intake data were available for survey years 2007–2008, 2009–2010, and 2011–2012 only; vitamin D intake is not considered a reliable estimate of status	Vitamin D intake was analyzed, but serum data were considered a better indicator of status
Serum 25(OH)D data were available for 2005–2006 survey years only and for individuals ages 1 year and older	25(OH)D status was estimated for this survey period and subgroups ages 1 year and older only

NOTES: NHANES = National Health and Nutrition Examination Survey; non-WIC = WIC-eligible nonparticipants; WIC = individuals participating in WIC.
* The typical age distribution for WIC participation is 18–34 years (USDA/FNS, 2013).

analyze WIC participants[4] and WIC-eligible nonparticipants in subgroups of women (ages 14 to 50 years, eligible by being pregnant, breastfeeding

[4] Capturing WIC participation is dependent upon accurate reporting in NHANES. The committee's comparison of the weighted total number of recipients reporting WIC as well as extensive experience with reporting of programs like WIC suggest that WIC use is underreported. There is also a challenge in identifying the low-income group as eligible; the concept of income reported in NHANES does not correspond to state-level income requirements for eligibility. Some individuals may be income ineligible but may still legitimately participate in the program if adjunctively or automatically eligible due to participation in Medicaid, Temporary Assistance for Needy Families (TANF), or the Supplemental Nutrition Assistance Program (SNAP).

TABLE J-6 NHANES Survey Years Applied for Each Analytical Subgroup

Subgroup	Survey Years Analyzed	Rationale
Women	2005–2012	Survey years were combined to increase sample size and allow for separation by physiological state; no postpartum variable is available in NHANES 2005–2006, so for these women, the data span NHANES 2007–2012
Formula-fed infants	2005–2008; 2011–2012	Sample size allows for examination of pre- and post-2009 food package changes
Breastfed infants	2009–2012*	Survey years were combined to increase sample size; the starting year of 2009 was chosen because sometime during this year, states issued jarred infant food meats
Children	2005–2008; 2011–2012	Sample size allows for examination of pre- and post-2009 food package changes

NOTES: NHANES = National Health and Nutrition Examination Survey.

* This group includes some WIC participants receiving the pre-2009 food package because the committee was unable to divide the 2009–2010 NHANES survey dataset. As a result, the 2009–2010 NHANES release was included in the post-2009 food package change analysis to ensure adequacy of sample sizes.

or postpartum), infants (formula fed or breastfed), and children (ages 1 to less than 2 years, and ages 2 to less than 5 years). These subgroups allow for comparison of nutrient and food intake of all individuals who participate in WIC as well as individuals who qualify but do not participate in the program. A third subgroup of women was included in the analyses: those who were low-income, but not WIC-eligible because they were not pregnant, breastfeeding, or postpartum. Inspection of the data in the survey years of interest (2005 through 2012) indicated that modification of these initially outlined population subgroups was required. Table J-5 details the limitations of NHANES for developing these initially designed population subsets and the modifications made to accommodate the limitations. Table J-6 details the survey years that were ultimately applied.

The committee first examined the subgroup sizes for women to determine the final analytical subgroups, as these were likely to be small. As shown in Table J-7, the sample sizes for eligible non-WIC-participating women that were breastfeeding or postpartum were 16 and 4, respectively. Therefore, these groups were not further examined.

Following careful consideration of these limitations and sample sizes, the committee designed the final population subgroups that would be analyzed for this report (see Table J-8). Subgroups identified as eligible, but non-WIC-participating reported incomes less than or equal to 185 percent of the poverty-to-income ratio (PIR) (based on PIR guidelines in HHS,

TABLE J-7 Sample Sizes for Subgroups of Women in the Combined NHANES 2005–2012 Dataset

Subgroup		N
1[a]	WIC, P[b]	165
2[a]	WIC, any BF	27
3[a]	WIC, PP	62
4	WIC, not 1, 2, or 3[c]	90
5[a]	Non-WIC, P[d]	87
6	Non-WIC, any BF	16
7	Non-WIC, PP	4
8[a]	Non-WIC, not 5, 6, or 7	2,611

NOTES: BF = breastfeeding (intensity unknown); N = sample size; P = pregnant; PP = postpartum.

[a] Analyses were carried out only for these subgroups.

[b] WIC subgroups included individuals of any income level that self-reported as WIC participants.

[c] Women in this subgroup self-reported as participating in WIC, but were not P, BF, or PP.

[d] Non-WIC indicates women who were at or below 185 percent of the federal poverty level, but did not identify as WIC participants.

2015 and USDA/FNS, 2015). The WIC subgroups include only individuals reported as being on WIC in the NHANES survey (these individuals may or may not have a PIR less than or equal to 185 percent). There are two reasons for inclusion of any income level in the WIC group: (1) income could change within the certification period, but the individual remains in the program at the new income level, and (2) the objective is primarily to evaluate the effect of the food package, not the effect of income. Table J-8 also includes sample sizes for the 2005–2008 analysis, for which results are also presented later in this appendix.

Challenges with Dietary Intake Assessment of Breastfeeding Women

Inasmuch as NHANES samples women and children separately, no dyadic data are available for breastfeeding women and their infants. NHANES is able to identify which women are breastfeeding but not the intensity of their breastfeeding or, more directly, the amount of milk they are producing. The DRIs for breastfeeding women are for those who are exclusively breastfeeding. Therefore, when women produce less milk than exclusively breastfeeding women at that same duration of breastfeeding, their caloric needs will be overestimated. For this report, intakes of women coded as "breastfeeding" in NHANES were compared to the DRIs for

TABLE J-8 NHANES Sample Sizes of Population Subgroups Selected for Nutrient and Food Intake Analyses: Phases I and II

	Sample Sizes					
	NHANES 2005–2008		NHANES 2011–2012		NHANES 2005–2012[a]	
Population Subgroup	Nutrients	Foods	Nutrients	Foods	Nutrients	Foods
WIC						
Women, pregnant	—	—	—	—	165	139
Women, breastfeeding	—	—	—	—	27	25
Women, postpartum	—	—	—	—	62	54
Infants, FF, 0 to less than 6 months	204	—[b]	93	—	—	—
Infants, FF, 6 to less than 12 months	252	—[b]	98	—	—	—
Infants, BF, 6 to less than 12 months	—	—	—	39[c]	39	39
Children, 1 to less than 2 years	311	263	96	81	—	—
Children, 2 to less than 5 years	474	402	263	228	—	—
Eligible, Non-WIC[d]						
Women, pregnant	—	—	—	—	87	58
Infants, FF, 0 to less than 6 months	21	19	15	—	—	—
Infants, FF, 6 to less than 12 months	35	31	16	—	—	—
Infants, BF, 6 to less than 12 months	—	—	—	68[c]	8	8
Children, 1 to less than 2 years	106	82	41	25	—	—
Children, 2 to less than 5 years	397	329	217	148	—	—
Low-Income, Ineligible[e]						
Women, not pregnant, BF, or postpartum	—	—	—	—	2,611	1,983

NOTES: — = data not analyzed except where indicated; BF = breastfed/breastfeeding; FF = formula-fed; NHANES = National Health and Nutrition Examination Survey.
Food intake was not analyzed for infants because there exist only intake recommendations for specific types of foods and consumption of formula complicates assessment of intake. Non-WIC breastfeeding and postpartum women were not analyzed due to small sample sizes. Sample sizes differ between the nutrient and food intake analyses because at least 2 days of intake data are required to estimate usual intakes for food.

TABLE J-8 Continued

[a] Except for BF infants, for which NHANES survey years are 2009–2012.
[b] Data are available in the phase I report (NASEM, 2016), but are not included in this appendix.
[c] Intake of meat only was evaluated for these infants. Data are presented in Chapter 4.
[d] Eligible, non-WIC indicates individuals who reported income at or below 185 percent of the federal poverty level but did not identify as WIC participants in the NHANES survey.
[e] Women were categorized as ineligible if they reported income below 185 percent of the federal poverty level but did not meet the WIC physiological requirements.
SOURCE: USDA/ARS, 2005–2012.

breastfeeding women, and to a 2,600-kcal food pattern (which may be high for a woman who is minimally breastfeeding). Therefore, the proportion of breastfeeding women whose intakes are inadequate and the proportion with food-group intakes below that recommended will also be overestimated.

Limitations of Small Sample Sizes

As indicated in Table J-8 some of the sample sizes were small. The committee determined that means for subgroups other than women were adequately precise, despite sample sizes as small as 19. For example, to estimate mean usual intake of calcium for infants ages 0 to less than 6

TABLE J-9 Design Effects for Usual Intake of Specific Nutrients

Population Subgroup	Design Effect						
	Energy	Calcium	Fiber	Potassium	Vitamin B12	Vitamin A	Protein
Pregnant, WIC	4.58	1.43	4.07	2.85	1.62	2.47	1.78
Breastfeeding, WIC	2.54	3.72	2.03	3.53	1.69	2.58	2.51
Postpartum, WIC	1.30	1.37	0.85	0.82	1.06	1.00	1.08
Nonpregnant, nonlactating, WIC	1.68	1.12	2.59	1.98	1.41	1.01	1.69
Pregnant, eligible non-WIC	1.80	1.96	1.53	1.40	1.79	1.77	1.58
Ineligible	2.14	2.11	3.04	1.30	0.95	1.53	1.29

NOTES: "Eligible" indicates women with household incomes below 185 percent of the poverty-to-income ratio that are pregnant, breastfeeding, or postpartum. "Ineligible" indicates women with household incomes in this category that are not eligible by physiological state.

months, a minimum sample size of about 20 infants is required to obtain an estimate that is no more than 20 mg below or above the true mean with 95 percent certainty. For zinc, a minimum of 12 infants is required to estimate the mean usual intake within 0.2 mg of the true value. This is because the estimated variance of usual intake tends to be small, in particular for infants and the design effect (DE) for infants is also small (below 2 for most nutrients). For quantities (i.e., "% Inadequacy") other than means, the required sample sizes are significantly larger.

For women, some samples remained small and the variance of usual intakes tend to be large. Furthermore, in the case of women, estimated DEs tended to be larger than for children, especially in some of the subdomains. Table J-9 shows estimated DEs for seven nutrients, by subdomain. Note that the DE can be larger than 4 in some specific cases, but in general is between 1.8 and 2.5. To generate more robust nutrient intake estimates of the ratio of the within- to the between-person variance in intake, the method of Jahns et al. (2005) was applied. In this method, the variance ratio estimated from the subgroup intake data is combined with a ratio estimate obtained from the group of all women. To do this, an estimate of within-person variance (external variance) is generated using PC-SIDE to assess intake information of all low-income, pregnant, lactating, or postpartum women in all survey years. An internal ratio estimate is obtained separately for each subgroup. A new within- to between-person variance ratio is then computed as a weighted average of the external and internal variance ratio estimates. On average, the external variance was weighted by 100, and the internal variance was weighted by the number of women in the subgroup who provided 2 days of information. When this number is small (as in the case of pregnant or lactating women in 2011–2012), the external variance plays a larger role in the combined estimate. The resulting estimates are less subject to the large degree of variability in the within-person variance estimate that can be introduced by a small sample size. Both means and the "% Inadequacy" have improved reliability.

For the analysis of episodically consumed foods, small samples add enormous challenges. Neither the National Cancer Institute (NCI) method (Dekkers et al., 2014) nor SPADE (used here and described below) results in reliable estimates of distributions of usual food intake when the sample size is small and the proportion of zero consumption is large. In many cases, the programs fail to converge, and no estimation beyond the usual intake mean is possible. Further, neither of the two approaches (NCI or SPADE) permit combining an external and an internal within-person variance estimate when estimating the intake distribution, so the approach followed for nutrients (described above) cannot be implemented for foods. Consequently, with the small sample sizes that were available for women, and the large proportion of zero intakes observed for many of the food subgroups, estimates of the proportion of usual intakes of foods below recommendations are less reliable. Estimates of mean food intake are, however, considered precise with the sample sizes available for this report (Dekkers et al., 2014).

Methods for Evaluation of Food Group and Subgroup Intakes

Food group and subgroup intakes among WIC participating women, infants, and children were evaluated relative to the DGA recommended intakes or other dietary guidance as appropriate. To estimate the distribution of dietary components consumed episodically (food groups and subgroups), SPADE, a method similar to NCI, was implemented. Estimation of usual intake requires two observations; therefore, sample sizes are smaller for food intake compared to nutrient analyses. One consequence of the small sample sizes is that the standard error values are large.

Rationale for Not Conducting Statistical Comparisons

As stated previously, data generated include the subcategories of WIC participants and non-WIC participants as well as pre-2009 and post-2009. WIC participants were not statistically compared to nonparticipants because interpretation of any differences is complicated by the potential for underlying differences between the two groups or selection bias. These comparisons could also be affected by challenges with correct identification of survey respondents as participating in WIC.

Similarly, statistical comparisons of pre- to post-2009 intake data were considered inappropriate. For women and breastfed infants, small sample sizes required the committee to collapse multiple survey years (see Table J-6); therefore, presented results do not uniquely represent pre- or post-2009 intake data. For other subgroups, any detected differences before and after 2009 cannot necessarily be attributed to changes in the food packages.[5] Additionally, the NHANES design is a repeated cross-sectional survey that does not allow for longitudinal analysis at any level (i.e., individual, state, or locality).

---

[5] For example, as discussed in more depth in Chapter 2, adoption of the new food package in 2009 took place at the end of a recession and at a time when families were facing the worst labor market since the recession of the early 1980s. The American Recovery and Reinvestment Act of 2009 provided the funds necessary to increase the maximum benefit level of the Supplemental Nutrition Assistance Program (SNAP) by about 15 percent (EOPUS, 2014). Because SNAP recipients that meet age and physiological state requirements for WIC are automatically income eligible for WIC and, therefore, many WIC participants also receive SNAP benefits, food expenditures and consumption may have changed among those who were receiving both benefits.

Tasks Specific to Infant Formulas

In addition to the science supporting functional ingredients in infant formulas, the IOM committee was asked to evaluate three additional aspects of infant formulas in the food packages: energy concentration, iron concentration, and volume provided. The three tasks and the evaluation approach are outlined in Table J-10.

Results of the Nutrient and Food Group Intake Analyses

In the tables that follow, results of the nutrient intake and food group intake analyses that were conducted for all analytical subgroups are presented.

TABLE J-10 Tasks Related to Infant Formula Requirements in the Food Packages and the Approach

Aspect for Evaluation	Information Collection Strategy	Information in Phase I*	Information in This Report
The current required minimum energy level of 20 kcal/ 100 milliliters	Literature review	Summary of evidence	Summary of literature review; summary of evidence; findings and conclusions (see Appendix Q)
The current WIC minimum iron requirement of 1.5 mg per 100 kcal formula	Current FDA requirements for infant formula; iron DRI for infants; iron intake of infants; EER for infants	Comparison of iron intake with requirements and anticipated iron intake given the EER of WIC-participating infants from NHANES 2005–2008	Comparison of iron intake with requirements and anticipated iron intake given the EER of WIC-participating infants from NHANES 2011–2012 (see Chapter 4, Appendix Q)
The current maximum allowances of infant formula in the food packages	EER calculations for the relevant infant population in NHANES	EER results for WIC infants from NHANES 2005–2008 and comparison to current infant food package energy content	EER results for WIC-participating infants from NHANES 2011–2012 and comparison to current infant food package energy content (see Chapter 4, Appendix Q)

NOTES: DRI = Dietary Reference Intake; EER = Estimated Energy Requirement; NHANES = National Health and Nutrition Examination Survey.
* NASEM, 2016.

TABLE J-11 Usual Intake Distributions of Energy Intake for Women Ages 19 to 50 Years

Participant Category	N	Kcal (SE) 10th	25th	Median	Mean	75th	90th
WIC, Pregnant, 2005–2012	165	1,677 (109)	1,980 (80)	2,333 (67)	2,360 (43)	2,710 (92)	3,079 (142)
WIC, Breastfeeding, 2005–2012	27	1,551 (209)	1,790 (164)	2,088 (143)	2,129 (92)	2,423 (208)	2,760 (328)
WIC, Postpartum, 2007–2012	62	1,242 (135)	1,483 (107)	1,788 (95)	1,832 (62)	2,133 (138)	2,480 (218)
Eligible Non-WIC, Pregnant, 2005–2012	87	1,558 (129)	1,839 (106)	2,212 (98)	2,298 (69)	2,662 (154)	3,147 (263)
Nonpregnant Postpartum or Breastfeeding Non-WIC, 2005–2012	2,611	1,279 (23)	1,536 (18)	1,849 (16)	1,893 (10)	2,202 (22)	2,563 (36)

NOTES: See additional notes following Table J-18.

TABLE J-12 Usual Intake Distributions of Energy Intake for Infants Ages 0 to Less Than 12 Months

Participant Category	N	Kcal (SE) 10th	25th	Median	Mean	75th	90th
0 to Less Than 6 months: WIC, 2005–2008	204	501 (27)	592 (18)	693 (15)	705 (12)	804 (22)	922 (38)
0 to Less Than 6 Months: Eligible Non-WIC, 2005–2008	21	492 (44)	548 (38)	629 (37)	659 (34)	738 (66)	865 (124)
0 to Less Than 6 Months: WIC, 2011–2012	93	492 (32)	574 (25)	677 (21)	6920 (17)	794 (31)	911 (50)
0 to Less Than 6 Months: Eligible Non-WIC, 2011–2012	15	563 (91)	640 (60)	724 (43)	722 (32)	805 (57)	877 (83)
6 to Less Than 12 Months: WIC, 2005–2008	252	672 (30)	792 (21)	941 (20)	978 (17)	1,128 (33)	1,337 (56)
6 to Less Than 12 Months: Eligible Non-WIC, 2005–2008	35	689 (65)	786 (52)	914 (48)	941 (37)	1,066 (75)	1,228 (125)
6 to Less Than 12 Months: WIC, 2011–2012	98	660 (48)	771 (38)	910 (34)	928 (22)	1,066 (48)	1,222 (74)
6 to Less Than 12 Months: Eligible Non-WIC, 2011–2012	16	644 (72)	714 (66)	827 (71)	884 (60)	993 (140)	1,199 (279)

NOTES: See additional notes following Table J-18.

TABLE J-13 Usual Intake Distributions of Energy Intake for Children Ages 1 to Less Than 2 Years

		Kcal (SE)					
Participant Category	N	10th	25th	Median	Mean	75th	90th
WIC, 2005–2008	311	951 (35)	1,098 (28)	1,284 (26)	1,314 (17)	1,498 (37)	1,716 (59)
Eligible Non-WIC, 2005–2008	106	978 (71)	1,152 (56)	1,367 (49)	1,395 (33)	1,608 (70)	1,848 (110)
WIC, 2011–2012	96	878 (63)	1,032 (49)	1,221 (42)	1,243 (30)	1,430 (60)	1,637 (93)
Eligible Non-WIC, 2011–2012	41	869 (107)	1,011 (80)	1,181 (66)	1,196 (41)	1,365 (94)	1,544 (145)

NOTES: See additional notes following Table J-18.

TABLE J-14 Usual Intake Distributions of Energy Intake for Children Ages 2 to Less Than 5 Years

		Kcal (SE)					
Participant Category	N	10th	25th	Median	Mean	75th	90th
WIC, 2005–2008	474	1,108 (35)	1,281 (27)	1,495 (24)	1,534 (17)	1,743 (35)	2,007 (60)
Eligible Non-WIC, 2005–2008	397	1,093 (38)	1,267 (28)	1,471 (23)	1,493 (17)	1,695 (33)	1,921 (54)
WIC, 2011–2012	263	1,114 (45)	1,282 (32)	1,479 (28)	1,509 (21)	1,702 (41)	1,939 (70)
Eligible Non-WIC, 2011–2012	217	1,247 (56)	1,407 (42)	1,599 (36)	1,614 (20)	1,804 (49)	2,001 (73)

NOTES: See additional notes following Table J-18.

TABLE J-15 Distributions of Estimated Energy Requirements for Women Ages 19 to 50 Years

		Kcal (SE)					
Participant Category	N	10th	25th	Median	Mean	75th	90th
WIC, Pregnant, 2005–2012	165	2,353 (24)	2,464 (22)	2,612 (22)	2,679 (24)	2,849 (42)	3,095 (80)
WIC, Any Breastfeeding, 2005–2012	27	2,339 (55)	2,420 (42)	2,530 (36)	2,557 (38)	2,670 (63)	2,820 (111)
WIC, Postpartum, 2007–2012	62	2,059 (35)	2,156 (27)	2,350 (23)	2,379 (33)	2,602 (44)	2,765 (111)
Eligible Non-WIC, Pregnant, 2005–2012	87	2,305 (40)	2,417 (30)	2,556 (24)	2,576 (24)	2,716 (38)	2,876 (63)
Nonpregnant Postpartum or Breastfeeding Non-WIC, 2005–2012	2,611	1,956 (7)	2,063 (5)	2,203 (5)	2,245 (5)	2,379 (8)	2,586 (16)

NOTES: See additional notes following Table J-18.

TABLE J-16 Distributions of Estimated Energy Requirements for Infants Ages 0 to Less Than 12 Months

		Kcal (SE)					
Participant Category	N*	10th	25th	Median	Mean	75th	90th
0 to Less Than 6 Months: WIC, 2005–2008	298	435 (13)	502 (9)	581 (7)	594 (8.6)	665 (10)	743 (16)
0 to Less Than 6 Months: Eligible Non-WIC, 2005–2008	70	383 (29)	456 (21)	542 (16)	547 (32.7)	633 (23)	720 (37)
0 to Less Than 6 Months: WIC, 2011–2012	93	508 (18)	557 (13)	617 (10)	623 (10)	682 (16)	747 (26)
0 to Less Than 6 Months: Eligible Non-WIC, 2011–2012	15	504 (49)	545 (30)	584 (18)	577 (14)	615 (20)	639 (26)
6 to Less Than 12 Months: WIC, 2005–2008	306	593 (12)	658 (9)	733 (7)	744 (7.2)	811 (9)	885 (15)
6 to Less Than 12 Months: Eligible Non-WIC, 2005–2008	59	578 (26)	638 (18)	708 (14)	713 (15)	781 (20)	850 (32)
6 to Less Than 12 Months: WIC, 2011–2012	98	616 (18)	666 (13)	727 (10)	734 (10)	794 (16)	860 (25)
6 to Less Than 12 Months: Eligible Non-WIC, 2011–2012	16	586 (65)	640 (43)	699 (30)	698 (22)	757 (42)	809 (62)

NOTES: See additional notes following Table J-18.

* Sample sizes for 2005–2008 are higher than those presented in Table J-8 because individuals with missing or incomplete food intake information can still be included in the estimation of EER for which only age and weight are required.

TABLE J-17 Distributions of Estimated Energy Requirements for Children Ages 1 to Less Than 2 Years

		Kcal (SE)					
Participant Category	N*	10th	25th	Median	Mean	75th	90th
WIC, 2005–2008	316	745 (16)	825 (10)	906 (7)	925 (8.8)	996 (12)	1,106 (25)
Eligible Non-WIC, 2005–2008	134	745 (20)	815 (15)	901 (12)	945 (14.3)	996 (18)	1,092 (30)
WIC, 2011–2012	96	819 (24)	886 (17)	962 (12)	966 (12)	1,033 (17)	1,110 (33)
Eligible Non-WIC, 2011–2012	41	865 (43)	921 (22)	971 (15)	977 (16)	1,025 (26)	1,096 (58)

NOTES: See additional notes following Table J-18.
* Sample sizes for 2005–2008 are higher than those presented in Table J-8 because individuals with missing or incomplete food intake information can still be included in the estimation of EER for which only age, height, weight and physical activity level are required.

TABLE J-18 Distributions of Estimated Energy Requirements for Children Ages 2 to Less Than 5 Years

		kcal (SE)					
Participant Category	N*	10th	25th	Median	Mean	75th	90th
WIC, 2005–2008	528	1,068 (21)	1,181 (11)	1,306 (8)	1,295 (8)	1,422 (9)	1,506 (15)
Eligible Non-WIC, 2005–2008	479	1,058 (25)	1,210 (15)	1,349 (8)	1,326 (10)	1,444 (9)	1,543 (19)
WIC, 2011–2012	263	1,362 (13)	1,428 (10)	1,517 (9)	1,532 (9)	1,620 (14)	1,723 (23)
Eligible Non-WIC, 2011–2012	217	1,376 (21)	1,473 (15)	1,569 (9)	1,569 (10)	1,651 (13)	1,743 (25)

NOTES: See additional notes following this table.
* Sample sizes for 2005–2008 are higher than those presented in Table J-8 because individuals with missing or incomplete food intake information can still be included in the estimation of EER for which only age, height, weight and physical activity level are required.
NOTES for Tables J-11 through J-18: kcal = kilocalories; N = sample size; SE = standard error. Sample sizes for calculation of EER are larger than for other analyses because a report of food intake is not required.
SOURCES: USDA/ARS, 2005–2012. EERs were calculated using the Dietary Reference Intake report method (IOM, 2002/2005).

TABLE J-19 Usual Intake Distributions of Selected Macronutrients for Pregnant WIC-Participating Women Ages 19 to 50 Years, NHANES 2005–2012

	Percentiles and Means (SE)					
Nutrient and Reported Units	10th	25th	Median	Mean	75th	90th
Carbohydrates (% of kcal)	46.5 (1.36)	49.8 (0.96)	53.4 (0.75)	53.3 (0.41)	56.9 (0.93)	60.1 (1.29)
Fiber (g/d)	11.4 (1.00)	14.3 (0.77)	18.0 (0.70)	18.9 (0.52)	22.5 (1.12)	27.5 (2.02)
Total fat (% of kcal)	27.3 (0.98)	29.8 (0.72)	32.5 (0.58)	32.6 (0.32)	35.3 (0.75)	37.9 (1.06)
Saturated fat (% of kcal)	9.0 (0.44)	10.0 (0.32)	11.1 (0.26)	11.1 (0.13)	12.3 (0.33)	13.3 (0.47)
Saturated fat (g/d)	20.4 (1.5)	24.5 (1.2)	29.4 (1.0)	30.1 (0.6)	34.9 (1.5)	40.6 (2.4)
Protein (g/kg/d)	0.8 (0.05)	0.9 (0.04)	1.1 (0.04)	1.1 (0.03)	1.3 (0.06)	1.6 (0.09)

NOTES: N = 165. See additional notes following Table J-39.

TABLE J-20 Usual Intake Distributions of Selected Macronutrients for Pregnant Eligible Non-WIC-Participating Women Ages 19 to 50 Years, NHANES 2005–2012

	Percentiles and Mean (SE)					
Nutrient and Reported Units	10th	25th	Median	Mean	75th	90th
Carbohydrates (% of kcal)	46.1 (1.68)	49.3 (1.21)	52.9 (0.97)	53.0 (0.58)	56.6 (1.26)	60.0 (1.82)
Fiber (g/d)	11.1 (1.09)	13.4 (0.88)	16.5 (0.80)	17.0 (0.54)	20.0 (1.20)	23.7 (1.96)
Total fat (% of kcal)	27.8 (1.46)	30.6 (1.05)	33.6 (0.81)	33.5 (0.46)	36.6 (0.97)	39.0 (1.24)
Saturated fat (% of kcal)	9.0 (0.46)	9.9 (0.34)	11.0 (0.28)	11.0 (0.17)	12.1 (0.38)	13.1 (0.57)
Saturated fat (g/d)	17.8 (1.9)	22.0 (1.6)	27.5 (1.5)	28.7 (1.0)	34.1 (2.3)	41.1 (3.9)
Protein (g/kg/d)	0.8 (0.08)	0.9 (0.07)	1.2 (0.06)	1.2 (0.04)	1.4 (0.10)	1.7 (0.16)

NOTES: N = 87. See additional notes following Table J-39.

TABLE J-21 Usual Intake Distributions of Selected Macronutrients for Breastfeeding WIC-Participating Women Ages 19 to 50 Years, NHANES 2005–2012

	Percentiles and Mean (SE)					
Nutrient and Reported Units	10th	25th	Median	Mean	75th	90th
Carbohydrates (% of kcal)	41.9 (3.39)	45.5 (2.41)	49.7 (1.89)	49.8 (1.21)	54.0 (2.55)	58.0 (3.79)
Fiber (g/d)	11.3 (1.96)	13.4 (1.45)	16.0 (1.18)	16.2 (0.76)	18.7 (1.67)	21.4 (2.58)
Total fat (% of kcal)	26.7 (2.73)	29.5 (1.87)	32.7 (1.40)	32.7 (0.90)	35.8 (1.87)	38.7 (2.73)
Saturated fat (% of kcal)	8.9 (1.21)	10.2 (0.83)	11.6 (0.63)	11.6 (0.39)	13.0 (0.77)	14.2 (1.05)
Saturated fat (g/d)	17.3 (3.7)	21.7 (3.1)	27.5 (2.9)	28.6 (1.8)	34.3 (4.3)	41.3 (6.9)
Protein (g/kg/d)	0.8 (0.13)	0.9 (0.10)	1.1 (0.08)	1.1 (0.05)	1.3 (0.13)	1.5 (0.20)

NOTES: N = 27. See additional notes following Table J-39.

TABLE J-22 Usual Intake Distributions of Selected Macronutrients for Postpartum WIC-Participating Women Ages 19 to 50 Years, NHANES 2007–2012

	Percentiles and Mean (SE)					
Nutrient and Reported Units	10th	25th	Median	Mean	75th	90th
Carbohydrates (% of kcal)	44.1 (2.91)	48.7 (1.93)	53.6 (1.51)	53.9 (1.03)	58.8 (2.13)	64.2 (3.54)
Fiber (g/d)	6.3 (1.26)	8.6 (1.05)	11.7 (0.97)	12.2 (0.63)	15.2 (1.43)	18.8 (2.28)
Total fat (% of kcal)	24.1 (2.37)	27.8 (1.62)	31.7 (1.21)	31.4 (0.71)	35.3 (1.43)	38.4 (1.91)
Saturated fat (% of kcal)	7.2 (0.80)	8.5 (0.58)	10.0 (0.47)	9.9 (0.28)	11.5 (0.61)	12.9 (0.86)
Saturated fat (g/d)	11.9 (1.9)	15.3 (1.6)	19.8 (1.5)	20.5 (0.9)	24.9 (2.1)	30.1 (3.3)
Protein (g/kg/d)	0.5 (0.07)	0.6 (0.06)	0.8 (0.05)	0.8 (0.03)	1.0 (0.08)	1.2 (0.13)

NOTES: N = 62. See additional notes following Table J-39.

TABLE J-23 Usual Intake Distributions of Selected Macronutrients for Nonpregnant, Postpartum, or Breastfeeding Eligible Non-WIC-Participating Women Ages 19 to 50 Years, NHANES 2005–2012

	Percentiles and Mean (SE)					
Nutrient and Reported Units	10th	25th	Median	Mean	75th	90th
Carbohydrates (% of kcal)	44.3 (0.40)	48.0 (0.28)	52.1 (0.22)	52.1 (0.12)	56.2 (0.29)	60.0 (0.42)
Fiber (g/d)	7.5 (0.20)	9.9 (0.17)	13.1 (0.16)	14.0 (0.11)	17.1 (0.26)	21.6 (0.45)
Total fat (% of kcal)	26.1 (0.32)	28.9 (0.23)	32.0 (0.18)	32.0 (0.09)	35.0 (0.23)	37.8 (0.32)
Saturated fat (% of kcal)	8.0 (0.12)	9.1 (0.09)	10.4 (0.08)	10.5 (0.04)	11.8 (0.10)	13.0 (0.14)
Saturated fat (g/d)	13.4 (0.4)	17.1 (0.3)	21.9 (0.3)	22.9 (0.2)	27.6 (0.4)	33.7 (0.7)
Protein (g/kg/d)	0.6 (0.01)	0.7 (0.01)	0.9 (0.01)	1.0 (0.01)	1.2 (0.02)	1.4 (0.03)

NOTES: N = 2,611. See additional notes following Table J-39.

TABLE J-24 Usual Intake Distributions of Selected Macronutrients for WIC-Participating Infants Ages 0 to Less Than 6 Months, NHANES 2005–2008

	Percentiles and Mean (SE)					
Nutrient and Reported Units	10th	25th	Median	Mean	75th	90th
Carbohydrates (% of kcal)	42.0 (0.25)	43.2 (0.26)	45.4 (0.34)	46.8 (0.35)	49.0 (0.70)	53.6 (1.33)
Total fat (% of kcal)	38.3 (1.24)	42.4 (0.64)	45.6 (0.33)	44.5 (0.32)	47.8 (0.29)	49.1 (0.29)
Saturated fat (% of kcal)	14.5 (0.50)	16.1 (0.23)	17.5 (0.21)	17.6 (0.19)	19.3 (0.30)	20.7 (0.25)
Protein (g/kg/d)	1.6 (0.10)	2.0 (0.07)	2.4 (0.06)	2.4 (0.05)	2.8 (0.09)	3.3 (0.15)

NOTES: N = 204. See additional notes following Table J-39.

TABLE J-25 Usual Intake Distributions of Selected Macronutrients for Eligible Non-WIC-Participating Infants Ages 0 to Less Than 6 Months, NHANES 2005–2008

	Percentiles and Mean (SE)					
Nutrient and Reported Units	10th	25th	Median	Mean	75th	90th
Carbohydrates (% of kcal)	42.2 (1.48)	43.5 (1.26)	45.4 (1.25)	45.8 (0.69)	47.6 (2.03)	50.1 (3.40)
Total fat (% of kcal)	40.0 (3.70)	43.1 (2.01)	45.7 (1.19)	45.1 (0.85)	47.8 (1.27)	49.5 (1.73)
Saturated fat (% of kcal)	15.3 (1.36)	16.6 (0.90)	17.8 (0.65)	17.7 (0.40)	19.0 (0.77)	20.0 (1.03)
Protein (g/kg/d)	1.8 (0.25)	2.0 (0.16)	2.3 (0.14)	2.5 (0.19)	2.8 (0.31)	3.5 (0.79)

NOTES: N = 21. See additional notes following Table J-39.

TABLE J-26 Usual Intake Distributions of Selected Macronutrients for WIC-Participating Infants Ages 0 to Less Than 6 Months, NHANES 2011–2012

	Percentiles and Mean (SE)					
Nutrient and Reported Units	10th	25th	Median	Mean	75th	90th
Carbohydrates (% of kcal)	42.3 (0.39)	43.3 (0.33)	44.8 (0.35)	45.5 (0.33)	47.0 (0.67)	49.7 (1.32)
Total fat (% of kcal)	41.3 (1.42)	44.1 (0.71)	46.3 (0.36)	45.6 (0.34)	47.8 (0.34)	48.9 (0.43)
Saturated fat (% of kcal)	15.0 (0.74)	16.7 (0.39)	18.4 (0.39)	19.0 (0.38)	20.7 (0.57)	23.4 (1.67)
Protein (g/kg/d)	1.5 (0.12)	1.9 (0.10)	2.3 (0.09)	2.4 (0.08)	2.8 (0.15)	3.4 (0.25)

NOTES: N = 93. See additional notes following Table J-39.

TABLE J-27 Usual Intake Distributions of Selected Macronutrients for Eligible Non-WIC-Participating Infants Ages 0 to Less Than 6 Months, NHANES 2011–2012

	Percentiles and Mean (SE)					
Nutrient and Reported Units	10th	25th	Median	Mean	75th	90th
Carbohydrates (% of kcal)	41.6 (2.12)	43.4 (1.49)	45.6 (1.15)	45.8 (0.87)	47.9 (1.68)	50.1 (2.65)
Total fat (% of kcal)	41.5 (2.59)	43.5 (1.27)	45.1 (0.73)	44.9 (0.70)	46.5 (1.07)	48.0 (2.03)
Saturated fat (% of kcal)	16.8 (0.81)	17.5 (0.55)	18.3 (0.41)	18.3 (0.31)	19.1 (0.59)	19.8 (0.90)
Protein (g/kg/d)	2.1 (0.19)	2.3 (0.16)	2.6 (0.15)	2.6 (0.12)	2.9 (0.27)	3.3 (0.51)

NOTES: N = 204. See additional notes following Table J-39.

TABLE J-28 Usual Intake Distributions of Selected Macronutrients for WIC-Participating Infants Ages 6 to Less Than 12 Months, NHANES 2005–2008

	Percentiles and Mean (SE)					
Nutrient and Reported Units	10th	25th	Median	Mean	75th	90th
Carbohydrates (% of kcal)	45.3 (0.94)	48.9 (0.63)	52.8 (0.48)	52.8 (0.38)	56.7 (0.64)	60.4 (1.00)
Fiber (g/d)	1.9 (0.24)	3.0 (0.21)	4.6 (0.22)	5.1 (0.19)	6.6 (0.37)	9.0 (0.68)
Total fat (% of kcal)	30.4 (0.88)	33.8 (0.58)	37.3 (0.42)	37.0 (0.32)	40.6 (0.50)	43.3 (0.67)
Saturated fat (% of kcal)	11.4 (0.4)	13.1 (0.3)	14.9 (0.2)	14.7 (0.2)	16.8 (0.3)	18.4 (0.4)
Protein (g/kg/d)	1.6 (0.09)	2.1 (0.08)	2.7 (0.09)	2.9 (0.08)	3.6 (0.17)	4.7 (0.28)

NOTES: N = 252. See additional notes following Table J-39.

TABLE J-29 Usual Intake Distributions of Selected Macronutrients for Eligible Non-WIC-Participating Infants Ages 6 to Less Than 12 Months, NHANES 2005–2008

	Percentiles and Mean (SE)					
Nutrient and Reported Units	10th	25th	Median	Mean	75th	90th
Carbohydrates (% of kcal)	45.2 (2.08)	48.3 (1.55)	52.2 (1.30)	52.6 (1.02)	56.3 (1.87)	60.5 (2.92)
Fiber (g/d)	1.8 (0.51)	2.7 (0.47)	4.0 (0.49)	4.5 (0.43)	5.8 (0.85)	7.9 (1.55)
Total fat (% of kcal)	30.3 (2.13)	33.2 (1.37)	36.2 (0.93)	35.9 (0.71)	38.9 (1.07)	41.0 (1.40)
Saturated fat (% of kcal)	11.9 (0.7)	13.3 (0.5)	14.9 (0.4)	15.1 (0.48)	16.5 (0.5)	18.0 (0.8)
Protein (g/kg/d)	1.6 (0.26)	2.1 (0.24)	2.8 (0.25)	3.2 (0.28)	3.9 (0.49)	5.3 (1.01)

NOTES: N = 35. See additional notes following Table J-39.

TABLE J-30 Usual Intake Distributions of Selected Macronutrients for WIC-Participating Infants Ages 6 to Less Than 12 Months, NHANES 2011–2012

	Percentiles and Mean (SE)					
Nutrient and Reported Units	10th	25th	Median	Mean	75th	90th
Carbohydrates (% of kcal)	47.4 (1.14)	50.1 (0.82)	53.2 (0.65)	53.2 (0.46)	56.3 (0.84)	59.1 (1.21)
Fiber (g/d)	1.9 (0.42)	3.0 (0.38)	4.7 (0.37)	5.1 (0.29)	6.8 (0.60)	9.0 (1.00)
Total fat (% of kcal)	30.3 (1.34)	33.5 (0.90)	36.8 (0.66)	36.6 (0.49)	40.0 (0.79)	42.7 (1.07)
Saturated fat (% of kcal)	11.7 (0.57)	13.1 (0.42)	14.6 (0.35)	14.7 (0.24)	16.3 (0.46)	17.8 (0.68)
Protein (g/kg/d)	1.7 (0.14)	2.0 (0.12)	2.6 (0.13)	2.8 (0.11)	3.4 (0.22)	4.3 (0.42)

NOTES: N = 98. See additional notes following Table J-39.

TABLE J-31 Usual Intake Distributions of Selected Macronutrients for Eligible Non-WIC-Participating Infants Ages 6 to Less Than 12 Months, NHANES 2011–2012

	Percentiles and Mean (SE)					
Nutrient and Reported Units	10th	25th	Median	Mean	75th	90th
Carbohydrates (% of kcal)	47.7 (3.24)	50.4 (2.12)	53.3 (1.49)	53.1 (1.05)	56.0 (1.93)	58.4 (2.76)
Fiber (g/d)	2.8 (1.00)	3.7 (0.79)	4.9 (0.69)	5.1 (0.48)	6.3 (1.05)	7.7 (1.72)
Total fat (% of kcal)	30.2 (4.75)	33.7 (2.12)	36.1 (1.04)	35.5 (1.05)	37.9 (1.39)	40.0 (2.74)
Saturated fat (% of kcal)	11.6 (1.44)	12.9 (1.05)	14.4 (0.84)	14.5 (0.58)	16.0 (1.19)	17.5 (1.83)
Protein (g/kg/d)	1.7 (0.26)	2.0 (0.28)	2.5 (0.35)	3.0 (0.39)	3.5 (0.86)	4.8 (2.1)

NOTES: N = 16. See additional notes following Table J-39.

TABLE J-32 Usual Intake Distributions of Selected Macronutrients for WIC-Participating Children Ages 1 to Less Than 2 Years, NHANES 2005–2008

	Percentiles and Mean (SE)					
Nutrient and Reported Units	10th	25th	Median	Mean	75th	90th
Carbohydrates (% of kcal)	45.8 (0.93)	49.1 (0.68)	52.8 (0.55)	52.9 (0.32)	56.6 (0.71)	60.1 (1.01)
Fiber (g/d)	4.8 (0.30)	6.0 (0.23)	7.5 (0.21)	7.8 (0.14)	9.2 (0.31)	11.0 (0.51)
Total fat (% of kcal)	26.7 (0.85)	29.7 (0.59)	33.0 (0.45)	32.9 (0.27)	36.1 (0.54)	38.8 (0.73)
Saturated fat (% of kcal)	11.4 (0.4)	13.1 (0.3)	14.9 (0.2)	13.6 (0.16)	16.8 (0.3)	18.4 (0.4)
Protein (g/kg/d)	3.1 (0.14)	3.6 (0.11)	4.4 (0.10)	4.5 (0.07)	5.2 (0.14)	6.0 (0.22)

NOTES: N = 311. See additional notes following Table J-39.

TABLE J-33 Usual Intake Distributions of Selected Macronutrients for Eligible Non-WIC-Participating Children Ages 1 to Less Than 2 Years, NHANES 2005–2008

	Percentiles and Mean (SE)					
Nutrient and Reported Units	10th	25th	Median	Mean	75th	90th
Carbohydrates (% of kcal)	48.0 (1.35)	50.5 (0.97)	53.4 (0.78)	53.5 (0.42)	56.4 (1.02)	59.1 (1.48)
Fiber (g/d)	5.3 (0.73)	6.9 (0.55)	8.9 (0.49)	9.2 (0.33)	11.2 (0.74)	13.6 (1.27)
Total fat (% of kcal)	26.5 (1.32)	29.5 (0.93)	32.9 (0.73)	33.0 (0.49)	36.4 (0.95)	39.5 (1.37)
Saturated fat (% of kcal)	11.9 (0.7)	13.3 (0.5)	14.9 (0.4)	13.2 (0.28)	16.5 (0.5)	18.0 (0.8)
Protein (g/kg/d)	3.0 (0.25)	3.6 (0.20)	4.3 (0.17)	4.4 (0.11)	5.1 (0.25)	5.9 (0.38)

NOTES: N = 106. See additional notes following Table J-39.

TABLE J-34 Usual Intake Distributions of Selected Macronutrients for WIC-Participating Children Ages 1 to Less Than 2 Years, NHANES 2011–2012

	Percentiles and Mean (SE)					
Nutrient and Reported Units	10th	25th	Median	Mean	75th	90th
Carbohydrates (% of kcal)	45.1 (1.57)	48.3 (1.16)	52.1 (0.96)	52.3 (0.58)	56.0 (1.28)	59.7 (1.88)
Fiber (g/d)	4.4 (0.69)	6.1 (0.53)	8.3 (0.44)	8.5 (0.33)	10.6 (0.62)	12.8 (0.93)
Total fat (% of kcal)	27.1 (1.48)	30.2 (1.03)	33.5 (0.79)	33.4 (0.49)	36.7 (0.96)	39.5 (1.33)
Saturated fat (% of kcal)	10.1 (0.69)	11.6 (0.51)	13.4 (0.41)	13.5 (0.27)	15.3 (0.53)	17.0 (0.77)
Protein (g/kg/d)	2.8 (0.23)	3.4 (0.18)	4.0 (0.15)	4.1 (0.10)	4.7 (0.21)	5.4 (0.32)

NOTES: N = 96. See additional notes following Table J-39.

TABLE J-35 Usual Intake Distributions of Selected Macronutrients for Eligible Non-WIC-Participating Children Ages 1 to Less Than 2 Years, NHANES 2011–2012

	Percentiles and Mean (SE)					
Nutrient and Reported Units	10th	25th	Median	Mean	75th	90th
Carbohydrates (% of kcal)	42.7 (2.58)	46.0 (1.75)	49.6 (1.30)	49.5 (0.82)	53.1 (1.65)	56.2 (2.35)
Fiber (g/d)	4.6 (1.03)	6.1 (0.83)	8.0 (0.72)	8.2 (0.47)	10.1 (1.07)	12.2 (1.71)
Total fat (% of kcal)	29.7 (1.97)	32.2 (1.40)	34.9 (1.09)	35.0 (0.66)	37.8 (1.48)	40.5 (2.22)
Saturated fat (% of kcal)	10.2 (1.11)	11.7 (0.78)	13.4 (0.61)	13.4 (0.39)	15.1 (0.81)	16.7 (1.19)
Protein (g/kg/d)	2.9 (0.38)	3.4 (0.28)	4.0 (0.23)	4.1 (0.15)	4.7 (0.32)	5.3 (0.49)

NOTES: N = 41. See additional notes following Table J-39.

TABLE J-36 Usual Intake Distributions of Selected Macronutrients for WIC-Participating Children Ages 2 to Less Than 5 Years, NHANES 2005–2008

	Percentiles and Mean (SE)					
Nutrient and Reported Units	10th	25th	Median	Mean	75th	90th
Carbohydrates (% of kcal)	49.0 (0.70)	51.9 (0.51)	55.3 (0.41)	55.3 (0.23)	58.6 (0.52)	61.7 (0.73)
Fiber (g/d)	6.2 (0.31)	7.8 (0.25)	10.0 (0.24)	10.5 (0.18)	12.6 (0.37)	15.5 (0.65)
Total fat (% of kcal)	26.4 (0.58)	29.0 (0.41)	31.8 (0.33)	31.8 (0.19)	34.6 (0.41)	37.1 (0.57)
Saturated fat (% of kcal)	9.7 (0.2)	10.7 (0.2)	12.0 (0.1)	11.7 (0.09)	13.2 (0.2)	14.4 (0.2)
Protein (g/kg/d)	2.3 (0.09)	2.8 (0.07)	3.4 (0.07)	3.5 (0.04)	4.1 (0.09)	4.8 (0.15)

NOTES: N = 474. See additional notes following Table J-39.

TABLE J-37 Usual Intake Distributions of Selected Macronutrients for Eligible Non-WIC-Participating Children Ages 2 to Less Than 5 Years, NHANES 2005–2008

	Percentiles and Mean (SE)					
Nutrient and Reported Units	10th	25th	Median	Mean	75th	90th
Carbohydrates (% of kcal)	48.6 (0.76)	51.3 (0.54)	54.3 (0.43)	54.3 (0.23)	57.3 (0.57)	60.2 (0.83)
Fiber (g/d)	5.9 (0.32)	7.5 (0.25)	9.5 (0.23)	9.8 (0.17)	11.8 (0.34)	14.2 (0.57)
Total fat (% of kcal)	27.8 (0.65)	30.1 (0.46)	32.6 (0.36)	32.6 (0.18)	35.1 (0.45)	37.3 (0.62)
Saturated fat (% of kcal)	9.0 (0.3)	10.0 (0.2)	11.1 (0.2)	12.1 (0.08)	12.3 (0.2)	13.4 (0.3)
Protein (g/kg/d)	2.3 (0.10)	2.7 (0.07)	3.3 (0.06)	3.4 (0.05)	3.9 (0.10)	4.6 (0.17)

NOTES: N = 397. See additional notes following Table J-39.

TABLE J-38 Usual Intake Distributions of Selected Macronutrients for WIC-Participating Children Ages 2 to Less Than 5 Years, NHANES 2011–2012

	Percentiles and Mean (SE)					
Nutrient and Reported Units	10th	25th	Median	Mean	75th	90th
Carbohydrates (% of kcal)	50.4 (0.90)	52.7 (0.64)	55.2 (0.50)	55.1 (0.23)	57.6 (0.62)	59.8 (0.86)
Fiber (g/d)	7.9 (0.46)	9.5 (0.37)	11.7 (0.34)	12.0 (0.21)	14.1 (0.49)	16.6 (0.76)
Total fat (% of kcal)	26.7 (0.75)	29.0 (0.54)	31.6 (0.43)	31.6 (0.24)	34.2 (0.55)	36.6 (0.77)
Saturated fat (% of kcal)	8.9 (0.31)	9.8 (0.23)	10.8 (0.19)	10.9 (0.10)	12.0 (0.25)	13.0 (0.36)
Saturated fat (g/d)	11.9 (0.7)	14.5 (0.6)	18.0 (0.5)	18.6 (0.4)	22.0 (0.8)	26.2 (1.2)
Protein (g/kg/d)	2.3 (0.12)	2.8 (0.09)	3.4 (0.08)	3.5 (0.06)	4.0 (0.12)	4.7 (0.21)

NOTES: N = 263. See additional notes following Table J-39.

TABLE J-39 Usual Intake Distributions of Selected Macronutrients for Eligible Non-WIC-Participating Children Ages 2 to Less Than 5 Years, NHANES 2011–2012

	Percentiles and Mean (SE)					
Nutrient and Reported Units	10th	25th	Median	Mean	75th	90th
Carbohydrates (% of kcal)	51.0 (1.02)	53.2 (0.72)	55.6 (0.57)	55.7 (0.26)	58.2 (0.77)	60.6 (1.18)
Fiber (g/d)	7.7 (0.48)	9.3 (0.38)	11.2 (0.34)	11.4 (0.21)	13.3 (0.48)	15.4 (0.75)
Total fat (% of kcal)	28.1 (0.83)	30.0 (0.57)	32.2 (0.45)	32.2 (0.22)	34.3 (0.59)	36.4 (0.85)
Saturated fat (% of kcal)	9.3 (0.40)	10.3 (0.29)	11.5 (0.24)	11.6 (0.12)	12.7 (0.32)	13.9 (0.48)
Saturated fat (g/d)	14.8 (0.9)	17.2 (0.7)	20.4 (0.7)	21.0 (0.4)	24.2 (1.0)	28.1 (1.6)
Protein (g/kg/d)	2.4 (0.14)	2.8 (0.10)	3.2 (0.09)	3.3 (0.05)	3.8 (0.13)	4.3 (0.19)

NOTES: N = 217. See additional notes following this table.
NOTES for Tables J-19 through J-39: g/d = grams per day; g/kg/d = grams per kilogram per day; kcal = kilocalories; SE = standard error.
SOURCE: USDA/ARS, 2005–2012.

TABLE J-40 Usual Intake Distributions of Selected Micronutrients for Pregnant WIC-Participating Women Ages 19 to 50 Years, NHANES 2005–2012

Nutrient	Percentiles and Mean (SE)			
	10th	25th	Median	Mean
Calcium (mg/d)	871 (67)	1,043 (51)	1,247 (42)	1,260 (24)
Copper (mg/d)	1.1 (0.06)	1.2 (0.05)	1.4 (0.05)	1.4 (0.02)
Iron (mg/d)	12.6 (0.84)	14.7 (0.70)	17.4 (0.66)	17.9 (0.28)
Magnesium (mg/d)	241 (13.7)	227 (10.8)	312 (9.5)	326 (5.4)
Phosphorus (mg/d)	1,157 (65)	1,321 (49)	1,514 (41)	1,526 (23)
Selenium (μg/d)	97 (5.7)	109 (4.4)	122 (3.8)	123 (1.6)
Zinc (mg/d)	8.5 (0.58)	10.0 (0.46)	11.8 (0.41)	12.0 (0.23)
Potassium (mg/d)	2,176 (133)	2,525 (104)	2,952 (90)	2,997 (52)
Sodium (mg/d)	2,666 (163)	3,072 (124)	3,556 (106)	3,603 (59)
Vitamin A (μg RAE/d)	480 (41)	577 (32)	700 (30)	729 (17)
Retinol (μg/d)	357 (37)	445 (28)	558 (26)	587 (16)
Vitamin E mg (αTOC/d)	4.8 (0.39)	5.9 (0.33)	7.2 (0.37)	7.5 (0.18)
Vitamin C (mg/d)	58 (8.0)	81 (7.3)	116 (7.6)	126 (4.8)
Thiamin (mg/d)	1.3 (0.09)	1.5 (0.07)	1.8 (0.06)	1.8 (0.03)
Riboflavin (mg/d)	1.7 (0.11)	2.0 (0.09)	2.4 (0.07)	2.4 (0.04)
Niacin (mg/d)	17.4 (1.2)	20.6 (0.96)	24.4 (0.83)	24.7 (0.45)
Vitamin B6 (mg/d)	1.5 (0.10)	1.8 (0.08)	2.2 (0.07)	2.2 (0.04)
Folate (μg DFE/d)	454 (32.3)	531 (25.8)	631 (24.8)	651 (13.1)
Vitamin B12 (mg/d)	3.8 (0.36)	4.7 (0.34)	6.1 (0.38)	6.7 (0.23)
Choline (mg/d)	289 (16)	320 (12)	358 (11)	362.4 (4.7)

NOTES: N = 165. See additional notes following Table J-44.

75th	90th	EAR or AI* (NPNL/P/BF)	% Inadeq (SE)	UL	% > UL (SE)
1,462 (57)	1,665 (84)	800	6.1 (5.5)	2,500	<0.01 (<0.01)
1.6 (0.07)	1.8 (0.13)	0.7/0.8/1.0	0.2 (0.8)	10	0
20.7 (0.99)	24.1 (1.62)	8.1/22.0/6.5	82.0 (8.6)	45	0
370 (13.3)	418 (20.3)	255/290/255	32.2 (6.7)	580	NE
1,743 (58)	1,911 (80)	580	0	4,000	0
137 (5.2)	151 (7.7)	45/49/59	0	400	0
13.8 (0.57)	15.9 (0.87)	6.8/9.5/10.4	19.5 (8.0)	40	0
3,423 (125)	3,877 (189)	4,700/4,700/5,100*	NA	ND	—
4,083 (147)	4,599 (225)	1,500*	NA	2,300	96.9 (4.0)
847 (46)	1,013 (83)	500/550/900	20.1 (9.0)	NA	—
695 (41)	852 (75)	NA	NA	3,000	0
8.8 (0.48)	10.5 (0.78)	12/12/2016	95.8 (4.9)	1000	NE
160 (12.3)	210 (21.4)	60/70/100	17.1 (7.1)	2,000	0
2.1 (0.08)	2.3 (0.12)	0.9/1.2/1.2	4.7 (5.9)	ND	—
2.7 (0.11)	3.1 (0.15)	0.9/1.2/1.2	0.4 (1.0)	ND	—
28.5 (1.1)	32.5 (1.7)	11/14/2013	2.2 (3.2)	35	NE
2.6 (0.11)	3.0 (0.17)	1.1/1.6/1.7	12.2 (6.7)	100	0
752 (37.6)	878 (59)	320/520/450	22.4 (8.9)	1,000	NE
8.0 (0.63)	10.4 (1.2)	2.0/2.2/2.4	0.3 (0.8)	ND	—
400 (16)	442 (24)	425/450/550	—	3,500	0

TABLE J-41 Usual Intake Distributions of Selected Micronutrients for Pregnant Eligible Non-WIC-Participating Women Ages 19 to 50 Years, NHANES 2005–2012

	Percentiles and Mean (SE)			
Nutrient	10th	25th	Median	Mean
Calcium (mg/d)	699 (71)	828 (56)	992 (50)	1,016 (28)
Copper (mg/d)	0.91 (0.09)	1.1 (0.06)	1.3 (0.06)	1.3 (0.04)
Iron (mg/d)	11.8 (1.0)	13.7 (0.87)	16.2 (0.84)	16.9 (0.48)
Magnesium (mg/d)	207 (17)	241 (14)	286 (13)	296 (8.3)
Phosphorus (mg/d)	978 (85)	1,139 (68)	1,346 (61)	1,383 (36)
Selenium (μg/d)	82 (8.0)	96 (6.3)	113 (5.6)	115 (3.0)
Zinc (mg/d)	8.1 (0.68)	9.4 (0.57)	11.2 (0.53)	11.5 (0.32)
Potassium (mg/d)	1,877 (159)	2,189 (127)	2,591 (113)	2,664 (71)
Sodium (mg/d)	2,548 (257)	3,016 (199)	3,591 (172)	3,655 (96)
Vitamin A (μg RAE/d)	433 (57)	535 (47)	673 (45)	721 (29)
Retinol (μg/d)	269 (44)	351 (37)	463 (35)	488 (20)
Vitamin E mg (αTOC/d)	4.7 (0.55)	5.8 (0.46)	7.2 (0.43)	7.5 (0.26)
Vitamin C (mg/d)	45 (10.1)	65 (9.3)	95 (9.7)	105 (5.9)
Thiamin (mg/d)	1.2 (0.11)	1.4 (0.09)	1.7 (0.08)	1.7 (0.04)
Riboflavin (mg/d)	1.4 (0.13)	1.7 (0.11)	1.9 (0.09)	2.0 (0.05)
Niacin (mg/d)	16 (1.7)	20 (1.4)	24 (1.3)	24 (0.72)
Vitamin B6 (mg/d)	1.3 (0.11)	1.6 (0.09)	1.9 (0.09)	1.9 (0.05)
Folate (μg DFE/d)	454 (32)	531 (26)	631 (25)	651 (13)
Vitamin B12 (mg/d)	3.2 (0.41)	3.9 (0.35)	4.9 (0.33)	2.7 (0.17)
Choline (mg/d)	218 (20)	257 (17)	308 (15)	318 (9.1)

NOTES: N = 87. See additional notes following Table J-44.

75th	90th	EAR or AI* (NPNL/P/BF)	% Inadeq (SE)	UL	% > UL (SE)
1,178 (73)	1,366 (116)	800	21.1 (11.3)	2,500	0
1.5 (0.11)	1.9 (0.22)	0.7/0.8/1.0	4.1 (6.0)	10	0
19.3 (1.3)	22.8 (2.3)	8.1/22.0/6.5	87.5 (11.5)	45	0
341 (21)	399 (35)	255/290/255	52.1 (7.3)	350	NE
1,587 (93)	1,837 (151)	580	0	3,500	0
133 (8.1)	152 (12.7)	45/49/59	0.1 (0.5)	400	0
13.0 (0.78)	15.5 (1.4)	6.8/9.5/10.4	26.0 (10.4)	40	0
3,058 (172)	3,588 (284)	4,700/4,700/5,100*	NA	ND	—
4,224 (243)	4,845 (373)	1,500*	0.2 (0.7)	2,300	94.8 (7.3)
852 (77)	1,065 (148)	500/550/900	27.6 (11.0)	NA	—
597 (55)	740 (91)	NA	NA	3,000	0
8.9 (0.67)	10.7 (1.1)	12/12/2016	99.6 (1.3)	1000	NE
134 (16.1)	178 (25.2)	60/70/100	29.2 (10.1)	2,000	0
2.0 (0.13)	2.3 (0.29)	0.9/1.2/1.2	8.3 (0.1)	ND	—
2.4 (0.14)	2.7 (0.23)	0.9/1.2/1.2	2.4 (4.6)	ND	—
28 (1.9)	33 (3.0)	11/14/2013	3.0 (5.6)	35	NE
2.2 (0.14)	2.6 (0.27)	1.1/1.6/1.7	26.8 (10.4)	100	0
752 (37)	878 (59)	320/520/450	29.5 (11.7)	1,000	NE
6.0 (0.51)	7.3 (0.85)	2.0/2.2/2.4	0.89 (2.82)	ND	—
368 (23)	431 (38)	425/450/550	NA	3,500	0

TABLE J-42 Usual Intake Distributions of Selected Micronutrients for Breastfeeding WIC-Participating Women Ages 19 to 50 Years, NHANES 2005–2012

	Percentiles and Mean (SE)			
Nutrient	10th	25th	Median	Mean
Calcium (mg/d)	783 (138)	879 (113)	1,066 (104)	1,106 (61)
Copper (mg/d)	0.89 (0.14)	1.0 (0.11)	1.2 (0.09)	1.2 (0.05)
Iron (mg/d)	11.8 (1.6)	13.3 (1.41)	15.6 (1.3)	16.1 (0.77)
Magnesium (mg/d)	199 (32.4)	231 (26)	274 (23.4)	284 (14.2)
Phosphorus (mg/d)	1,041 (158)	1,200 (126)	1,405 (113)	1,443 (66)
Selenium (μg/d)	83 (9.7)	93 (7.4)	105 (6.3)	105 (3.5)
Zinc (mg/d)	8.0 (1.5)	9.4 (1.1)	11.1 (0.91)	11.2 (0.49)
Potassium (mg/d)	2,045 (364)	2,408 (277)	2,846 (235)	2,885 (130)
Sodium (mg/d)	2,5085 (289)	2,805 (237)	3,191 (222)	3,266 (124)
Vitamin A (μg RAE/d)	459 (105)	573 (93)	726 (88)	746 (44)
Retinol (μg/d)	297 (78.7)	379 (66)	488 (62)	512 (35)
Vitamin E mg (αTOC/d)	4.9 (0.81)	5.8 (0.73)	7.0 (0.76)	7.4 (0.45)
Vitamin C (mg/d)	65 (22.8)	89 (21.1)	124 (22.2)	135 (12.4)
Thiamin (mg/d)	1.2 (0.23)	1.4 (0.18)	1.7 (0.16)	1.7 (0.08)
Riboflavin (mg/d)	1.6 (0.29)	1.9 (0.23)	2.3 (0.21)	2.4 (0.12)
Niacin (mg/d)	15.0 (2.8)	17.7 (2.1)	21.1 (1.9)	21.4 (0.99)
Vitamin B6 (mg/d)	1.3 (0.27)	1.6 (0.24)	2.0 (0.23)	2.1 (0.14)
Folate (μg DFE/d)	360 (72)	441 (69)	568 (80)	635 (54)
Vitamin B12 (mg/d)	3.3 (0.85)	4.2 (0.75)	5.5 (0.75)	5.8 (0.45)
Choline (mg/d)	289 (32)	320 (23)	355 (18)	355.6 (10.1)

NOTES: N = 27. See additional notes following Table J-44.

75th	90th	EAR or AI* (NPNL/P/BF)	% Inadeq (SE)	UL	% > UL (SE)
1,289 (162)	1,527 (273)	800	15.8 (19.9)	2,500	0
1.4 (0.14)	1.6 (0.22)	0.7/0.8/1.0	21.8 (19.9)	10	0
18.4 (2.0)	21.4 (3.4)	8.1/22.0/6.5	0	45	0
326 (37.9)	381 (66)	255/290/255	38.7 (15.4)	350	NE
1,645 (172)	1,894 (285)	580	0	3,500	0
117 (8.7)	130 (13.2)	45/49/59	0.1 (0.9)	400	0
12.9 (1.2)	14.5 (1.7)	6.8/9.5/10.4	38.5 (15.9)	40	0
3,319 (325)	3,775 (492)	4,700/4,700/5,100*	NA	ND	—
3,644 (330)	4,120 (534)	1,500*	NA	2,300	96.1 (11.5)
900 (121)	1,064 (166)	500/550/900	75.0 (19.7)	NA	—
619 (95)	758 (156)	NA	NA	3,000	0
8.7 (1.2)	10.5 (2.2)	12/12/2016	99.4 (3.4)	1000	NE
170 (35.5)	221 (61)	60/70/100	32.8 (18.5)	2,000	0
2.0 (0.22)	2.3 (0.33)	0.9/1.2/1.2	9.8 (17.7)	ND	—
2.8 (0.32)	3.3 (0.53)	0.9/1.2/1.2	1.4 (6.0)	ND	—
24.7 (2.5)	28.2 (3.8)	11/14/2013	4.1 (11.7)	35	NE
2.5 (0.38)	3.1 (0.67)	1.1/1.6/1.7	29.7 (18.3)	100	0
753 (149)	990 (294)	320/520/450	26.8 (19.4)	1,000	NE
7.1 (1.21)	8.9 (2.11)	2.0/2.2/2.4	2.0 (7.6)	ND	—
391 (24)	423 (34)	425/450/550	NA	3,500	0

TABLE J-43 Usual Intake Distributions of Selected Micronutrients for Postpartum WIC-Participating Women Ages 19 to 50 Years, NHANES 2007–2012

	Percentiles and Mean (SE)			
Nutrient	10th	25th	Median	Mean
Calcium (mg/d)	496 (82)	624 (68)	789 (69)	816 (34)
Copper (mg/d)	0.52 (0.08)	0.65 (0.06)	0.82 (0.06)	0.84 (0.03)
Iron (mg/d)	7.6 (1.3)	9.7 (1.1)	12.6 (1.1)	13.5 (0.68)
Magnesium (mg/d)	139 (20.6)	172 (16.4)	213 (14.6)	218 (8.3)
Phosphorus (mg/d)	756 (103)	914 (80)	1,106 (69)	1,123 (37)
Selenium (μg/d)	59 (7.9)	71 (6.1)	85 (5.2)	86 (2.8)
Zinc (mg/d)	5.1 (0.84)	6.4 (0.70)	8.2 (0.65)	8.5 (0.37)
Potassium (mg/d)	1,252 (184)	1,541 (145)	1,898 (128)	1,940 (71)
Sodium (mg/d)	2,033 (218)	2,370 (174)	2,793 (157)	2,855 (87)
Vitamin A (μg RAE/d)	184 (48)	266 (44)	386 (46)	426 (28)
Retinol (μg/d)	139 (37)	203 (34)	298 (35)	326 (21)
Vitamin E mg (αTOC/d)	3.1 (0.56)	4.0 (0.46)	5.2 (0.42)	5.4 (0.23)
Vitamin C (mg/d)	30 (9.3)	47 (9.7)	74 (11.2)	85 (6.6)
Thiamin (mg/d)	0.76 (0.12)	0.95 (0.10)	1.2 (0.09)	1.2 (0.05)
Riboflavin (mg/d)	0.88 (0.16)	1.1 (0.13)	1.4 (0.12)	1.5 (0.07)
Niacin (mg/d)	12.0 (1.7)	14.7 (1.3)	18.0 (1.1)	18.3 (0.64)
Vitamin B6 (mg/d)	0.94 (0.14)	1.2 (0.11)	1.46 (0.10)	1.49 (0.06)
Folate (μg DFE/d)	225 (43)	292 (35)	382 (34)	409 (21)
Vitamin B12 (mg/d)	1.7 (0.45)	2.5 (0.43)	3.8 (0.48)	4.3 (0.32)
Choline (mg/d)	147 (25)	187 (21)	238 (19)	246.7 (10.6)

NOTES: N = 62. See additional notes following Table J-44.

		EAR or AI*	% Inadeq		
75th	90th	(NPNL/P/BF)	(SE)	UL	% > UL (SE)
979 (92)	1174 (145)	800	51.7 (9.7)	2,500	0
1.0 (0.08)	1.2 (0.14)	0.7/0.8/1.0	32.4 (11.0)	10	0
16.4 (1.8)	20.6 (3.1)	8.1/22.0/6.5	13.3 (11.9)	45	<0.1 (0.04)
259 (20.8)	305 (32.2)	255/290/255	77.6 (12.6)	350	NE
1,313 (94)	1,512 (140)	580	2.2 (5.2)	3,500	0
101 (6.9)	116 (10.3)	45/49/59	2.1 (5.1)	400	0
10.3 (0.96)	12.4 (1.5)	6.8/9.5/10.4	30.2 (11.5)	40	0
2,293 (179)	2,682 (273)	4,700/4,700/5,100*	NA	ND	—
3,274 (226)	3,757 (351)	1,500*	NA	2,300	78.7 (13.3)
543 (76)	719 (132)	500/550/900	69.4 (11.7)	—	—
418 (57)	553 (99)	NA	NA	3,000	0
6.5 (0.60)	7.8 (0.93)	12/12/2016	99.8 (0.9)	1000	NE
112 (19.1)	156 (32.6)	60/70/100	37.5 (10.7)	2,000	0
1.5 (0.13)	1.8 (0.22)	0.9/1.2/1.2	20.3 (12.5)	ND	—
1.8 (0.18)	2.3 (0.29)	0.9/1.2/1.2	10.8 (11.4)	ND	—
21.6 (1.6)	25.0 (2.4)	11/14/2013	6.3 (9.4)	35	NE
1.71 (0.14)	2.1 (0.23)	1.1/1.6/1.7	19.7 (12.7)	100	0
495 (56)	627 (105)	320/520/450	32.6 (11.6)	1,000	NE
5.5 (0.86)	7.6 (1.6)	2.0/2.2/2.4	14.3 (12.3)	ND	—
297 (28)	358 (45)	425/450/550	NA	3,500	0

TABLE J-44 Usual Intake Distributions of Selected Micronutrients for Nonpregnant, Postpartum, or Breastfeeding Non-WIC-Participating Women Ages 19 to 50 Years, NHANES 2005–2012

	Percentiles and Mean (SE)			
Nutrient	10th	25th	Median	Mean
Calcium (mg/d)	498 (12)	633 (10)	812 (10)	852 (6)
Copper (mg/d)	0.70 (0.01)	0.85 (0.01)	1.0 (0.01)	1.1 (0.01)
Iron (mg/d)	8.1 (0.16)	9.9 (0.13)	12.3 (0.13)	12.8 (0.08)
Magnesium (mg/d)	158 (3.0)	195 (2.5)	243 (2.4)	253 (1.6)
Phosphorus (mg/d)	766 (14)	926 (11)	1,127 (11)	1,163 (6.5)
Selenium (µg/d)	63 (1.3)	76 (1.0)	92 (0.95)	94 (0.51)
Zinc (mg/d)	6.4 (0.13)	7.7 (0.11)	9.3 (0.10)	9.7 (0.05)
Potassium (mg/d)	1,431 (25)	1,758 (23)	2,178 (22)	2,248 (13)
Sodium (mg/d)	1,947 (39)	2,379 (31)	2,918 (28)	3,013 (18)
Vitamin A (µg RAE/d)	246 (7.7)	332 (7.1)	461 (8.1)	531 (5.8)
Retinol (µg/d)	111 (58)	167 (55)	251 (59)	281 (35)
Vitamin E mg (αTOC/d)	3.7 (0.09)	4.7 (0.08)	6.0 (0.08)	6.5 (0.05)
Vitamin C (mg/d)	28 (1.2)	42 (1.2)	66 (1.5)	78 (0.97)
Thiamin (mg/d)	0.88 (0.02)	1.0 (0.01)	1.3 (0.01)	1.3 (0.01)
Riboflavin (mg/d)	1.1 (0.02)	1.3 (0.02)	1.7 (0.02)	1.7 (0.01)
Niacin (mg/d)	13 (0.28)	16 (0.23)	20 (0.21)	21 (0.12)
Vitamin B6 (mg/d)	1.0 (0.02)	1.2 (0.02)	1.6 (0.02)	1.7 (0.01)
Folate (µg DFE/d)	273 (6.4)	341 (5.5)	433 (5.6)	459 (3.2)
Vitamin B12 (mg/d)	2.5 (0.07)	3.1 (0.06)	3.9 (0.06)	4.2 (0.03)
Choline (mg/d)	173 (3.7)	210 (3.0)	259 (2.8)	268 (1.6)

NOTES: N = 2,611. See additional notes following this table.
NOTES for Tables J-40 through J-44: * = an AI value; — = not applicable due to no recommendation; % Inadeq = percentage of individuals with usual intake below the EAR; αTOC = α-tocopherol; AI = Adequate Intake; EAR = Estimated Average Requirement; NA = not applicable; ND = not determined; NE = not evaluated; NPNL/P/BF = nonpregnant, nonbreastfeeding/pregnant/breastfeeding; RAE = retinol activity equivalents; SE = standard error; UL = Tolerable Upper Limit. The ULs for folate, vitamin E, niacin, and magnesium represent intake from pharmacological agents only and do not include food intake. Vitamin D is not included because intake is a poor reflection of status. For percent inadequate calculations, the approach of IOM (2000b) was applied in which, when combining groups with different EARs, intakes in one of the groups are rescaled so they can be compared to the EAR of the other group. One value indicates that the EAR is the same across groups.

75th	90th	EAR or AI* (NPNL/P/BF)	% Inadeq (SE)	UL	% > UL (SE)
1,028 (15)	1,258 (24)	800	48.3 (1.3)	2,500	0
1.2 (0.01)	1.6 (0.03)	0.7/0.8/1.0	10.2 (1.5)	10	0
15.2 (0.20)	18.3 (0.34)	8.1/22.0/6.5	10.1 (1.6)	45	0
300 (3.6)	362 (6.0)	255/290/255	61.0 (1.3)	350	NE
1,362 (16)	1,606 (25)	580	0	3,500	0
110 (1.3)	129 (2.1)	45/49/59	1.1 (0.5)	400	0
11.4 (0.15)	13.5 (0.25)	6.8/9.5/10.4	14.4 (2.1)	40	0
2,660 (31)	3,153 (49)	4,700/4,700/5,100*	NA	ND	—
3,536 (41)	4,189 (69)	1,500*	2.4 (0.7)	2,300	78.3 (1.7)
650 (15.0)	897 (29.6)	500/550/900	56.4 (1.5)	NA	—
363 (99)	492 (178)	NA	NA	3,000	0
7.8 (0.13)	9.8 (0.24)	12/12/2016	96.4 (1.1)	1000	NE
101 (2.6)	144 (4.8)	60/70/100	43.7 (1.4)	2,000	0
1.6 (0.02)	1.9 (0.03)	0.9/1.2/1.2	11.4 (1.8)	ND	—
2.1 (0.03)	2.6 (0.05)	0.9/1.2/1.2	4.3 (1.0)	ND	—
24 (0.31)	29 (0.53)	11/14/2013	2.9 (1.0)	35	NE
2.0 (0.03)	2.4 (0.05)	1.1/1.6/1.7	13.6 (2.1)	100	0
548 (8.6)	676 (14.8)	320/520/450	19.8 (2.1)	1,000	NE
4.9 (0.10)	6.2 (0.19)	2.0/2.2/2.4	3.2 (1.5)	ND	—
316 (4.2)	376 (6.7)	425/450/550	NA	3,500	0

TABLE J-45 Usual Intake Distributions of Selected Micronutrients for WIC-Participating Infants Ages 0 to Less Than 6 Months, NHANES 2005–2008

	Percentiles and Mean (SE)								
Nutrient	10th	25th	Median	Mean	75th	90th	AI	UL	% > UL (SE)
Calcium (mg/d)	433 (24)	515 (17)	610 (15)	625 (11)	718 (22)	834 (38)	200	1,000	2.2 (1.8)
Copper (mg/d)	0.5 (0.02)	0.6 (0.02)	0.7 (0.01)	0.7 (0.01)	0.8 (0.02)	0.9 (0.04)	0.2	ND	—
Iron (mg/d)	9.5 (0.58)	11.4 (0.38)	13.9 (0.44)	15.5 (0.45)	18.2 (0.94)	23.8 (1.83)	0.27	40	<0.01
Magnesium (mg/d)	44 (2.7)	55 (2.1)	70 (2.3)	77 (2.2)	93 (4.5)	121 (8.2)	30	ND	—
Phosphorus (mg/d)	241 (15)	297 (11)	367 (11)	388 (9)	461 (18)	567 (31)	100	ND	—
Selenium (µg/d)	12 (0.6)	14 (0.5)	17 (0.5)	18 (0.4)	21 (0.7)	25 (1.2)	15	45	<0.01
Zinc (mg/d)	4.2 (0.26)	5.1 (0.17)	6.0 (0.14)	6.2 (0.12)	7.1 (0.22)	8.3 (0.39)	2	4	92.2 (3.5)
Potassium (mg/d)	540 (30)	649 (21)	787 (20)	821 (17)	967 (34)	1,160 (54)	400	ND	—
Sodium (mg/d)	155 (8)	184 (6)	221 (6)	236 (6)	270 (11)	333 (22)	120	ND	—
Vitamin A (µg RAE/d)	461 (24.4)	532 (16.8)	614 (14.3)	625 (9.7)	705 (21.5)	802 (36.8)	400	NA	—
Retinol (µg/d)	426 (19)	483 (13)	558 (13)	573 (9)	650 (20)	748 (33)	NA	600	39.2 (2.9)
Vitamin E mg (αTOC/d)	5.7 (0.29)	6.7 (0.18)	7.8 (0.19)	8.2 (0.16)	9.4 (0.34)	11.3 (0.56)	4	ND	—
Vitamin C (mg/d)	52 (3.3)	64 (2.3)	79 (2.2)	83 (2.0)	98 (3.8)	120 (6.9)	40	ND	—
Thiamin (mg/d)	0.5 (0.03)	0.6 (0.02)	0.7 (0.03)	0.8 (0.03)	1.0 (0.05)	1.3 (0.10)	0.2	ND	—
Riboflavin (mg/d)	0.7 (0.05)	0.9 (0.03)	1.1 (0.03)	1.1 (0.03)	1.3 (0.05)	1.6 (0.09)	0.3	ND	—
Niacin (mg/d)	5.7 (0.37)	7.0 (0.25)	8.7 (0.28)	9.8 (0.30)	11.5 (0.61)	15.3 (1.19)	2	ND	—
Vitamin B6 (mg/d)	0.3 (0.02)	0.4 (0.01)	0.5 (0.01)	0.5 (0.01)	0.6 (0.02)	0.7 (0.04)	0.1	ND	—
Folate (µg DFE/d)	129.9 (6.3)	150.2 (4.1)	174.5 (3.9)	179.9 (3.1)	205.6 (6.5)	239.0 (10.4)	65	ND	—
Vitamin B12 (mg/d)	1.3 (0.08)	1.5 (0.05)	1.8 (0.04)	1.9 (0.03)	2.1 (0.06)	2.5 (0.11)	0.4	ND	—
Choline (mg/d)	65 (3.5)	76 (2.2)	90 (2.5)	97 (2.2)	113 (5.0)	140 (8.9)	125	ND	—

NOTES: N = 204. See additional notes following Table J-60.

TABLE J-46 Usual Intake Distributions of Selected Micronutrients for Eligible Non-WIC-Participating Infants Ages 0 to Less Than 6 Months, NHANES 2005–2008

	Percentiles and Mean (SE)								
Nutrient	10th	25th	Median	Mean	75th	90th	AI	UL	% > UL (SE)
Calcium (mg/d)	382 (51)	449 (43)	546 (41)	582 (41)	675 (76)	829 (146)	200	1,000	3.4 (5.8)
Copper (mg/d)	0.5 (0.04)	0.5 (0.04)	0.6 (0.04)	0.6 (0.03)	0.7 (0.07)	0.8 (0.12)	0.2	ND	—
Iron (mg/d)	9.3 (1.28)	10.9 (1.12)	13.2 (1.16)	14.1 (1.02)	16.4 (2.11)	20.2 (4.06)	0.27	40	<0.01
Magnesium (mg/d)	38 (5.7)	46 (5.2)	59 (5.7)	68 (7.0)	80 (12.3)	107 (27.2)	30	ND	—
Phosphorus (mg/d)	217 (29)	257 (27)	323 (29)	365 (35)	426 (63)	565 (136)	100	ND	—
Selenium (μg/d)	12 (1.3)	14 (1.0)	16 (0.8)	16 (0.6)	18 (1.1)	19 (1.7)	15	45	<0.01
Zinc (mg/d)	4.1 (0.44)	4.7 (0.35)	5.4 (0.32)	5.5 (0.26)	6.2 (0.51)	7.1 (0.88)	2	4	92.8 (10.0)
Potassium (mg/d)	510 (65)	593 (54)	713 (52)	754 (46)	874 (95)	1,062 (181)	400	ND	—
Sodium (mg/d)	156 (13)	171 (10)	196 (15)	215 (13)	251 (33)	309 (51)	120	ND	—
Vitamin A (μg RAE/d)	415 (40.0)	466 (36.4)	545 (39.2)	584 (36.9)	660 (75.3)	804 (148.7)	400	NA	—
Retinol (μg/d)	387 (69.3)	461 (42.5)	536 (32.4)	552 (32.1)	623 (55.8)	735 (116.0)	NA	600	30.4 (9.8)
Vitamin E mg (αTOC/d)	4.8 (0.83)	5.9 (0.71)	7.6 (0.69)	8.2 (0.72)	9.8 (1.30)	12.5 (2.57)	4	ND	—
Vitamin C (mg/d)	58 (9.7)	67 (8.1)	79 (7.9)	82 (4.8)	94 (12.6)	111 (21.7)	40	ND	—
Thiamin (mg/d)	0.4 (0.07)	0.5 (0.06)	0.7 (0.07)	0.7 (0.07)	0.9 (0.13)	1.1 (0.26)	0.2	ND	—
Riboflavin (mg/d)	0.7 (0.07)	0.8 (0.06)	0.9 (0.05)	1.0 (0.04)	1.1 (0.08)	1.2 (0.14)	0.3	ND	—
Niacin (mg/d)	4.8 (0.78)	5.9 (0.74)	7.7 (0.84)	9.0 (1.03)	10.6 (1.83)	14.7 (4.11)	2	ND	—
Vitamin B6 (mg/d)	0.3 (0.04)	0.4 (0.03)	0.4 (0.03)	0.5 (0.03)	0.5 (0.06)	0.6 (0.12)	0.1	ND	—
Folate (μg DFE/d)	112.6 (21.2)	135.9 (13.2)	159.8 (10.2)	165.5 (10.42)	188.3 (17.8)	225.0 (37.3)	65	ND	—
Vitamin B12 (mg/d)	1.1 (0.18)	1.3 (0.15)	1.7 (0.15)	1.8 (0.14)	2.1 (0.27)	2.6 (0.51)	0.4	ND	—
Choline (mg/d)	68 (6.5)	74 (5.5)	83 (5.6)	86 (3.4)	94 (9.2)	106 (15.9)	125	ND	—

NOTES: N = 21. See additional notes following Table J-60.

TABLE J-47 Usual Intake Distributions of Selected Micronutrients for WIC-Participating Infants Ages 0 to Less Than 6 Months, NHANES 2011–2012

	Percentiles and Mean (SE)								
Nutrient	10th	25th	Median	Mean	75th	90th	AI	UL	% > UL (SE)
Calcium (mg/d)	429 (29)	513 (26)	637 (26)	689.7 (26.3)	808 (49)	1,016 (94)	200	1,000	10.8 (4.9)
Copper (mg/d)	0.44 (0.03)	0.51 (0.02)	0.61 (0.02)	0.62 (0.02)	0.71 (0.03)	0.81 (0.04)	0.2	ND	—
Iron (mg/d)	8.8 (0.67)	10.7 (0.57)	13.4 (0.58)	14.8 (0.6)	17.2 (1.1)	22.3 (2.4)	0.27	40	0.6 (0.9)
Magnesium (mg/d)	46 (3.3)	56 (2.9)	70 (3.3)	77.5 (3.1)	93 (6.6)	120 (11.4)	30	ND	—
Phosphorus (mg/d)	220 (18)	265 (16)	355 (18)	401.0 (19.6)	477 (35)	635 (74)	100	ND	—
Selenium (μg/d)	11 (0.75)	13 (0.63)	16 (0.6)	16.9 (0.6)	20 (1.0)	24 (1.8)	15	45	0.07 (0.2)
Zinc (mg/d)	3.8 (0.26)	4.6 (0.21)	5.5 (0.19)	5.7 (0.2)	6.6 (0.3)	7.8 (0.51)	2	4	87.6 (5.1)
Potassium (mg/d)	541 (36)	638 (30)	769 (28)	805.6 (24.5)	934 (47)	1,116 (82)	400	ND	—
Sodium (mg/d)	148 (12)	180 (10.2)	223 (9.9)	236.6 (8.3)	279 (16.4)	342 (29)	120	ND	—
Vitamin A (μg RAE/d)	433 (31)	510 (22)	601 (19)	620.0 (16.9)	708 (30)	828 (55)	400	NA	—
Retinol (μg/d)	402 (27)	473 (21)	562 (18)	575 (15)	663 (26)	765 (42)	NA	600	50.3 (5.3)
Vitamin E mg (αTOC/d)	5.2 (0.33)	6.1 (0.67)	7.3 (0.24)	7.5 (0.2)	8.7 (0.37)	10.1 (0.61)	4	ND	—
Vitamin C (mg/d)	50 (3.3)	59 (2.8)	71 (2.8)	75.4 (2.5)	88 (4.8)	107 (8.7)	40	ND	—
Thiamin (mg/d)	0.42 (0.04)	0.52 (0.03)	0.66 (0.03)	0.74 (0.04)	0.86 (0.06)	1.1 (0.13)	0.2	ND	—
Riboflavin (mg/d)	0.65 (0.05)	0.8 (0.04)	0.99 (0.04)	1.06 (0.04)	1.28 (0.08)	1.5 (0.15)	0.3	ND	—
Niacin (mg/d)	5.2 (0.39)	6.3 (0.31)	7.9 (0.38)	9.1 (0.4)	10.8 (0.87)	14.5 (1.7)	2	ND	—
Vitamin B6 (mg/d)	0.31 (0.02)	0.36 (0.02)	0.44 (0.02)	0.47 (0.02)	0.55 (0.03)	0.67 (0.05)	0.1	ND	—
Folate (μg DFE/d)	123 (7.6)	143 (5.9)	168 (5.1)	171.5 (4.1)	196 (7.5)	224 (12.1)	65	ND	—
Vitamin B12 (mg/d)	1.2 (0.09)	1.5 (0.07)	1.8 (0.07)	1.9 (0.1)	2.2 (0.11)	2.7 (0.19)	0.4	ND	—
Choline (mg/d)	64 (5.3)	79 (4.6)	101 (4.6)	109.3 (4.5)	130 (8.2)	165 (15.5)	125	ND	—

NOTES: N = 93. See additional notes following Table J-60.

TABLE J-48 Usual Intake Distributions of Selected Micronutrients for Eligible Non-WIC-Participating Infants Ages 0 to Less Than 6 Months, NHANES 2011–2012

	Percentiles and Mean (SE)								
Nutrient	10th	25th	Median	Mean	75th	90th	AI	UL	% > UL (SE)
Calcium (mg/d)	512 (43)	553 (36)	605 (34)	632 (28)	690 (64)	781 (119)	200	1,000	0.8 (3.4)
Copper (mg/d)	0.49 (0.09)	0.56 (0.06)	0.65 (0.04)	0.66 (0.03)	0.74 (0.06)	0.83 (0.1)	0.2	ND	—
Iron (mg/d)	9.9 (1.3)	11.1 (0.99)	12.6 (0.82)	12.8 (0.62)	14.3 (1.3)	16 (2.1)	0.27	40	0.11 (0.21)
Magnesium (mg/d)	64 (7.7)	71 (5.4)	78 (4.1)	79 (3.0)	87 (5.9)	94 (9.2)	30	ND	—
Phosphorus (mg/d)	252 (29)	279 (22)	313 (16)	322 (19)	342 (29)	399 (81)	100	ND	—
Selenium (μg/d)	13 (1.2)	14 (0.96)	16 (0.89)	16 (0.72)	18 (1.6)	20 (2.9)	15	45	0.03 (0.08)
Zinc (mg/d)	4.7 (0.5)	5.2 (0.42)	5.9 (0.42)	6.1 (0.36)	6.8 (0.78)	8 (1.5)	2	4	99.3 (3.0)
Potassium (mg/d)	632 (108)	726 (74)	833 (55)	836 (41)	943 (77)	1,043 (118)	400	ND	—
Sodium (mg/d)	193 (25)	213 (16)	234 (11)	232 (7.9)	254 (14)	271 (21)	120	ND	—
Vitamin A (μg RAE/d)	497 (65)	555 (51)	633 (44)	651 (34)	728 (74)	830 (130)	400	NA	—
Retinol (μg/d)	460 (62)	519 (52)	606 (51)	640 (14)	725 (95)	865 (184)	NA	600	ND
Vitamin E mg (αTOC/d)	5.6 (1.5)	7.0 (1.1)	8.8 (0.94)	9.0 (0.73)	10.8 (1.5)	12.8 (2.5)	4	ND	—
Vitamin C (mg/d)	66 (5.8)	72 (5.3)	21 (5.6)	85 (4.9)	94 (11)	110 (22)	40	ND	—
Thiamin (mg/d)	0.48 (0.11)	0.58 (0.09)	0.71 (0.07)	0.73 (0.05)	0.86 (0.1)	1.0 (0.17)	0.2	ND	—
Riboflavin (mg/d)	0.67 (0.21)	0.85 (0.13)	1.0 (0.08)	1.0 (0.06)	1.2 (0.1)	1.3 (0.13)	0.3	ND	—
Niacin (mg/d)	5.7 (1.2)	6.7 (0.85)	8.0 (0.66)	8.1 (0.51)	9.4 (1.0)	10.7 (1.6)	2	ND	—
Vitamin B6 (mg/d)	0.37 (0.07)	0.43 (0.05)	0.5 (0.04)	0.51 (0.03)	0.58 (0.05)	0.66 (0.09)	0.1	ND	—
Folate (μg DFE/d)	144 (19)	162 (15)	186 (13)	192 (11)	216 (23)	249 (41)	65	ND	—
Vitamin B12 (mg/d)	1.3 (0.16)	1.5 (0.13)	1.7 (0.13)	1.7 (0.1)	1.9 (0.23)	2.3 (0.44)	0.4	ND	—
Choline (mg/d)	87 (6.8)	94 (6.1)	104 (4.6)	105 (4.3)	112 (7.4)	129 (23)	125	ND	—

NOTES: N = 15. See additional notes following Table J-60.

TABLE J-49 Usual Intake Distributions of Selected Micronutrients for WIC-Participating Infants Ages 6 to Less Than 12 Months, NHANES 2005–2008

	Percentiles and Mean (SE)			
Nutrient	10th	25th	Median	Mean
Calcium (mg/d)	496 (25)	593 (19)	719 (19)	752 (14)
Copper (mg/d)	0.5 (0.02)	0.6 (0.02)	0.7 (0.01)	0.8 (0.01)
Iron (mg/d)	9.2 (0.69)	12 (0.54)	15.7 (0.49)	16.5 (0.40)
Magnesium (mg/d)	75 (3.9)	92 (3.3)	116 (3.1)	122 (2.6)
Phosphorus (mg/d)	354 (20)	442 (17)	573 (18)	618 (15)
Selenium (μg/d)	19 (1.2)	24 (1.1)	32 (1.2)	35 (1.0)
Zinc (mg/d)	4.7 (0.27)	5.7 (0.20)	7.0 (0.18)	7.3 (0.15)
Potassium (mg/d)	862 (42)	1,041 (34)	1,278 (32)	1,353 (29)
Sodium (mg/d)	259 (21)	378 (26)	611 (35)	780 (36)
Vitamin A (μg RAE/d)	438 (25.6)	538 (20.1)	661 (17.7)	676 (12.3)
Retinol (μg/d)	340 (20)	420 (16)	516 (13)	524 (9)
Vitamin E mg (αTOC/d)	4.4 (0.39)	6.1 (0.31)	8.0 (0.23)	8.0 (0.18)
Vitamin C (mg/d)	72 (5.1)	90 (3.9)	112 (3.6)	119 (2.7)
Thiamin (mg/d)	0.6 (0.04)	0.8 (0.03)	1.0 (0.03)	1.0 (0.02)
Riboflavin (mg/d)	1.0 (0.05)	1.2 (0.04)	1.4 (0.04)	1.5 (0.03)
Niacin (mg/d)	7.1 (0.47)	9.1 (0.39)	11.8 (0.36)	12.3 (0.28)
Vitamin B6 (mg/d)	0.5 (0.03)	0.6 (0.02)	0.8 (0.02)	0.8 (0.02)
Folate (μg DFE/d)	149 (7.84)	180 (6.08)	223 (6.26)	239 (5.29)
Vitamin B12 (mg/d)	1.4 (0.09)	1.8 (0.07)	2.4 (0.08)	2.6 (0.07)
Choline (mg/d)	89 (5.1)	110 (4.2)	140 (4.3)	149 (3.3)

NOTES: N = 252. See additional notes following Table J-60.

75th	90th	EAR or AI*	% Inadeq (SE)	UL	% > UL (SE)
883 (31)	1,058 (49)	260*	NA	1,500	0.4 (0.44)
0.9 (0.02)	1 (0.04)	0.22*	NA	ND	—
20 (0.77)	24.8 (1.35)	6.9	5 (2)	40	0.4 (0.40)
145 (4.8)	176 (8.2)	75*	NA	ND	—
755 (32)	955 (50)	275*	NA	ND	—
44 (2.1)	57 (3.4)	20*	NA	60	7.6 (2.86)
8.5 (0.28)	10.3 (0.52)	2.5	0.3 (0.4)	5	86.1 (3.86)
1,577 (53)	1,930 (101)	700*	NA	ND	—
1,000 (73)	1,520 (143)	370*	NA	ND	—
798 (25.1)	934 (38.7)	500*	NA	NA	—
620 (18)	720 (27)	NA	NA	600	29.2 (4.15)
9.8 (0.29)	11.6 (0.50)	5*	NA	ND	—
140 (6.0)	174 (11.7)	50*	NA	ND	—
1.2 (0.04)	1.5 (0.08)	0.3*	NA	ND	—
1.7 (0.06)	2.1 (0.10)	0.4*	NA	ND	—
14.9 (0.54)	18.1 (0.89)	4*	NA	ND	—
1.0 (0.04)	1.2 (0.08)	0.3*	NA	ND	—
281 (11.1)	349 (20.1)	80	0.25 (0.31)	ND	—
3.2 (0.15)	4.1 (0.25)	0.5*	NA	ND	—
179 (7.2)	221 (11.6)	150*	NA	ND	—

TABLE J-50 Usual Intake Distributions of Selected Micronutrients for Eligible Non-WIC-Participating Infants Ages 6 to Less Than 12 Months, NHANES 2005–2008

	Percentiles and Mean (SE)			
Nutrient	10th	25th	Median	Mean
Calcium (mg/d)	400 (69)	528 (64)	734 (70)	858 (83)
Copper (mg/d)	0.5 (0.05)	0.5 (0.04)	0.6 (0.03)	0.6 (0.02)
Iron (mg/d)	7.2 (1.54)	9.8 (1.28)	13.4 (1.17)	14.1 (1.00)
Magnesium (mg/d)	74 (9.7)	91 (8.4)	115 (8.2)	124 (7.9)
Phosphorus (mg/d)	334 (51)	429 (49)	586 (55)	690 (67)
Selenium (μg/d)	18 (2.59)	22 (2.44)	29 (2.73)	34 (2.94)
Zinc (mg/d)	4.9 (0.47)	5.6 (0.37)	6.4 (0.32)	6.5 (0.22)
Potassium (mg/d)	796 (121)	1,007 (102)	1,301 (96)	1,389 (90)
Sodium (mg/d)	236 (56)	345 (57)	531 (66)	667 (85)
Vitamin A (μg RAE/d)	515 (70.0)	620 (54.3)	749 (46.6)	764 (34.3)
Retinol (μg/d)	329 (61.2)	426 (44.8)	539 (35.5)	544 (28.6)
Vitamin E mg (αTOC/d)	2.9 (0.61)	4.0 (0.53)	5.5 (0.51)	5.9 (0.44)
Vitamin C (mg/d)	35 (12.5)	56 (10.9)	85 (10.4)	92 (8.1)
Thiamin (mg/d)	0.6 (0.08)	0.7 (0.07)	0.9 (0.06)	0.9 (0.05)
Riboflavin (mg/d)	0.9 (0.14)	1.1 (0.13)	1.5 (0.13)	1.7 (0.13)
Niacin (mg/d)	6.9 (0.82)	8.0 (0.69)	9.5 (0.67)	9.9 (0.44)
Vitamin B6 (mg/d)	0.5 (0.06)	0.6 (0.04)	0.7 (0.04)	0.7 (0.03)
Folate (μg DFE/d)	136 (19.0)	158 (15.4)	184 (14.0)	189 (7.44)
Vitamin B12 (mg/d)	1.2 (0.24)	1.7 (0.24)	2.4 (0.28)	3.1 (0.38)
Choline (mg/d)	86 (11.4)	106 (10.4)	136 (11.1)	151 (11.0)

NOTES: N = 35. See additional notes following Table J-60.

75th	90th	EAR or AI*	% Inadeq (SE)	UL	% > UL (SE)
1,046 (144)	1,461 (311)	260*	NA	1,500	9.2 (6.93)
0.7 (0.04)	0.8 (0.06)	0.22*	NA	ND	—
17.6 (1.86)	22.1 (3.15)	6.9	7 (6)	40	0.1 (0.31)
147 (14.6)	184 (27.6)	75*	NA	ND	—
831 (117)	1,168 (259)	275*	NA	ND	—
41 (5.47)	55 (11.53)	20*	NA	60	7.5 (7.25)
7.3 (0.46)	8.2 (0.72)	2.5	0	5	88.5 (11.45)
1,674 (164)	2,094 (298)	700*	NA	ND	—
830 (144)	1,249 (325)	370*	NA	ND	—
892 (66.7)	1,032 (104.1)	500*	NA	NA	—
656 (48.7)	765 (73.1)	NA	NA	600	36.1 (8.90)
7.3 (0.84)	9.4 (1.48)	5*	NA	ND	—
120 (16.3)	156 (27.2)	50*	NA	ND	—
1.1 (0.10)	1.3 (0.18)	0.3*	NA	ND	—
2.0 (0.25)	2.7 (0.49)	0.4*	NA	ND	—
11.3 (1.06)	13.4 (1.81)	4*	NA	ND	—
0.9 (0.06)	1.0 (0.09)	0.3*	NA	ND	—
215 (20.4)	247 (32.5)	80	0.01 (0.13)	ND	—
3.7 (0.63)	5.6 (1.47)	0.5*	NA	ND	—
179 (20.9)	233 (41.7)	150*	NA	ND	—

TABLE J-51 Usual Intake Distributions of Selected Micronutrients for WIC-Participating Infants Ages 6 to Less Than 12 Months, NHANES 2011–2012

	Percentiles and Mean (SE)			
Nutrient	10th	25th	Median	Mean
Calcium (mg/d)	524 (42)	630 (34)	766 (31)	788.6 (22.4)
Copper (mg/d)	0.54 (0.04)	0.62 (0.03)	0.72 (0.02)	0.73 (0.02)
Iron (mg/d)	9.1 (1.2)	12.3 (0.95)	16.4 (0.86)	17.6 (0.8)
Magnesium (mg/d)	84 (6.9)	101 (5.7)	123 (5.2)	126.9 (3.6)
Phosphorus (mg/d)	345 (33)	436 (28)	561 (27)	595.3 (22.4)
Selenium (µg/d)	17 (1.7)	22 (1.6)	30 (1.7)	32.9 (1.5)
Zinc (mg/d)	4.6 (0.37)	5.5 (0.30)	6.6 (0.27)	6.8 (0.2)
Potassium (mg/d)	859 (61)	1,015 (52)	1,224 (49)	1,276 (37)
Sodium (mg/d)	269 (35)	374 (35)	547 (41)	656.3 (43.0)
Vitamin A (µg RAE/d)	426 (38)	527 (32)	664 (21)	698.3 (24.1)
Retinol (µg/d)	351 (30)	425 (23)	515 (20)	524 (14)
Vitamin E mg (αTOC/d)	4.9 (0.55)	6.3 (0.42)	7.9 (0.36)	8.1 (0.3)
Vitamin C (mg/d)	66 (6.4)	81 (5.1)	100 (4.6)	102.4 (3.0)
Thiamin (mg/d)	0.63 (0.06)	0.79 (0.05)	1.0 (0.05)	1.07 (0.04)
Riboflavin (mg/d)	0.95 (0.08)	1.1 (0.06)	1.4 (0.06)	1.50 (0.05)
Niacin (mg/d)	7.1 (0.84)	9.3 (0.71)	12.3 (0.66)	12.9 (0.5)
Vitamin B6 (mg/d)	0.5 (0.04)	0.6 (0.04)	0.75 (0.04)	0.81 (0.03)
Folate (µg DFE/d)	156 (14)	187 (11)	227 (10)	237.2 (7.5)
Vitamin B12 (mg/d)	1.3 (0.12)	1.7 (0.11)	2.1 (0.11)	2.30 (0.09)
Choline (mg/d)	85 (7.2)	104 (6.2)	130 (6.1)	137.5 (4.8)

NOTES: N = 98. See additional notes following Table J-60.

75th	90th	EAR or AI*	% Inadeq (SE)	UL	% > UL (SE)
922 (45)	1,083 (72)	260*	NA	1,500	0.5 (0.9)
0.83 (0.03)	0.92 (0.04)	0.22*	NA	ND	—
21.5 (1.4)	27.6 (2.7)	6.9	4.2 (3.4)	40	1.5 (1.7)
148 (7.7)	175 (12.3)	75*	NA	ND	—
717 (43)	889 (75)	275*	NA	ND	—
40 (3.0)	52 (5.7)	20*	NA	60	5.4 (4.1)
7.9 (0.39)	9.2 (0.62)	2.5	0.08 (0.2)	5	84.5 (7.4)
1,480 (77)	1,758 (132)	700*	NA	ND	—
812 (82)	1,168 (174)	370*	NA	ND	—
832 (49)	1,014 (83)	500*	NA	NA	—
614 (28)	710 (43)	NA	NA	600	28.1 (6.0)
9.7 (0.49)	11.4 (0.75)	5*	NA	ND	—
121 (6.5)	172 (11.1)	50*	NA	ND	—
1.3 (0.08)	1.6 (0.13)	0.3*	NA	ND	—
1.7 (0.1)	2.1 (0.16)	0.4*	NA	ND	—
15.9 (1.0)	19.6 (1.6)	4*	NA	ND	—
0.95 (0.07)	1.2 (0.12)	0.3*	NA	ND	—
275 (16)	331 (30.2)	80*	NA	ND	—
2.7 (0.17)	3.4 (0.31)	0.5*	NA	ND	—
162 (9.9)	199 (17.5)	150*	NA	ND	—

TABLE J-52 Usual Intake Distributions of Selected Micronutrients for Eligible Non-WIC-Participating Infants Ages 6 to Less Than 12 Months, NHANES 2011–2012

Nutrient	Percentiles and Mean (SE)			
	10th	25th	Median	Mean
Calcium (mg/d)	620 (97)	708 (83)	833 (82)	875 (59)
Copper (mg/d)	0.49 (0.07)	0.56 (0.05)	0.63 (0.04)	0.64 (0.03)
Iron (mg/d)	8.6 (2.6)	10.5 (1.9)	13.6 (1.6)	13.9 (1.1)
Magnesium (mg/d)	87 (17.3)	103 (13.2)	122 (11.1)	125 (7.9)
Phosphorus (mg/d)	337 (94)	427 (83)	564 (83)	627 (72)
Selenium (µg/d)	13 (3.8)	17 (3.8)	24 (4.6)	30 (4.8)
Zinc (mg/d)	5.0 (0.34)	5.3 (0.28)	5.7 (0.26)	5.8 (0.18)
Potassium (mg/d)	922 (142)	1,057 (121)	1,253 (120)	1,329 (96)
Sodium (mg/d)	256 (81)	341 (86)	508 (114)	688 (149)
Vitamin A (µg RAE/d)	568 (99)	659 (86)	819 (98)	961 (155)
Retinol (µg/d)	406 (74)	463 (40)	513 (28)	515 (23)
Vitamin E mg (αTOC/d)	4.6 (1.4)	5.9 (1.0)	7.5 (0.89)	7.7 (0.62)
Vitamin C (mg/d)	55 (11.5)	64 (7.6)	73 (5.4)	73 (3.3)
Thiamin (mg/d)	0.61 (0.13)	0.72 (0.1)	0.87 (0.08)	0.89 (0.05)
Riboflavin (mg/d)	1.1 (0.12)	1.2 (0.11)	1.4 (0.11)	1.4 (0.09)
Niacin (mg/d)	6.9 (1.7)	8.4 (1.3)	10.2 (1.1)	10.3 (0.69)
Vitamin B6 (mg/d)	0.54 (0.09)	0.63 (0.07)	0.74 (0.06)	1.76 (0.04)
Folate (µg DFE/d)	108 (32)	137 (24)	171 (20)	175 (12)
Vitamin B12 (mg/d)	1.8 (0.3)	2.2 (0.28)	2.6 (0.32)	2.9 (0.28)
Choline (mg/d)	79 (18)	97 (16)	123 (16)	135 (14)

NOTES: N = 16. See additional notes following Table J-60.

75th	90th	EAR or AI*	% Inadeq (SE)	UL	% > UL (SE)
996 (141)	1,184 (256)	260*	NA	1,500	1.9 (7.4)
0.71 (0.06)	0.79 (0.09)	0.22*	NA	ND	—
16.7 (2.3)	19.7 (3.7)	6.9	3.6 (10.3)	40	0.11 (0.21)
145 (16.9)	167 (27.8)	75*	NA	ND	—
757 (162)	994 (329)	275*	NA	ND	—
36 (10.3)	52 (24)	20*	NA	60	6.8 (13.9)
6.2 (0.4)	6.8 (0.68)	2.5	0	5	90.2 (17.1)
1,519 (218)	1,832 (416)	700*	NA	ND	—
815 (288)	1,305 (750)	370*	NA	ND	—
1,042 (219)	1,413 (607)	500*	NA	NA	—
565 (44)	628 (84)	NA	NA	600	ND
9.3 (1.3)	11 (2.1)	5*	NA	ND	—
82 (6.5)	89 (8.7)	50*	NA	ND	—
1.0 (0.12)	1.2 (0.19)	0.3*	NA	ND	—
1.6 (0.21)	1.9 (0.4)	0.4*	NA	ND	—
12.1 (1.5)	14 (2.3)	4*	NA	ND	—
0.87 (0.1)	1.0 (0.16)	0.3*	NA	ND	—
208 (28)	243 (42)	80*	NA	ND	—
3.1 (0.53)	4.3 (1.3)	0.5*	NA	ND	—
160 (32)	207 (66)	150*	NA	ND	—

TABLE J-53 Usual Intake Distributions of Selected Micronutrients for WIC-Participating Children Ages 1 to Less Than 2 Years, NHANES 2005–2008

Nutrient	Percentiles and Mean (SE)			
	10th	25th	Median	Mean
Calcium (mg/d)	655 (34)	808 (29)	1,018 (28)	1,053 (19)
Copper (mg/d)	0.5 (0.02)	0.6 (0.02)	0.7 (0.01)	0.7 (0.01)
Iron (mg/d)	5.8 (0.36)	7.3 (0.31)	9.4 (0.30)	9.9 (0.20)
Magnesium (mg/d)	129 (5.1)	149 (3.8)	173 (3.3)	177 (2.3)
Phosphorus (mg/d)	698 (29)	826 (24)	1,000 (24)	1,029 (16)
Selenium (μg/d)	45 (2.0)	53 (1.6)	62 (1.4)	63 (0.9)
Zinc (mg/d)	5.0 (0.23)	5.9 (0.19)	7.2 (0.18)	7.4 (0.12)
Potassium (mg/d)	1,471 (58)	1,699 (46)	1,983 (40)	2,021 (26)
Sodium (mg/d)	1,131 (60)	1,373 (48)	1,685 (44)	1,756 (31)
Vitamin A (μg RAE/d)	339 (20.8)	413 (17.2)	510 (16.0)	534 (9.9)
Retinol (μg/d)	265 (17)	332 (14)	425 (15)	450 (10)
Vitamin E mg (αTOC/d)	2.1 (0.12)	2.6 (0.10)	3.2 (0.10)	3.4 (0.07)
Vitamin C (mg/d)	36 (3.87)	55 (3.82)	84 (4.24)	97 (3.35)
Thiamin (mg/d)	0.8 (0.03)	0.9 (0.03)	1.1 (0.03)	1.1 (0.01)
Riboflavin (mg/d)	1.4 (0.06)	1.6 (0.05)	1.9 (0.05)	2.0 (0.03)
Niacin (mg/d)	8.1 (0.44)	9.9 (0.37)	12.1 (0.34)	12.5 (0.21)
Vitamin B6 (mg/d)	0.8 (0.04)	1.0 (0.03)	1.2 (0.03)	1.2 (0.02)
Folate (μg DFE/d)	197 (12.0)	243 (10.5)	306 (10.4)	324 (6.45)
Vitamin B12 (mg/d)	2.8 (0.15)	3.4 (0.13)	4.3 (0.13)	4.5 (0.08)
Choline (mg/d)	143 (6.8)	171 (5.7)	208 (5.3)	215 (3.5)

NOTES: N = 311. See additional notes following Table J-60.

75th	90th	EAR or AI*	% Inadeq (SE)	UL	% > UL (SE)
1,261 (40)	1,498 (60)	500	2.2 (1.58)	2,500	0.1 (0.11)
0.8 (0.02)	1.0 (0.05)	0.26	0	1	0
11.8 (0.47)	14.6 (0.80)	3	0	40	0
200 (5.0)	230 (8.6)	65	0	65	NE
1,202 (33)	1,399 (50)	380	0.2 (0.2)	3,000	0
73 (2.0)	83 (3.1)	17	0	90	5.0 (3.25)
8.6 (0.27)	10.1 (0.44)	2.5	0	7	53.3 (3.66)
2,301 (57)	2,618 (88)	3,000*	NA	ND	—
2,058 (69)	2,468 (119)	1,000*	NA	1,500	65.0 (4.01)
626 (24.6)	755 (43.9)	210	0.5 (0.7)	NA	—
540 (22)	664 (38)	NA	NA	600	16.3 (4.89)
4.0 (0.16)	4.9 (0.29)	5	91.2 (4.36)	200	NE
125 (7.42)	174 (13.64)	13	0.6 (0.60)	400	0
1.3 (0.04)	1.5 (0.06)	0.4	0	ND	—
2.3 (0.07)	2.7 (0.10)	0.4	0	ND	—
14.6 (0.49)	17.3 (0.79)	5	0.3 (0.5)	10	NE
1.4 (0.04)	1.6 (0.07)	0.4	0	30	0
386 (16.3)	474 (27.9)	120	0.4 (0.6)	300	NE
5.3 (0.19)	6.4 (0.32)	0.7	0	ND	—
251 (8.0)	296 (12.9)	200*	NA	1,000	0

TABLE J-54 Usual Intake Distributions of Selected Micronutrients for Eligible Non-WIC-Participating Children Ages 1 to Less Than 2 Years, NHANES 2005–2008

Nutrient	Percentiles and Mean (SE)			
	10th	25th	Median	Mean
Calcium (mg/d)	680 (67)	815 (50)	980 (43)	1,010 (28)
Copper (mg/d)	0.5 (0.04)	0.6 (0.03)	0.7 (0.03)	0.7 (0.02)
Iron (mg/d)	6.8 (0.63)	8 (0.44)	9.4 (0.37)	9.6 (0.24)
Magnesium (mg/d)	136 (10.3)	155 (7.6)	178 (6.5)	182 (3.8)
Phosphorus (mg/d)	723 (61)	858 (46)	1,020 (39)	1,042 (26)
Selenium (μg/d)	41 (3.9)	51 (3.1)	64 (2.6)	66 (1.9)
Zinc (mg/d)	5.7 (0.43)	6.4 (0.30)	7.2 (0.24)	7.3 (0.13)
Potassium (mg/d)	1,492 (106)	1,715 (83)	1,993 (73)	2,032 (44)
Sodium (mg/d)	1,021 (123)	1,352 (97)	1,768 (84)	1,820 (63)
Vitamin A (μg RAE/d)	332 (37.4)	414 (28.2)	515 (25.1)	539 (17.8)
Retinol (μg/d)	267 (31)	335 (23)	418 (21)	435 (14)
Vitamin E mg (αTOC/d)	2.5 (0.25)	3.0 (0.20)	3.7 (0.18)	3.8 (0.11)
Vitamin C (mg/d)	48 (7.84)	65 (7.01)	90 (7.02)	97 (4.31)
Thiamin (mg/d)	0.8 (0.06)	0.9 (0.04)	1.1 (0.04)	1.1 (0.02)
Riboflavin (mg/d)	1.3 (0.12)	1.6 (0.08)	1.8 (0.07)	1.9 (0.04)
Niacin (mg/d)	8.1 (0.76)	9.8 (0.56)	12.0 (0.48)	12.4 (0.36)
Vitamin B6 (mg/d)	0.8 (0.07)	1.0 (0.06)	1.2 (0.05)	1.2 (0.03)
Folate (μg DFE/d)	217 (21.3)	260 (16.9)	314 (15.0)	322 (8.41)
Vitamin B12 (mg/d)	2.6 (0.30)	3.2 (0.20)	3.9 (0.17)	4.1 (0.13)
Choline (mg/d)	142 (10.8)	168 (8.8)	201 (8.1)	208 (5.4)

NOTES: N = 106. See additional notes following Table J-60.

	75th	90th	EAR or AI*	% Inadeq (SE)	UL	% > UL (SE)
	1,170 (66)	1,376 (116)	500	1.6 (2.9)	2,500	0.03 (0.12)
	0.8 (0.04)	1.0 (0.09)	0.26	0	1	0
	11 (0.58)	12.8 (1.04)	3	1 (1)	40	0
	204 (9.8)	232 (16.8)	65	0	65	NE
	1,201 (57)	1,388 (94)	380	0.1 (0.3)	3,000	0
	78 (3.7)	92 (5.7)	17	0.1 (0.2)	90	11.6 (5.59)
	8.1 (0.35)	9.0 (0.59)	2.5	0	7	56.5 (8.37)
	2,307 (106)	2,623 (168)	3,000*	—	ND	—
	2,230 (121)	2,685 (188)	1,000*	—	1,500	66.4 (5.71)
	636 (40.5)	774 (74.3)	210	1.1 (2.0)	NA	—
	515 (32)	623 (58)	NA	NA	600	12.2 (7.79)
	4.5 (0.27)	5.3 (0.42)	5	85.1 (8.88)	200	NE
	121 (11.40)	156 (19.79)	13	0.02 (0.08)	400	0
	1.2 (0.05)	1.4 (0.09)	0.4	0	ND	—
	2.1 (0.10)	2.4 (0.17)	0.4	0	ND	—
	14.5 (0.74)	17.2 (1.30)	5	0.8 (1.3)	10	NE
	1.4 (0.08)	1.6 (0.12)	0.4	0	30	0
	375 (21.6)	436 (34.1)	120	0.1 (0.5)	300	NE
	4.8 (0.27)	5.7 (0.50)	0.7	0.04 (0.15)	ND	—
	240 (12.3)	282 (20.3)	200*	NA	1,000	0

TABLE J-55 Usual Intake Distributions of Selected Micronutrients for WIC-Participating Children Ages 1 to Less Than 2 Years, NHANES 2011–2012

	Percentiles and Mean (SE)			
Nutrient	10th	25th	Median	Mean
Calcium (mg/d)	624 (67)	768 (52)	946 (45)	964 (28)
Copper (mg/d)	0.41 (0.04)	0.51 (0.03)	0.65 (0.03)	0.67 (0.02)
Iron (mg/d)	4.8 (0.61)	6.4 (0.51)	8.6 (0.48)	9.1 (0.38)
Magnesium (mg/d)	125 (10.1)	149 (7.7)	177 (6.5)	179 (4.4)
Phosphorus (mg/d)	683 (56)	809 (43)	961 (36)	973 (24)
Selenium (µg/d)	43 (3.7)	51 (2.3)	61 (2.3)	62 (1.5)
Zinc (mg/d)	4.5 (0.38)	5.4 (0.31)	6.5 (0.27)	6.7 (0.18)
Potassium (mg/d)	1,375 (101)	1,599 (76)	1,864 (63)	1,881 (41)
Sodium (mg/d)	1,070 (96)	1,311 (76)	1,615 (67)	1,660 (49.8)
Vitamin A (µg RAE/d)	316 (38)	402 (32)	510 (27)	526 (18)
Retinol (µg/d)	252 (34)	334 (28)	439 (25)	454 (17)
Vitamin E mg (αTOC/d)	2.2 (0.26)	3.8 (0.21)	3.8 (0.21)	4.0 (0.16)
Vitamin C (mg/d)	33 (5.7)	47 (4.9)	66 (5.0)	73 (4.0)
Thiamin (mg/d)	0.6 (0.05)	0.74 (0.04)	0.93 (0.04)	0.95 (0.03)
Riboflavin (mg/d)	1.1 (0.1)	1.3 (0.08)	1.6 (0.07)	1.7 (0.04)
Niacin (mg/d)	6.6 (0.71)	8.1 (0.59)	10.5 (0.51)	10.8 (0.35)
Vitamin B6 (mg/d)	0.73 (0.06)	0.88 (0.05)	1.1 (0.04)	1.1 (0.03)
Folate (µg DFE/d)	170 (19)	218 (16)	281 (15)	293 (10)
Vitamin B12 (mg/d)	2.4 (0.28)	3.0 (0.23)	3.9 (0.2)	4.0 (0.14)
Choline (mg/d)	140 (13)	169 (10.3)	206 (9.1)	211.0 (6.0)

NOTES: N = 96. See additional notes following Table J-60.

75th	90th	EAR or AI*	% Inadeq (SE)	UL	% > UL (SE)
1,140 (63)	1,329 (95)	500	3.2 (4.2)	2,500	0
0.81 (0.04)	0.98 (0.07)	0.26	0.7 (1.1)	1	8.6 (5.3)
11.3 (0.75)	14.1 (1.2)	3	1.7 (2.0)	40	0
207 (8.8)	236 (13.3)	65	0.07 (0.2)	65	NE
1,125 (49)	1,281 (74)	380	0.1 (0.4)	3,000	0
71 (3.1)	81 (4.7)	17	0	90	3.4 (4.2)
7.8 (0.39)	9.0 (0.62)	2.5	0.09 (0.3)	7	39.2 (6.8)
2,144 (86)	2,410 (127)	3,000*	NA	ND	—
1,960 (97)	2,306 (154)	1,000*	NA	1,500	58.6 (6.0)
627 (38)	748 (67)	210	1.2 (2.3)	—	—
558 (36)	667 (56)	NA	NA	600	18.5 (7.5)
4.9 (0.33)	6.1 (0.56)	5	76.1 (6.8)	200	NE
91 (8.8)	123 (17.4)	13	0.5 (1.1)	400	0
1.1 (0.05)	1.3 (0.09)	0.4	1.1 (1.5)	ND	—
2.0 (0.09)	2.3 (0.15)	0.4	0	ND	—
13 (0.79)	15.5 (1.1)	5	2.5 (3.1)	10	NE
1.3 (0.06)	1.5 (0.1)	0.4	0.2 (0.5)	30	0
355 (22)	432 (36)	120	2.0 (2.7)	300	NE
4.8 (0.29)	5.8 (0.45)	0.7	0.02 (0.06)	ND	—
248 (12.9)	289 (20.1)	200*	NA	1,000	0

TABLE J-56 Usual Intake Distributions of Selected Micronutrients for Eligible Non-WIC-Participating Children Ages 1 to Less Than 2 Years, NHANES 2011–2012

	Percentiles and Mean (SE)			
Nutrient	10th	25th	Median	Mean
Calcium (mg/d)	588 (93)	727 (73)	900 (63)	923 (43)
Copper (mg/d)	0.43 (0.05)	0.51 (0.04)	0.59 (0.03)	0.62 (0.03)
Iron (mg/d)	6.1 (0.85)	7.3 (0.74)	9.1 (0.74)	9.7 (0.52)
Magnesium (mg/d)	113 (16.5)	137 (13)	168 (11.3)	172 (7.7)
Phosphorus (mg/d)	691 (96)	820 (67)	965 (51)	966 (33.5)
Selenium (μg/d)	46 (5.9)	54 (4.4)	64 (3.7)	65 (2.4)
Zinc (mg/d)	5.5 (0.52)	6.2 (0.38)	7.0 (0.31)	7.1 (0.19)
Potassium (mg/d)	1,131 (171)	1,386 (135)	1,709 (118)	1,758 (81)
Sodium (mg/d)	1,181 (141)	1,383 (116)	1,657 (109)	1,729 (76)
Vitamin A (μg RAE/d)	348 (51.4)	418 (37)	499 (30)	503 (19)
Retinol (μg/d)	297 (43)	356 (33)	429 (27)	436 (17)
Vitamin E mg (αTOC/d)	2.5 (0.52)	3.3 (0.44)	4.3 (0.42)	4.6 (0.29)
Vitamin C (mg/d)	40 (10.8)	56 (8.9)	76 (8.2)	80 (5.3)
Thiamin (mg/d)	0.75 (0.09)	0.87 (0.07)	1.0 (0.07)	1.1 (0.004)
Riboflavin (mg/d)	1.2 (0.16)	1.4 (0.11)	1.7 (0.09)	1.7 (0.06)
Niacin (mg/d)	7.5 (1.2)	9.3 (1.0)	11.7 (0.97)	12.4 (0.68)
Vitamin B6 (mg/d)	0.75 (0.1)	0.92 (0.08)	1.1 (0.08)	1.2 (0.68)
Folate (μg DFE/d)	218 (29)	259 (24)	312 (21)	321 (14)
Vitamin B12 (mg/d)	2.7 (0.44)	3.3 (0.32)	4.0 (0.26)	4.1 (0.17)
Choline (mg/d)	144 (26)	181 (19)	224 (16)	227 (10)

NOTES: N = 41. See additional notes following Table J-60.

75th	90th	EAR or AI*	% Inadeq (SE)	UL	% > UL (SE)
1,094 (92)	1,288 (145)	500	4.3 (7.0)	2,500	0
0.7 (0.06)	0.84 (0.12)	0.26	0.2 (0.9)	1	3.7 (6.9)
11.4 (1.3)	14.1 (2.4)	3	0	40	0
203 (16.8)	238 (26.9)	65	0.3 (1.0)	65	NE
1,110 (68)	1,242 (99)	380	0.2 (1.0)	3,000	0
75 (5.2)	85 (7.9)	17	0	90	6.2 (9.1)
7.9 (0.42)	8.7 (0.64)	2.5	0	7	50.7 (10.0)
2,077 (175)	2,448 (280)	3,000*	NA	ND	—
1,995 (178)	2,367 (312)	1,000*	NA	1,500	64.4 (11.2)
584 (41)	664 (62)	210	0.4 (1.6)	NA	—
508 (39)	585 (60)	NA	NA	600	8.1 (10.5)
5.6 (0.68)	7.1 (1.2)	5	64.1 (11.2)	200	NE
101 (12.6)	126 (20.8)	13	0.2 (1.0)	400	0
1.2 (0.11)	1.4 (0.21)	0.4	0	ND	—
2.0 (0.13)	2.2 (0.21)	0.4	0	ND	—
14.7 (1.6)	18.1 (2.8)	5	0.7 (2.3)	10	NE
1.4 (0.13)	1.7 (0.24)	0.4	<0.01	30	0
374 (32)	438 (53)	120	<0.01	300	NE
4.8 (0.35)	5.5 (0.53)	0.7	NA	ND	—
271 (22)	305 (33)	200*	NA	1,000	0

TABLE J-57 Usual Intake Distributions of Selected Micronutrients for WIC-Participating Children Ages 2 to Less Than 5 Years, NHANES 2005–2008

	Percentiles and Mean (SE)			
Nutrient	10th	25th	Median	Mean
Calcium (mg/d)	549 (26)	686 (22)	869 (21)	908 (14)
Copper (mg/d)	0.6 (0.02)	0.7 (0.02)	0.8 (0.01)	0.8 (0.01)
Iron (mg/d)	7.3 (0.32)	8.9 (0.27)	11.1 (0.26)	11.6 (0.17)
Magnesium (mg/d)	133 (4.61)	157 (3.78)	190 (3.50)	196 (2.44)
Phosphorus (mg/d)	701 (26.43)	834 (20.53)	1,000 (18.47)	1,032 (13.09)
Selenium (µg/d)	48 (1.73)	56 (1.40)	67 (1.28)	69 (0.78)
Zinc (mg/d)	5.9 (0.23)	7.0 (0.18)	8.3 (0.17)	8.6 (0.11)
Potassium (mg/d)	1,417 (54.12)	1,693 (41.98)	2,040 (37.94)	2,114 (27.91)
Sodium (mg/d)	1,430 (57.97)	1,721 (46.05)	2,091 (42.13)	2,168 (29.32)
Vitamin A (µg RAE/d)	328 (17.04)	403 (13.56)	499 (12.71)	525 (8.12)
Retinol (µg/d)	283 (14.60)	345 (11.64)	425 (10.75)	442 (6.35)
Vitamin E mg (αTOC/d)	2.6 (0.11)	3.2 (0.10)	4.0 (0.10)	4.3 (0.08)
Vitamin C (mg/d)	45 (3.69)	66 (3.48)	98 (3.78)	113 (3.11)
Thiamin (mg/d)	0.9 (0.03)	1.0 (0.03)	1.2 (0.02)	1.3 (0.02)
Riboflavin (mg/d)	1.3 (0.05)	1.6 (0.04)	1.9 (0.04)	1.9 (0.02)
Niacin (mg/d)	10.6 (0.43)	12.6 (0.35)	15.1 (0.32)	15.5 (0.19)
Vitamin B6 (mg/d)	1.0 (0.04)	1.2 (0.03)	1.5 (0.03)	1.5 (0.02)
Folate (µg DFE/d)	261 (13.3)	327 (11.4)	417 (11.2)	439 (7.14)
Vitamin B12 (mg/d)	2.9 (0.14)	3.5 (0.11)	4.3 (0.10)	4.5 (0.07)
Choline (mg/d)	145 (5.9)	175 (4.9)	214 (4.6)	223 (3.2)

NOTES: N = 474. For percent inadequate calculations, the approach of IOM (2000b) was applied in which, when combining groups with different EARs, intakes in one of the groups are rescaled so they can be compared to the EAR of the other group. One value indicates that the EAR is the same across groups. See additional notes following Table J-60.

75th	90th	EAR or AI* (Ages 1–3/ Age 4)	% Inadeq (SE)	UL (Ages 1–3/ Age 4)	% > UL (SE)
1,087 (31)	1,317 (51)	500/800	16.7 (2.99)	2,500	0.1 (0.07)
1.0 (0.02)	1.2 (0.05)	0.26/0.34	0.1 (0.07)	1/3	15.5 (3.13)
13.7 (0.39)	16.4 (0.63)	3.0/4.1	0	40	0
227 (5.19)	266 (8.38)	65/110	0.6 (0.5)	65/110	NE
1,195 (27.91)	1,403 (47.56)	380/405	0.1 (0.2)	3,000	0
79 (1.85)	91 (2.92)	17/23	0	90/150	6.6 (2.77)
9.9 (0.26)	11.8 (0.46)	2.5/4.0	0.1 (0.1)	7/12	54.3 (2.96)
2,451 (58.46)	2,900 (102.27)	3,000/3,800*	NA	ND	—
2,529 (63.97)	3,000 (108.98)	1,000/1,200*	—	1,500/1,900	82.4 (3.59)
617 (20.26)	751 (36.81)	210/275	1.5 (1.4)	NA	—
519 (16.31)	621 (27.99)	NA	NA	600/900	12.1 (4.51)
5.0 (0.17)	6.4 (0.33)	5.0/6.0	79.2 (3.62)	200/300	NE
143 (6.76)	198 (13.22)	13/22	0.6 (0.5)	400/650	0.4 (0.37)
1.5 (0.03)	1.7 (0.06)	0.4/0.5	0	ND	—
2.2 (0.05)	2.6 (0.08)	0.4/0.5	0	ND	—
18.0 (0.45)	21.0 (0.71)	5.0/6.0	0	10/15	NE
1.8 (0.05)	2.1 (0.07)	0.4/0.5	0	30/40	0
526 (17.1)	645 (28.6)	120/160	0	300/400	NE
5.2 (0.16)	6.3 (0.30)	0.7/1.0	0	ND	—
261 (7.1)	313 (12.1)	200/250*	NA	1,000	0

TABLE J-58 Usual Intake Distributions of Selected Micronutrients for Eligible Non-WIC-Participating Children Ages 2 to Less Than 5 Years, NHANES 2005–2008

	Percentiles and Mean (SE)			
Nutrient	10th	25th	Median	Mean
Calcium (mg/d)	522 (27)	661 (22)	838 (20)	866 (14)
Copper (mg/d)	0.6 (0.02)	0.7 (0.02)	0.8 (0.02)	0.8 (0.01)
Iron (mg/d)	7.3 (0.31)	8.7 (0.25)	10.4 (0.24)	10.8 (0.15)
Magnesium (mg/d)	123 (5.1)	147 (3.7)	176 (3.2)	180 (2.4)
Phosphorus (mg/d)	682 (28)	813 (21)	971 (18)	996 (13)
Selenium (µg/d)	49 (2.20)	58 (1.64)	69 (1.41)	70 (0.90)
Zinc (mg/d)	5.6 (0.24)	6.6 (0.20)	8.0 (0.19)	8.3 (0.12)
Potassium (mg/d)	1,214 (54)	1,472 (42)	1,792 (37)	1,847 (27)
Sodium (mg/d)	1,448 (68)	1,765 (53)	2,152 (45)	2,191 (30)
Vitamin A (µg RAE/d)	322 (19.8)	406 (16.1)	514 (14.9)	536 (9.2)
Retinol (µg/d)	265 (16)	329 (13)	409 (11)	422 (7)
Vitamin E mg (αTOC/d)	2.8 (0.14)	3.3 (0.11)	4.0 (0.10)	4.1 (0.06)
Vitamin C (mg/d)	39 (3.68)	54 (3.36)	77 (3.44)	83 (2.01)
Thiamin (mg/d)	0.8 (0.04)	1.0 (0.03)	1.2 (0.02)	1.2 (0.02)
Riboflavin (mg/d)	1.2 (0.05)	1.5 (0.04)	1.8 (0.04)	1.8 (0.03)
Niacin (mg/d)	10.4 (0.48)	12.3 (0.36)	14.7 (0.31)	15.1 (0.20)
Vitamin B6 (mg/d)	0.9 (0.04)	1.0 (0.03)	1.3 (0.03)	1.3 (0.02)
Folate (µg DFE/d)	253 (14.4)	315 (11.7)	397 (11.0)	417 (7.27)
Vitamin B12 (mg/d)	2.7 (0.16)	3.4 (0.13)	4.3 (0.12)	4.4 (0.07)
Choline (mg/d)	142 (6.4)	168 (5.2)	203 (5.0)	210 (2.9)

NOTES: N = 397. For percent inadequate calculations, the approach of IOM (2000b) was applied in which, when combining groups with different EARs, intakes in one of the groups are rescaled so they can be compared to the EAR of the other group. One value indicates that the EAR is the same across groups. See additional notes following Table J-60.

		EAR or AI*		UL	
75th	90th	(Ages 1–3/ Age 4)	% Inadeq (SE)	(Ages 1–3/ Age 4)	% > UL (SE)
1,040 (29)	1,245 (46)	500/800	21.9 (3.04)	2,500	0
0.9 (0.02)	1.1 (0.04)	0.26/0.34	0.3 (0.3)	1/3	11.5 (3.21)
12.5 (0.35)	14.7 (0.56)	3.0/4.1	0	40	0
207 (4.7)	241 (7.8)	65/110	2.5 (1.2)	65/110	NE
1,151 (27)	1,339 (45)	380/405	0.3 (0.3)	3,000	0
81 (2.03)	94 (3.29)	17/23	0	90/150	5.9 (2.94)
9.6 (0.27)	11.3 (0.44)	2.5/4.0	0.7 (0.6)	7/12	45.4 (2.98)
2,160 (55)	2,546 (92)	3,000/3,800*	NA	ND	—
2,575 (63)	2,985 (95)	1,000/1,200*	NA	1,500/1,900	83.7 (3.75)
641 (22.4)	777 (37.4)	210/275	2.5 (1.9)	NA	—
500 (16)	595 (27)	NA	NA	600/900	9.4 (4.30)
4.8 (0.15)	5.6 (0.23)	5.0/6.0	87.6 (5.42)	200/300	NE
105 (5.50)	137 (9.40)	13/22	1 (1)	400/650	0
1.4 (0.03)	1.6 (0.06)	0.4/0.5	0.2 (0.3)	ND	—
2.1 (0.05)	2.5 (0.09)	0.4/0.5	0	ND	—
17.4 (0.45)	20.2 (0.73)	5.0/6.0	0.1 (0.2)	10/15	NE
1.6 (0.05)	1.9 (0.08)	0.4/0.5	0.2 (0.3)	30/40	0
495 (17.0)	604 (30.0)	120/160	0	300/400	NE
5.2 (0.17)	6.3 (0.29)	0.7/1.0	0	ND	—
245 (7.7)	289 (12.0)	200/250*	NA	1,000	0

TABLE J-59 Usual Intake Distributions of Selected Micronutrients for WIC-Participating Children Ages 2 to Less Than 5 Years, NHANES 2011–2012

	Percentiles and Mean (SE)			
Nutrient	10th	25th	Median	Mean
Calcium (mg/d)	590 (41)	753 (33)	961 (30)	994 (21)
Copper (mg/d)	0.54 (0.02)	0.64 (0.02)	0.76 (0.02)	0.78 (0.01)
Iron (mg/d)	8.1 (0.46)	9.6 (0.36)	11.4 (0.32)	11.7 (0.19)
Magnesium (mg/d)	150 (6.5)	174 (4.8)	203 (4.1)	207 (3.0)
Phosphorus (mg/d)	758 (37)	901 (29)	1,081 (26)	1,105 (17.7)
Selenium (μg/d)	52 (2.4)	60 (1.8)	70 (1.7)	72 (1.0)
Zinc (mg/d)	5.9 (0.31)	6.9 (0.24)	8.1 (0.21)	8.2 (0.12)
Potassium (mg/d)	1,536 (69)	1,780 (52)	2,071 (45)	2,110 (29)
Sodium (mg/d)	1,476 (70)	1,755 (58)	2,118 (54)	2,190 (38)
Vitamin A (μg RAE/d)	324 (25)	416 (20)	532 (18)	547 (11)
Retinol (μg/d)	276 (20)	351 (16)	443 (14)	452 (8.8)
Vitamin E mg (αTOC/d)	3.2 (0.2)	4.0 (0.17)	5.0 (0.16)	5.2 (0.1)
Vitamin C (mg/d)	59 (5.1)	73 (4.3)	92 (4.1)	96 (1.9)
Thiamin (mg/d)	0.85 (0.04)	0.99 (0.03)	1.2 (0.04)	1.2 (0.02)
Riboflavin (mg/d)	1.2 (0.06)	1.4 (0.05)	1.7 (0.4)	1.7 (0.03)
Niacin (mg/d)	11 (0.56)	13 (0.44)	15 (0.4)	15 (0.21)
Vitamin B6 (mg/d)	1.0 (0.05)	1.2 (0.04)	1.4 (0.03)	1.5 (0.02)
Folate (μg DFE/d)	261 (16)	322 (13)	401 (12)	416 (8)
Vitamin B12 (mg/d)	2.8 (0.19)	3.4 (0.15)	4.2 (0.13)	4.3 (0.07)
Choline (mg/d)	153 (8.2)	183 (6.7)	221 (6.2)	228 (3.9)

NOTES: N = 263. For percent inadequate calculations, the approach of IOM (2000b) was applied in which, when combining groups with different EARs, intakes in one of the groups are rescaled so they can be compared to the EAR of the other group. One value indicates that the EAR is the same across groups. See additional notes following Table J-60.

75th	90th	EAR or AI* (Ages 1–3/ Age 4)	% Inadeq (SE)	UL (Ages 1–3/ Age 4)	% > UL (SE)
1,200 (43)	1,441 (68)	500/800	2.0 (1.4)	2,500	4.8 (2.5)
0.91 (0.03)	1.0 (0.04)	0.26/0.34	0	1/3	9.8 (5.4)
13.5 (0.49)	15.8 (0.82)	3.0/4.1	0	40	0
236 (6.1)	270 (10.2)	65/110	0	65/110	NE
1,283 (37)	1,485 (57)	380/405	0.02 (0.04)	3,000	0
82 (2.5)	95 (4.1)	17/23	0	90/150	11.0 (5.8)
9.5 (0.3)	10.8 (0.46)	2.5/4.0	0	7/12	95.0 (3.5)
2,396 (64)	2,730 (105)	3,000/3,800*	NA	ND	—
2,546 (80)	2,995 (131)	1,000/1,200*	0	1,500/1,900	65.2 (4.0)
663 (25)	793 (39)	210/275	0.9 (1.0)	NA	—
544 (19)	641 (29)	NA	NA	600/900	15.1 (4.9)
6.2 (0.24)	7.4 (0.4)	5.0/6.0	34.9 (4.5)	200/300	NE
114 (6.0)	137 (9.6)	13/22	0	400/650	0.1 (0.3)
1.4 (0.04)	1.6 (0.07)	0.4/0.5	0	ND	—
2.0 (0.06)	2.4 (0.09)	0.4/0.5	0	ND	—
18 (0.57)	20 (0.88)	5.0/6.0	0	10/15	NE
1.7 (0.05)	1.9 (0.09)	0.4/0.5	0	30/40	0
494 (19)	592 (30)	120/160	0	300/400	NE
5.0 (0.17)	5.8 (0.26)	0.7/1.0	0	ND	—
266 (9.1)	313 (14.4)	200/250*	NA	1,000	0

TABLE J-60 Usual Intake Distributions of Selected Micronutrients for Eligible Non-WIC-Participating Children Ages 2 to Less Than 5 Years, NHANES 2011–2012

	Percentiles and Mean (SE)			
Nutrient	10th	25th	Median	Mean
Calcium (mg/d)	583 (49)	745 (40)	953 (36)	986 (23)
Copper (mg/d)	0.56 (0.03)	0.66 (0.02)	0.77 (0.02)	0.79 (0.01)
Iron (mg/d)	7.9 (0.49)	9.1 (0.4)	10.8 (0.36)	11 (0.18)
Magnesium (mg/d)	156 (7.1)	175 (5.4)	199 (4.6)	201 (2.5)
Phosphorus (mg/d)	797 (42)	918 (32)	1,069 (29)	1,088 (16)
Selenium (μg/d)	58 (3.1)	64 (2.3)	70 (1.9)	71 (0.69)
Zinc (mg/d)	6.1 (0.36)	7.0 (0.28)	8.0 (0.25)	8.1 (0.11)
Potassium (mg/d)	1,517 (77)	1,744 (57)	2,013 (48)	2,031 (28)
Sodium (mg/d)	1,783 (92)	1,987 (69)	2,227 (57)	2,242 (25)
Vitamin A (μg RAE/d)	395 (34)	471 (27)	567 (24)	583 (11)
Retinol (μg/d)	291 (29)	372 (24)	476 (21)	493 (11)
Vitamin E mg (αTOC/d)	4.1 (0.28)	4.7 (0.22)	5.5 (0.2)	5.6 (0.08)
Vitamin C (mg/d)	40 (4.9)	56 (4.5)	80 (4.7)	88 (3.0)
Thiamin (mg/d)	0.93 (0.05)	1.0 (0.04)	1.2 (0.03)	1.2 (0.02)
Riboflavin (mg/d)	1.2 (0.07)	1.4 (0.06)	1.7 (0.06)	1.8 (0.03)
Niacin (mg/d)	12 (0.68)	14 (0.51)	16 (0.45)	16 (0.22)
Vitamin B6 (mg/d)	1.0 (0.06)	1.2 (0.05)	1.4 (0.04)	1.4 (0.02)
Folate (μg DFE/d)	295 (21)	341 (16)	399 (15)	408 (6.4)
Vitamin B12 (mg/d)	3.0 (0.15)	3.5 (0.12)	4.3 (0.12)	4.4 (0.08)
Choline (mg/d)	159 (8.8)	179 (6.9)	205 (6.4)	210 (2.9)

NOTES: N = 217. For percent inadequate calculations, the approach of IOM (2000b) was applied in which, when combining groups with different EARs, intakes in one of the groups are rescaled so they can be compared to the EAR of the other group. See additional notes following this table.

75th	90th	EAR or AI* (Ages 1–3/ Age 4)	% Inadeq (SE)	UL (Ages 1–3/Age 4)	% > UL (SE)
1,191 (52)	1,432 (83)	500/800	2.1 (1.9)	2,500	3.2 (2.6)
0.91 (0.03)	1.0 (0.06)	0.26/0.34	0	1/3	9.2 (7.7)
12.7 (0.55)	14.7 (0.9)	3.0/4.1	0	40	0
224 (6.4)	249 (9.8)	65/110	0	65/110	NE
1,239 (41)	1,408 (63)	380/405	0	3,000	0
77 (2.6)	84 (3.9)	17/23	0	90/150	5.3 (9.0)
9.2 (0.35)	10.3 (0.55)	2.5/4.0	0	7/12	95.7 (5.0)
2,298 (65)	2,569 (97)	3,000/3,800*	NA	ND	—
2,481 (77)	2,721 (114)	1,000/1,200*	NA	1,500/1,900	82.2 (10.9)
677 (36)	793 (60)	210/275	0.05 (0.2)	NA	—
597 (31)	719 (50)	NA	NA	600/900	24.4 (7.5)
6.4 (0.28)	7.3 (0.45)	5.0/6.0	17.4 (11.8)	200/300	NE
112 (7.7)	148 (13.7)	13/22	0.04 (0.12)	400/650	0.21 (0.44)
1.4 (0.05)	1.6 (0.08)	0.4/0.5	0	ND	—
2.1 (0.08)	2.4 (0.13)	0.4/0.5	0	ND	—
18 (0.66)	20 (1.1)	5.0/6.0	0	10/15	NE
1.6 (0.07)	1.8 (0.11)	0.4/0.5	0	30/40	0
466 (22)	535 (36)	120/160	0	300/400	NE
5.2 (0.17)	6.1 (0.26)	0.7/1.0	0	ND	—
236 (9.6)	268 (14.9)	200/250*	NA	1,000	0

NOTES for Tables J-45 through J-60: — = not applicable due to no recommendation; % Inadeq = percentage of individuals with usual intake below the EAR; αTOC = α-tocopherol; AI = Adequate Intake; DFE = dietary folate equivalents; EAR = Estimated Average Requirement; NA = not available (data were inadequate to estimate); NA = not applicable; ND = not determined; NE = not evaluated; RAE = retinol activity equivalents; SE = standard error; UL = Tolerable Upper Intake Level. The ULs for folate, vitamin E, niacin, and magnesium represent intake from pharmacological agents only and do not include food intake. Vitamin D is not included because intake is a poor reflection of status.

Subgroup definitions are as follows:

WIC: the subgroup of individuals reporting participation in WIC regardless of income level

Eligible non-WIC: the subgroup of individuals with incomes less than or equal to 185 percent of poverty who did not report participation in WIC

* Adequate Intake value.

SOURCES: Intake data are from NHANES 2005–2012 (USDA/ARS, 2005–2012). Intake recommendations from Dietary Reference Intake reports (IOM, 1997, 1998, 2000a, 2001, 2002/2005, 2005, 2011b).

TABLE J-61 Distributions of Serum 25-Hydroxy Vitamin D of WIC Participants, NHANES 2005–2006

		25(OH)D Percentiles and Means (nmol/L) (SE)						
WIC Participant Category	N	10th	25th	Median	Mean	75th	90th	% < 40 nmol/L*
Women, P	120	41 (3.5)	52 (2.6)	66 (2.3)	72.8 (2.9)	83 (4.6)	111 (10.5)	8.6 (3.6)
Women, BF	19	33 (7.8)	42 (5.6)	53 (4.3)	54 (3.9)	65 (6.7)	77 (11.1)	21.2 (12.2)
Women, PP	38	37 (7.5)	49 (4.7)	62 (3.1)	61 (2.8)	73 (4.0)	82 (5.8)	12.6 (7.6)
Children, 1 to <2 Years	101	55.2 (3.4)	64.3 (2.2)	74.3 (1.6)	74.0 (1.4)	83.9 (2.1)	92.5(3.2)	1.1 (1.2)
Children, 2 to <5 Years	201	49 (2.0)	57 (1.5)	67 (1.2)	68.9 (1.2)	79 (2.0)	91 (3.3)	2.1 (1.3)

NOTES: 25(OH)D = 25-hydroxy-vitamin D; BF = breastfeeding, nonpregnant WIC-participating women; N = sample size; P = pregnant WIC-participating women; PP = WIC-participating women who are 6 months postpartum, not pregnant, and not breastfeeding; SE = standard error. Distributions were adjusted according to the method of Jahns et al. (2005), borrowing within-person variance from NHANES 2001–2002, for which two serum values were obtained. Serum data for 25(OH)D were only available in NHANES 2005–2006.

* A serum 25(OH)D level of 40 nmol/L was established by the Institute of Medicine (2011b) as an average requirement that meets the needs of approximately half the population, used to establish EARs for dietary intake of vitamin D.

SOURCE: USDA/ARS, 2005–2006.

TABLE J-62 Food Group Intake Distributions of Pregnant WIC-Participating Women Ages 19 to 50 Years, NHANES 2005–2012

		Percentiles and Mean (SE)		
Food Group	N	10th	25th	Median
Total fruit (c-eq/d)	101	0.24 (0.19)	0.57 (0.18)	1.23 (0.16)
Whole fruit (c-eq/d)	75	0.11 (0.17)	0.27 (0.17)	0.65 (0.17)
Fruit juice (c-eq/d)	54	0.14 (0.05)	0.30 (0.07)	0.59 (0.10)
Total vegetables (c-eq/d)	122	0.62 (0.13)	0.91 (0.11)	1.33 (0.09)
Dark green vegetables (c-eq/wk)	5	0.09 (0.19)	0.20 (0.19)	0.44 (0.19)
Total red and orange vegetables (c-eq/wk)	94	0.91 (0.17)	1.45 (0.19)	2.32 (0.21)
Beans and peas Computed as vegetables (c-eq/wk)	9	NA	NA	NA
Total starchy vegetables (c-eq/wk)	46	1.25 (0.38)	2.36 (0.58)	4.72 (0.98)
Other vegetables (c-eq/wk)	94	0.61 (0.33)	1.22 (0.36)	2.41 (0.39)
Total grains (oz-eq/d)	138	4.92 (0.45)	6.11 (0.38)	7.62 (0.35)
Whole grains (oz-eq/d)	46	0.34 (0.11)	0.56 (0.10)	0.83 (0.12)
Refined grains (oz-eq/d)	138	4.46 (0.36)	5.52 (0.31)	6.86 (0.32)
Total protein foods (oz-eq/d)	137	2.97 (0.39)	3.90 (0.320	5.10 (0.26)
Meat, poultry, and eggs (not seafood) (oz-eq/wk)	135	17.28 (2.20)	22.55 (1.94)	29.33 (1.65)
Seafood (oz-eq/wk)	5	0.12 (1.07)	0.69 (1.22)	2.85 (1.27)
Nuts, seeds, and soy (oz-eq/wk)	23	0.12 (0.18)	0.51 (0.34)	1.60 (0.51)
Total dairy (c-eq/d)	132	1.18 (0.21)	1.58 (0.15)	2.10 (0.11)
Oils (g-eq/d)	129	9.81 (1.56)	14.08 (1.40)	20.11 (1.33)
Solid fats (g-eq/d)	137	22.36 (3.31)	29.68 (2.50)	39.14 (1.77)
Added sugars (g-eq/d)	134	34.83 (6.27)	56.38 (6.08)	88.89 (6.34)

NOTES: N = 139. The reference food intake pattern used was 2,600 kcals, which was approximately the calculated EER for pregnant women in NHANES 2005–2012. See additional notes following Table J-74.

Mean	75th	90th	Recommended Intake	% Below Recommended Intake (SE)
1.73 (0.15)	2.34 (0.20)	3.83 (0.34)	2.00	69.05 (6.60)
1.14 (0.16)	1.41 (0.20)	2.68 (0.33)	1.00	64.38 (12.08)
0.72 (0.10)	0.98 (0.15)	1.47 (0.23)	1.00	75.76 (7.11)
1.44 (0.08)	1.84 (0.11)	2.39 (0.18)	3.50	98.93 (0.28)
0.66 (0.18)	0.88 (0.27)	1.50 (0.56)	2.50	97.41 (3.65)
2.73 (0.22)	3.55 (0.29)	5.05 (0.46)	7.00	97.02 (1.51)
NA	NA	NA	2.50	NA
7.72 (1.71)	9.32 (1.93)	17.03 (4.04)	7.00	65.16 (8.02)
3.29 (0.39)	4.37 (0.50)	7.07 (0.79)	5.50	83.07 (4.81)
7.84 (0.35)	9.32 (0.45)	11.03 (0.67)	9.00	71.00 (5.61)
0.85 (0.11)	1.11 (0.16)	1.35 (0.22)	4.50	100.00 (0.01)
7.06 (0.33)	8.39 (0.43)	9.92 (0.63)	4.50	10.42 (3.87)
5.30 (0.25)	6.48 (0.28)	7.88 (0.40)	6.50	75.30 (5.08)
30.38 (1.55)	37.06 (1.78)	44.81 (2.53)	31.00	56.08 (5.41)
5.47 (1.24)	7.53 (2.17)	14.27 (5.01)	10.00	82.14 (8.73)
2.34 (0.53)	3.38 (0.91)	5.55 (1.38)	5.00	87.21 (6.61)
2.21 (0.10)	2.73 (0.16)	3.38 (0.29)	3.00	82.49 (6.88)
21.79 (1.34)	27.66 (1.70)	35.84 (2.53)	34.00	87.57 (3.74)
				% Above Recommended Intake (SE)
40.68 (1.71)	50.00 (2.19)	60.98 (3.60)	<28.9	76.87 (6.17)
100.02 (6.53)	131.45 (8.28)	179.20 (11.94)	<65	68.27 (5.08)

TABLE J-63 Food Group Intake Distributions of Pregnant, Eligible Non-WIC-Participating Women Ages 19 to 50 Years, NHANES 2005–2012

		Percentiles and Mean (SE)		
Food Group	N	10th	25th	Median
Total fruit (c-eq/d)	40	0.22 (0.08)	0.46 (0.12)	0.94 (0.17)
Whole fruit (c-eq/d)	18	0.07 (0.05)	0.26 (0.09)	0.63 (0.17)
Fruit juice (c-eq/d)	28	0.07 (0.05)	0.15 (0.08)	0.31 (0.13)
Total vegetables (c-eq/d)	53	0.76 (0.14)	1.11 (0.11)	1.58 (0.11)
Dark green vegetables (c-eq/wk)	4	0.00 (NA)	0.03 (NA)	0.35 (NA)
Total red and orange vegetables (c-eq/wk)	35	1.48 (0.31)	2.04 (0.33)	2.84 (0.34)
Beans and peas Computed as vegetables (c-eq/wk)	8	0.03 (0.20)	0.14 (0.23)	0.48 (0.27)
Total starchy vegetables (c-eq/wk)	25	0.73 (0.48)	1.70 (0.62)	3.18 (0.98)
Other vegetables (c-eq/wk)	43	1.33 (0.40)	2.09 (0.43)	3.31 (0.46)
Total grains (oz-eq/d)	58	4.75 (0.64)	5.83 (0.46)	7.21 (0.39)
Whole grains (oz-eq/d)	16	0.06 (0.10)	0.16 (0.12)	0.35 (0.15)
Refined grains (oz-eq/d)	57	4.28 (0.65)	5.40 (0.50)	6.80 (0.42)
Total protein foods (oz-eq/d)	56	3.42 (0.59)	4.35 (0.42)	5.54 (0.36)
Meat, poultry, and eggs (not seafood) (oz-eq/wk)	55	16.75 (4.48)	22.62 (3.51)	30.35 (2.40)
Seafood (oz-eq/wk)	2	1.09 (NA)	2.08 (NA)	4.09 (NA)
Nuts, seeds, and soy (oz-eq/wk)	9	0.04 (0.56)	0.27 (0.61)	1.29 (1.01)
Total dairy (c-eq/d)	56	1.11 (0.20)	1.44 (0.16)	1.88 (0.14)
Oils (g-eq/d)	54	13.32 (6.27)	17.58 (4.76)	23.51 (3.02)
Solid fats (g-eq/d)	58	26.21 (3.63)	32.20 (2.93)	40.24 (2.26)
Added sugars (g-eq/d)	57	40.55 (14.09)	61.83 (10.26)	91.61 (6.88)

NOTES: N = 58. The reference food intake pattern used was 2,600 kcals, which was approximately the calculated EER for pregnant women in NHANES 2005–2012. See additional notes following Table J-74.

Mean	75th	90th	Recommended Intake	% Below Recommended Intake (SE)
1.32 (0.21)	1.74 (0.28)	2.87 (0.46)	2.00	79.81 (5.45)
0.80 (0.18)	1.15 (0.28)	1.76 (0.41)	1.00	69.26 (10.55)
0.43 (0.11)	0.57 (0.17)	0.93 (0.27)	1.00	91.49 (7.31)
1.69 (0.12)	2.16 (0.17)	2.77 (0.26)	3.50	97.23 (0.65)
0.97 (NA)	1.41 (NA)	3.03 (NA)	2.50	86.44 NA
3.10 (0.34)	3.87 (0.44)	5.05 (0.77)	7.00	98.12 (2.67)
0.77 (0.18)	1.13 (0.31)	1.95 (0.78)	2.50	94.81 (5.44)
3.71 (0.81)	5.06 (1.24)	7.28 (1.56)	7.00	88.70 (9.93)
3.87 (0.47)	5.04 (0.62)	7.13 (1.08)	5.50	79.51 (5.47)
7.45 (0.42)	8.81 (0.65)	10.44 (1.06)	9.00	77.31 (10.02)
0.50 (0.16)	0.67 (0.24)	1.12 (0.39)	4.50	99.95 (0.35)
6.98 (0.42)	8.36 (0.56)	9.90 (0.84)	4.50	12.35 (6.50)
5.71 (0.37)	6.88 (0.56)	8.22 (0.88)	6.50	68.86 (10.55)
31.68 (2.16)	39.28 (2.87)	48.32 (5.05)	31.00	52.10 (8.10)
6.31 (NA)	7.88 (NA)	13.75 (NA)	10.00	82.22 NA
3.87 (1.58)	4.21 (2.21)	10.09 (4.25)	5.00	78.44 (10.64)
1.96 (0.14)	2.39 (0.19)	2.92 (0.31)	3.00	91.36 (4.65)
25.13 (2.64)	30.90 (3.31)	39.00 (6.38)	34.00	82.13 (17.12)
				% Above Recommended Intake
42.17 (2.16)	50.03 (2.74)	60.58 (4.56)	<28.9	84.01 (8.08)
98.86 (6.79)	127.96 (9.78)	166.40 (17.13)	<65	72.41 (9.91)

TABLE J-64 Food Group Intake Distributions of Breastfeeding, WIC-Participating Women Ages 19 to 50 Years, NHANES 2005–2012

		Percentiles and Mean (SE)		
Food Group	N	10th	25th	Median
Total fruit (c-eq/d)	18	0.38 (0.08)	0.65 (0.14)	1.12 (0.22)
Whole fruit (c-eq/d)	14	0.03 (0.10)	0.10 (0.12)	0.34 (0.18)
Fruit juice (c-eq/d)	7	0.18 (0.10)	0.38 (0.17)	0.90 (0.36)
Total vegetables (c-eq/d)	25	1.69 (0.19)	1.69 (0.13)	1.69 (0.16)
Dark green vegetables (c-eq/wk)	1	NA	NA	NA
Total red and orange vegetables (c-eq/wk)	22	1.25 (0.49)	1.93 (0.41)	2.89 (0.37)
Beans and peas Computed as vegetables (c-eq/wk)	1	NA	NA	NA
Total starchy vegetables (c-eq/wk)	11	1.29 (0.49)	2.04 (0.58)	3.38 (0.75)
Other vegetables (c-eq/wk)	19	2.60 (0.69)	3.12 (0.59)	3.79 (0.52)
Total grains (oz-eq/d)	25	4.44 (0.81)	5.30 (0.57)	6.44 (0.54)
Whole grains (oz-eq/d)	10	0.00 (0.02)	0.01 (0.04)	0.22 (0.19)
Refined grains (oz-eq/d)	25	4.21 (0.83)	5.04 (0.55)	6.11 (0.52)
Total protein foods (oz-eq/d)	24	3.19 (0.97)	4.08 (0.70)	5.20 (0.43)
Meat, poultry, and eggs (not seafood) (oz-eq/wk)	22	16.80 (7.11)	23.22 (5.13)	31.47 (3.02)
Seafood (oz-eq/wk)	1	NA	NA	NA
Nuts, seeds, and soy (oz-eq/wk)	1	NA	NA	NA
Total dairy (c-eq/d)	23	0.67 (0.43)	1.20 (0.37)	2.02 (0.39)
Oils (g-eq/d)	20	19.13 (3.81)	19.13 (2.9)	19.13 (2.71)
Solid fats (g-eq/d)	25	20.21 (3.71)	27.45 (3.39)	37.57 (4.28)
Added sugars (g-eq/d)	25	41.85 (7.71)	63.28 (8.56)	93.22 (10.82)

NOTES: N = 25. The reference food intake pattern used was 2,600 kcals, which was approximately the calculated EER for breastfeeding women in NHANES 2005–2012. See additional notes following Table J-74.

Mean	75th	90th	Recommended Intake	% Below Recommended Intake (SE)
1.40 (0.28)	1.84 (0.38)	2.77 (0.67)	2.00	78.67 (6.21)
1.11 (0.36)	1.04 (0.37)	2.65 (0.89)	1.00	74.15 (9.28)
2.03 (1.59)	2.13 (0.90)	4.61 (2.59)	1.00	53.14 (12.90)
1.69 (0.18)	1.69 (0.29)	1.69 (0.46)	3.50	50.00 (16.08)
NA	NA	NA	2.50	NA
3.15 (0.36)	4.09 (0.49)	5.38 (0.74)	7.00	97.40 (9.75)
NA	NA	NA	2.50	NA
4.41 (1.06)	5.56 (1.22)	8.67 (2.51)	7.00	83.84 (6.82)
3.89 (0.54)	4.55 (0.70)	5.32 (1.12)	5.50	92.12 (10.24)
6.72 (0.65)	7.83 (1.02)	9.34 (1.75)	9.00	87.58 (16.02)
0.46 (0.14)	0.99 (0.30)	1.21 (0.29)	4.50	100.00 (0.00)
6.32 (0.63)	7.38 (1.05)	8.69 (1.78)	4.50	14.43 (16.75)
5.34 (0.39)	6.44 (0.44)	7.67 (0.78)	6.50	75.95 (12.35)
32.70 (2.78)	40.83 (3.04)	50.16 (5.54)	31.00	48.55 (12.62)
NA	NA	NA	10.00	NA
NA	NA	NA	5.00	NA
2.32 (0.43)	3.12 (0.64)	4.35 (1.04)	3.00	72.86 (13.09)
19.13 (3.24)	19.13 (5.14)	19.13 (9.14)	34.00	50.00 (15.83)
				% Above Recommended Intake (SE)
40.35 (4.87)	50.20 (7.04)	64.03 (10.92)	<28.9	71.49 (8.32)
100.55 (11.43)	129.80 (14.92)	168.55 (20.16)	<65	73.61 (7.05)

TABLE J-65 Food Group Intake Distributions of Postpartum, WIC-Participating Women Ages 19 to 50 Years, NHANES 2005–2012

		Percentiles and Mean (SE)		
Food Group	N	10th	25th	Median
Total fruit (c-eq/d)	20	0.08 (0.05)	0.21 (0.08)	0.52 (0.16)
Whole fruit (c-eq/d)	6	0.02 (NA)	0.05 (NA)	0.12 (NA)
Fruit juice (c-eq/d)	12	0.02 (0.02)	0.06 (0.04)	0.22 (0.12)
Total vegetables (c-eq/d)	43	0.44 (0.19)	0.62 (0.13)	0.87 (0.09)
Dark green vegetables (c-eq/wk)	2	0.00 (NA)	0.01 (NA)	0.18 (NA)
Total red and orange vegetables (c-eq/wk)	31	0.58 (0.30)	1.01 (0.29)	1.82 (0.27)
Beans and peas Computed as vegetables (c-eq/wk)	1	NA	NA	NA
Total starchy vegetables (c-eq/wk)	14	0.35 (0.21)	0.64 (0.23)	1.16 (0.27)
Other vegetables (c-eq/wk)	29	0.74 (0.50)	1.26 (0.46)	2.21 (0.44)
Total grains (oz-eq/d)	53	4.06 (0.83)	5.31 (0.62)	6.97 (0.47)
Whole grains (oz-eq/d)	15	0.04 (0.06)	0.18 (0.09)	0.58 (0.15)
Refined grains (oz-eq/d)	52	3.45 (0.91)	4.65 (0.68)	6.27 (0.50)
Total protein foods (oz-eq/d)	51	2.25 (0.46)	3.26 (0.39)	4.63 (0.36)
Meat, poultry, and eggs (not seafood) (oz-eq/wk)	49	15.59 (3.93)	21.10 (2.83)	28.34 (2.23)
Seafood (oz-eq/wk)	1	NA	NA	NA
Nuts, seeds, and soy (oz-eq/wk)	7	0.11 (0.27)	0.34 (0.29)	0.96 (0.34)
Total dairy (c-eq/d)	48	0.95 (0.40)	1.23 (0.33)	1.62 (0.23)
Oils (g-eq/d)	50	10.72 (3.41)	14.19 (2.49)	18.99 (1.77)
Solid fats (g-eq/d)	52	17.28 (4.92)	23.93 (3.70)	32.72 (2.45)
Added sugars (g-eq/d)	54	40.74 (18.84)	61.15 (13.59)	90.82 (8.19)

NOTES: N = 54. The reference food intake pattern used was 2,300 kcals, which was approximately the calculated EER for postpartum women in NHANES 2005–2012. See additional notes following Table J-74.

				% Below
Mean	75th	90th	Recommended Intake	Recommended Intake (SE)
0.85 (0.28)	1.11 (0.36)	2.02 (0.72)	2.00	89.87 (6.70)
0.24 (NA)	0.29 (NA)	0.59 (NA)	1.00	96.13 (NA)
0.54 (0.31)	0.61 (0.34)	1.38 (0.82)	1.00	84.64 (8.92)
0.94 (0.09)	1.19 (0.14)	1.54 (0.24)	3.00	99.87 (25.10)
0.67 (NA)	0.90 (NA)	2.10 (NA)	2.00	89.15 (NA)
2.41 (0.30)	3.13 (0.42)	4.95 (0.83)	6.00	93.90 (7.08)
NA	NA	NA	2.00	NA
1.52 (0.31)	1.99 (0.39)	3.10 (0.74)	6.00	98.79 (1.69)
2.92 (0.48)	3.76 (0.63)	5.92 (1.20)	5.00	85.38 (9.29)
7.30 (0.47)	8.93 (0.66)	10.96 (1.09)	7.50	57.63 (9.78)
0.68 (0.11)	1.06 (0.23)	1.45 (0.26)	3.75	100.00 (0.29)
6.64 (0.49)	8.23 (0.64)	10.30 (1.06)	3.75	13.22 (9.71)
4.93 (0.36)	6.27 (0.46)	7.99 (0.66)	6.25	74.71 (7.82)
29.64 (2.26)	36.77 (3.23)	45.37 (5.05)	29.50	53.94 (12.98)
NA	NA	NA	9.50	NA
1.97 (0.86)	2.33 (0.81)	4.74 (2.23)	5.00	90.74 (6.51)
1.70 (0.20)	2.08 (0.20)	2.57 (0.34)	3.00	95.96 (10.31)
20.26 (1.74)	24.94 (2.26)	31.42 (3.68)	30.00	87.64 (22.52)
				% Above Recommended Intake (SE)
34.33 (2.26)	42.97 (2.60)	53.42 (4.34)	<25.6	70.44 (11.75)
99.92 (7.73)	128.72 (12.67)	170.57 (24.53)	<57.5	77.98 (13.20)

TABLE J-66 Food Group Intake Distributions of Nonpregnant, Postpartum, or Breastfeeding Non-WIC-Participating Women Ages 19 to 50 Years, NHANES 2005–2012

		Percentiles and Mean (SE)		
Food Group	N	10th	25th	Median
Total fruit (c-eq/d)	986	0.11 (0.02)	0.27 (0.03)	0.69 (0.05)
Whole fruit (c-eq/d)	422	0.07 (0.01)	0.16 (0.01)	0.34 (0.02)
Fruit juice (c-eq/d)	598	0.03 (0.00)	0.08 (0.01)	0.19 (0.01)
Total vegetables (c-eq/d)	1,737	0.62 (0.02)	0.86 (0.02)	1.19 (0.02)
Dark green vegetables (c-eq/wk)	101	0.09 (0.03)	0.20 (0.04)	0.44 (0.04)
Total red and orange vegetables (c-eq/wk)	1,152	0.76 (0.07)	1.27 (0.07)	2.15 (0.08)
Beans and peas Computed as vegetables (c-eq/wk)	124	0.09 (0.03)	0.23 (0.04)	0.52 (0.04)
Total starchy vegetables (c-eq/wk)	611	1.22 (0.10)	1.75 (0.09)	2.48 (0.09)
Other vegetables (c-eq/wk)	1,221	1.03 (0.09)	1.70 (0.09)	2.86 (0.09)
Total grains (oz-eq/d)	1,927	3.33 (0.10)	4.34 (0.09)	5.64 (0.07)
Whole grains (oz-eq/d)	488	0.10 (0.01)	0.23 (0.02)	0.47 (0.02)
Refined grains (oz-eq/d)	1,899	2.87 (0.09)	3.82 (0.08)	5.06 (0.07)
Total protein foods (oz-eq/d)	1,886	2.62 (0.11)	3.49 (0.09)	4.65 (0.07)
Meat, poultry, and eggs (not seafood) (oz-eq/wk)	1,818	11.42 (0.87)	17.36 (0.74)	26.53 (0.51)
Seafood (oz-eq/wk)	71	0.42 (0.17)	1.00 (0.21)	2.24 (0.19)
Nuts, seeds, and soy (oz-eq/wk)	276	0.26 (0.05)	0.67 (0.08)	1.66 (0.14)
Total dairy (c-eq/d)	1,740	0.56 (0.04)	0.84 (0.03)	1.25 (0.03)
Oils (g-eq/d)	1,848	9.16 (0.42)	12.76 (0.38)	17.85 (0.35)
Solid fats (g-eq/d)	1,941	17.04 (0.68)	22.53 (0.56)	29.83 (0.48)
Added sugars (g-eq/d)	1,935	32.89 (1.86)	52.07 (1.58)	81.12 (1.49)

NOTES: N = 1,983. The reference food intake pattern used was 2,200 kcals, which was approximately the calculated EER for this subgroup of women in NHANES 2005–2012. See additional notes following Table J-74.

Mean	75th	90th	Recommended Intake	% Below Recommended Intake (SE)
1.42 (0.06)	1.64 (0.08)	3.40 (0.15)	2.00	79.89 (1.46)
0.46 (0.02)	0.63 (0.03)	1.00 (0.05)	1.00	90.11 (1.29)
0.31 (0.02)	0.41 (0.02)	0.73 (0.04)	1.00	95.00 (0.83)
1.27 (0.02)	1.59 (0.03)	2.02 (0.04)	3.00	99.18 (0.12)
0.65 (0.04)	0.87 (0.06)	1.46 (0.14)	2.00	95.31 (1.50)
2.68 (0.09)	3.49 (0.13)	5.25 (0.24)	6.00	93.18 (1.06)
0.75 (0.03)	1.03 (0.05)	1.72 (0.11)	2.00	93.01 (1.28)
2.69 (0.10)	3.40 (0.14)	4.43 (0.23)	6.00	97.90 (0.85)
3.54 (0.10)	4.61 (0.12)	6.88 (0.23)	5.00	78.67 (1.39)
5.85 (0.07)	7.13 (0.09)	8.63 (0.14)	7.00	73.17 (1.64)
0.59 (0.02)	0.82 (0.03)	1.21 (0.06)	3.50	99.97 (0.03)
5.28 (0.07)	6.50 (0.09)	7.96 (0.13)	3.50	19.26 (1.47)
4.88 (0.07)	6.02 (0.10)	7.43 (0.16)	6.00	74.71 (1.83)
30.28 (0.45)	39.08 (0.67)	53.88 (1.45)	28.00	53.60 (1.53)
3.17 (0.19)	4.32 (0.27)	7.12 (0.68)	9.00	94.53 (1.72)
2.93 (0.23)	3.60 (0.28)	6.91 (0.61)	5.00	83.60 (1.91)
1.39 (0.03)	1.79 (0.04)	2.40 (0.06)	3.00	96.24 (0.40)
19.26 (0.35)	24.20 (0.43)	31.14 (0.66)	29.00	86.55 (1.16)
				% Above Recommended Intake (SE)
31.32 (0.48)	38.47 (0.64)	47.45 (1.00)	<24	68.79 (2.16)
91.44 (1.59)	119.51 (2.25)	163.03 (3.65)	<55	72.45 (1.55)

TABLE J-67 Food Group Intake Distributions of WIC-Participating Children Ages 1 to Less Than 2 Years, NHANES 2005–2008

Food Group	N	Percentiles and Mean (SE)					
		10th	25th	Median	Mean	75th	90th
Total fruit (c-eq/d)	231	0.55 (0.10)	0.84 (0.08)	1.26 (0.06)	1.39 (0.06)	1.79 (0.09)	2.37 (0.15)
Whole fruit (c-eq/d)	156	0.09 (0.04)	0.20 (0.04)	0.44 (0.05)	0.66 (0.05)	0.87 (0.07)	1.50 (0.12)
Fruit juice (c-eq/d)	178	0.17 (0.09)	0.34 (0.07)	0.64 (0.04)	0.84 (0.04)	1.12 (0.06)	1.75 (0.13)
Total vegetables (c-eq/d)	229	0.27 (0.05)	0.36 (0.04)	0.49 (0.03)	0.52 (0.02)	0.64 (0.03)	0.80 (0.05)
Dark green vegetables (c-eq/wk)	7	0.00 (0.01)	0.00 (0.01)	0.03 (0.02)	0.13 (0.03)	0.12 (0.02)	0.35 (0.08)
Total red and orange vegetables (c-eq/wk)	142	0.38 (0.11)	0.63 (0.11)	1.06 (0.10)	1.33 (0.10)	1.73 (0.14)	2.61 (0.26)
Beans and peas computed as vegetables (c-eq/wk)	21	0.00 (0.01)	0.03 (0.03)	0.18 (0.05)	0.35 (0.03)	0.52 (0.05)	0.97 (0.14)
Total starchy vegetables (c-eq/wk)	118	0.57 (0.31)	0.94 (0.26)	1.61 (0.21)	2.09 (0.19)	2.68 (0.27)	4.16 (0.51)
Other vegetables (c-eq/wk)	108	0.26 (0.10)	0.48 (0.12)	0.92 (0.17)	1.37 (0.25)	1.72 (0.32)	2.97 (0.60)
Total grains (oz-eq/d)	259	1.68 (0.16)	2.21 (0.12)	2.89 (0.09)	3.02 (0.09)	3.69 (0.12)	4.51 (0.21)
Whole grains (oz-eq/d)	122	0.13 (0.02)	0.21 (0.02)	0.34 (0.03)	0.39 (0.03)	0.52 (0.04)	0.72 (0.08)
Refined grains (oz-eq/d)	257	1.41 (0.16)	1.88 (0.12)	2.50 (0.08)	2.62 (0.08)	3.23 (0.12)	4.00 (0.20)
Total protein foods (oz-eq/d)	240	0.83 (0.18)	1.27 (0.14)	1.93 (0.09)	2.13 (0.09)	2.77 (0.13)	3.70 (0.22)
Meat, poultry, and eggs (not seafood) (oz-eq/wk)	236	5.31 (1.19)	8.18 (0.88)	12.40 (0.63)	13.72 (0.62)	17.80 (0.89)	23.75 (1.52)
Seafood (oz-eq/wk)	1	NA	NA	NA	NA	NA	NA
Nuts, seeds, and soy (oz-eq/wk)	31	0.03 (0.04)	0.15 (0.09)	0.49 (0.14)	0.84 (0.13)	1.14 (0.24)	2.08 (0.34)
Total dairy (c-eq/d)	259	1.32 (0.12)	1.85 (0.10)	2.55 (0.08)	2.67 (0.08)	3.35 (0.11)	4.16 (0.15)
Oils (g-eq/d)	236	3.03 (0.67)	4.73 (0.55)	7.32 (0.44)	8.27 (0.42)	10.78 (0.54)	14.74 (0.86)
Solid fats (g-eq/d)	262	15.62 (1.20)	20.29 (0.96)	26.29 (0.85)	27.25 (0.85)	33.17 (1.09)	40.11 (1.57)
Added sugars (g-eq/d)	254	12.28 (2.97)	19.59 (2.29)	30.77 (1.62)	34.87 (1.53)	45.66 (2.09)	62.64 (3.68)

NOTES: N = 263. See additional notes following Table J-74.

TABLE J-68 Food Group Intake Distributions of Eligible Non-WIC-Participating Children Ages 1 to Less Than 2 Years, NHANES 2005–2008

Food Group	N	Percentiles and Mean (SE)					
		10th	25th	Median	Mean	75th	90th
Total fruit (c-eq/d)	73	0.40 (0.20)	0.71 (0.17)	1.22 (0.12)	1.43 (0.10)	1.91 (0.11)	2.72 (0.18)
Whole fruit (c-eq/d)	53	0.09 (0.09)	0.20 (0.10)	0.44 (0.10)	0.70 (0.09)	0.90 (0.11)	1.60 (0.15)
Fruit juice (c-eq/d)	59	0.10 (0.05)	0.24 (0.06)	0.55 (0.07)	0.82 (0.08)	1.09 (0.11)	1.87 (0.18)
Total vegetables (c-eq/d)	73	0.21 (0.07)	0.35 (0.06)	0.54 (0.05)	0.61 (0.05)	0.80 (0.06)	1.10 (0.10)
Dark green vegetables (c-eq/wk)	4	0.00 (NA)	0.00 (NA)	0.03 (NA)	0.27 (NA)	0.23 (NA)	0.78 (NA)
Total red and orange vegetables (c-eq/wk)	55	0.29 (0.17)	0.55 (0.15)	1.03 (0.13)	1.38 (0.14)	1.82 (0.19)	2.88 (0.36)
Beans and peas computed as vegetables (c-eq/wk)	2	0.14 (NA)	0.22 (NA)	0.34 (NA)	0.37 (NA)	0.50 (NA)	0.66 (NA)
Total starchy vegetables (c-eq/wk)	38	1.04 (0.14)	1.49 (0.19)	2.20 (0.27)	2.57 (0.35)	3.24 (0.44)	4.54 (0.80)
Other vegetables (c-eq/wk)	34	0.27 (0.22)	0.48 (0.27)	0.93 (0.37)	1.51 (0.47)	1.81 (0.57)	3.29 (1.05)
Total grains (oz-eq/d)	79	1.39 (0.28)	2.12 (0.23)	3.14 (0.19)	3.38 (0.17)	4.38 (0.21)	5.69 (0.33)
Whole grains (oz-eq/d)	34	0.10 (0.03)	0.18 (0.04)	0.33 (0.06)	0.41 (0.07)	0.55 (0.10)	0.83 (0.16)
Refined grains (oz-eq/d)	78	1.05 (0.35)	1.71 (0.27)	2.66 (0.19)	2.95 (0.17)	3.88 (0.20)	5.21 (0.35)
Total protein foods (oz-eq/d)	76	0.84 (0.27)	1.30 (0.19)	1.96 (0.13)	2.15 (0.14)	2.80 (0.21)	3.71 (0.36)
Meat, poultry, and eggs (not seafood) (oz-eq/wk)	72	5.44 (2.14)	8.17 (1.46)	12.14 (0.86)	13.31 (0.85)	17.15 (1.33)	22.62 (2.39)
Seafood (oz-eq/wk)	1	NA	NA	NA	NA	NA	NA
Nuts, seeds, and soy (oz-eq/wk)	8	0.27 (0.49)	0.53 (0.49)	0.99 (0.51)	1.29 (0.50)	1.70 (0.63)	2.70 (0.98)
Total dairy (c-eq/d)	79	1.08 (0.19)	1.64 (0.16)	2.38 (0.14)	2.53 (0.14)	3.26 (0.17)	4.16 (0.24)
Oils (g-eq/d)	72	4.22 (0.77)	5.97 (0.70)	8.47 (0.69)	9.20 (0.72)	11.63 (0.94)	15.09 (1.44)
Solid fats (g-eq/d)	80	14.08 (2.83)	19.59 (2.06)	26.64 (1.44)	27.63 (1.38)	34.58 (1.84)	42.44 (2.97)
Added sugars (g-eq/d)	80	12.13 (4.74)	21.21 (3.98)	36.13 (3.48)	43.04 (3.51)	57.32 (4.69)	82.79 (7.59)

NOTES: N = 82. See additional notes following Table J-74.

TABLE J-69 Food Group Intake Distributions of WIC-Participating Children Ages 1 to Less Than 2 Years, NHANES 2011–2012

		Percentiles and Mean (SE)					
Food Group	N	10th	25th	Median	Mean	75th	90th
Total fruit (c-eq/d)	72	0.49 (0.10)	0.78 (0.10)	1.20 (0.11)	1.36 (0.12)	1.77 (0.16)	2.41 (0.27)
Whole fruit (c-eq/d)	46	0.11 (0.07)	0.22 (0.08)	0.44 (0.08)	0.62 (0.07)	0.81 (0.09)	1.34 (0.15)
Fruit juice (c-eq/d)	61	0.16 (0.09)	0.32 (0.08)	0.62 (0.08)	0.83 (0.10)	1.10 (0.15)	1.75 (0.29)
Total vegetables (c-eq/d)	58	0.23 (0.09)	0.32 (0.07)	0.44 (0.04)	0.47 (0.04)	0.59 (0.06)	0.76 (0.11)
Dark green vegetables (c-eq/wk)	4	0.00 (NA)	0.01 (NA)	0.04 (NA)	0.14 (NA)	0.16 (NA)	0.39 (NA)
Total red and orange vegetables (c-eq/wk)	36	0.19 (0.17)	0.39 (0.20)	0.85 (0.25)	1.57 (0.30)	1.82 (0.38)	3.56 (0.70)
Beans and peas computed as vegetables (c-eq/wk)	6	0.37 (0.15)	0.61 (0.14)	0.99 (0.13)	1.11 (0.14)	1.48 (0.20)	2.01 (0.32)
Total starchy vegetables (c-eq/wk)	21	0.05 (0.17)	0.15 (0.16)	0.37 (0.12)	0.45 (0.12)	0.68 (0.18)	0.99 (0.34)
Other vegetables (c-eq/wk)	28	0.27 (0.15)	0.42 (0.14)	0.65 (0.14)	0.78 (0.15)	1.00 (0.21)	1.44 (0.36)
Total grains (oz-eq/d)	79	1.85 (0.39)	2.45 (0.25)	3.23 (0.17)	3.36 (0.18)	4.13 (0.33)	5.03 (0.55)
Whole grains (oz-eq/d)	36	0.09 (0.09)	0.19 (0.11)	0.41 (0.15)	0.83 (0.20)	0.92 (0.24)	1.88 (0.47)
Refined grains (oz-eq/d)	78	1.67 (0.39)	2.14 (0.23)	2.74 (0.13)	2.83 (0.14)	3.42 (0.31)	4.10 (0.54)
Total protein foods (oz-eq/d)	73	1.03 (0.26)	1.42 (0.17)	1.94 (0.13)	2.05 (0.13)	2.56 (0.21)	3.21 (0.33)
Meat, poultry, and eggs (not seafood) (oz-eq/wk)	69	4.84 (1.98)	7.59 (1.33)	11.69 (0.83)	12.98 (0.83)	16.94 (1.30)	22.71 (2.27)
Seafood (oz-eq/wk)	0	NA	NA	NA	NA	NA	NA
Nuts, seeds, and soy (oz-eq/wk)	11	0.16 (0.20)	0.36 (0.23)	0.72 (0.27)	0.81 (0.27)	1.19 (0.40)	1.61 (0.55)
Total dairy (c-eq/d)	80	1.42 (0.27)	1.85 (0.18)	2.40 (0.12)	2.48 (0.12)	3.03 (0.19)	3.65 (0.31)
Oils (g-eq/d)	73	4.47 (1.62)	6.01 (1.17)	8.11 (0.68)	8.62 (0.60)	10.67 (0.78)	13.40 (1.53)
Solid fats (g-eq/d)	80	14.82 (2.93)	19.22 (2.02)	25.10 (1.68)	26.37 (1.72)	32.14 (2.66)	39.56 (4.16)
Added sugars (g-eq/d)	80	15.11 (6.64)	22.69 (4.53)	34.12 (2.72)	38.35 (2.69)	49.38 (4.49)	66.99 (8.30)

NOTES: N = 81. See additional notes following Table J-74.

TABLE J-70 Food Group Intake Distributions of Eligible Non-WIC-Participating Children Ages 1 to Less Than 2 Years, NHANES 2011–2012

		Percentiles and Mean (SE)					
Food Group	N	10th	25th	Median	Mean	75th	90th
Total fruit (c-eq/d)	20	0.51 (0.31)	0.74 (0.25)	1.06 (0.18)	1.16 (0.16)	1.48 (0.20)	1.93 (0.35)
Whole fruit (c-eq/d)	15	0.08 (0.19)	0.19 (0.15)	0.42 (0.12)	0.63 (0.11)	0.85 (0.13)	1.45 (0.22)
Fruit juice (c-eq/d)	14	0.08 (0.25)	0.18 (0.25)	0.43 (0.30)	0.87 (0.38)	0.98 (0.49)	2.02 (0.88)
Total vegetables (c-eq/d)	18	0.19 (0.13)	0.32 (0.10)	0.53 (0.09)	0.63 (0.09)	0.83 (0.14)	1.20 (0.27)
Dark green vegetables (c-eq/wk)	0	NA	NA	NA	NA	NA	NA
Total red and orange vegetables (c- eq/wk)	13	1.11 (0.20)	1.11 (0.18)	1.11 (0.17)	1.11 (0.19)	1.11 (0.26)	1.11 (0.48)
Beans and peas computed as vegetables (c-eq/wk)	0	NA	NA	NA	NA	NA	NA
Total starchy vegetables (c-eq/wk)	8	0.40 (0.37)	0.73 (0.39)	1.31 (0.39)	1.58 (0.40)	2.14 (0.54)	3.14 (0.88)
Other vegetables (c-eq/wk)	5	0.15 (NA)	0.48 (NA)	1.14 (NA)	1.22 (NA)	1.91 (NA)	2.42 (NA)
Total grains (oz-eq/d)	24	1.83 (0.37)	2.40 (0.35)	3.12 (0.34)	3.24 (0.33)	3.95 (0.37)	4.79 (0.45)
Whole grains (oz-eq/d)	12	0.10 (0.05)	0.19 (0.07)	0.36 (0.10)	0.50 (0.14)	0.64 (0.18)	1.07 (0.33)
Refined grains (oz-eq/d)	24	1.74 (0.31)	2.18 (0.30)	2.75 (0.30)	2.83 (0.29)	3.39 (0.33)	4.04 (0.41)
Total protein foods (oz-eq/d)	22	1.34 (0.30)	1.80 (0.28)	2.43 (0.37)	2.56 (0.39)	3.17 (0.55)	3.95 (0.76)
Meat, poultry, and eggs (not seafood) (oz-eq/wk)	21	7.58 (2.10)	10.45 (1.95)	14.43 (2.44)	15.45 (2.59)	19.34 (3.62)	24.62 (5.14)
Seafood (oz-eq/wk)	2	0.00 (NA)	0.00 (NA)	0.00 (NA)	0.81 (NA)	0.16 (NA)	2.76 (NA)
Nuts, seeds, and soy (oz-eq/wk)	5	0.10 (NA)	0.18 (NA)	0.33 (NA)	0.41 (NA)	0.55 (NA)	0.83 (NA)
Total dairy (c-eq/d)	25	1.11 (0.18)	1.48 (0.16)	1.98 (0.15)	2.09 (0.15)	2.58 (0.18)	3.22 (0.23)
Oils (g-eq/d)	25	6.49 (2.00)	7.85 (1.56)	9.60 (1.10)	9.89 (1.02)	11.60 (1.15)	13.65 (1.91)
Solid fats (g-eq/d)	25	12.52 (2.50)	17.12 (2.34)	22.92 (2.38)	23.65 (2.39)	29.38 (2.84)	35.72 (3.61)
Added sugars (g-eq/d)	25	21.53 (8.19)	26.77 (6.09)	33.62 (3.86)	34.94 (3.71)	41.67 (5.19)	50.04 (9.94)

NOTES: N = 25. See additional notes following Table J-74.

TABLE J-71 Food Group Intake Distributions of WIC-Participating Children Ages 2 to Less Than 5 Years, NHANES 2005–2008

		Percentiles and Mean (SE)		
Food Group	N	10th	25th	Median
Total fruit (c-eq/d)	335	0.48 (0.09)	0.81 (0.07)	1.35 (0.05)
Fruit juice (c-eq/d)	259	0.16 (0.07)	0.33 (0.06)	0.67 (0.05)
Whole fruit (c-eq/d)	209	0.12 (0.06)	0.26 (0.06)	0.56 (0.05)
Total vegetables (c-eq/d)	347	0.28 (0.05)	0.43 (0.04)	0.64 (0.02)
Dark green vegetables (c-eq/wk)	12	0.02 (0.02)	0.05 (0.03)	0.12 (0.03)
Total red and orange vegetables (c-eq/wk)	218	0.40 (0.14)	0.69 (0.12)	1.24 (0.10)
Beans and peas computed as vegetables (c-eq/wk)	26	0.05 (0.03)	0.13 (0.05)	0.33 (0.05)
Total starchy vegetables (c-eq/wk)	149	0.70 (0.27)	1.28 (0.30)	2.46 (0.33)
Other vegetables (c-eq/wk)	191	0.30 (0.09)	0.59 (0.11)	1.21 (0.13)
Total grains (oz-eq/d)	398	2.52 (0.21)	3.25 (0.15)	4.18 (0.10)
Whole grains (oz-eq/d)	160	0.16 (0.02)	0.25 (0.02)	0.38 (0.02)
Refined grains (oz-eq/d)	393	2.20 (0.24)	2.89 (0.16)	3.77 (0.10)
Total protein foods (oz-eq/d)	378	1.69 (0.20)	2.23 (0.13)	2.93 (0.08)
Meat, poultry, and eggs (not seafood) (oz-eq/wk)	365	10.22 (1.02)	13.56 (0.68)	17.95 (0.51)
Seafood (oz-eq/wk)	6	0.14 (0.18)	0.33 (0.19)	0.68 (0.15)
Nuts, seeds, and soy (oz-eq/wk)	59	0.18 (0.08)	0.43 (0.12)	1.05 (0.22)
Total dairy (c-eq/d)	394	1.09 (0.13)	1.49 (0.08)	2.00 (0.06)
Oils (g-eq/d)	382	5.44 (0.73)	7.88 (0.53)	11.37 (0.41)
Solid fats (g-eq/d)	401	18.38 (0.98)	22.61 (0.73)	27.90 (0.68)
Added sugars (g-eq/d)	398	28.76 (3.03)	39.95 (2.31)	55.35 (1.83)

NOTES: N = 402. The reference food intake pattern used was 1,300 kcals. See additional notes following Table J-74.

Mean	75th	90th	Recommended Intake	% Below Recommended Intake (SE)
1.57 (0.05)	2.09 (0.07)	2.94 (0.13)	1.25	45.45 (4.92)
0.94 (0.05)	1.25 (0.07)	2.05 (0.15)	0.625	47.34 (6.36)
0.88 (0.05)	1.12 (0.07)	1.98 (0.14)	0.625	54.17 (5.75)
0.71 (0.03)	0.91 (0.04)	1.22 (0.08)	1.5	95.93 (0.99)
0.19 (0.03)	0.25 (0.04)	0.45 (0.09)	1	98.63 (1.20)
1.63 (0.10)	2.12 (0.13)	3.33 (0.24)	3	87.23 (2.60)
0.50 (0.04)	0.68 (0.06)	1.18 (0.13)	0.5	64.54 (3.55)
3.79 (0.43)	4.67 (0.53)	8.21 (1.18)	3.5	64.40 (5.28)
1.90 (0.16)	2.37 (0.20)	4.21 (0.41)	2.5	76.77 (2.98)
4.32 (0.10)	5.24 (0.15)	6.30 (0.25)	4.5	58.41 (5.16)
0.43 (0.03)	0.55 (0.04)	0.75 (0.06)	2.25	99.99 (0.01)
3.91 (0.10)	4.78 (0.16)	5.80 (0.28)	2.25	10.81 (2.09)
3.05 (0.08)	3.75 (0.14)	4.57 (0.26)	3.5	68.46 (7.15)
18.76 (0.55)	23.08 (0.98)	28.33 (1.70)	16.5	41.65 (4.60)
0.90 (0.09)	1.24 (0.16)	1.97 (0.45)	5	99.79 (0.68)
1.81 (0.29)	2.28 (0.40)	4.26 (0.74)	2.5	77.57 (4.98)
2.10 (0.06)	2.61 (0.10)	3.24 (0.17)	2.5	71.09 (7.80)
12.41 (0.46)	15.80 (0.76)	20.67 (1.35)	17	79.81 (5.10)
				% Above Recommended Intake (SE)
28.61 (0.72)	33.84 (1.06)	39.75 (1.63)	<14.4	97.36 (0.43)
59.10 (1.87)	74.14 (2.76)	94.15 (4.62)	<32.5	85.62 (2.29)

TABLE J-72 Food Group Intake Distributions of Eligible Non-WIC-Participating Children Ages 2 to Less Than 5 Years, NHANES 2005–2008

		Percentiles and Mean (SE)		
Food Group	N	10th	25th	Median
Total fruit (c-eq/d)	250	0.39 (0.06)	0.67 (0.06)	1.12 (0.06)
Fruit juice (c-eq/d)	166	0.13 (0.03)	0.26 (0.04)	0.53 (0.05)
Whole fruit (c-eq/d)	176	0.13 (0.06)	0.27 (0.06)	0.58 (0.06)
Total vegetables (c-eq/d)	291	0.32 (0.06)	0.45 (0.04)	0.64 (0.03)
Dark green vegetables (c-eq/wk)	6	0.01 (0.04)	0.04 (0.04)	0.11 (0.05)
Total red and orange vegetables (c-eq/wk)	202	0.58 (0.08)	0.91 (0.08)	1.44 (0.08)
Beans and peas computed as vegetables (c-eq/wk)	13	0.84 (0.13)	1.28 (0.11)	1.90 (0.13)
Total starchy vegetables (c-eq/wk)	122	0.22 (0.06)	0.47 (0.10)	1.08 (0.17)
Other vegetables (c-eq/wk)	150	0.04 (0.05)	0.10 (0.06)	0.24 (0.05)
Total grains (oz-eq/d)	324	2.74 (0.18)	3.53 (0.13)	4.53 (0.10)
Whole grains (oz-eq/d)	133	0.12 (0.04)	0.23 (0.05)	0.48 (0.07)
Refined grains (oz-eq/d)	322	2.47 (0.16)	3.18 (0.12)	4.08 (0.09)
Total protein foods (oz-eq/d)	315	1.84 (0.19)	2.32 (0.12)	2.92 (0.08)
Meat, poultry, and eggs (not seafood) (oz-eq/wk)	306	10.36 (0.91)	13.43 (0.68)	17.41 (0.56)
Seafood (oz-eq/wk)	8	0.00 (0.05)	0.05 (0.11)	0.35 (0.18)
Nuts, seeds, and soy (oz-eq/wk)	50	0.57 (0.21)	0.93 (0.24)	1.58 (0.27)
Total dairy (c-eq/d)	323	1.01 (0.09)	1.41 (0.07)	1.95 (0.05)
Oils (g-eq/d)	312	7.29 (0.95)	9.28 (0.65)	11.88 (0.42)
Solid fats (g-eq/d)	327	18.17 (1.15)	22.95 (0.96)	28.90 (0.83)
Added sugars (g-eq/d)	328	34.44 (3.57)	46.32 (2.69)	62.40 (2.10)

NOTES: N = 329. The reference food intake pattern used was 1,300 kcals. See additional notes following Table J-74.

Mean	75th	90th	Recommended Intake	% Below Recommended Intake (SE)
1.32 (0.06)	1.75 (0.08)	2.50 (0.14)	1.25	56.37 (3.62)
0.81 (0.08)	1.03 (0.10)	1.79 (0.19)	0.625	56.53 (4.63)
0.91 (0.06)	1.16 (0.08)	2.08 (0.16)	0.625	52.99 (5.60)
0.69 (0.03)	0.87 (0.04)	1.12 (0.08)	1.5	98.11 (7.02)
0.21 (0.04)	0.27 (0.05)	0.52 (0.14)	1	97.54 (2.08)
1.71 (0.09)	2.21 (0.13)	3.15 (0.23)	3	88.37 (2.54)
2.07 (0.14)	2.67 (0.20)	3.50 (0.33)	0.5	90.02 (3.62)
2.06 (0.30)	2.40 (0.34)	4.77 (0.73)	3.5	76.12 (4.19)
0.31 (0.04)	0.45 (0.07)	0.70 (0.16)	2.5	78.91 (6.17)
4.67 (0.10)	5.66 (0.14)	6.79 (0.23)	4.5	49.35 (4.04)
0.79 (0.08)	0.97 (0.10)	1.77 (0.17)	2.25	93.66 (1.37)
4.22 (0.10)	5.11 (0.14)	6.14 (0.22)	2.25	6.79 (1.01)
3.00 (0.08)	3.60 (0.14)	4.27 (0.24)	3.5	71.93 (7.22)
18.08 (0.56)	21.99 (0.82)	26.65 (1.31)	16.5	44.22 (5.09)
0.94 (0.16)	1.28 (0.21)	2.80 (0.69)	5	97.80 (2.27)
2.03 (0.31)	2.60 (0.40)	4.01 (0.79)	2.5	73.21 (6.47)
2.05 (0.05)	2.57 (0.07)	3.21 (0.11)	2.5	72.74 (3.23)
12.36 (0.42)	14.91 (0.67)	18.03 (1.17)	17	86.21 (7.40)
				% Above Recommended Intake (SE)
29.63 (0.81)	35.51 (0.91)	42.02 (1.22)	<14.4	96.56 (0.61)
66.04 (2.09)	81.77 (2.89)	102.24 (4.65)	<32.5	91.83 (0.65)

TABLE J-73 Food Group Intake Distributions of WIC-Participating Children Ages 2 to Less Than 5 Years, NHANES 2011–2012

		Percentiles and Mean (SE)		
Food Group	N	10th	25th	Median
Total fruit (c-eq/d)	209	0.69 (0.10)	0.97 (0.08)	1.37 (0.06)
Whole fruit (c-eq/d)	137	0.29 (0.06)	0.45 (0.06)	0.71 (0.06)
Fruit juice (c-eq/d)	166	0.22 (0.10)	0.36 (0.07)	0.59 (0.04)
Total vegetables (c-eq/d)	194	0.31 (0.04)	0.43 (0.03)	0.61 (0.03)
Dark green vegetables (c-eq/wk)	5	0.00 (NA)	0.03 (NA)	0.13 (NA)
Total red and orange vegetables (c-eq/wk)	130	0.34 (0.08)	0.60 (0.09)	1.08 (0.10)
Beans and peas computed as vegetables (c-eq/wk)	27	0.01 (0.01)	0.06 (0.04)	0.33 (0.07)
Total starchy vegetables (c-eq/wk)	80	1.11 (0.13)	1.61 (0.15)	2.42 (0.20)
Other vegetables (c-eq/wk)	94	0.35 (0.09)	0.67 (0.14)	1.34 (0.24)
Total grains (oz-eq/d)	226	3.12 (0.28)	3.81 (0.19)	4.67 (0.14)
Whole grains (oz-eq/d)	115	0.15 (0.09)	0.29 (0.08)	0.58 (0.07)
Refined grains (oz-eq/d)	224	2.47 (0.34)	3.11 (0.23)	3.92 (0.12)
Total protein foods (oz-eq/d)	218	1.65 (0.27)	2.20 (0.18)	2.93 (0.12)
Meat, poultry, and eggs (not seafood) (oz-eq/wk)	212	8.63 (1.63)	12.38 (1.13)	17.52 (0.74)
Seafood (oz-eq/wk)	5	0.08 (0.19)	0.26 (0.23)	0.70 (0.26)
Nuts, seeds, and soy (oz-eq/wk)	32	0.36 (0.17)	0.74 (0.21)	1.40 (0.27)
Total dairy (c-eq/d)	221	1.00 (0.10)	1.40 (0.08)	1.94 (0.07)
Oils (g-eq/d)	221	8.98 (1.20)	11.16 (0.85)	13.97 (0.59)
Solid fats (g-eq/d)	227	15.15 (1.66)	19.29 (1.19)	24.67 (0.87)
Added sugars (g-eq/d)	226	25.64 (2.58)	35.44 (2.15)	48.58 (1.82)

NOTES: N = 228. The reference food intake pattern used was 1,300 kcals. See additional notes following Table J-74.

Mean	75th	90th	Recommended Intake	% Below Recommended Intake (SE)
1.47 (0.06)	1.85 (0.08)	2.37 (0.13)	1.25	42.58 (7.20)
0.83 (0.06)	1.07 (0.07)	1.52 (0.13)	0.625	42.49 (5.84)
0.71 (0.04)	0.93 (0.07)	1.33 (0.13)	0.625	52.95 (10.78)
0.65 (0.03)	0.82 (0.05)	1.06 (0.09)	1.50	98.67 (1.13)
0.28 (NA)	0.38 (NA)	0.76 (NA)	1.00	94.28 (NA)
1.43 (0.11)	1.86 (0.14)	2.94 (0.26)	3.00	90.49 (2.19)
0.62 (0.07)	0.93 (0.14)	1.68 (0.27)	0.50	58.82 (3.47)
2.88 (0.35)	3.62 (0.40)	5.18 (0.94)	3.50	73.14 (4.39)
2.13 (0.41)	2.62 (0.49)	4.70 (1.00)	2.50	73.40 (7.45)
4.76 (0.15)	5.61 (0.23)	6.52 (0.37)	4.50	44.99 (7.13)
0.86 (0.07)	1.10 (0.10)	1.87 (0.18)	2.25	93.34 (1.68)
4.03 (0.11)	4.82 (0.18)	5.72 (0.35)	2.25	6.55 (12.84)
3.06 (0.12)	3.77 (0.19)	4.63 (0.33)	3.50	67.99 (8.01)
18.69 (0.73)	23.72 (1.15)	30.21 (2.00)	16.50	45.08 (1.70)
1.01 (0.20)	1.44 (0.29)	2.37 (0.65)	5.00	99.52 (7.61)
1.73 (0.27)	2.38 (0.41)	3.54 (0.59)	2.50	77.28 (5.02)
2.04 (0.07)	2.57 (0.10)	3.21 (0.16)	2.50	72.82 (8.39)
14.44 (0.58)	17.20 (0.84)	20.50 (1.42)	17.00	73.74 (8.39)
				% Above recommended intake
25.62 (0.88)	30.90 (1.30)	37.29 (2.16)	<14.4	91.96 (1.85)
51.24 (1.77)	64.12 (2.05)	80.21 (2.88)	<32.5	80.09 (3.04)

TABLE J-74 Food Group Intake Distributions of Eligible Non-WIC-Participating Children Ages 2 to Less Than 5 Years, NHANES 2011–2012

		Percentiles and Mean (SE)		
Food Group	N	10th	25th	Median
Total fruit (c-eq/d)	125	0.39 (0.11)	0.68 (0.10)	1.13 (0.09)
Whole fruit (c-eq/d)	89	0.14 (0.09)	0.28 (0.09)	0.55 (0.08)
Fruit juice (c-eq/d)	88	0.07 (0.05)	0.16 (0.08)	0.38 (0.10)
Total vegetables (c-eq/d)	125	0.36 (0.04)	0.48 (0.04)	0.65 (0.04)
Dark green vegetables (c-eq/wk)	5	0.38 (NA)	0.62 (NA)	1.04 (NA)
Total red and orange vegetables (c-eq/wk)	80	0.34 (0.06)	0.58 (0.07)	1.00 (0.10)
Beans and peas computed as vegetables (c-eq/wk)	10	0.04 (0.08)	0.11 (0.09)	0.24 (0.08)
Total starchy vegetables (c-eq/wk)	57	1.00 (0.27)	1.44 (0.24)	2.07 (0.28)
Other vegetables (c-eq/wk)	67	0.97 (0.13)	1.43 (0.20)	2.16 (0.32)
Total grains (oz-eq/d)	148	3.25 (0.19)	3.90 (0.17)	4.73 (0.18)
Whole grains (oz-eq/d)	76	0.13 (0.04)	0.25 (0.05)	0.51 (0.07)
Refined grains (oz-eq/d)	147	2.66 (0.18)	3.30 (0.18)	4.12 (0.18)
Total protein foods (oz-eq/d)	144	1.68 (0.15)	2.27 (0.14)	3.03 (0.15)
Meat, poultry, and eggs (not seafood) (oz-eq/wk)	140	8.00 (0.86)	12.00 (0.85)	17.65 (0.98)
Seafood (oz-eq/wk)	5	0.00 (NA)	0.00 (NA)	0.02 (NA)
Nuts, seeds, and soy (oz-eq/wk)	29	0.73 (0.30)	1.35 (0.34)	2.41 (0.49)
Total dairy (c-eq/d)	145	1.07 (0.11)	1.48 (0.10)	2.03 (0.11)
Oils (g-eq/d)	145	7.61 (0.86)	10.51 (0.78)	14.49 (0.82)
Solid fats (g-eq/d)	147	17.90 (1.56)	22.30 (1.37)	27.91 (1.25)
Added sugars (g-eq/d)	146	32.37 (4.23)	44.06 (3.37)	60.21 (3.33)

NOTES: N = 148. The reference food intake pattern used was 1,300 kcals. See additional notes following this table.
NOTES for Tables J-62 through J-74: c-eq = cup-equivalents; d = day; g-eq = gram-equivalents; N = sample size; NA = data not available; oz-eq = ounce-equivalents; SE = standard error; wk = week. NA = estimate could not be obtained because the Statistical Program for Age-adjusted Dietary Assessment (SPADE) requires more than two observations per group with two non-zero intakes in order to estimate a within-person variance, or, for median standard errors, a sample size of 30 is required to estimate this value from mean standard error.
SOURCES: Intake data are from NHANES 2005–2012 (USDA/ARS, 2005–2012). Reference values are the USDA food patterns from the *Dietary Guidelines for Americans* 2015–2020 (USDA/HHS, 2016).

Mean	75th	90th	Recommended Intake	% Below Recommended Intake (SE)
1.32 (0.09)	1.76 (0.12)	2.47 (0.20)	1.25	55.66 (5.88)
0.75 (0.07)	0.99 (0.13)	1.61 (0.19)	0.625	55.73 (9.23)
0.65 (0.10)	0.83 (0.08)	1.54 (0.16)	0.625	66.24 (8.00)
0.68 (0.04)	0.85 (0.06)	1.06 (0.09)	1.50	99.10 (1.03)
1.32 (NA)	1.70 (NA)	2.59 (NA)	1.00	93.29 (NA)
1.30 (0.15)	1.68 (0.20)	2.61 (0.40)	3.00	93.06 (3.08)
0.30 (0.06)	0.42 (0.08)	0.64 (0.20)	0.50	81.33 (8.42)
2.24 (0.31)	2.86 (0.45)	3.71 (0.69)	3.50	87.20 (7.81)
2.55 (0.48)	3.22 (0.58)	4.58 (1.12)	2.50	59.68 (6.89)
4.88 (0.19)	5.70 (0.25)	6.70 (0.37)	4.50	42.90 (4.83)
0.78 (0.09)	0.99 (0.11)	1.74 (0.21)	2.25	94.18 (1.71)
4.26 (0.18)	5.07 (0.22)	6.05 (0.30)	2.25	4.24 (2.07)
3.15 (0.16)	3.90 (0.21)	4.79 (0.29)	3.50	64.63 (5.02)
19.12 (1.05)	24.64 (1.43)	32.09 (2.11)	16.50	45.00 (4.60)
0.67 (NA)	0.38 (NA)	1.97 (NA)	5.00	96.66 (NA)
2.94 (0.51)	3.94 (0.78)	5.82 (1.15)	2.50	51.98 (12.57)
2.13 (0.11)	2.66 (0.14)	3.31 (0.19)	2.50	69.49 (5.81)
15.42 (0.87)	19.30 (1.20)	24.38 (1.84)	17.00	64.33 (5.07)
				% Above Recommended Intake (SE)
28.80 (1.23)	34.33 (1.45)	40.82 (2.00)	<14.4	96.68 (1.50)
64.32 (3.52)	80.10 (5.02)	101.53 (7.66)	<32.5	89.86 (1.01)

DIET QUALITY OF WIC SUBGROUPS

The committee was tasked with evaluating the diet quality of WIC-eligible subpopulations using the Healthy Eating Index–2010 (HEI–2010) and one additional index of the committee's choosing. This appendix describes the methods applied in these analyses.

The Healthy Eating Index–2010

Because it is based on the DGA food patterns, which apply only to individuals ages 2 and older, the HEI–2010 was likewise applied only to individuals ages 2 year and older (Guenther et al., 2013). The HEI–2010 was designed to measure compliance with the key recommendations in the 2010 *Dietary Guidelines for Americans* (DGA). The HEI–2010 has not yet been updated to reflect the 2015–2020 DGA. The HEI–2010 covers 12 components as shown in Table J-75. Adequate consumption of all components except refined grains, sodium, and empty calories raises scores. Over-consumption of these three components lowers scores. A perfect overall score for the HEI–2010 is 100. Subscores for the components can be up to 20, with the ranges for each individual component being 0 to 5, 0 to 10, or 0 to 20. The HEI–2010 is the only metric in this report that applies the 2010 DGA as a point of comparison. Only data from the first 24-hour recall was used to calculate HEI–2010.[6]

Nutrient-Based Diet Quality Index

As described in the phase I report (NASEM, 2016), options for a second index were considered by the committee based on its evaluation of the literature on existing diet quality indexes other than the HEI–2010 and with consideration to three criteria: (1) the index can be applied to adults and children, (2) 24-hour recall data are applied, and (3) the index is based on a metric other than comparison to the DGA. After reviewing potential indexes, the committee determined that responding to the task

[6] The committee computed the distribution of HEI–2010 scores using the HEI–2010 Statistical Analysis System (SAS) macros that were posted by the National Cancer Institute (NCI, 2016). At the time these analyses were conducted, NCI had not yet updated the code to compute the HEI–2010; therefore, in cooperation with researchers at NCI, the macros were modified as appropriate. The updated macros now available through NCI are essentially identical to those used for the analyses in this report. The HEI–2010 SAS macros were used to implement the ratio method (Freedman et al., 2008), and provide a mean score with its standard error (SE) for each of the 12 HEI–2010 components as well as for the total score. The SE is computed using a Monte Carlo approach that permits accounting for the complex survey design of NHANES. For the time being, the NCI macros use only the first 24-hour recall for each person.

TABLE J-75 HEI–2010 Components and Scoring System

HEI–2010 Component[a]	Maximum	Standard for Maximum Score	Standard for Minimum Score of Zero
	Adequacy		
Total fruit[b]	5	≥0.8 c-eq / 1,000 kcal	No fruit
Whole fruit[c]	5	≥0.4 c-eq / 1,000 kcal	No whole fruit
Total vegetables[d]	5	≥1.1 c-eq / 1,000 kcal	No vegetables
Greens and beans[d]	5	≥0.2 c-eq / 1,000 kcal	No dark-green vegetables, beans, or peas
Whole grains	10	≥1.5 c-eq / 1,000 kcal	No whole grains
Dairy[e]	10	≥1.3 c-eq / 1,000 kcal	No dairy
Total protein foods[f]	5	≥2.5 c-eq / 1,000 kcal	No protein foods
Seafood and plant proteins[f,g]	5	≥0.8 c-eq / 1,000 kcal	No seafood or plant proteins
Fatty acids[h]	10	(PUFAs + MUFAs) / SFAs ≥2.5	(PUFAs + MUFAs) / SFAs ≤1.2
	Moderation		
Refined grains	10	≤1.8 oz-eq / 1,000 kcal	≥4.3 oz-eq / 1,000 kcal
Sodium	10	≤1.1 g / 1,000 kcal	≥2.0 g / 1,000 kcal
Empty calories[i]	20	≤19% of energy	≥50% of energy

NOTES: c-eq = cup-equivalent; kcal = kilocalorie; oz-eq = ounce-equivalent; MUFAs = monounsaturated fatty acids; PUFAs = polyunsaturated fatty acids; SFAs = saturated fatty acids.

[a] Intakes between the minimum and maximum standards are scored proportionately.

[b] Includes 100 percent fruit juice.

[c] Includes all forms except juice.

[d] Includes any beans and peas not counted as total protein foods.

[e] Includes all milk products such as fluid milk, yogurt, and cheese, and fortified soy beverages.

[f] Beans and peas are included here (not with vegetables) when the total protein foods standard is otherwise not met.

[g] Includes seafood, nuts, seeds, soy products (other than beverages) as well as beans and peas counted as Total Protein Foods.

[h] Ratio of poly- and monounsaturated fatty acids (PUFAs and MUFAs) to saturated fatty acids (SFAs).

[i] Calories from solid fats, alcohol, and added sugars; threshold for counting alcohol is >13 g / 1,000 kcal.

SOURCE: Guenther et al., 2013.

TABLE J-76 Summary of Mean HEI–2010 Scores for Women Ages 19 to 50 Years, NHANES 2005–2012

HEI–2010 Component	Maximum Score	Pregnant WIC (N = 169)	Pregnant Non-WIC (N = 90)	Any Breastfeeding WIC (N = 54)	Postpartum WIC (N = 62)	Nonpregnant, Breastfeeding, or Postpartum, Non-WIC (N = 2,666)
		Mean Score (SE)				
Adequacy						
Total vegetables	5	2.66 (0.32)	3.20 (0.37)	3.16 (0.40)	2.50 (0.34)	3.13 (0.06)
Greens and beans	5	2.11 (0.88)	2.12 (1.04)	2.62 (1.12)	2.14 (1.04)	2.61 (0.14)
Total fruit	5	4.50 (0.37)	3.81 (0.51)	4.62 (0.52)	3.90 (1.23)	2.50 (0.10)
Whole fruit	5	3.84 (0.41)	3.71 (0.69)	4.95 (0.23)	2.19 (0.50)	2.78 (0.12)
Whole grains	10	2.08 (0.29)	1.46 (0.38)	2.80 (0.82)	2.31 (0.63)	1.83 (0.09)
Dairy	10	7.30 (0.50)	6.52 (0.62)	7.87 (0.89)	5.54 (0.79)	5.68 (0.11)
Total protein foods	5	4.87 (0.19)	4.85 (0.23)	4.96 (0.12)	4.97 (0.09)	5.0 (0.0)
Seafood and plant proteins	5	3.63 (0.64)	3.71 (0.77)	2.84 (0.84)	2.37 (0.88)	3.08 (0.13)
Fatty acids	10	3.57 (0.54)	3.99 (0.60)	2.86 (0.62)	4.79 (0.67)	4.32 (0.14)
Moderation						
Sodium	10	5.76 (0.71)	5.22 (0.59)	5.40 (0.56)	5.23 (0.74)	4.61 (0.11)
Refined grains	10	5.78 (0.49)	4.48 (0.60)	5.79 (1.03)	5.63 (0.88)	5.86 (0.14)
Empty calories	20	10.94 (1.01)	11.48 (0.72)	12.73 (1.36)	10.26 (1.48)	10.74 (0.26)
Total HEI–2010 Score	100	57.04 (2.35)	54.55 (2.84)	60.60 (3.30)	51.83 (3.26)	52.13 (0.60)

NOTES: HEI–2010 = Healthy Eating Index–2010; N = sample size; SE = standard error. Sample sizes may differ from other analyses because the methodology uses reported intake on day 1 only.

TABLE J-77 Summary of Mean HEI–2010 Scores for Children Ages 2 to Less Than 5 Years, NHANES 2011–2012

HEI–2010 Component	Maximum Score	WIC, 2005–2008 (N = 477)	Eligible Non-WIC, 2005–2008 (N = 448)	WIC, 2011–2012 (N = 263)	Eligible Non-WIC, 2011–2012 (N = 216)
		Mean Score (SE)			
Adequacy					
Total vegetables	5	2.2 (0.10)	2.1 (0.10)	2.1 (0.18)	1.8 (0.13)
Greens and beans	5	0.3 (0.12)	0.7 (0.18)	1.1 (0.76)	0.5 (0.21)
Total fruit	5	5.0 (0.00)	5.0 (0.08)	5.0 (0.05)	5.0 (0.12)
Whole fruit	5	5.0 (0.07)	5.0 (0.03)	5.0 (0.08)	4.9 (0.20)
Whole grains	10	1.8 (0.15)	2.2 (0.29)	3.1 (0.35)	2.5 (0.33)
Dairy	10	10.0 (0.01)	9.9 (0.15)	10.0 (0.09)	9.9 (0.33)
Total protein foods	5	4.1 (0.13)	4.3 (0.15)	4.4 (0.21)	3.9 (0.40)
Seafood and plant proteins	5	2.2 (0.22)	2.7 (0.37)	3.0 (0.43)	2.2 (0.63)
Fatty acids	10	2.1 (0.22)	2.2 (0.23)	3.6 (0.50)	2.8 (0.63)
Moderation					
Sodium	10	6.7 (0.25)	5.9 (0.25)	6.1 (0.24)	6.7 (0.42)
Refined grains	10	7.4 (0.31)	6.6 (0.26)	6.8 (0.45)	6.7 (0.39)
Empty calories	20	13.2 (0.34)	12.0 (0.41)	14.7 (0.64)	12.8 (0.68)
Total HEI–2010 Score	100	59.8 (0.66)	58.7 (1.08)	65.0 (0.86)	59.6 (1.61)

NOTES: HEI–2010 = Healthy Eating Index–2010; N = sample size; SE = standard error. Sample sizes may differ from other analyses because the methodology uses reported intake on day 1 only.

would require an index that focuses mainly on nutrient content to provide a contrast to the food-group focus of the HEI–2010. However, the committee found that existing nutrient-based indexes could not be applied directly for two reasons. First, they could not be applied because they use daily values based on a 2,000-calorie diet as reference standards for nutrient intake rather than age-appropriate DRI values. Second, they do not necessarily include all of the nutrients and dietary components the committee was interested in assessing, based on current knowledge about nutrients of concern in the diets of young children and women of childbearing age (noted in the DGA) and the committee's assessment of the nutrient intakes of WIC-eligible populations. The committee developed an adapted nutrient-based diet quality (NBDQ) index based on the mean probability of adequacy for the nine shortfall nutrients, calculated for each individual (see Box 3-2).[7]

The index examined the following "positive" nutrients included in the DGA as shortfall nutrients and nutrients of concern:

- Potassium
- Dietary fiber
- Calcium
- Iron
- Vitamin C
- Folate
- Vitamin A
- Vitamin E
- Magnesium

The index is the mean percentage adequacy for these nine nutrients, calculated for each individual. Thus, the NBDQ can take on values between 0 and 100 for a person.

- For nutrients with an EAR: the *percentage adequacy* was calculated for each individual for each day. To do this, the method described in IOM (2000b) was applied using the DRI for assessment of intake of individuals and groups and z-scores were computed for each respondent as follows:
    a. Usual intake at the individual level was first estimated as the best linear unbiased predictor (BLUP) of intake. The BLUP has the smallest prediction error variance among all linear predictors.

[7] There are ample precedents for the use of a composite nutrient adequacy index. Mean adequacy ratios have been used for many years and have more recently been updated to reflect the DRIs. The NDBQ is essentially the same as the indexes used in several published studies (Foote et al., 2004; Murphy et al., 2006).

b. The difference between the individual's estimated usual intake of the nutrient and the EAR for the nutrient was then computed.
c. A z-score was computed as the ratio of the difference to the standard error of that difference.
d. Finally, the probability of observing a z-value that was at least as large as the one we observed for the individual was computed and multiplied by 100. These calculations were repeated for all the nutrients included in the index. The possible range is from 0 to 100.

- For the nutrients with an AI value (potassium and dietary fiber), reasonable intake ranges based on the AI were applied, to assign 0, 25, 50 and 100 percentage adequacy as follows:
  a. Intake equal to or above the AI, percentage adequacy = 100
  b. Intake below the AI but equal to or above 75 of the AI, percentage adequacy = 75
  c. Intake below 75 percentage of the AI but equal to or above 50 percent of the AI, percentage adequacy = 50
  d. Intake below 50 percent of the AI but equal to or above 25 percent of the AI, percentage adequacy = 25
  e. Intake below 25 percent of the AI, percentage adequacy = 0
- The mean percentage adequacy for each individual was calculated by averaging the nutrient-wise percentage adequacy.
- The mean percentage adequacy for population subgroups was then calculated using individual survey weights.

  Initial descriptive statistics were generated to validate the index:
  a. As a first step, the mean and standard deviation of the index were evaluated.
  b. Second, the association of the index with energy intake was examined.

This approach is very similar to that published by Verger et al. (2012), except that the NBDQ includes only shortfall nutrients as defined by the 2015 DGA. When tracked with energy intake, the association between the NBDQ index and energy intake was not strong, which suggests that the index is a summary measure that predicts dietary quality beyond simply being a measure of overall energy intakes. NBDQ was applied to all subpopulations excluding infants.

Additional Adjustments for Within-Person Variance

One challenge with calculating the NBDQ is that within-person variance in intake must be estimated for each person although it is known that this within-person variance may not be constant across population subgroups or even across individuals within population subgroups. Given only 1 or 2 days of intake information for each person, it is not possible to estimate within-person variances at the individual level with confidence.

Instead of attempting to compute a within-person variance in intake for each person individually, a hierarchical model was applied to intake data. This allows for estimation of individual and subpopulation-level variances more precisely by using information across individuals and across groups. As a result, an individual's estimated within-person variance in intake is based not only on the individual's 2 days of data but also on the measurements taken on other individuals. The resulting estimate "shrinks" an individual's naïve estimate (based on the person's 2 days) toward the group's mean. In this light, the estimated variances are similar (in terms of methodology) to the estimated usual intakes that are obtained using the ISU (Nusser et al., 1996), the NCI (Dekkers et al., 2014), or other methods.

Once having these estimated within-person variances, the analysis proceeded as described in the 2000 IOM report (2000b) with two minor differences: first, the best linear unbiased predictor was used to estimate the person's usual intake of a nutrient, and second, the statistic was compared to a t-distribution to account for the fact that the within-person variances in intake are estimates.

For results of the NBDQ analysis, see Chapter 4, Tables 4-30 and 4-31.

REFERENCES

Beaton, G. H. 1994. Approaches to analysis of dietary data: Relationship between planned analyses and choice of methodology. *American Journal of Clinical Nutrition* 59(1 Suppl):253s–261s.

Butte, N. F., W. W. Wong, T. A. Wilson, A. L. Adolph, M. R. Puyau, and I. F. Zakeri. 2014. Revision of dietary reference intakes for energy in preschool-age children. *American Journal of Clinical Nutrition* 100(1):161–167.

Carriquiry, A. L. 1999. Assessing the prevalence of nutrient inadequacy. *Public Health Nutrition* 2(1):23–33.

Cashman, K. D. 2012. The role of vitamers and dietary-based metabolites of vitamin D in prevention of vitamin D deficiency. *Food and Nutrition Research* 56.

Cashman, K. D., K. M. Seamans, A. J. Lucey, E. Stocklin, P. Weber, M. Kiely, and T. R. Hill. 2012. Relative effectiveness of oral 25-hydroxyvitamin D3 and vitamin D3 in raising wintertime serum 25-hydroxyvitamin D in older adults. *American Journal of Clinical Nutrition* 95(6):1350–1356.

CDC (Centers for Disease Control and Prevention). 2014. *National Health and Nutrition Examination Survey: Sample design, 2011–2014.* http://www.cdc.gov/nchs/data/series/sr_02/sr02_162.pdf (accessed December 21, 2016).

Dekkers, A. L., J. Verkaik-Kloosterman, C. T. van Rossum, and M. C. Ocke. 2014. SPADE, a new statistical program to estimate habitual dietary intake from multiple food sources and dietary supplements. *Journal of Nutrition* 144(12):2083–2091.

EOPUS (Executive Office of the President of the United States). 2014. The economic impact of the American Recovery and Reinvestment Act five years later: Final report to Congress. https://www.gpo.gov/fdsys/pkg/ERP-2014/pdf/ERP-2014-chapter3.pdf (accessed March 1, 2017).

Foote, J. A., S. P. Murphy, L. R. Wilkens, P. P. Basiotis, and A. Carlson. 2004. Dietary variety increases the probability of nutrient adequacy among adults. *Journal of Nutrition* 134(7):1779–1785.

Freedman, L. S., P. M. Guenther, S. M. Krebs-Smith, P. S. Kott. 2008. A population's mean Healthy Eating Index-2005 scores are best estimated by the score of the population ratio when one 24-hour recall is available. *Journal of Nutrition* 138(9):1725–1729.

Fuller, W. 2009. *Sampling statistics*. Hoboken, NJ: John Wiley & Sons.

Guenther, P. M., K. O. Casavale, J. Reedy, S. I. Kirkpatrick, H. A. Hiza, K. J. Kuczynski, L. L. Kahle, and S. M. Krebs-Smith. 2013. Update of the Healthy Eating Index: HEI-2010. *Journal of the Academy of Nutrition and Dietetics* 113(4):569–580.

HHS (U.S. Department of Health and Human Services). 2015. 2015 Federal poverty guidelines. http://aspe.hhs.gov/2015-poverty-guidelines (accessed December 21, 2016).

IOM (Institute of Medicine). 1997. *Dietary Reference Intakes for calcium, phosphorus, magnesium, vitamin D, and fluoride*. Washington, DC: National Academy Press.

IOM. 1998. *Dietary Reference Intakes for thiamin, riboflavin, niacin, vitamin B6, folate, vitamin B12, pantothenic acid, biotin, and choline*. Washington, DC: National Academy Press.

IOM. 2000a. *Dietary Reference Intakes for vitamin C, vitamin E, selenium, and carotenoids*. Washington, DC: National Academy Press.

IOM. 2000b. *Dietary Reference Intakes: Applications in dietary assessment*. Washington, DC: National Academy Press.

IOM. 2001. *Dietary Reference Intakes for vitamin A, vitamin K, arsenic, boron, chromium, copper, iodine, iron, manganese, molybdenum, nickel, silicon, vanadium, and zinc*. Washington, DC: National Academy Press.

IOM. 2002/2005. *Dietary Reference Intakes for energy, carbohydrate, fiber, fat, fatty acids, cholesterol, protein and amino acids*. Washington, DC: The National Academies Press.

IOM. 2003. *Dietary Reference Intakes: Applications in dietary planning*. Washington, DC: The National Academies Press.

IOM. 2005. *Dietary Reference Intakes for water, potassium, sodium, chloride, and sulfate*. Washington, DC: The National Academies Press.

IOM. 2006. *WIC food packages: Time for a change*. Washington, DC: The National Academies Press.

IOM. 2011a. *Child and Adult Care Food Program: Aligning dietary guidance for all*. Washington, DC: The National Academies Press.

IOM. 2011b. *Dietary Reference Intakes for calcium and vitamin D*. Washington, DC: The National Academies Press.

IOM. 2015. *Review of WIC Food Packages: An evaluation of white potatoes in the cash value voucher: Letter Report*. Washington, DC: The National Academies Press.

Jahns, L., L. Arab, A. Carriquiry, B. M. Popkin. 2005. The use of external within-person variance estimates to adjust nutrient intake distributions over time and across populations. *Public Health Nutrition* 8(1):69–76.

Murphy, S. P., J. A. Foote, L. R. Wilkens, P. P. Basiotis, A. Carlson, K. K. White, and K. M. Yonemori. 2006. Simple measures of dietary variety are associated with improved dietary quality. *Journal of the American Dietetic Association* 106(3):425–429.

NASEM (National Academies of Sciences, Engineering, and Medicine). 2016. *Review of WIC food packages: Proposed framework for revisions: Interim report*. Washington, DC: The National Academies Press. doi: 10.17226/21832.

NCI (National Cancer Institute). 2016. *HEI tools for researchers*. http://epi.grants.cancer.gov/hei/tools.html (accessed October 28, 2016).

Nusser, S. M., A. L. Carriquiry, K. W. Dodd, and W. A. Fuller. 1996. A semiparametric transformation approach to estimating usual daily intake distributions. *Journal of the American Statistical Association* 91(436):1440–1449.

Taylor, C. L., A. L. Carriquiry, R. L. Bailey, C. T. Sempos, and E. A. Yetley. 2013. Appropriateness of the probability approach with a nutrient status biomarker to assess population inadequacy: A study using vitamin D. *American Journal of Clinical Nutrition* 97(1):72–78.

USDA/ARS (U.S. Department of Agriculture/Agricultural Research Service). 2005–2012. *What We Eat in America, NHANES 2005–2012*. Beltsville, MD: USDA/ARS. http://www.cdc.gov/nchs/nhanes/wweia.htm (accessed December 21, 2016).

USDA/ARS. 2014. *Food Patterns Equivalents Database 2011–2012: Methodology and user guide*. Beltsville, MD: USDA/ARS. http://www.ars.usda.gov/SP2UserFiles/Place/80400530/pdf/fped/FPED_1112.pdf (accessed December 21, 2016).

USDA/FNS (U.S. Department of Agriculture/Food and Nutrition Service). 2012. *Special Supplemental Nutrition Program for Women, Infants, and Children (WIC) erroneous payments to vendors: Annual estimates for FY 2011*. Alexandria, VA: USDA/FNS. http://www.fns.usda.gov/sites/default/files/WICErroneousPayment_2011.pdf (accessed December 21, 2016).

USDA/FNS. 2013. *WIC participant and program characteristics 2012: Final report*. Alexandria, VA: USDA/FNS. http://www.fns.usda.gov/sites/default/files/WICPC2012.pdf (accessed December 21, 2016).

USDA/FNS. 2014. *National and state-level estimates of the Special Supplemental Nutrition Program for Women, Infants, and Children (WIC) eligibles and program reach*. 2011, Vol I. Alexandria, VA: USDA/FNS. http://www.fns.usda.gov/sites/default/files/WICEligibles2011Volume1.pdf (accessed December 21, 2016).

USDA/FNS. 2015. WIC income eligibility guidelines. http://www.fns.usda.gov/wic/wic-income-eligibility-guidelines (accessed December 21, 2016).

USDA/HHS (U.S. Department of Agriculture/U.S. Department of Health and Human Services). 2016. *2015–2020 Dietary Guidelines for Americans*. Washington, DC: U.S. Government Printing Office. https://health.gov/dietaryguidelines/2015 (accessed December 21, 2016).

Verger, E. O., F. Mariotti, B. A. Holmes, D. Paineau, and J. F. Huneau. 2012. Evaluation of a diet quality index based on the probability of adequate nutrient intake (PANDIET) using national French and US dietary surveys. *PloS One* 7(8):e42155.

Appendix K

Study Design Strategies for Reducing the Effects of Selection Bias in Studies Comparing WIC Participants to Others

In Chapter 4, the committee reviewed study designs that could to some degree ameliorate the challenges to evaluating the effects of the Special Supplemental Nutrition Program for Women, Infants, and Children (WIC). In particular, specific types of study designs that could address the problem of selection bias, or other biases due to reverse causation or measurement error, were reviewed. In this appendix, the committee defines these types of study designs, and proposes ways that the U.S. Department of Agriculture's Food and Nutrition Service (USDA-FNS) could apply these designs to the evaluation of the WIC program.

REGRESSION DISCONTINUITY

A regression discontinuity (RD) design compares people who are just below an eligibility threshold for a program or treatment with those who are just above it. Because the likelihood of an individual falling just above or below a threshold is not affected by self-selection, this method yields high internal validation,[1] provided that these individuals do not manipulate their presence below or above the threshold (the method typically includes tests for this). The types of thresholds that are relevant to WIC and can potentially be used in RD designs include (1) income eligibility, (2) age after which one can no longer participate in the program, and (3) age at which the value of the program changes (i.e., the value of the food package

[1] Internal validation can be indicative of causality regarding the relationship between WIC participation and measured outcomes.

changes). Versions of this design, which rely on comparing individuals with incomes just below and just above the eligibility threshold for WIC participation, require researchers to use the measure of income that is applied by the program. Similarly, versions of the design which rely on age thresholds require researchers to identify age thresholds relevant to the program (e.g. age 5 when children are no longer eligible for WIC). RD designs yield unbiased estimates of the impact of WIC, provided that the identifying assumptions are satisfied for individuals that are right at the eligibility thresholds.[2] However, RD designs are not necessarily applicable to the WIC participants with the most need, who might have lower income-to-poverty ratios and may be affected differently by WIC.

Potential USDA-FNS Applications for WIC

Research studies could target comparisons at 185 percent of poverty, at age 5 when eligibility ends, and at eligibility/takeup at 1 year when formula is no longer provided. Research examining comparisons at the income threshold would compare WIC participants near but below the top of the income threshold (170–185 percent) with non-WIC participants just above the income threshold (185–200 percent), while controlling for the income-to-poverty ratio.[3] Comparisons of the two age thresholds would involve what is known as a "fuzzy RD." At age 5, when children that meet the income criteria are no longer eligible, they would be compared to themselves at periods before and after program participation, while controlling for age. At age 1, some families may choose not to participate (particularly formula-feeding families) because the value of the package is reduced with the loss of formula. Thus, if one could follow families who use formula throughout the first year and into the second year, comparisons between families who fail to recertify before and after age 1 might be useful. The RD approach could be made more feasible if USDA-FNS encouraged states to make administrative data on health outcomes and precise income-to-poverty and age (in months or exact days) available for large numbers of potential WIC participants (including participants and nonparticipants). Another strategy could be to collect data on all Medicaid participants near

---

[2] Other assumptions for RD are either that the potential outcomes are continuous and have a number of continuous derivatives or that within some window close to the income eligibility threshold, the side of the threshold is randomly assigned. This is easy to test for income (i.e., are there more families with income levels just below the 185 percent of poverty threshold) and less necessary for age (i.e., age is generally well-captured in administrative data).

[3] The income-to-poverty ratio is the ratio of family income to the federal poverty guideline. It is this ratio which must be below 1.85 for families to be eligible for WIC.

these same WIC age and income thresholds as all Medicaid recipients are adjunctively eligible for WIC. These data will provide estimates that have high internal validity for those near the age or income thresholds (and can be indicative of causality) but may not be externally valid for those far from the age or income thresholds.

COMPARISON GROUP

In a comparison group (CG) design, WIC participants are usually compared with income-eligible nonparticipants. In contrast to RD studies, these designs can be applied to groups of the lowest-income WIC participants. However, a major drawback of CG designs is that it is not possible to know if the analysis has accounted for all unobservable differences between the two groups. The analysis can be made more robust by including an additional comparison between the treatment and control groups when program changes are taking place in what is known as a differences-in-differences or interrupted-time-series design (i.e., a series of observations over time interrupted by introduction of an intervention). Thus, studies in which program changes are implemented randomly across locations are best suited for this design.

Potential USDA-FNS Applications for WIC

Application of this approach could be optimized if the timing and scope of rule changes in WIC and other programs affecting WIC use were made available. The period of new food package implementation offers one such opportunity. Larger sample sizes and access to linked WIC administrative data on WIC eligibility and participation would allow for useful outcomes as long as nonparticipants are somehow included. It is also key to have data on individuals who are potentially eligible but not enrolling in the program. This approach relies on assumptions of common trends and the absence of changes in the composition of the comparison and treatment groups after treatment.

INSTRUMENTAL VARIABLES

The instrumental variables (IV) approach considers a population of participants and nonparticipants whose decision to participate was based on a factor that is: strongly correlated with participation, cannot be directly related to the outcome, and only affects the outcome through participation. An example is distance of residence from the WIC clinic (ideally combined with variation in locations of clinics driven by clinics closing and opening). Distance (particularly driven by openings and closings) plausibly affects use of WIC but should not otherwise have direct effects on dietary intake. Although this is a sound method for obtaining causal estimates, it can have low external validity (i.e., results will not be generalizable). Some researchers who have tried to use IV to estimate the impact of WIC have concluded that they were unable to identify an instrument that works well to predict WIC use.

Potential USDA-FNS Applications for WIC

As an example of how IV has been applied to evaluate WIC, Rossin-Slater (2013) used, as the instrument, whether a mother resided close to a WIC clinic at the timing of conception of her oldest child. Controlling for mothers' fixed characteristics, this instrument proved to be a strong predictor of WIC participation in Texas during a period when many clinics were opening or closing. This type of instrument (relying on distance to a location where eligibility for a program is assessed) is common in the evaluation of the effects of other programs. Another IV application would rely on state differences in assessment of eligibility by income (e.g., disregards family units, the way that eligibility is assessed for the other programs such as Temporary Assistance for Needy Families, Supplemental Nutrition Assistance Program [SNAP] and Medicaid, which confer automatic WIC eligibility). For example, Ziliak (2016) demonstrated that states where SNAP uses broad-based categorical eligibility (which raises the gross income threshold for eligibility) have higher SNAP participation. This might permit use of these SNAP rules for IV estimation.

FIXED EFFECTS

The fixed effects (FE) approach uses variation in WIC participation across time, time and place, siblings within a family, or other variables, to estimate effects. This approach has some disadvantages, including lack of control for unobserved factors associated with participation in WIC that change over time (e.g., shocks to the economy) and lack of sufficiently detailed longitudinal data on participation over time and on outcomes.

Potential USDA-FNS Applications for WIC

This approach would be made more useful by encouraging more sharing of WIC administrative data and WIC data from other data systems, including data on families with not all siblings enrolled, as well as data from locations where program changes affect eligibility and enrollment.

REFERENCES

Rossin-Slater, M. 2013. WIC in your neighborhood: New evidence on the impacts of geographic access to clinics. *Journal of Public Economics* 102(C):51–69.

Ziliak, J. 2016. Why Are So Many Americans on Food Stamps? The Role of the Economy, Policy, and Demographics (Chapter 1). In *SNAP matters: How food stamps affect health and well-being*, edited by J. Bartfeld, C. Gundersen, T. Smeeting, and J. Ziliak. Stanford, CA: Stanford University Press. Pp. 18–48.

Appendix L

Gap Analysis

The committee conducted a gap analysis to determine the average intake of a nutrient that would be needed to ensure an acceptable level of inadequacy in a population (for this report, 5 percent of the population subgroup or less). For nutrients with an Estimated Averaged Requirement (EAR) and for which intake was inadequate, the gap is the difference between the EAR and the 5th percentile of intake; for nutrients with an Adequate Intake (AI) and for which intake was below the AI, the gap is the difference between the AI and the median intake; for sodium, for which there is excess intake, the gap is the difference between the Tolerable Upper Intake Level (UL) and the 95th percentile of intake. For added sugars and saturated fat, the gap is the difference between the upper limit (the value that is 10 percent of the associated kcal pattern) and the 95th percentile of intake. Two gaps were evaluated for nutrients with an EAR: the gap to shift the subgroup to 5 percent inadequacy or less and to 10 percent inadequacy or less.

Results of the gap analysis for nutrients that were categorized as higher, middle, or lower priority in Chapter 5, Tables 5-2 through 5-6 are presented below in Tables L-1 through L-6. Within each priority group, nutrients are ordered from the highest to lowest percent of inadequacy. Nutrients for which intakes exceeded a recommended upper limit (sodium, saturated fat, and added sugars) are presented last in the order. The gap was not evaluated for nutrients for which intakes exceeding the UL were not of concern, as described in Chapter 4. Meeting the gap identified for the nutrients that were evaluated did not result in any subgroups with nutrient intakes over the UL.

TABLE L-1 Gap Analysis Summary for Pregnant WIC-Participating Women

		5th Percentile		10th Percentile		Median			95th Percentile	
Nutrient	EAR/AI*	Intake	Gap	Intake	Gap	Intake	Gap	UL	Intake	Gap
Higher Priority										
Iron (mg/d)	22	11.5	10.5	12.6	9.4	—	—	45	26.5	—
Choline (mg/d)	450*	—	—	—	—	348	102	3,500	469	—
Potassium (mg/d)	4,700*	—	—	—	—	2,952	1,748	—	—	—
Fiber (g/d)	28*	—	—	—	—	18	10	—	—	—
Sodium (mg/d)	1,500*	—	—	—	—	3,566	0	2,300	4,930	2,630
Saturated fat (g/d)	—	—	—	—	—	—	—	29	44	15
Added sugars (g/d)	—	—	—	—	—	—	—	65	212	147
Middle Priority										
Folate (μg DFE/d)	520	412	108	454	66	—	—	—	—	—
Lower Priority										
Magnesium (mg/d)	290	221	69	241	49	—	—	—	—	—
Vitamin A (μg RAE/d)	550	426	124	480	70	—	—	—	—	—
Zinc (mg/d)	9.5	7.7	1.8	8.5	1	—	—	40	17.2	—
Vitamin C (mg/d)	70	46	24	58	12	—	—	2,000	244	—
Vitamin B6 (mg/d)	1.6	1.4	0.2	1.6	0.1	—	—	100	3.3	—
Serum Vitamin D (nmol/L)	40	36	4	41	0	—	—	—	—	—
Calcium (mg/d)	800	773	27	871	0	—	—	2,500	1,791	—

NOTES: N = 165. — = not applicable; AI = Adequate Intake; DFE = dietary folate equivalents; EAR = Estimated Average Requirement; RAE = retinol activity equivalents; UL = Tolerable Upper Intake Level. For nutrients with an AI, the median and gap between the median and AI are indicated. For nutrients with an EAR, 5th and 10th percentile gaps are evaluated. Shaded nutrients are nutrients to limit; for these, the gaps to reduce the prevalence of excessive intake to 5 percent were evaluated. For sodium, this is the 95th percentile gap compared to the UL. For saturated fat and added sugar, the 95th percentile intakes are compared to the *Dietary Guidelines for Americans* upper limit of 10 percent of kcal.

* Values with an asterisk are AIs; otherwise, EARs are indicated in this column.

SOURCES: IOM, 1998, 2000, 2001, 2002/2005, 2005, 2011; USDA/ARS, 2005–2012; USDA/HHS, 2016.

TABLE L-2 Gap Analysis Summary for Breastfeeding WIC-Participating Women

Nutrient	EAR/AI *	5th Percentile		10th Percentile		Median		UL	95th Percentile	
		Intake	Gap	Intake	Gap	Intake	Gap		Intake	Gap
Higher Priority										
Potassium (mg/d)	5,100*	—	—	—	—	2,846	2,254	—	—	—
Fiber (g/d)	29*	—	—	—	—	16	13	—	—	—
Sodium (mg/d)	1,500*	—	—	—	—	3,191	0	2,300	4,439	2,139
Saturated fat (g/d)	—	—	—	—	—	—	—	29	46	17
Added sugars (g/d)	—	—	—	—	—	—	—	65	194	129
Middle Priority										
Folate (μg DFE/d)	450	323	127	360	90	—	—	—	—	—
Serum Vitamin D (nmol/L)	40	28	12	33	7	—	—	—	—	—
Calcium (mg/d)	800	664	136	738	62	—	—	2,500	1,689	—
Lower Priority										
Vitamin A (μg RAE/d)	900	402	498	459	441	—	—	—	—	—
Magnesium (mg/d)	255	182	73	199	56	—	—	—	—	—
Zinc (mg/d)	10.4	7.1	3.3	8	2.4	—	—	40	15.4	—
Vitamin C (mg/d)	100	53	47	65	35	—	—	2,000	257	—
Vitamin B6 (mg/d)	1.7	1.2	0.5	1.3	0.4	—	—	100	3.5	—
Copper (mg/d)	1	0.8	0.2	0.9	0.1	—	—	10	1.7	—
Thiamin (mg/d)	1.2	1.1	0.1	1.2	0	—	—	—	—	—

NOTES: N = 27. — = not applicable; AI = Adequate Intake; DFE = dietary folate equivalents; EAR = Estimated Average Requirement; RAE = retinol activity equivalents; UL = Tolerable Upper Intake Level. For nutrients with an AI, the median and gap between the median and AI are indicated. For nutrients with an EAR, 5th and 10th percentile gaps are evaluated. Shaded nutrients are nutrients to limit; for these, the gaps to reduce the prevalence of excessive intake to 5 percent were evaluated. For sodium, this is the 95th percentile gap compared to the UL. For saturated fat and added sugar, the 95th percentile intakes are compared to the *Dietary Guidelines for Americans* upper limit of 10 percent of kcal.

* Values with an asterisk are AIs; otherwise, EARs are indicated in this column.

SOURCES: IOM, 1998, 2000, 2001, 2002/2005, 2005, 2011; USDA/ARS, 2005–2012; USDA/HHS, 2016.

TABLE L-3 Gap Analysis Summary for Postpartum WIC-Participating Women

		5th Percentile		10th Percentile		Median			95th Percentile	
Nutrient	EAR/AI*	Intake	Gap	Intake	Gap	Intake	Gap	UL	Intake	Gap
Higher Priority										
Calcium (mg/d)	800	429	371	496	304	—	—	2,500	1,301	—
Potassium (mg/d)	4,700*	—	—	—	—	1,898	2,802	—	—	—
Fiber (g/d)	25*	—	—	—	—	12	13	—	—	—
Sodium (mg/d)	1,500*	—	—	—	—	2,793	0	2,300	4,071	1,771
Added sugars (g/d)	—	—	—	—	—	—	—	58	199	142
Middle Priority										
Folate (μg DFE/d)	320	189	131	225	95	—	—	—	—	—
Serum Vitamin D (nmol/L)	40	30	10	37	3	—	—	—	—	—
Iron (mg/d)	8.1	6.5	1.6	7.6	0.5	—	—	45	23.5	21.5
Saturated fat (g/d)	—	—	—	—	—	—	—	26	34	8

Lower Priority										
Magnesium (mg/d)	265	121	144	139	126	—	—	—	—	—
Vitamin A (μg RAE/d)	500	145	355	184	316	—	—	—	—	—
Vitamin C (mg/d)	60	23	37	30	30	—	—	2,000	186	—
Copper (mg/d)	0.7	0.5	0.3	0.5	0.2	—	—	10	1.3	—
Zinc (mg/d)	6.8	4.3	2.5	5.1	1.7	—	—	40	13.9	—
Thiamin (mg/d)	0.9	0.7	0.2	0.8	0.1	—	—	—	—	—
Vitamin B6 (mg/d)	1.1	0.8	0.3	0.9	0.2	—	—	100	2.3	—
Vitamin B12 (mg/d)	2.0	1.4	0.6	1.7	0.3	—	—	—	—	—
Riboflavin (mg/g)	0.9	0.8	0.2	0.9	0	—	—	—	—	—
Niacin (mg/d)	11	10.6	0.4	12.0	0	—	—	—	—	—

NOTES: N = 62. — = not applicable; AI = Adequate Intake; DFE = dietary folate equivalents; EAR = Estimated Average Requirement; RAE = retinol activity equivalents; UL = Tolerable Upper Intake Level. For nutrients with an AI, the median and gap between the median and AI are indicated. For nutrients with an EAR, 5th and 10th percentile gaps are evaluated. Shaded nutrients are nutrients to limit; for these, the gaps to reduce the prevalence of excessive intake to 5 percent were evaluated. For sodium, this is the 95th percentile gap compared to the UL. For saturated fat and added sugar, the 95th percentile intakes are compared to the *Dietary Guidelines for Americans* upper limit of 10 percent of kcal.

* Values with an asterisk are AIs; otherwise, EARs are indicated in this column.

SOURCES: IOM, 1997, 1998, 2000, 2001, 2002/2005, 2005, 2011; USDA/ARS, 2005–2012; USDA/HHS, 2016.

TABLE L-4 Gap Analysis Summary for Breastfed WIC-Participating Infants

		5th Percentile		10th Percentile	
Nutrient	EAR	Intake	Gap	Intake	Gap
Iron (mg/d)	6.9	2.1	4.8	3.1	3.8
Zinc (mg/d)	2.5	0.5	2.0	0.9	1.6

NOTES: N = 39. EAR = Estimated Average Requirement; UL = Tolerable Upper Intake Level.
SOURCES: IOM, 2001; USDA/ARS, 2009–2012.

TABLE L-5 Gap Analysis Summary for WIC-Participating Children Ages 1 to Less Than 2 Years: Nutrients with Inadequacy or Excess Greater Than 50 Percent

		Median			95th Percentile	
Nutrient	AI, 1–3 y	Intake	Gap	UL	Intake	Gap
Potassium (mg/d)	3,000	1,864	1,136	—	—	—
Fiber (g/d)	19	8	11	—	—	—
Sodium (mg/d)	1,000	1,615	0	1,500	2,306	806

NOTES: N = 96. — = not applicable (UL gap only evaluated for sodium, for which intakes exceed the UL); AI = Adequate Intake; UL = Tolerable Upper Intake Level. The shaded nutrient (sodium) is a nutrient to limit.
SOURCES: IOM, 2005, 2002/2005; USDA/ARS, 2011–2012.

TABLE L-6 Gap Analysis Summary for WIC-Participating Children Ages 2 to Less Than 5 Years: Nutrients with Inadequacy or Excess Greater Than 50 Percent

			Median					95th Percentile		
Nutrient	AI, 1–3 Years	AI, 4–5 Years	Intake	Gap, 2–3 Years	Gap, 4–5 Years	UL, 1–3 Years	UL, 4–5 Years	Intake	Gap, 2–3 Years	Gap, 4–5 Years
Potassium (mg/d)	3,000	3,800	2,071	929	1,729	—	—	—	—	—
Fiber (g/d)	19	25	12	7	13	—	—	—	—	—
Sodium (mg/d)	1,000	1,200	2,118	0	0	1,500	1,900	2,995	1,495	1,095
Saturated fat (g/d)	—	—	—	—	—	14	14	29	15	15
Added sugars (g/d)	—	—	—	—	—	32	32	91	59	59

NOTES: N = 263. — = not applicable; AI = Adequate Intake; UL = Tolerable Upper Intake Level. Shaded nutrients are nutrients to limit; for these, the gaps to reduce the prevalence of excessive intake to 5 percent were evaluated. For sodium, this is the 95th percentile gap compared to the UL. For saturated fat and added sugar, the 95th percentile intakes are compared to the *Dietary Guidelines for Americans* upper limit of 10 percent of kcal.
SOURCES: IOM, 2005, 2002/2005; USDA/ARS, 2011–2012; USDA/HHS, 2016.

REFERENCES

IOM (Institute of Medicine). 1997. *Dietary Reference Intakes for calcium, phosphorus, magnesium, vitamin D, and fluoride*. Washington, DC: National Academy Press.

IOM. 1998. *Dietary Reference Intakes for thiamin, riboflavin, niacin, vitamin B6, folate, vitamin B12, pantothenic acid, biotin, and choline*. Washington, DC: National Academy Press.

IOM. 2000. *Dietary Reference Intakes for vitamin C, vitamin E, selenium, and carotenoids*. Washington, DC: National Academy Press.

IOM. 2001. *Dietary Reference Intakes for vitamin A, vitamin K, arsenic, boron, chromium, copper, iodine, iron, manganese, molybdenum, nickel, silicon, vanadium, and zinc*. Washington, DC: National Academy Press.

IOM. 2002/2005. *Dietary Reference Intakes for energy, carbohydrate, fiber, fat, fatty acids, cholesterol, protein and amino acids*. Washington, DC: The National Academies Press.

IOM. 2005. *Dietary Reference Intakes for water, potassium, sodium, chloride, and sulfate*. Washington, DC: The National Academies Press.

IOM. 2011. *Dietary Reference Intakes for calcium and vitamin D*. Washington, DC: The National Academies Press.

USDA/ARS (U.S. Department of Agriculture/Agriculture Research Service). 2005–2012. *What We Eat in America, NHANES 2005–2012*. http://www.cdc.gov/nchs/nhanes/wweia.htm (accessed November 29, 2016).

USDA/ARS. 2009–2012. *What We Eat in America, NHANES 2009–2012*. http://www.cdc.gov/nchs/nhanes/wweia.htm (accessed November 29, 2016).

USDA/ARS. 2011–2012. *What We Eat in America, NHANES 2011–2012*. http://www.cdc.gov/nchs/nhanes/wweia.htm (accessed November 29, 2016).

USDA/HHS (U.S. Department of Agriculture/U.S. Department of Health and Human Services). 2016. *2015–2020 Dietary Guidelines for Americans*. https://health.gov/dietaryguidelines/2015 (accessed August 29, 2016).

Appendix M

Behavioral Approaches in WIC as a Potential Action

The decision tree in Chapter 5, Figure 5-1, includes behavioral approaches as a possible option for addressing low consumption of nutrients or food groups. Behavioral approaches may overcome some challenges that prevent individuals from making the choice that best aligns with the *Dietary Guidelines for Americans* (DGA). These approaches to reducing cognitive load (the amount of information that must be processed at one time) have been demonstrated to improve individual food choice behavior.

Consumers frequently behave in ways (e.g., make decisions about foods) that contradict standard assumptions of economic theory (Just and Payne, 2009). Individuals often exhibit biases, a prime example being loss aversion (Kahneman and Tversky, 1984), when making choices. Loss aversion refers to the tendency to treat losses differently than gains, that is, people will pay less for an object they do not already have compared to what they will accept to give that object up. People also exhibit a tendency to remain within the status quo, even if choosing an alternative action seems clearly better. The implication for the Special Supplemental Nutrition Program for Women, Infants, and Children (WIC) is that there may be ways to frame food package choices to influence participant decisions, for example to make the breastfeeding package the status quo or "default" choice, or alternatively, to make it clear that when one chooses the partial or nonbreastfeeding package, the mother receives less food. There is evidence to suggest that, when individuals select new goods, they tend to focus on utilitarian characteristics (functional features of a good; an example for food is "healthful"). However, when individuals decide what to give up, they focus instead on hedonic characteristics (experiential features of a good; an example for food is taste) (Dhar and Wertenbroch, 2000; USDA/ERS, 2007). Thus, individuals might be willing to consider healthfulness when adding foods to their diet, but be less willing to give up a food that is perceived as tasting good. In the context of WIC, an example would be a greater willingness to add low-fat yogurt compared to giving up higher-fat milk. The U.S. Department of Agriculture's Economic Research Service (USDA-ERS) also reviewed research showing that specific cues (i.e., appearance, brand, name, price, and information) can influence product choices, which may be relevant for the labeling of food items (USDA/ERS, 2007).

Additionally, there is considerable evidence from the field of behavioral economics that the present time is valued more than future time and that individuals respond differently when asked what they would trade "now" for $10 provided in 2 weeks compared to what they would trade 1 month from now for $10 provided in 6 weeks (Loewenstein, 1988).[1] In the context of this decision being faced by a new WIC woman participant, the trade-off would be what the participant might receive now compared to the value of what would be received later. The choice now is the value of 806 fluid ounces of formula right away and less food in her package compared to the value of the breastfeeding package now (extra food in the package for the mother and nothing for the infant). The option (choice) later in the period of 6 to 12 months from now is the relatively lower value of the formula package but no benefits for the mother compared to the value of the breastfeeding package (maternal food and some additional food [meats] for the infant). The participant might be inclined to select the breastfeeding package at higher rates than if she had made the decision at some point before the baby was born, over both choices that occur in the future. Recommitment has been suggested as a strategy to address this tendency, or present bias. In the WIC program, periodic WIC office visits and breastfeeding peer counseling offer participants continuing opportunity for (re)commitment.

Although the field of behavioral economics is relatively new, there is evidence from intervention studies that indicates that incentives can induce behavior change. For example, the Health Incentives Pilot study conducted in Massachusetts provided Supplemental Nutrition Assistance Program recipients with an additional benefit of 30 cents for every dollar spent on specific vegetables and fruits. Participants who received the benefits consumed 26 percent more of the targeted vegetables and fruits compared to the group that did not receive the extra benefit (USDA/FNS, 2014). A number of other behavioral economics studies of potential relevance to

[1] There is a body of literature that suggests food assistance recipients consume more of their allotment right around the time the benefits are disbursed (e.g., Wilde and Ranney, 2000). One explanation for this is that recipients have a high personal discount rate and value the present much more than the future.

WIC are currently under way, funded through the Behavioral Economics Research Center at Duke University (BECR, 2016). Outcomes of this and future work may yield practically applicable strategies for improving WIC participant redemption and intake of foods provided in the food packages.

REFERENCES

BECR (Behavioral Economics Research Center at Duke University). 2016. *Funded 2015 WIC white papers*. https://becr.sanford.duke.edu/funding/wic (accessed August 30, 2016).

Dhar, R., and K. Wertenbroch. 2000. Consumer choice between hedonic and utilitarian goods. *Journal of Marketing Research* 37(1):60–71.

Just, D. R., and C. R. Payne. 2009. Obesity: Can behavioral economics help? *Annals of Behavioral Medicine* 38(Suppl 1):S47–S55.

Kahneman, D., and A. Tversky. 1984. Choices, values, and frames. *American Psychologist* 39(4):341–350.

Loewenstein, G. F. 1988. Frames of mind in intertemporal choice. *Management Science* 34(2):200–214.

USDA/ERS (U.S. Department of Agriculture/Economic Research Service). 2007. Could behavioral economics help improve diet quality for nutrition assistance program participants? Washington, DC: USDA/ERS. http://ben.cornell.edu/pdfs/USDA-BeEcon.pdf (accessed December 21, 2016).

USDA/FNS (U.S. Department of Agriculture/Food and Nutrition Service). 2014. Evaluation of the healthy incentives pilot (HIP): Final report. http://www.fns.usda.gov/sites/default/files/HIP-Final.pdf (accessed December 21, 2016).

Wilde, P. E., and C. K. Ranney. 2000. The monthly food stamp cycle: Shopping frequency and food intake decisions in an endogenous switching regression framework. *American Journal of Agricultural Economics* 82(1):200–213.

Appendix N

Comparison of Current and Revised Food Packages

TABLES

TABLE N-1 Comparison of the Current and Revised Food Packages for Young Infants, Full Nutrition Benefits and Maximum Monthly Allowances (Food Package I)

	Current Food Package I	Revised Food Package I
Partially breastfed infants[a]		
Infant formula	*Birth through 1 month of age:* 104 fl oz reconstituted powder	*Birth through 1 month of age:* Up to 364 fl oz[b,c]
	1 month through 3 months of age: About 384 fl oz of iron-fortified formula[b] (example: 52 oz of powdered formula) FNB = 364 fl oz; MMA = 388 fl oz reconstituted liquid concentrate or 384 fl oz RTF or 435 fl oz reconstituted powder [12 fl oz of formula per day]	*1 month through 3 months of age:* Up to 364 fl oz (no change to FNB or MMA)[b,c]
	4 months through 5 months of age: About 442 fl oz of iron-fortified formula[b] (example: 221 fl oz of liquid concentrate) FNB = 442 fl oz; MMA = 460 fl oz, reconstituted liquid concentrate or 474 fl oz RTF or 522 fl oz reconstituted powder [14 fl oz of formula per day]	*4 months through 5 months of age:* Up to 442 fl oz (no change to FNB or MMA)[b,c]
Fully formula fed infants[a]		
Infant formula	*Birth through 3 months of age:* About 806 fl oz of iron-fortified formula[b] (example: 403 fl oz of liquid concentrate) FNB = 806 fl oz; MMA = 823 fl oz, reconstituted liquid concentrate or 832 fl oz RTF or 870 fl oz reconstituted powder [26 fl oz of formula per day]	*Birth through 3 months of age:* Up to 806 fl oz (no change to FNB or MMA)[b,c]
	4 months through 5 months of age: About 884 fl oz of iron-fortified formula[b] (example: 442 fl oz of liquid concentrate) FNB = 884 fl oz; MMA = 896 fl oz, reconstituted liquid concentrate or 913 fl oz RTF or 960 fl oz reconstituted powder [29 fl oz of formula per day]	*4 months through 5 months of age:* Up to 884 fl oz (no change to FNB or MMA)[b,c]
Participant eligibility		
Partially breastfed infants[a]		
	Birth through 5 months of age	No change
Fully formula fed infants[a]		
	Birth through 5 months of age	No change

TABLE N-1 Continued

NOTES: fl oz = fluid ounce(s); FNB = full nutrition benefit; MMA = maximum monthly allowance; RTF = ready-to-feed.

[a] Infants are certified without respect to the feeding method to be used; however, the amount of formula prescribed for infants will vary depending on the WIC staff assessment of needs.

[b] The number of reconstituted fl oz of formula refers to the amount as prepared according to directions on the container.

[c] Following a detailed assessment of the needs of the mother–infant dyad by WIC staff, infants may be issued the quantity of formula needed to support any level of breastfeeding, up to the full nutrition benefit. The corresponding MMA amounts that account for the form of formula (ready-to-feed and concentrate) are unchanged from those presented in the Final Rule. Infant formula amounts for all infants should be individually tailored to the amounts that meet their nutritional needs.

TABLE N-2 Comparison of the Current and Revised Food Packages for Older Infants, Full Nutrition Benefits and Maximum Monthly Allowances (Food Package II)

	Current Food Package II	Revised Food Package II
Fully breastfed infants[a]		
Food group		
Vegetables and fruits	256 oz of jarred infant food vegetables and fruits [8.5 oz per day]	128 oz of jarred infant food vegetables and fruits *or* 64 oz of jarred infant food vegetables and fruits and $10 CVV *or* 0 oz of jarred infant food vegetables and fruits and $20 CVV[c] [4.3 or 2.1 oz per day in jar form]
Grains	24 oz of iron-fortified infant cereal [0.80 oz per day]	16 oz of iron-fortified infant cereal [0.53 oz per day]
Total protein foods	77.5 oz of infant food meat [2.6 oz per day]	40 ounces of infant food meat[d] [1.3 ounces per day]
Partially breastfed infants[a]		
Specialty food		
Infant formula	About 312 fl oz of iron-fortified formula[b] (example: 156 fl oz of liquid concentrate) FNB = 312 fl oz; MMA = 315 fl oz, reconstituted liquid concentrate or 338 fl oz RTF or 384 fl oz reconstituted powder [10 fl oz of formula per day]	Up to 312 fl oz of infant formula (no change in FNB or MMA)[b,e] [10 fl oz of formula per day]
Food group		
Vegetables and fruits	128 oz of jarred infant food vegetables and fruits [4.3 oz per day]	128 oz of jarred infant food vegetables and fruits *or* 64 oz of jarred infant food vegetables and fruits and $10 CVV *or* 0 oz of jarred infant food vegetables and fruits and $20 CVV[c] [4.3 or 2.1 oz per day in jar form]
Grains	24 oz of iron-fortified infant cereal [0.80 oz per day]	8 oz of iron-fortified infant cereal [0.27 oz per day]

TABLE N-2 Continued

	Current Food Package II	Revised Food Package II
Fully formula fed infants[a]		
Specialty food		
Infant formula	About 624 fl oz of iron- fortified formula[b] (example: 312 fl oz of liquid concentrate) FNB = 624 fl oz; MMA = 630 fl oz, reconstituted liquid concentrate or 643 fl oz RTF or 696 fl oz reconstituted powder [20 fl oz of formula per day]	Up to 624 fl oz of formula (no change in FNB or MMA)[b,e] [20 fl oz of formula per day]
Food group		
Fruits and vegetables	128 oz of jarred infant food vegetables and fruits [4.3 oz per day]	128 oz of jarred infant food vegetables and fruits *or* 64 oz of jarred infant food vegetables and fruits and $10 CVV *or* 0 oz of jarred infant food vegetables and fruits and $20 CVV[c] [4.3 or 2.1 oz per day in jar form]
Grains	24 oz of iron-fortified infant cereal [0.80 oz per day]	8 oz of infant cereal [0.27 oz per day]
Participant eligibility		
	Infants, 6 through 11 months of age	No change

NOTES: CVV = cash value voucher; fl oz = fluid ounce(s); FNB = full nutrition benefit; MMA = maximum monthly allowance; oz = ounce(s); RTF = ready-to-feed.

[a] Infants are certified without respect to the feeding method to be used; however, the amount of formula prescribed for infants will vary depending on whether they are fully breastfed, partially breastfed, or fully formula fed.

[b] The number of reconstituted fl oz of formula refers to the amount as prepared according to directions on the container.

[c] Depending upon the amount of infant food vegetables and fruits selected for food package II for infants, $0, $10, or $20 can be provided as CVV.

[d] Participants may substitute 10 oz of infant food meat with 10 oz of canned fish meeting WIC specifications for this food category.

[e] Following a detailed assessment of the needs of the mother–infant dyad by WIC staff, infants may be issued the quantity of formula needed to support any level of breastfeeding, up to the full nutrition benefit, which is the amount specified. The corresponding MMA amounts that account for the form of formula (ready-to-feed and concentrate) are unchanged from those presented in the Final Rule. Infant formula amounts for all infants should be individually tailored to the amounts that meet their nutritional needs.

TABLE N-3 Comparison of the Current and Revised Food Packages for Participants with Special Dietary Needs, Maximum Monthly Allowances (Food Package III)

	Current Food Package III	Revised Food Package III
Specialty food		
WIC formula*	About 455 fl oz of liquid concentrate	Up to 455 fl oz of liquid concentrate, if appropriate (no change)
Food group		
Other WIC foods	Participants receive up to the MMA of foods from the life stage-appropriate package	Amounts and types of foods in the life-stage package are provided as appropriate
Participant eligibility		
	Infants, children, and women	No change

NOTES: fl oz = fluid ounce(s); MMA = maximum monthly allowance.

* WIC formula means infant formula, exempt infant formula, or WIC-eligible nutritionals. Powder and ready-to-feed may be substituted at rates that provide comparable nutritive value.

TABLE N-4 Comparison of the Current and Revised Food Packages for Children, Maximum Monthly Allowances (Food Package IV)

	Current Food Package IV	Revised Food Package IV
Food group		
Vegetables and fruits	$8 CVV for vegetables and fruits [0.5 c-eq per day] 1 lb of legumes (or peanut butter as noted below) [0.13 oz-eq per day] 128 fl oz of vitamin C-rich juice [4.3 fl oz per day]	$12 CVV for vegetables and fruits [0.7 c-eq per day] 1 lb every 3 months of legumes[a,b] [0.08 oz-eq per day] 64 fl oz of vitamin C-rich juice [2.1 fl oz per day] *or* $3 addition to CVV for vegetables and fruits in place of juice
Dairy (milk)	16 qt of milk, with allowed substitutions [2.1 c-eq per day] • 1-year-old: whole milk (3.5%–4% milk fat) • 2- to 4-year-old: (1% milk fat or less)	IV-A: 12 qt of milk for 1-year-old children, option to substitute additional qt of yogurt[c,d,g,h] [1.5 c-eq per day] IV-B: 14 qt of milk for 2- through 4-year-old children, option to substitute additional qt of yogurt[e,f,g,h,i] [1.9 c-eq per day] No change in % milk fat
Grains	36 oz of iron-fortified breakfast cereal [1.2 oz-eq per day] 2 lb of whole grain bread or other whole grain options [1.1 oz-eq per day]	36 oz of iron-fortified whole-grain breakfast cereal[j] [1.2 oz-eq per day] 16–24 oz of whole wheat bread or other whole grain options[k] [maximum 0.8 oz-eq per day]
Total protein foods	1 dozen eggs [0.4 oz-eq per day] 18 oz of peanut butter (or legumes as noted above) [0.6 oz-eq per day]	1 dozen eggs[l] [0.4 oz-eq per day] 16–18 oz every 3 months of peanut butter[b] [maximum 0.4 oz-eq per day] 10 oz every 3 months of fish [0.1 oz-eq per day]
Participant eligibility		
	Children, 1 through 4 years of age	No change

continued

TABLE N-4 Continued

NOTES: c-eq = cup-equivalents; CVV = cash value voucher; oz-eq = ounce-equivalents.

[a] States are required to offer both dry legumes (1 lb) and canned legumes (64 oz or four 15–16 oz cans). Legumes are provided 1 month per quarter (or once every 3 months).

[b] Legumes and peanut butter must be provided and are not interchangeable. Participants may be issued legumes (1 lb dry or 64 oz [four 15–16 oz cans]) in place of peanut butter in the case of a peanut allergy.

[c] Whole milk is the standard milk for issuance to 1-year-old children (12 through 23 months). At a state agency option, fat-reduced milks may be issued to 1-year-old children for whom overweight or obesity is a concern. The need for fat-reduced milks for 1-year-old children must be based on an individual nutritional assessment and consultation with the child's health care provider if necessary, as established by state agency policy (current policy is unchanged).

[d] Children receiving food package IV-A may substitute 1 lb of cheese and 1 qt of yogurt (30 to 32 oz are allowed at the discretion of the state agency) for 4 qt of milk or 2 qt of yogurt for 2 qt of milk. State agencies do not have the option to issue additional amounts of cheese or yogurt beyond these maximums even with medical documentation. At state agency option, low-fat or nonfat yogurt may be issued to 1-year-old children for whom overweight and obesity is a concern. The need for low-fat or nonfat yogurt for 1-year-old children must be based on an individual nutritional assessment and consultation with the child's health care provider if necessary, as established by state agency policy.

[e] Low-fat (1 percent) or nonfat milks are the standard milk for issuance to children ≥24 months of age. Reduced fat (2 percent) milk is authorized only for participants with certain conditions, including but not limited to, underweight and maternal weight loss during pregnancy. The need for reduced fat (2 percent) milk must be based on an individual nutritional assessment as established by state agency policy (no change from the Final Rule).

[f] Children receiving food package IV-B may substitute 1 lb of cheese and 1 qt of yogurt for 4 qt of milk, or 2 qt of yogurt for 2 qt of milk. State agencies do not have the option to issue additional amounts of cheese or yogurt beyond these maximums even with medical documentation.

[g] For children, issuance of tofu and soy-based beverage as substitutes for milk must be based on an individual nutritional assessment and consultation with the participant's health care provider if necessary, as established by state agency policy. Such determination can be made for situations that include, but are not limited to, milk allergy, lactose intolerance, and vegan diets. Soy-based beverage may be substituted for milk for children on a qt for qt basis up to the total maximum allowance of milk. Tofu may be substituted for milk for children at the rate of 1 lb of tofu per 1 qt of milk.

[h] Evaporated milk may be substituted at the rate of 16 fl oz of evaporated milk per 32 fl oz of fluid milk or a 1:2 fluid ounce substitution ratio. Dry milk may be substituted at an equal reconstituted rate to fluid milk.

[i] Low-fat or nonfat yogurts are the only types of yogurt authorized for children ≥24 months of age or women. Soy-based yogurt or soy-based cheese substitutes are authorized yogurt and cheese options for individuals with a milk allergy or who consume a vegan diet.

[j] All breakfast cereals on the state agency's authorized food list must meet the whole grain-rich criteria as described in Chapter 6, Table 6-4.

[k] Whole wheat bread must be authorized. State agencies have the option to also authorize brown rice, bulgur, oatmeal, whole grain barley, cornmeal (including blue), corn masa flour, whole wheat macaroni (pasta) products, soft corn or whole wheat tortillas, buckwheat, corn masa flour, or teff in the range specified.

[l] A substitution of dry legumes (1 lb) or canned legumes (64 oz or four 15–16 oz cans) for each 1 dozen eggs is permitted for individuals with an egg allergy or who consume a vegan diet.

TABLE N-5 Comparison of the Current and Revised Food Packages for Pregnant Women and Partially Breastfeeding Women, Maximum Monthly Allowances (Food Package V)

	Current Food Package V	Revised Food Packages V-A and V-B
Food group		
Vegetables and fruits	$11 CVV for vegetables and fruits [0.7 c-eq per day] 1 lb of legumes [0.25 oz-eq per day] 144 fl oz of vitamin C-rich juice [4.8 fl oz per day]	CVV for vegetables and fruits: V-A: $15 [0.9 c-eq per day] V-B: $25 [1.5 c-eq per day] 2 lb every 3 months of legumes[a,b] [0.17 oz-eq per day] 64 fl oz of vitamin C-rich juice [2.1 fl oz per day] *or* $3 addition to the CVV for vegetables and fruits in place of juice
Dairy (milk)	22 qt of milk, 1% milk fat or less, with allowed substitutions [2.9 c-eq per day]	16 qt of milk, option to substitute additional qt of yogurt[c,d,e,f] [2.1 c-eq per day] No change in % milk fat
Grains	36 oz of iron-fortified breakfast cereal [1.2 oz-eq per day] 1 lb of whole grain bread or other whole grain options [0.5 oz-eq per day]	36 oz of iron-fortified whole grain breakfast cereal [1.2 oz-eq per day] 16–24 oz of whole wheat bread or other whole grain options[g] [maximum 0.8 oz-eq per day]
Total protein foods	1 dozen eggs [0.4 oz-eq per day] 18 oz of peanut butter [0.6 oz-eq per day]	1 dozen eggs[b] [0.4 oz-eq per day] 16–18 oz every 3 months of peanut butter[b] [maximum 0.4 oz-eq per day] V-A: 10 oz every 3 months of fish [0.1 oz-eq per day] V-B: 30 oz every 3 months of fish [0.3 oz-eq per day]
Participant eligibility		
Length of eligibility		
Eligibility during pregnancy		No change
	Throughout pregnancy	
Eligibility after giving birth		No change
	Up to 1 year postpartum	
Description of breastfeeding		
Definition of breastfeeding:		Definition of breastfeeding:
	Breastfeeding an average of once per day	No change

continued

TABLE N-5 Continued

Current Food Package V	Revised Food Packages V-A and V-B
Definition of partially breastfeeding:	Definition of partially breastfeeding:
Breastfeeding and requesting formula in amounts that do not exceed approximately half the amount of formula allowed for a fully formula-fed infant	No change

NOTES: c-eq = cup-equivalents; CVV = cash value voucher; oz-eq = ounce-equivalents.

[a] Two pounds of dry legumes or 128 oz (eight 15–16 oz cans) of canned legumes are provided once per quarter (once every 3 months).

[b] Legumes and peanut butter must be provided and are not interchangeable. Participants may be issued legumes (1 lb dry or 64 oz [four 15–16 oz cans]) in place of peanut butter in the case of a peanut allergy.

[c] Low-fat (1%) or nonfat milks are the standard milk for issuance to women. Reduced fat (2%) milk is authorized only for participants with certain conditions, including but not limited to, underweight and maternal weight loss during pregnancy. The need for reduced fat (2%) milk must be based on an individual nutritional assessment as established by state agency policy (no change from the current policy).

[d] Evaporated milk may be substituted at the rate of 16 fl oz of evaporated milk per 32 fl oz of fluid milk or a 1:2 fluid ounce substitution ratio. Dry milk may be substituted at an equal reconstituted rate to fluid milk.

[e] For women receiving food package V, two substitution options are available for milk: 1 lb of cheese and 1 qt of yogurt (30 to 32 oz are allowed at the discretion of the state agency) may substitute for 4 qt of milk or 2 qt of yogurt may substitute for 2 qt of milk. Low-fat or nonfat yogurts are the only types of yogurt authorized for women. State agencies do not have the option to issue additional amounts of cheese or yogurt beyond these maximums even with medical documentation. Soy-based yogurt or soy-based cheese substitutes are authorized yogurt and cheese options for individuals with a milk allergy or who consume a vegan diet.

[f] For women, soy-based beverage may be substituted for milk on a quart-for-quart basis up to the total maximum allowance of milk. Tofu may be substituted for milk at the rate of 1 lb of tofu per 1 qt of milk. Additional amounts of tofu may be substituted, up to the maximum allowances for fluid milk, for lactose intolerance or other reasons, as established by state agency policy.

[g] Whole wheat bread must be authorized. State agencies have the option to also authorize brown rice, bulgur, oatmeal, whole grain barley, cornmeal (including blue), corn masa flour, whole wheat macaroni (pasta) products, soft corn or whole wheat tortillas, buckwheat, corn masa flour, or teff in the range specified.

[h] A substitution of dry legumes (1 lb) or canned legumes (64 oz or four 15–16 oz cans) for each 1 dozen eggs is permitted for individuals with an egg allergy or who consume a vegan diet.

TABLE N-6 Comparison of the Current and Revised Food Packages for Nonbreastfeeding Postpartum Women, Maximum Monthly Allowances (Food Package VI)

	Current Food Package VI	Revised Food Package VI
Food group		
Vegetables and fruits	$11 CVV for vegetables and fruits [0.7 c-eq per day] 1 lb of legumes (or peanut butter as noted below) [0.25 oz-eq per day] 96 fl oz of vitamin C-rich juice [3.2 fl oz per day]	$15 CVV for vegetables and fruits [0.9 c-eq per day] 2 lb every 3 months of legumes[a,b] [0.17 oz-eq per day] *and* No juice
Dairy (milk)	16 qt of milk, 1% milk fat or less, with allowed substitutions [2.1 c-eq per day]	No change in amount or % milk fat, option to substitute additional qt of yogurt[c,d,e,f] [2.1 c-eq per day]
Grains	36 oz of iron-fortified breakfast cereal [1.2 oz-eq per day]	36 oz of iron-fortified whole grain breakfast cereal [1.2 oz-eq per day]
Total protein foods	1 dozen eggs [0.4 oz-eq per day] 18 oz of peanut butter (or legumes as noted above) [0.6 oz-eq per day]	1 dozen eggs[g] [0.4 oz-eq per day] 16–18 oz every 3 months of peanut butter[b] [maximum 0.4 oz-eq per day] 10 oz every 3 months of fish [0.1 oz-eq per day]
Participant eligibility		
Length of eligibility		
	Up to 6 months after delivery	No change

NOTES: c-eq = cup-equivalents; CVV = cash value voucher; oz-eq = ounce-equivalents.

[a] States are required to offer both dry legumes and canned legumes. Two lb of dry legumes or 128 oz (eight 15–16 oz cans) of canned legumes are provided once per quarter (once every 3 months).

[b] Legumes and peanut butter must be provided and are not interchangeable. Participants may be issued legumes (1 lb dry or 64 oz [four 15–16 oz cans]) in place of peanut butter in the case of a peanut allergy.

[c] Low-fat (1%) or nonfat milks are the standard milk for issuance to women. Reduced fat (2%) milk is authorized only for participants with certain conditions, including but not limited to, underweight and maternal weight loss during pregnancy. The need for reduced fat (2%) milk must be based on an individual nutritional assessment as established by state agency policy (no change from the current policy).

[d] Evaporated milk may be substituted at the rate of 16 fl oz of evaporated milk per 32 fl oz of fluid milk or a 1:2 fluid ounce substitution ratio. Dry milk may be substituted at an equal reconstituted rate to fluid milk.

continued

TABLE N-6 Continued

[e] For women receiving food package VI, two substitution options are available for milk: 1 lb of cheese and 1 qt of yogurt (30 to 32 oz are allowed at the discretion of the state agency) may substitute for 4 qt of milk or 2 qt of yogurt may substitute for 2 qt of milk. Low-fat or nonfat yogurts are the only types of yogurt authorized for women. State agencies do not have the option to issue additional amounts of cheese or yogurt beyond these maximums even with medical documentation. Soy-based yogurt or soy-based cheese substitutes are authorized yogurt and cheese options for individuals with a milk allergy or who consume a vegan diet.

[f] For women, soy-based beverage may be substituted for milk on a quart-for-quart basis up to the total maximum allowance of milk. Tofu may be substituted for milk at the rate of 1 lb of tofu per 1 qt of milk. Additional amounts of tofu may be substituted, up to the maximum allowances for fluid milk, for lactose intolerance or other reasons, as established by state agency policy.

[g] A substitution of dry legumes (1 lb) or canned legumes (64 oz or four 15–16 oz cans) for each 1 dozen eggs is permitted for individuals with an egg allergy or who consume a vegan diet.

TABLE N-7 Comparison of the Current and Revised Food Packages for Fully Breastfeeding Women, Maximum Monthly Allowances (Food Package VII)

	Current Food Package VII	Revised Food Package VII
Food group		
Vegetables and fruits	$11 CVV for vegetables and fruits [0.7 c-eq per day] 1 lb of legumes [0.25 oz-eq per day] 144 fl oz of vitamin C-rich juice [4.8 fl oz per day]	$35 in CVV for vegetables and fruits [2.1 c-eq per day] 2 lb every 3 months of legumes[a,b] [0.17 oz-eq per day] 64 fl oz of vitamin C-rich juice [2.1 fl oz per day] *or* $3 addition to CVV for fresh vegetables and fruits in place of juice
Dairy (milk)	24 qt of milk, 1% milk fat or less, with allowed substitutions [3.2 c-eq per day] 1 lb of cheese [about 0.5 oz per day]	16 qt of milk, option to substitute additional qt of yogurt[c,d,e,f] [2.1 c-eq per day] No change in % milk fat No cheese, except through milk substitutions[e]
Grains	36 oz of iron-fortified breakfast cereal [1.2 oz-eq per day] 1 lb of whole grain bread or other whole grain options [0.5 oz-eq per day]	36 oz of iron-fortified whole grain breakfast cereal [1.2 oz-eq per day] 16–24 oz of whole wheat bread or other whole grain options[g] [maximum 0.8 oz-eq per day]
Total protein foods	2 dozen eggs [0.8 oz-eq per day] 18 oz of peanut butter [0.6 oz-eq per day] 30 oz canned fish [1 oz-eq per day]	2 dozen eggs[h] [0.8 oz-eq per day] 16 to 18 oz every 3 months of peanut butter[b] [maximum 0.4 oz-eq per day] 60 oz every 3 months of fish [0.7 oz-eq per day]
Participant eligibility		
Length of eligibility		
	Up to 12 months after delivery	Up to 12 months after delivery

continued

TABLE N-7 Continued

NOTES: c-eq = cup-equivalents; CVV = cash value voucher; oz-eq = ounce-equivalents.

[a] States are required to offer both dry legumes and canned legumes. Two lb of dry legumes or 128 oz (eight 15–16 oz cans) of canned legumes are provided once per quarter (once every 3 months).

[b] Legumes and peanut butter must be provided and are not interchangeable. Participants may be issued legumes (1 lb dry or 64 oz [four 15–16 oz cans]) in place of peanut butter in the case of a peanut allergy.

[c] Low-fat (1%) or nonfat milks are the standard milk for issuance to women. Reduced fat (2%) milk is authorized only for participants with certain conditions, including but not limited to, underweight and maternal weight loss during pregnancy. The need for reduced fat (2%) milk must be based on an individual nutritional assessment as established by state agency policy (no change from the current policy).

[d] Evaporated milk may be substituted at the rate of 16 fl oz of evaporated milk per 32 fl oz of fluid milk or a 1:2 fluid ounce substitution ratio. Dry milk may be substituted at an equal reconstituted rate to fluid milk.

[e] For women receiving food package VII, three substitution options are available for milk: 1 lb of cheese and 1 qt of yogurt (30 to 32 oz are allowed at the discretion of the state agency) may substitute for 4 qt of milk, 2 qt of yogurt may substitute for 2 qt of milk, or 2 lb of cheese may substitute for 6 qt of milk. Low-fat or nonfat yogurts are the only types of yogurt authorized for women. State agencies do not have the option to issue additional amounts of cheese or yogurt beyond these maximums even with medical documentation. Soy-based yogurt or soy-based cheese substitutes are authorized yogurt and cheese options for individuals with a milk allergy or who consume a vegan diet.

[f] For women, soy-based beverage may be substituted for milk on a quart-for-quart basis up to the total maximum allowance of milk. Tofu may be substituted for milk at the rate of 1 lb of tofu per 1 qt of milk. Additional amounts of tofu may be substituted, up to the maximum allowances for fluid milk, for lactose intolerance or other reasons, as established by state agency policy.

[g] Whole wheat bread must be authorized. State agencies have the option to also authorize brown rice, bulgur, oatmeal, whole-grain barley, cornmeal (including blue), corn masa flour, whole wheat macaroni (pasta) products, soft corn or whole wheat tortillas, buckwheat, corn masa flour, or teff in the range specified.

[h] A substitution of dry legumes (1 lb) or canned legumes (64 oz or four 15–16 oz cans) for each 1 dozen eggs is permitted for individuals with an egg allergy or who consume a vegan diet.

Appendix O

Specific Nutrient Comparisons

TABLE O-1 Nutrients in 1/4 Cup-Equivalent of Example Infant Food Vegetables and Canned or Frozen Counterparts

Nutrient	Infant Food Peas	Fresh, Boiled Peas	Frozen, Boiled Peas	Canned Peas	Infant Food Carrots	Fresh, Boiled Carrots	Canned Carrots
Energy (kcal)	22	37	34	30	9	13	9
Protein (g)	1.4	2.3	2.3	1.9	0.3	0.3	0.2
Total fat (g)	0.2	0.1	0.1	0.2	0.0	0.1	0.1
Saturated fat (g)	0.03	0.02	0.02	0.03	0.01	0.01	0.01
Carbohydrate (g)	3.7	6.8	6.2	5.5	2.2	3.0	2.0
Dietary fiber (g)	0.9	2.4	2.0	1.8	0.6	1.1	0.5
Total sugar (g)	0.9	2.6	1.9	1.8	1.3	1.3	0.9
Calcium (mg)	8	12	11	9	8	11	9
Iron (mg)	0.4	0.7	0.7	0.4	0.1	0.1	0.2
Magnesium (mg)	8	17	10	8	3	4	3
Phosphorus (mg)	22	51	34	29	7	11	9
Potassium (mg)	47	119	48	76	71	85	65
Sodium (mg)	2	1	32	1	25	21	15
Zinc (mg)	0.2	0.5	0.3	0.3	0.1	0.1	0.1
Copper (mg)	0.03	0.08	0.05	0.04	0.02	0.01	0.04
Selenium (µg)	0.1	0.8	0.5	0.8	0.1	0.3	0.1
Vitamin C (mg)	0.3	6.2	4.3	4.2	2.1	1.3	1
Thiamin (mg)	0.04	0.11	0.12	0.05	0.01	0.02	0.01
Riboflavin (mg)	0.03	0.07	0.04	0.03	0.01	0.02	0.01
Niacin (mg)	0.5	0.9	0.6	0.3	0.2	0.2	0.2
Vitamin B6 (mg)	0.01	0.09	0.05	0.03	0.03	0.06	0.04
Folate, DFE (µg)	12.3	27.5	25.8	19.3	5.0	5.0	3.0
Choline (mg)	14.1	13.0	12.0	NR	2.5	3.2	NR
Vitamin B12 (µg)	0	0	0	0	0	0	0
Vitamin A, RAE (µg)	5	18	46	12	208	309	202
Retinol (µg)	0	0	0	0	0	0	0
Vitamin E (mg)	0.01	0.06	0.01	0.01	0.19	0.37	0.27
Vitamin D (µg)	0	0	0	0	0	0	0

NOTES: NR = not reported.
SOURCE: USDA/ARS, 2016.

TABLE O-2 Nutrients in 1/4 Cup-Equivalent of Example Infant Food Fruits and Canned or Frozen Counterparts

Nutrient	Infant Food Bananas	Fresh, Raw Bananas	Infant Food Applesauce	Applesauce	Boiled Apples	Infant Food Peaches	Canned Peaches[a]	Frozen Peaches[b]
Energy (kcal)	34	34	12	12	15	25	24	24
Protein (g)	0.4	0.4	0.1	0.1	0.1	0.4	0.2	1.0
Total fat (g)	0.1	0.1	0.1	0.0	0.1	0.1	0.1	0.0
Saturated fat (g)	0.03	0.04	0.01	0.00	0.02	0.01	0.00	0.00
Carbohydrate (g)	8.0	8.6	3.1	3.2	3.8	5.6	6.1	6.0
Dietary fiber (g)	0.6	1.0	0.5	0.3	0.7	0.5	0.3	1.0
Total sugar (g)	4.3	4.6	2.8	2.7	3.0	4.5	4.1	5.0
Calcium (mg)	1.5	2.0	1.0	1.0	1.0	2.0	1.0	4.0
Iron (mg)	0.1	0.1	0.1	0.1	0.1	0.1	0.1	0.0
Magnesium (mg)	9.8	10.0	1.0	1.0	1.0	3.0	2.0	6.0
Phosphorus (mg)	7.5	8.3	2.0	1.0	2.0	6.0	4.0	13.0
Potassium (mg)	108.8	134.3	20.0	21.0	24.0	76.0	34.0	107.0
Sodium (mg)	0.8	0.5	0.0	1.0	0.0	2.0	3.0	0.0
Zinc (mg)	0.02	0.06	0.01	0.01	0.01	0.04	0.06	0.00
Copper (mg)	0.02	0.03	0.01	0.01	0.01	0.01	0.01	0.04
Selenium (μg)	0.4	0.4	0.1	0.0	0.0	0.0	NR	0.0
Vitamin C (mg)	8.2	3.3	10.9	6.0	0.1	17.9	1.0	59.0
Thiamin (mg)	0.01	0.01	0.00	0.01	0.00	0.01	0.01	0.00
Riboflavin (mg)	0.02	0.03	0.01	0.01	0.00	0.03	0.01	0.00

continued

TABLE O-2 Continued

Nutrient	Infant Food Bananas	Fresh, Raw Bananas	Infant Food Applesauce	Applesauce	Boiled Apples	Infant Food Peaches	Canned Peaches[a]	Frozen Peaches[b]
Niacin (mg)	0.2	0.2	0.0	0.0	0.0	0.6	0.2	1.0
Vitamin B6 (mg)	0.1	0.1	0.0	0.0	0.0	0.0	0.0	0.0
Folate, DFE (μg)	6.5	7.5	1.0	1.0	0.0	8.0	3.0	3.0
Choline (mg)	1.5	3.7	1.0	0.6	0.9	3.3	NR	4.0
Vitamin B12 (μg)	0	0	0	0	0	0	NR	0
Vitamin A, RAE (μg)	0	1	0	0	1	13	10	9
Retinol (μg)	0	0	0	0	0	0	NR	NR
Vitamin E (mg)	0.10	0.04	0.17	0.05	0.01	0.77	0.48	0.00
Vitamin D (μg)	0	0	0	0	0	0	NR	0

NOTES: NR = not reported.
[a] Canned in light syrup.
[b] Data from Supertracker.
SOURCES: USDA, 2016; USDA/ARS, 2016.

TABLE O-3 Comparison of Iron, Zinc, Sodium, and Fat Content Across Water- and Oil-Packed Varieties Compared to Jarred Infant Food Meat; Cost per Ounce; Sizes Available

Product	Iron (mg/oz)	Zinc (mg/oz)	Cost ($/oz)	Sodium (mg/oz)	Total Fat (gm/oz)	Saturated Fat (gm/oz)	Sizes (oz)
Infant food meat composite[a]	0.30	0.52	0.40	13	1.55	1.13	2.5
Canned fish composite[b]	0.42	0.20	0.20	77	0.44	0.09	
Tuna, light in water	0.46	0.20	0.19	70	0.27	0.06	5, 12
Tuna, light in oil	0.39	0.26	NA	118	2.33	0.44	5, 12
Salmon, pink in water	0.18	0.22	0.31	114	1.41	0.25	5, 14.75

NOTES: NA = not available in redemption data provided to the committee.

[a] A composite of commonly consumed jarred infant food meats (beef, chicken, turkey, ham), based on the assumptions outlined in Appendix R.

[b] A composite of tuna and salmon, based on redemption of fish species by WIC participants as outlined in Appendix R.

SOURCE: USDA/ARS, 2016.

REFERENCES

USDA (U.S. Department of Agriculture). 2016. Supertracker home. https://www.supertracker.usda.gov (accessed September 14, 2016).

USDA/ARS (U.S. Department of Agriculture/Agriculture Research Service). 2016. *USDA National Nutrient Database for Standard Reference, release 28*. http://www.ars.usda.gov/ba/bhnrc/ndl (accessed September 14, 2016).

Appendix P

Food Specification Detail

TABLE P-1 Proposed Specifications for Foods in the Revised WIC Food Packages[a]

Category/Food	Food Package and Affected Participant Group, Considering the Proposed Food Package Revisions	Selected Current Specifications	Proposed Change to the Specifications[b]	Rationale[c]
Infant formulas	I, II Infants	All authorized infant formulas must (1) meet the definition for an infant formula in section 201(z) of the Federal Food, Drug, and Cosmetic Act (21 U.S.C. 321(z)) and meet the requirements for an infant formula under section 412 of the Federal Food, Drug and Cosmetic Act, as amended (21 U.S.C. 350a) and the regulations at 21 C.F.R. Parts 106 and 107; (2) be designed for enteral digestion via oral or tube feeding; (3) provide at least 10 mg iron per liter (at least 1.5 mg iron/100 kilocalories) at standard dilution; (4) provide at least 67 kilocalories per 100 milliliters (approximately 20 kilocalories per fluid ounce) at standard dilution; (5) not require the addition of any ingredients other than water prior to being served in a liquid state	No change from current specifications	Lack of sufficient evidence to support a change related to required energy concentration; other specifications were considered appropriate
Infant foods	II Infants			
Infant cereals		Infant cereal must contain a minimum of 45 mg of iron per 100 g of dry cereal	No change from current specifications	NA
Infant food fruits		Any variety of single ingredient commercial infant food fruit without added sugars, starches, or salt (i.e., sodium). Texture may range from strained through diced	No change from current specifications	NA

Infant food vegetables		Any variety of single ingredient commercial infant food vegetables without added sugars, starches, or salt (i.e., sodium). Texture may range from strained through diced	No change from current specifications	NA
Infant food meats		Any variety of commercial infant food meat or poultry, as a single major ingredient, with added broth or gravy Added sugars or salt (i.e., sodium) are not allowed. Texture may range from pureed through diced	No change from current specifications	NA
Vegetables and Fruits Purchased with the CVV	II Infants	Any variety of fresh whole or cut fruit without added sugars Any variety of fresh whole or cut vegetable, without added sugars, fats, or oils (as defined in 21 C.F.R. 101.95)	Fresh, frozen, or canned forms of vegetables and fruits meeting other specifications may be purchased	Fresh, frozen, and canned vegetables and fruits are suitable for infants and meet developmental needs when prepared appropriately
	IV, V-A, V-B, VI, VII Women and children	Any variety of fresh whole or cut fruit without added sugars Any variety of fresh whole or cut vegetable, without added sugars, fats, or oils (as defined in 21 C.F.R. 101.95) Any variety of canned fruits (must conform to FDA standard of identity [21 C.F.R. 145]) including applesauce, juice pack or water pack without added sugars, fats, oils, or salt (i.e., sodium). Any variety of frozen fruits without added sugars Any variety of canned or frozen vegetables (must conform to FDA standard of identity [21 C.F.R. 155]) without added sugars, fats, or oils. May be regular or lower in sodium	No change from current specifications	NA

continued

TABLE P-1 Continued

Category/Food	Food Package and Affected Participant Group, Considering the Proposed Food Package Revisions	Selected Current Specifications	Proposed Change to the Specifications[b]	Rationale[c]
		Any type of dried fruits or dried vegetable without added sugars, fats, oils, or salt (i.e., sodium)		
Milk and Milk Alternatives				
Cow's milk	IV, V-A, V-B, VI, VII Women and children	Must conform to FDA standard of identity for whole, reduced fat, low-fat, or nonfat milks (21 C.F.R. 131.110). Must be pasteurized and contain at least 400 IU of vitamin D per quart (100 IU per cup) and 2000 IU of vitamin A per quart (500 IU per cup) May be flavored or unflavored. May be fluid, shelf stable, evaporated (21 C.F.R. 131.130), or dried (i.e., powdered) (21 C.F.R. 131.147). Cultured milks must conform to FDA standard of identity for cultured milk (21 C.F.R. 131.112—cultured buttermilk, kefir cultured milk, acidophilus cultured milk)	Only unflavored milk is permitted	Low-fat forms (for children 2 years of age and older, and women) align with CACFP provision of milk and with the DGA; requiring unflavored forms reduces inclusion of added sugars in the WIC food packages
Goat's milk	IV, V-A, V-B, VI, VII Women and children	Must be pasteurized and contain at least 400 IU of vitamin D per quart (100 IU per cup) and 2000 IU of vitamin A per quart (500 IU per cup). May be flavored or unflavored. May be fluid, shelf-stable, evaporated, or dried (i.e., powdered)	See above, as for cow's milk	See above, as for cow's milk

Soy-based beverage	IV, V-A, V-B, VI, VII Women and children	Must be fortified to meet the following nutrient levels: 276 mg calcium per cup, 8 g protein per cup, 500 IU vitamin A per cup, 100 IU vitamin D per cup, 24 mg magnesium per cup, 222 mg phosphorus per cup, 349 mg potassium per cup, 0.44 mg riboflavin per cup, and 1.1 mcg vitamin B12 per cup, in accordance with fortification guidelines issued by FDA	In addition, the total sugar content of soy-based beverages should be as low as possible, not to exceed 12 g per 8 oz serving	Soy-based beverages are available in the marketplace that contain 12 g or less of total sugars per serving; sugars in soy-based beverages are 100 percent added; added sugars intakes are excessive in the WIC population, therefore it is prudent to apply a limit that considers nationwide availability of these products
Tofu	IV, V-A, V-B, VI, VII Women and children	Calcium-set tofu prepared with calcium salts (e.g., calcium sulfate). May not contain added fats, sugars, oils, or sodium	Must contain a minimum of 200 mg of calcium per 100 g of tofu (calcium-set is no longer part of the specification); retain the specification that tofu may not contain added fats, sugars, oils, or sodium	Tofu in the food packages serves as a milk substitution; as such, the revised specification ensures that tofu in the food packages provides an amount of calcium as close to that in a serving of milk as reasonable, considering marketplace options

continued

TABLE P-1 Continued

Category/Food	Food Package and Affected Participant Group, Considering the Proposed Food Package Revisions	Selected Current Specifications	Proposed Change to the Specifications[b]	Rationale[c]
Yogurt	IV, V-A, V-B, VI, VII Women and children	Must be pasteurized and conform to standards of identity for yogurt as listed in Table 4 of 7 C.F.R. 246.10(e)(12); may be plain or flavored with ≤40 grams of total sugars per 1 cup of yogurt.	Must contain ≤30 g total sugars per 8 oz serving (≤3.75 g total sugars per ounce); soy-based yogurt substitute must contain at least 250 mg of calcium and 6.5 g of protein per 8 oz serving	The availability of yogurts containing 30 g or less of total sugars per 8 oz serving has expanded substantially; this level is more closely aligned with the DGA; soy products meet the needs of individuals with a milk allergy or who consume a vegan diet
	IV-B, V-A, V-B, VI, VII Women and children	Only lowfat and nonfat yogurts are authorized for children 2 years of age and older and women	No change from current specifications	NA
	IV-A Children	Must be whole-milk yogurt	No change from current specifications	NA
Cheese	IV, V-A, V-B, VI, VII Women and children	Domestic cheese made from 100 percent pasteurized milk. Must conform to FDA standard of identity (21 C.F.R. Part 133); Monterey Jack, Colby, natural Cheddar, Swiss, Brick, Muenster, Provolone, part skim or whole Mozzarella,	In addition, soy-based cheese substitute (not soy curd cheese) is permitted and must contain at least 250 mg	Soy products meet the needs of individuals with a milk allergy or who consume a vegan diet

		pasteurized processed American, or blends of any of these cheeses are authorized Cheeses that are labeled low, free, reduced, less or light in the nutrients of sodium, fat or cholesterol are WIC-eligible	of calcium and 6.5 g of protein per 1.5 ounce serving	
Juice	IV, V-A, V-B, VII Women and children	Must be pasteurized 100% unsweetened fruit juice. Must conform to FDA standard of identity (21 C.F.R. Part 146) or vegetable juice must conform to FDA standard of identity (21 C.F.R. Part 156) and contain at least 30 mg of vitamin C per 100 mL of juice. With the exception of 100% citrus juices, state agencies must verify the vitamin C content of all state-approved juices. Juices that are fortified with other nutrients may be allowed at the state agency's option. Juice may be fresh, from concentrate, frozen, canned, or shelf stable Vegetable juice may be regular or lower in sodium	No change from current specifications	NA
Eggs	IV, V-A, V-B, VI, VII Women and children	Fresh shell domestic hens' eggs or dried eggs mix (must conform to FDA standard of identity in 21 C.F.R. 160.105) or pasteurized liquid whole eggs (must conform to FDA standard of identity in 21 C.F.R. 160.115). Hard boiled eggs, where readily available for purchase in small quantities, may be provided for homeless participants	No change from current specifications	NA

continued

TABLE P-1 Continued

Category/Food	Food Package and Affected Participant Group, Considering the Proposed Food Package Revisions	Selected Current Specifications	Proposed Change to the Specifications[b]	Rationale[c]
Breakfast cereal	IV, V-A, V-B, VI, VII Women and children	Must contain a minimum of 28 mg iron per 100 g dry cereal Must contain ≤21.2 g sucrose and other sugars per 100 g dry cereal (≤6 g per dry oz) At least half of the cereals authorized on a state agency's food list must have whole grain as the primary ingredient by weight AND meet labeling requirements for making a health claim as a "whole grain food with moderate fat content": (1) contain a minimum of 51% whole grains (using dietary fiber as the indicator); (2) meet the regulatory definitions for "low saturated fat" at 21 C.F.R. 101.62 (≤1 g saturated fat per RACC) and "low cholesterol" (≤20 mg cholesterol per RACC); (3) bear quantitative trans fat labeling; and (4) contain ≤6.5 g total fat per RACC and ≤0.5 g trans fat per RACC	All ready-to-eat cereals on a state agency's authorized food list must adhere to the whole grain-rich criteria[d] and conform to other current specifications (e.g., must be iron-fortified, must not exceed added sugars limitations)	Intake of whole grains is low in the WIC population; whole grain cereal options have expanded substantially since the last review; the same products should qualify while aligning with USDA guidance for CACFP, the National School Lunch and Breakfast Programs (USDA/FNS, 2016)

Whole grain options				
Whole wheat and whole grain bread	IV, V-A, V-B, VI, VII Women and children	Whole wheat bread must conform to FDA standard of identity (21 C.F.R. 136.180); whole grain bread must conform to FDA standard of identity (21 C.F.R. 136.110) (includes whole wheat or whole grain buns and rolls) AND Whole grain must be the primary ingredient by weight in all whole wheat or whole grain bread products Whole wheat and whole grain bread must meet labeling requirements for making a health claim as a "whole grain food with moderate fat content": (1) contain a minimum of 51% whole grains (using dietary fiber as the indicator); (2) meet the regulatory definitions for "low saturated fat" at 21 C.F.R. 101.62 (≤1 g saturated fat per RACC) and "low cholesterol" (≤20 mg cholesterol per RACC); (3) bear quantitative trans fat labeling; and (4) contain ≤6.5 g total fat per RACC and ≤0.5 g trans fat per RACC	Whole wheat bread: no change from current specifications; Whole grain bread is no longer permitted; only 100% whole wheat bread is permitted	Very few states offer whole grain bread options; identification of suitable whole grain breads (>50% whole grain) is challenging; restricting to 100% whole wheat bread is in alignment with most current state WIC authorized food lists and promotes intake of whole grains by WIC participants

continued

TABLE P-1 Continued

Category/Food	Food Package and Affected Participant Group, Considering the Proposed Food Package Revisions	Selected Current Specifications	Proposed Change to the Specifications[b]	Rationale[c]
Other whole grain options		Other whole unprocessed grains: Brown rice, bulgur (cracked wheat), oats, whole grain barley, and whole wheat macaroni (pasta) products without added sugars, fats, oils, or salt (i.e., sodium)	In addition, teff or buckwheat may be offered; cornmeal (including blue); and corn masa flour meeting specifications outlined below are allowed	Additional options provide culturally suitable alternatives; participants and WIC staff expressed an interest in addition of these grains
Tortillas		Soft corn or whole wheat tortillas may be allowed at the state agency's option. Soft corn tortillas made from ground masa flour (corn flour) using traditional processing methods are WIC-eligible, e.g., whole corn, corn (masa), whole ground corn, corn masa flour, masa harina, and white corn flour. For whole wheat tortillas, "whole wheat flour" must be the only flour listed in the ingredient list	In addition, once available in the marketplace, states are encouraged to offer tortillas made with folic acid-fortified corn masa flour	Folic acid is a nutrient of concern for pre-menopausal women; consumption of folic acid is lower among Hispanic compared to non-Hispanic women (Williams et al., 2015)
Whole wheat macaroni (pasta) products		Must conform to FDA standard of identity (21 C.F.R. 139.138) and have no added sugars, fats, oils, or salt (i.e., sodium). "Whole wheat flour" and/or "whole durum wheat flour" must be the only flours listed in the ingredient list. Other shapes and sizes that otherwise meet the FDA standard of identity for whole wheat macaroni	No change from current specifications	NA

		(pasta) products (139.138), and have no added sugars, fats, oils, or salt (i.e., sodium), are also authorized (e.g., whole wheat rotini, and whole wheat penne)		
Cornmeal		Not yet permitted	Add whole cornmeal (including blue) meeting the FDA standard of identity (21 C.F.R. 137.260) and that is in alignment with USDA specifications for cornmeal in school meal programs (USDA-CNP-01-2008) to current options	Provides a culturally suitable option; similar in nutritive value to some types of permitted corn tortillas
Corn masa flour		Not yet permitted	Add corn masa flour. Once available in the marketplace, states are encouraged to offer folic acid-fortified corn masa flour	Allowing this flour is in alignment with the allowance of tortillas made with corn masa flour; participants expressed an interest in this addition
Fish	IV, V-A, V-B, VI, VII Women and children	Canned only: Light tuna (must conform to FDA standard of identity [21 C.F.R. 161.190]); Salmon (must conform to FDA standard of identity [21 C.F.R. 161.170]); Sardines; Mackerel (N. Atlantic *Scomber scombrus*, or Chub Pacific *Scomber japonicas*; Jack Mackerel)	No changes to the species specified	NA

continued

TABLE P-1 Continued

Category/Food	Food Package and Affected Participant Group, Considering the Proposed Food Package Revisions	Selected Current Specifications	Proposed Change to the Specifications[b]	Rationale[c]
		May be packed in water or oil. Pack may include bones or skin. Added sauces and flavorings (e.g., tomato sauce, mustard, lemon) are authorized at the state agency's option. May be regular or lower in sodium content.	Canned fish may be water-packed, or contain added sauces and flavorings. All other specifications remain unchanged	Few states currently offer oil-packed fish so there is minimal effect on participant choice; water-packed varieties are more nutrient dense because water-packed fish is lower in energy but contains the same levels of key nutrients per serving
Mature legumes	IV, V-A, V-B, VI, VII Women and children	Any type of mature dry beans, peas, or lentils in dry-packaged or canned forms. Examples include but are not limited to black beans ("turtle beans"), black-eyed peas (cowpeas of the blackeye variety, "cow beans"), garbanzo beans (chickpeas), great northern beans, kidney beans, lima beans ("butter beans"), navy beans, pinto beans, soybeans, split peas, and lentils. All categories exclude soups. May not contain added sugars, fats, oils or meat as purchased. Canned legumes may be regular or lower in sodium content Baked beans may be provided for participants with limited cooking facilities	No change from current specifications	NA

Peanut butter	IV, V-A, V-B, VI, VII Women and children	Peanut butter and reduced fat peanut butter (must conform to FDA Standard of Identity [21 C.F.R. 164.150]); creamy or chunky, regular or reduced fat, salted or unsalted forms are allowed	No change from current specifications	NA
WIC-eligible nutritionals	I, II, IV, V-A, V-B, VI, VII Women, infants, and children	Certain enteral products that are specifically formulated to provide nutritional support for individuals with a qualifying condition, when the use of conventional foods is precluded, restricted, or inadequate. Such WIC-eligible nutritionals must serve the purpose of a food, meal, or diet (may be nutritionally complete or incomplete) and provide a source of calories and one or more nutrients; be designed for enteral digestion via an oral or tube feeding; and may not be a conventional food, drug, flavoring, or enzyme	No change from current specifications	NA

NOTES: CACFP = Child and Adult Care Food Program; C.F.R. = Code of Federal Regulations; CVV = cash value voucher; DGA = *Dietary Guidelines for Americans*; FDA = Food and Drug Administration; IU = international units; NA = not applicable; RACC = reference amount customarily consumed; RTE = ready-to-eat. Food packages: I = infants ages 0 to <6 months; II = infants ages 6 to <12 months; IV-A = children ages 1 to <2 years; IV-B = children 2 to < 5 years; V-A = pregnant women; V-B = partially breastfeeding women; VI = postpartum women; VII = fully breastfeeding women.

[a] See the Final Rule (USDA/FNS, 2014) for a detailed list of current food specifications. Some text in this table is updated from the original prepublication version.

[b] Details are provided only for the proposed change. Other components of the specification remain as detailed in the Final Rule.

[c] With some exceptions, rationale is only provided in cases where changes to the current specifications are proposed. Exceptions include cases where USDA-FNS specifically requested committee review of a specification.

[d] It is anticipated that changes to the whole grain-rich criteria in alignment with the FDA proposed changes to the RACCs used for food labeling would be applied to the WIC food packages.

SOURCES: For current specifications, see USDA/FNS, 2014, 2015.

REFERENCES

USDA/FNS (U.S. Department of Agriculture/Food and Nutrition Service). 2014. *Special Supplemental Nutrition Program for Women, Infants and Children (WIC): Revisions in the WIC food packages*. Final Rule. 7 C.F.R. § 246.

USDA/FNS. 2015. WIC policy memorandum #2015-3 to WIC state agency directors: Eligibility of white potatoes for purchase with the cash-value voucher. Alexandria, VA: USDA-FNS.

USDA/FNS. 2016. *Whole grain resource for the national school lunch and school breakfast programs*. http://www.fns.usda.gov/sites/default/files/WholeGrainResource.pdf (accessed November 11, 2016).

Williams, J., C. T. Mai, J. Mulinare, J. Isenburg, T. J. Flood, M. Ethen, B. Frohnert, and R. S. Kirby. 2015. Updated estimates of neural tube defects prevented by mandatory folic acid fortification—United States, 1995–2011. *Morbidity and Mortality Weekly Report* 64(1):1–5.

Appendix Q

Foods and Food Specifications That Were Reviewed, But Not Changed

INFANT FORMULA AMOUNTS AND SPECIFICATIONS

Infant Formula Amounts

The committee determined that the current full nutrition benefit amounts approximate the infant's energy needs, and the maximum monthly allowance appropriately accommodates package sizes of powdered formula products. The amounts currently provided were based on the Estimated Energy Requirement (EER) for infants in an Institute of Medicine (IOM) 2006 report. Although EERs calculated for Special Supplemental Nutrition Program for Women, Infants, and Children (WIC) participating infants using National Health and Nutrition Examination Survey (NHANES) 2011–2012 data were slightly higher, median EER is too imprecise to support a change to currently offered amounts. In addition, the committee did not receive any feedback either through public comments or from WIC staff in the March 31 workshop suggesting a need for adjustments in formula amounts.

Iron Content of WIC-Approved Infant Formulas

WIC infant formulas are required to provide at least 1.5 milligrams of iron per 100 kcal at standard dilution (USDA/FNS, 2014). The U.S. Food and Drug Administration (FDA)–required range for iron in infant formulas is 0.15–3 mg per 100 kcal.[1] The committee evaluated the iron content of

[1] 21 C.F.R. § 106–107.

formulas provided through WIC contracts by reviewing products from the three major WIC formula manufacturers. These formulas, considering the full nutrition benefit (FNB) amounts, provide iron in the range of 1.5–2 mg per 100 kcal. This amount of iron falls well within the FDA acceptable range, as would be expected. Infants that consume the full nutrition benefit of WIC-eligible formulas and/or foods would consume more than the Adequate Intake (AI), less than the Tolerable Upper Intake Level (UL), and older infants consuming infant cereals and vegetables and fruits would consume slightly less than the Estimated Average Requirement (EAR).

Recent published evidence comparing health outcomes at different levels of iron in infant formula is limited, as was described in the phase I report (NASEM, 2016). Some inconclusive evidence suggests that iron intake in infants is associated with long-term cognitive, motor, and social-emotional outcomes. Updated data are needed to understand the optimal level of infant formula iron, particularly in cases where the baseline iron status of infants is poor compared to cases where iron status is adequate.

In summary, eligible WIC formulas contain an amount of iron that supports the needs of infants ages 0 to less than 12 months, without exceeding the UL for this age group. Overall, inadequate evidence is available to support changing the concentration of iron that is currently required in WIC-eligible formulas.

Energy Density of WIC-Approved Infant Formulas

Formulas provided through WIC primary contracts must contain 20 kcal per ounce (kcal/oz) prepared at standard dilution with a state option to allow lower-energy formulas in cases of medically documented qualifying conditions (7 C.F.R. § 246.10[c][1][i]; USDA/FNS, 2014). In 2014, a 19 kcal/oz infant formula was introduced to the U.S. market with the rationale that the lower energy formula better reflects the energy density of human milk (Abbott Nutrition, 2015). States having infant formula contracts with companies that subsequently reduced the energy density of their products mid-contract were permitted to continue providing non-primary contract formulas to WIC participating infants with medical documentation (USDA/FNS, 2013).

Federal Regulations and Evidence Related to Lower-Energy Formulas[2]

The lower-energy 19 kcal/oz formulas, equivalent to 64.2 kcal/dL, fall at the lower end of the energy range of 63 to 71 kcal/dL that was recommended to the FDA by the American Academy of Pediatrics (AAP) committee

[2] Text in this section is updated from the original prepublication version.

on Nutrition (FDA, 1988). The most recent edition of the AAP nutrition handbook indicates that the energy density of human milk varies depending upon the mother, time of day, and fraction of milk (foremilk versus hind milk), and states that the energy density of preterm and term human milk is approximately 67 kcal/dL (20 kcal/oz) at 21 days of lactation (AAP, 2014).

Findings from a systematic review suggest adequate growth during infancy and early childhood with energy concentrations slightly below historical U.S. standards (Abrams et al., 2015). However, the six intervention studies included in this review were heterogeneous in design and did not follow participants past early childhood. The studies cited in Abrams et al. (2015) did not report the amount of formula consumed by the infants, so it is not possible to ascertain whether or not infants compensated for the lower energy density by increasing the amount of formula consumed. The AAP states that infants appear to satisfy energy needs by increasing the intake of foods if the diet is low in energy density (AAP, 2014). Therefore, one potential outcome of lower-energy density formulas is an increase in the cost of formula feeding without other benefits.

In summary, although there is some shorter-term evidence that lower-energy (19 kcal/oz) formulas promote adequate growth in infants, these products lack the extensive history of proven safe use and long-term outcomes associated with formulas containing 20 kcal/oz. Additional research is needed to assess long-term effects of infant formulas that are lower in energy density. The current WIC regulation therefore remains unchanged.

OTHER FOOD SPECIFICATIONS AND OPTIONS

Total Sugars in Breakfast Cereals

The current specification for WIC-approved ready-to-eat (RTE) cereals was unchanged, and remains 6 grams of sucrose and other sugars per dry ounce (USDA/FNS, 2014). RTE cereals have been reported to contribute between 3 and 8 percent of total added sugars intakes in various subgroups of the U.S. population (Reedy and Krebs-Smith, 2010; Huth et al., 2013; Keast et al., 2013; Drewnowski and Rehm, 2014; USDA/HHS, 2015) and approximately 8 percent of added sugars in the diets of low-income children (Reedy and Krebs-Smith, 2010).[3] This is more than the contribution of yogurts, but a relatively small amount compared to soft drinks and sodas (up to 33 percent [Huth et al., 2013]), grain-based desserts (up to 14 percent [Huth et al., 2013]), and other sugary foods and candies (up to 31 percent [USDA/HHS, 2015]).

---

[3] Low income was defined as between 131 and 185 percent of poverty. Data are from 2003–2004 NHANES, children ages 2 to 18 years.

RTE cereals are a dietary staple and a popular food, they are significant contributors to micronutrient intakes in the U.S. population (see Fulgoni and Buckley, 2015), are a source of whole-grains, and may promote the consumption of milk (Hill et al., 2012; Michels et al., 2016) and the associated vitamins D (Hill et al., 2012) or A (Affenito et al., 2013). The committee's analysis of NHANES 2011–2012 data indicated a high prevalence of low intake of a number of micronutrients as well as whole-grains among WIC participants, both of which may be provided in fortified RTE cereals. Because fortified cereals are significant contributors to the overall micronutrient content of WIC food package grain foods, it is likely important to ensure the continuing palatability of RTE breakfast cereals. The 2015–2020 *Dietary Guidelines for Americans* (DGA) note that the inclusion of some added sugars in foods, including whole grain foods, is one way to maintain palatability (USDA/HHS, 2016).

Retaining Fortified RTE Breakfast Cereals

The committee received several comments that RTE cereals are not consumed in some cultures. Fortified RTE cereals offer higher concentrations of nearly all nutrients compared to other whole grain products, so were retained as a separate food category (see Table Q-1). Of particular importance to the WIC population are folate and iron, which are not required fortificants in whole grain products, but are typically added to RTE breakfast cereals. Therefore, the retention of fortified RTE cereals was considered important to support intake of these priority nutrients.

Requiring Lower-Sodium Options

Although sodium intakes exceed upper limits in all WIC population subgroups, lower-sodium options remain encouraged but not required. Lower-sodium options may be more expensive than their regular counterparts. In addition, availability of lower-sodium options may be limited in some areas, and may be difficult for smaller vendors to stock. Given these possibilities and the lack of evidence to support a low administrative burden of adding a sodium restriction, a requirement for lower-sodium products is not recommended.

Allowing 2% Milk for Women and Children

The committee received many comments related to the change in the Final Rule that disallowed issuance of 2% milk to children and women (see Appendix D). Emerging evidence suggest that dairy fat intake is not associated with obesity or body weight (Kratz et al., 2013; Keast et al., 2015),

TABLE Q-1 Contribution to Amounts of Selected Nutrients per Day, Considering Specific Selection Scenarios for Grains per Month (0.53 oz/d)

Currently Available Grains	Fiber gm	Added Sugar g	Calcium mg	Iron mg	Magnesium mg	Phosphorus mg	Potassium mg	Sodium mg	Vitamin C mg	Folate µg DFE	Vitamin A µg RAE	Vitamin D IU
RTE cereal, composite (refined and whole)[a]	1	2	27	5	10	38	43	58	2	164	74	15
Oat O's	1	0	61	5	17	73	97	75	3	108	150	21
Whole wheat bread	1	0	24	0	11	32	38	69	0	6	0	0
Corn tortillas	1	0	12	0	11	47	28	7	0	16	0	0
Instant oatmeal, fortified	2	0	53	4	19	64	55	33	0	5	117	0
Whole-wheat pasta	1	0	4	1	19	52	66	1	0	10	—	0
Brown rice	1	0	5	0	22	40	41	1	0	3	0	0
Possible new grains												
Corn meal	1	0	1	1	19	36	43	5	0	4	2	0
Teff (grain)	1	0	27	1	28	65	65	2	—	—	0	—
Corn masa flour[b]	1	0	21	1	14	35	40	1	0	51	2	0
Buckwheat groats	2	0	3	0	35	52	70	0	0	5	0	0

NOTES: This table was generated as a means of comparing nutrient contributions of the same quantity of various grains on a per day basis. The unit applied is 16 oz per month because this is the maximum allowance of grains provided in the current WIC food packages. RTE = ready-to-eat.

[a] The cereal composite includes the top most commonly selected RTE cereals based on redemption data provided by states.

[b] Assumes 0.7 mg of folic acid added per pound of corn masa flour, or 475 µg DFE for corn tortillas, based on the new FDA Final Rule for voluntary addition of folic acid to corn masa flour and a typical tortilla recipe. Results do not account for losses during baking, estimated to be 20 percent (DSM, 2016).

SOURCE: USDA/ARS, 2016.

body mass index (Scharft et al., 2013), or metabolic health (Kratz et al., 2013) (see the phase I report [NASEM, 2016] for additional details). In the phase I report, the committee noted that the 2015 Dietary Guidelines Advisory Committee (DGAC) did not review this topic because studies evaluating the differential effects of dairy fat were just appearing in the published literature at the close of DGAC deliberations (personal communication, A. Lichtenstein, Tufts University, to the committee in their workshop held on March 12, 2015). The specifications for the fat content of milk in food packages IV through VII are unchanged for two reasons: (1) because the DGA continue to advise consumption of low-fat dairy products, and (2) because the committee was tasked by U.S. Department of Agriculture's Food and Nutrition Service (USDA-FNS) to align the WIC food packages with the DGA, which recommend fat-free or low-fat dairy for individuals 2 years of age and older. Furthermore, fat-free and low-fat dairy are the standard for other federal feeding programs including the Child and Adult Care Feeding Program (CACFP) (USDA/FNS, 2011) and the National School Nutrition Program (USDA/FNS, 2016), which includes school breakfast and lunch. The committee considered it important to provide a consistent message to children and families about the recommendations for fat in milk.

Individuals who commented had a preference for 2% milk, did not believe it was detrimental to health, and/or were concerned that the change was resulting in lower milk redemption and consumption by WIC participants. Data from Texas milk sales indicated that by 2015, there was a 17 percent drop in milk redemption compared to when 2% milk was allowed. This decrease was more than four times higher than the decline in WIC participation over the same time period (3 percent) (C. Frye, International Dairy Foods Association, as commented to the committee in their workshop held on March 31, 2016). National data were not available to permit the committee to evaluate changes in milk redemption before and after the October 1, 2014, change from up-to-2% milks to lower-fat milks. Should future DGA change the recommendation on fat levels of milk, or should conclusive evidence on the differential health effects of dairy fat compared to other types of saturated fats become available, USDA-FNS or a future committee may reconsider the requirement that fluid milk be fat free or low fat for children and women.

Vitamin D Fortification of Yogurts

Vitamin D is a DGA nutrient of public health concern, and vitamin D status was poor among women participating in WIC. Although some yogurts available in the marketplace are fortified with vitamin D, moving to near universal voluntary fortification (as is the case for milk) may improve vitamin D status of WIC participants (and the U.S. population broadly).

When market data indicate an increased availability of vitamin D-fortified yogurts that meet other WIC product specifications and cost requirements, it may be prudent to consider requiring that WIC-approved yogurts be fortified with vitamin D.

Allowing 100% Whole Grain Options Other Than Whole Wheat Bread

Although 100 percent whole grain breads other than wheat are available in the marketplace, identification of these products is complicated by the fact that some products labeled as "whole grain," may contain some proportion of whole grain or may be 100 percent whole grain (Oldways Whole Grain Council, 2017). Clear guidance and further investigation of the ability of WIC staff and participants to identify 100 percent whole grain products other than 100 percent whole wheat bread would facilitate the decision to expand the options for this WIC food category.

Further Reductions in Legumes and Peanut Butter

As noted in the report, available package sizes limited the degree to which these WIC foods could be further reduced without increasing cost because of turning to uncommonly available sizes. Further reductions in these items (mainly for children) may be possible with increasing availability of smaller package sizes with a proportional price reduction. Evaluation of the response of WIC participants to the initial reduction proposed in this review would also inform further changes.

Additional Fish Species and Wild Salmon

In addition to considering the inclusion of fish in additional food packages, USDA-FNS requested that the committee consider the inclusion of additional fish species, and the inclusion of wild salmon. Fish species currently allowed by the Final Rule in food package VII may be light tuna, salmon, sardines, and mackerel, and states are required to make at least two options available to participants (USDA/FNS, 2014).

The committee's requirements for expanding this list of approved species included: availability in a shelf-stable form (i.e., canned), nationwide availability, appropriate nutrient contribution (considering sodium and provision of omega-3 fatty acids), low in contaminants of particular relevance to growth and development, in a price range that permits cost-neutral adjustments to the food packages, and a likelihood of redemption and consumption. Considering these requirements, the committee did not identify fish species appropriate for addition to food packages other than those already permitted. Therefore, fish options continue to be at least two of light tuna, salmon, sardines, and mackerel.

Although a small amount of farmed salmon is marketed as canned, most canned salmon is wild,[4] removing the option to easily distinguish the two. Additionally, there is currently no requirement to label canned salmon as wild or farmed, so it may not be possible for state agencies to differentiate.[5] Finally, the committee did not find a substantial difference in risk–benefit for consumption of farmed compared to wild salmon (EPA/TERA, 1999; Foran et al., 2005; Health Canada, 2007; IOM, 2007; FAO/WHO, 2010; Loring et al., 2010; Sirot et al., 2012; FDA, 2014; USDA/HHS, 2015).

Substitutions: Cases Without Nutritionally Comparable Options

Milk Alternatives Other Than Soy Beverage

The committee considered inclusion of nonsoy milk alternatives such as almond, rice, or coconut milks. They were not considered suitable substitutes for milk because most such products do not confer the same key nutrients that the currently allowable milks or soy beverage are intended to supply, namely calcium, vitamin A, and vitamin D (USDA/ARS, 2016).

Fish and Vegans or Vegetarians

Although fish is not compatible with vegan or vegetarian diets, fish is included in the revised food packages specifically to provide long-chain omega-3 fatty acids. The committee did not identify another food that could supply this nutrient that also met the criteria for wide availability and nonperishability that also met cost-constraints. Therefore, no substitution is offered for fish in the food packages.

Jarred Infant Food Meat Substitutions

Similar to fish in food packages for women and children, jarred infant food meat plays a very specific nutritional role in the food packages, that being to serve as a source of highly bioavailable iron and zinc. The committee explored other options including legume-based infant foods, canned legumes, eggs, and mixed dinners. Iron bioavailability of legumes is approximately 2 percent owing to the non-heme form and presence of iron absorption inhibitors such as phytates (IOM, 2001). This is in contrast to the 40 percent absorption rate of iron from heme-containing foods (IOM,

---

[4] Personal Communication, National Fisheries Institute, December 9, 2015.

[5] The FDA requirement is that labels be truthful and not misleading, but a label specification for canned fish as wild or farmed is not currently required.

2001). Boiled eggs contain at least as much iron per ounce-equivalent as infant food meats (USDA/ARS, 2016). However, infant food meats contain a combination of heme and non-heme iron, while eggs contain only non-heme iron, the less bioavailable of the two forms (IOM, 2001).

The committee considered inclusion of infant meat dinners (which contain meat and vegetables), but similarly, the quantity of iron per ounce and/or the bioavailability of iron is significantly lower compared to single-ingredient products. Infants would need to consume an unreasonably large amount of legume-based or infant dinner products to achieve the same amount of iron intake in an equivalent volume of jarred infant food meats. Therefore, it was economically not feasible to provide the same amount of iron using these alternatives.

Food Package III: Substitutions for Restricted Diets or Cases in Which Human Milk Fortifier Is Needed

The committee received several comments about situations in which participants have medical conditions with very specific nutritional implications, such as in cases where an infant or child is required to follow a very-low protein diet and an exempt formula is needed, but other foods in the WIC packages are not suitable. While participants may feel short-changed on the quantity of items provided, the value of the special formulas is generally much higher than that of the food in the packages. It is also reiterated in this report that as for the current food packages, the revised food packages do not require issuance of foods that are not in alignment with the participant's prescribed diet. The committee received several comments related to the issuance of human milk fortifier (HMF) through WIC; however, there is no universal agreement on the use of this product (see, e.g., Zachariassen et al., 2011; Kreissl et al., 2013; Lafeber, 2013; Teller et al., 2016). HMF is needed only in very rare cases, and often human milk can be fortified with powdered infant formula for these medically fragile infants.

REFERENCES

AAP (American Academy of Pediatrics). 2014. *Pediatric nutrition.* 7th ed. Edited by R. E. Kleinman and F. R. Greer. Elk Grove Village, IL: American Academy of Pediatrics.

Abbott Nutrition. 2015. *Similac: Knowing means growing.* http://static.abbottnutrition.com/cms-prod/similac.com/img/sim-optigro-faq.pdf (accessed December 21, 2016).

Abrams, S. A., K. M. Hawthorne, and M. Pammi. 2015. A systematic review of controlled trials of lower-protein or energy-containing infant formulas for use by healthy full-term infants. *Advances in Nutrition* 6(2):178–188.

Affenito, S. G., D. Thompson, A. Dorazio, A. M. Albertson, A. Loew, and N. M. Holschuh. 2013. Ready-to-eat cereal consumption and the school breakfast program: Relationship to nutrient intake and weight. *Journal of School Health* 83(1):28–35.

Drewnowski, A., and C. D. Rehm. 2014. Consumption of added sugars among US children and adults by food purchase location and food source. *American Journal of Clinical Nutrition* 100(3):901–907.

DSM. 2016. *Fortification basics: Stability*. https://www.dsm.com/content/dam/dsm/nip/en_US/documents/stability.pdf (accessed October 18, 2016).

EPA/TERA (U.S. Environmental Protection Agency/Toxicology Excellence for Risk Assessment). 1999. *Comparative dietary risks: Balancing the risks and benefits of fish consumption*. http://www.tera.org/Publications/CDR%20Front%20Matter.pdf (accessed December 21, 2016).

FAO/WHO (Food and Agriculture Organization/World Health Organization). 2010. *Joint FAO/WHO expert consultation on the risks and benefits of fish consumption*. http://www.fao.org/docrep/014/ba0136e/ba0136e00.pdf (accessed December 21, 2016).

FDA (U.S. Food and Drug Administration). 1988. *Clinical testing of infant formulas with respect to nutritional suitability for term infants*. http://www.fda.gov/Food/GuidanceRegulation/GuidanceDocumentsRegulatoryInformation/InfantFormula/ucm170649.htm (accessed December 22, 2016).

FDA. 2014. *Fish: What pregnant women and parents should know*. http://www.fda.gov/food/foodborneillnesscontaminants/metals/ucm393070.htm (accessed December 22, 2016).

Foran, J. A., D. H. Good, D. O. Carpenter, M. C. Hamilton, B. A. Knuth, and S. J. Schwager. 2005. Quantitative analysis of the benefits and risks of consuming farmed and wild salmon. *Journal of Nutrition* 135(11):2639–2643.

Fulgoni, V. L., and R. B. Buckley. 2015. The contribution of fortified ready-to-eat cereal to vitamin and mineral intake in the U.S. population, NHANES 2007–2010. *Nutrients* 7(6):3949–3958.

Health Canada. 2007. *Human health risk assessment of mercury in fish and health benefits of fish consumption*. http://www.hc-sc.gc.ca/fn-an/pubs/mercur/merc_fish_poisson-eng.php (accessed December 22, 2016).

Hill, K. M., S. S. Jonnalagadda, A. M. Albertson, N. A. Joshi, and C. M. Weaver. 2012. Top food sources contributing to vitamin D intake and the association of ready-to-eat cereal and breakfast consumption habits to vitamin D intake in Canadians and United States Americans. *Journal of Food Science* 77(8):H170–H175.

Huth, P. J., V. L. Fulgoni, D. R. Keast, K. Park, and N. Auestad. 2013. Major food sources of calories, added sugars, and saturated fat and their contribution to essential nutrient intakes in the U.S. diet: Data from the National Health and Nutrition Examination Survey (2003–2006). *Nutrition Journal* 12:116.

IOM (Institute of Medicine). 2001. *Dietary Reference Intakes for vitamin A, vitamin K, arsenic, boron, chromium, copper, iodine, iron, manganese, molybdenum, nickel, silicon, vanadium, and zinc*. Washington, DC: National Academy Press.

IOM. 2006. *WIC food packages: Time for a change*. Washington, DC: The National Academies Press.

IOM. 2007. *Seafood choices: Balancing benefits and risks*. Washington, DC: The National Academies Press.

Keast, D. R., V. L. Fulgoni, 3rd, T. A. Nicklas, and C. E. O'Neil. 2013. Food sources of energy and nutrients among children in the United States: National Health and Nutrition Examination Survey 2003–2006. *Nutrients* 5(1):283–301.

Keast, D. R., K. M. Hill Gallant, A. M. Albertson, C. K. Gugger, and N. M. Holschuh. 2015. Associations between yogurt, dairy, calcium, and vitamin D intake and obesity among U.S. children aged 8–18 years: NHANES, 2005–2008. *Nutrients* 7(3):1577–1593.

Kratz, M., T. Baars, and S. Guyenet. 2013. The relationship between high-fat dairy consumption and obesity, cardiovascular, and metabolic disease. *European Journal of Nutrition* 52(1):1–24.

Kreissl, A., V. Zwiauer, A. Repa, C. Binder, N. Haninger, B. Jilma, A. Berger, and N. Haiden. 2013. Effect of fortifiers and additional protein on the osmolarity of human milk: Is it still safe for the premature infant? *Journal of Pediatric Gastroenterology and Nutrition* 57(4):432–437.

Lafeber, H. N. 2013. Fortification of human milk fed to preterm infants: Are our guidelines safe? *Journal of Pediatric Gastroenterology and Nutrition* 57(4):414.

Loring, P. A., L. K. Duffy, and M. S. Murray. 2010. A risk-benefit analysis of wild fish consumption for various species in Alaska reveals shortcomings in data and monitoring needs. *Science of the Total Environment* 408(20):4532–4541.

Michels, N., S. De Henauw, L. Beghin, M. Cuenca-Garcia, M. Gonzalez-Gross, L. Hallstrom, A. Kafatos, M. Kersting, Y. Manios, A. Marcos, D. Molnar, R. Roccaldo, A. M. Santaliestra-Pasias, M. Sjostrom, B. Reye, F. Thielecke, K. Widhalm, and M. Claessens. 2016. Ready-to-eat cereals improve nutrient, milk and fruit intake at breakfast in European adolescents. *European Journal of Nutrition* 55(2):771–779.

NASEM (National Academies of Sciences, Engineering, and Medicine). 2016. *Review of WIC food packages: Proposed framework for revisions: Interim report.* Washington, DC: The National Academies Press. doi: 10.17226/21832.

Oldways Whole Grain Council. 2017. *Identifying whole grain products.* https://wholegrainscouncil.org/whole-grains-101/identifying-whole-grain-products (accessed March 15, 2017).

Reedy, J., and S. M. Krebs-Smith. 2010. Dietary sources of energy, solid fats, and added sugars among children and adolescents in the United States. *Journal of the American Dietetic Association* 110(10):1477–1484.

Scharf, R. J., R. T. Demmer, and M. D. DeBoer. 2013. Longitudinal evaluation of milk type consumed and weight status in preschoolers. *Archives of Disease in Childhood* 98(5):335–340.

Sirot, V., J. C. Leblanc, and I. Margaritis. 2012. A risk-benefit analysis approach to seafood intake to determine optimal consumption. *British Journal of Nutrition* 107(12):1812–1822.

Teller, I. C., N. D. Embleton, I. J. Griffin, and R. M. van Elburg. 2016. Post-discharge formula feeding in preterm infants: A systematic review mapping evidence about the role of macronutrient enrichment. *Clinical Nutrition* 35(4):791–801.

USDA/ARS (U.S. Department of Agriculture/Agriculture Research Service). 2016. *USDA National Nutrient Database for Standard Reference, release 28.* http://www.ars.usda.gov/ba/bhnrc/ndl (accessed September 14, 2016).

USDA/FNS (U.S. Department of Agriculture/Food and Nutrition Service). 2011. *Policy memorandum CACFP 21-2011-revised: Child nutrition reauthorization 2010: Nutrition requirements for fluid milk and fluid milk substitutions in the child and adult care food program, questions and answers.* Alexandria, VA: USDA/FNS.

USDA/FNS. 2013. *WIC policy memorandum #2014-1 to WIC state agency directors: Changes to Abbott infant formula product line.* Alexandria, VA: USDA/FNS.

USDA/FNS. 2014. *Special Supplemental Nutrition Program for Women, Infants and Children (WIC): Revisions in the WIC food packages.* Final Rule, 7 C.F.R. § 246.

USDA/FNS. 2016. *School meals.* http://www.fns.usda.gov/school-meals/nutrition-standards-school-meals (accessed July 13, 2016).

USDA/HHS (U.S. Department of Agriculture/U.S. Department of Health and Human Services). 2015. The report of the Dietary Guidelines Advisory Committee on the Dietary Guidelines for Americans, 2015, to the secretary of agriculture and the secretary of health and human services. http://www.health.gov/dietaryguidelines/2015-scientific-report/PDFs/Scientific-Report-of-the-2015-Dietary-Guidelines-Advisory-Committee.pdf (accessed December 22, 2016).

USDA/HHS. 2016. *Dietary Guidelines for Americans 2015–2020.* https://health.gov/dietaryguidelines/2015 (accessed August 29, 2016).

Zachariassen, G., J. Faerk, C. Grytter, B. H. Esberg, J. Hjelmborg, S. Mortensen, H. Thybo Christesen, and S. Halken. 2011. Nutrient enrichment of mother's milk and growth of very preterm infants after hospital discharge. *Pediatrics* 127(4):e995–e1003.

Appendix R

Development of the Food Package Nutrient and Cost Profiles

To develop the nutrient and cost profiles of the food packages that are evaluated in this report, the committee created a series of linked spreadsheets representing the current and revised sets of food packages. These spreadsheets allowed the committee to determine the average per-participant cost difference between the current and revised packages to meet the charge of cost-neutrality. The basis for these profiles was a set of detailed assumptions based on the U.S. Department of Agriculture's Food and Nutrition Service (USDA-FNS) price and redemption dataset, the Special Supplemental Nutrition Program for Women, Infants, and Children (WIC) Food Package Report series, and information provided by individual states. The assumptions applied to develop composites for WIC food categories included ratios of substitution options based on available data or a conservative assumption. Assumptions also differed for some WIC food categories depending on the food package. All details are included in the tables that follow. Details related to costs at the program level are provided in Chapter 10, "The Regulatory Impact Analysis." Spreadsheets generated for this report were reviewed by the committee members, as well as internally cross-checked by staff. The regulatory impact analyses used the revised package data, with the base year of 2015 as the starting point, and therefore re-created the revised package cost profiles and compared them to the profiles that were created for the cost-neutral assessment.

TABLES

TABLE R-1 Cost Data and Assumptions Used in Analyses of Current and Revised Food Packages for Women and Children

Food Category	Cost per Unit	Data Source	Assumptions
Juice	$0.05/oz	FNS redemption data*	CPI inflation factor to 2015: 1.0085
Milk and milk alternatives	Fat-free and 1% milk: $0.82/qt	FNS redemption data*	CPI inflation factor to 2015: 0.9826
	Whole milk: $0.86/qt	FNS redemption data*	
	Soy milk: $1.82/qt	FNS redemption data*	
	Lactose-free milk: $1.63/qt	FNS redemption data*	
	Yogurt, lowfat: $3.22/qt	IRI 2014 qt-size yogurt	CPI inflation factor to 2015: 0.9960
	Yogurt, whole milk: $3.22/qt	IRI 2014 qt-size yogurt	
	Cheese: $5.33/lb	FNS redemption data*	
	Weighted mean, lowfat milk: $0.84/qt Weighted mean, whole milk: $0.87/qt	Quart prices for milk calculated by dividing gallon prices by 4	Lowfat milk weighting: 1% milk: 93% Nonfat milk: 4% Soymilk: 1% Lactose-free milk: 1% Tofu: <1% Whole milk weighting: Whole milk: 98% Lactose-free milk: 1% Tofu: <1%
	Current composite food package mean costs assuming full cheese/yogurt substitution: FP IV-A: $1.19 FP IV-B: $1.16 FP V: $1.08 FP VI: $1.16 FP VII: $1.06		FP IV-A uses weighted whole milk cost; all other packages use weighted lowfat milk cost.
	Revised composite food package mean costs assuming full cheese/yogurt substitution: FP IV-A: $1.29 FP IV-B: $1.20		Composite food package milk and milk alternative costs are weighted assuming maximum allowable substitutions of cheese and yogurt

continued

TABLE R-1 Continued

Food Category	Cost per Unit	Data Source	Assumptions
	FP V: $1.15 FP VI: $1.15 FP VII: $1.16		This is a conservative estimate; no data are available on substitution rate
Breakfast cereal	Current (redeemed cereals): $0.21/oz Revised (all whole grain): $0.23/oz	FNS redemption data*	CPI inflation factor to 2015: 1.0060
Cheese	$5.33/lb	FNS redemption data*	CPI inflation factor to 2015: 1.0390
Eggs	$2.17/dozen	FNS redemption data*	CPI inflation factor to 2015: 1.1576
Whole wheat bread and alternatives	Current: $2.35/lb	FNS redemption data*	Bread CPI inflation factor to 2015: 1.0061
	Revised: Whole wheat bread: $2.65/24 oz Corn tortillas: $2.26/24 oz Instant oatmeal: $4.14/24 oz Weighted mean cost: $2.67/24 oz	IRI 2014 calendar year for 24 oz container sizes	Bread alternatives CPI inflation factor to 2015: 1.0037
Canned fish	$0.20/oz	FNS redemption data*	CPI inflation factor to 2015: 1.0123
Legumes and peanut butter	Peanut butter: $2.29/18 oz jar	FNS redemption data*	CPI inflation factor to 2015: 0.9828
	Canned beans: $4.06 per 4 cans (4 cans substitute for 1 lb dry)	FNS redemption data*	CPI inflation factor to 2015: 1.0026
	Dry beans: $1.50/lb	FNS redemption data*	CPI inflation factor to 2015: 1.0471

Current: Weighted mean cost (weighted average of peanut butter and weighted legumes): $2.45 Unweighted mean cost (average of peanut butter and weighted legumes): $2.37	Current: legumes versus peanut butter: Legumes: 50% Peanut butter: 50%
Revised: Weighted mean cost (weighted average of peanut butter and weighted legumes): $2.48 Unweighted mean cost (average of peanut butter and weighted legumes): $2.43	Revised: Weighted mean of peanut butter and legumes used for FP V, VI, and VII (participants receive a 3-month rotation of legumes, legumes, peanut butter) Unweighted mean of peanut butter and legumes used for FP IV (participants receive a 3-month rotation of legumes, peanut butter, nothing)
	Current canned versus dry weighting: Canned: 37% Dry: 63% From six states average redemption*
	Revised canned versus dry weighting: Canned: 42% Dry: 58% 5% shift of dry to canned due to recommendation that states allow more canned options

continued

TABLE R-1 Continued

Food Category	Cost per Unit	Data Source	Assumptions
Fruit and vegetable composite (CVV)	\$0.55/c-eq	2013 ERS data on fruit and vegetable prices, updated with CPI adjustment to 2015	CPI inflation factor to 2015: 1.0380

NOTES: c-eq = cup equivalent; CPI = Consumer Price Index; CVV = cash value voucher; ERS = USDA's Economic Research Service; FNS = USDA's Food and Nutrition Service; FP = food package; IRI = Information Resources, Inc.,` Consumer Network data 2014; PC = WIC Participant and Program Characteristics Report. Food costs were found to be comparable to those reported in the fiscal year (FY) 2010 WIC Food Cost Report (USDA/FNS, 2013).

* FNS redemption data: The average prices of WIC foods redeemed in six states (Personal communication, K. Castellanos-Brown, USDA-FNS, April 7, 2016, and June 30, 2016) were adjusted for inflation to an average price for FY2015. The six-state prices provided were an average over the fiscal year August 2013 to July 2014. It was therefore assumed that the six-state average price was equivalent to the price for January 2014, the approximate midpoint of the August 2013 to July 2014 12-month period. This assumption is approximately equal to assuming the average of the nominal prices for the August to July 12-month period is equal to the price from redemption data. The average January 2014 price was then inflated to the average price for fiscal year 2015 using U.S. Bureau of Labor Statistics (BLS) CPI adjustments (see http://data.bls.gov/cgi-bin/dsrv?cu [accessed December 22, 2016]). This procedure was carried out using the FNS average prices for juice, milk, cheese, breakfast cereal, eggs, whole wheat bread and alternatives, canned fish, legumes, peanut butter, jarred infant fruits and vegetables, jarred infant food meat, and infant cereal. CPI inflation factors were matched to the closest BLS food category for each item.

TABLE R-2 Cost Data and Assumptions Used in Analyses of Current and Revised Food Packages for Infants

Food Category	Cost per Unit	Data Source	Assumptions
Formula	CPI-adjusted cost per prepared fl oz of formula without rebate: Powder: \$0.18/fl oz Liquid concentrate: \$0.19/fl oz Ready-to-feed: \$0.23/fl oz	Prescription percentages from PC 2014 Food Package Report Table II.2, which uses PC 2014 participant characteristics data. Scaled to 100%	Composite formula costs are weighted by form: Powder: 77.9% Liquid concentrate: 11.8% Ready-to-feed: 10.3% Using prescription percentages, assuming 100% redemption and use
	CPI-adjusted cost per prepared fl oz of formula with rebate: Powder: \$0.06/fl oz Liquid concentrate: \$0.07/fl oz Ready-to-feed: \$0.08/fl oz Composite formula cost with rebate: \$0.07/fl oz	IRI Consumer Network data 2014 Dilutions and preparation of formula: FNS WIC Works and Mead Johnson websites Source for % rebate: WIC Food Cost FY 2010 Report, Table 4	Before CPI-adjustment cost per *unprepared* ounce of formula: Powder: \$1.32/oz Liquid concentrate: \$0.38/oz Ready-to-feed: \$0.23/oz CPI-U inflation factor to 2015: 0.999965 Powder reconstitution: 12.9 oz powder per 94 fl oz Liquid concentrate reconstitution: 1:1 dilution at 20 kcal/fl oz (standard dilution) Rebate percentage: 64.58% Food package III infant formula costs include nonexempt only and are assumed to equal FP I and II infant formula costs

continued

TABLE R-2 Continued

Food Category	Cost per Unit	Data Source	Assumptions
Infant food cereal	$0.26/oz	FNS redemption data*	CPI inflation factor to 2015: 1.0110
Infant food vegetable and fruit composite	$0.16/oz	FNS redemption data*	A substitution of 1 banana per 4 oz of jarred infant fruits and vegetables is a currently available option that covers 30% of WIC participants (USDA/FNS, 2015). The effect of this substitution on cost was considered and calculated to be nominal; therefore, the substitution is omitted in the current food package cost estimate CPI inflation factor to 2015: 1.0110
Infant food meats	$0.40/oz	FNS redemption data*	CPI inflation factor to 2015: 1.0110

NOTES: CPI = Consumer Price Index; FP = food package; PC = WIC Participant and Program Characteristics Report. Values were multiplied by a redemption factor, based on FNS redemption data for current packages and projected values for revised packages (see Table R-5). Food costs based on redemption were found to be comparable to those reported in the FY 2010 WIC Food Cost Report (USDA/FNS, 2013). Note that the maximum amount of formula was assumed for the purpose of these analyses, although USDA/FNS supports provision of the least amount of formula possible or that is needed.

* FNS redemption data: The six-state average prices (Personal communication, K. Castellanos-Brown, USDA-FNS, April 7, 2016, and June 30, 2016) were adjusted for inflation to an average price for FY2015. The six-state prices provided were an average over the fiscal year August 2013 to July 2014. It was therefore assumed that the six-state average price was equivalent to the price for January 2014, the approximate midpoint of the August 2013 to July 2014 12-month period. This assumption is approximately equal to assuming the average of the nominal prices for the August to July 12-month period is equal to the price from redemption data. The average January 2014 price was then inflated to the average price for fiscal year 2015 using U.S. Bureau of Labor Statistics (BLS) CPI adjustments (see http://data.bls.gov/cgi-bin/dsrv?cu [accessed March 10, 2017]). CPI inflation factors were matched to the closest BLS food category for each item.

TABLE R-3 Assumptions Used in Nutrient Analyses of Current and Revised Food Packages for Infants

Food Category	Weighting and Assumptions*	Rationale	Products Included	NDB No.
Formula	Type weighting: Milk-based: 64.9% Soy-based: 19.0% Lactose-free: 11.6% Hydrolysate: 4.5%	Prescription percentages from PC 2014 Food Package Report Exhibit FP1, which uses PC 2008 participant characteristics data. Percentages in the report did not add to 100% as infants can be prescribed more than one type of formula. These percentages were scaled to 100% for weighting	Powder, routine: Enfamil Premium Infant Similac Advance Gerber Good Start Gentle Powder, soy: Enfamil ProSobee Isomil Advance Soy Gerber Good Start Soy	 33877 03950 33868 03826 03954 33872
	Assumes prescription equals redemption	Overall redemption of infant formula was 97% according to five states average redemption	Powder, milk-based lactose-free: Similac for Spit-Up Powder, hydrolysate Similac Expert Care Alimentum	 03999 03957
	Brand weighting: Mead Johnson: 43.7% Abbott: 42.7% Nestle-Gerber: 13.6%	WIC infant formula brand shares for 2015, determined by dividing total number of infants under each contract (obtained from state contracts with manufacturers) by total number of infants participating in WIC (obtained from USDA/FNS website) for each formula manufacturer	Ready-to-feed, routine: Enfamil Premium Infant Similac Advance Gerber Good Start Gentle Ready-to-feed, soy: Enfamil ProSobee Isomil Advance Soy Gerber Good Start Soy Ready-to-feed, milk-based lactose-free:	 33876 03949 03989 03823 03953 03987
	Form weighting: Powder: 77.9% Liquid concentrate: 11.8% Ready-to-feed: 10.3%	Prescription percentages from PC 2014 Food Package Report Table II.2, which uses PC 2014 participant characteristics data. Scaled to 100%.	Similac for Spit-Up Ready-to-feed, hydrolysate Similac Expert Care Alimentum	03993 03846

continued

TABLE R-3 Continued

Food Category	Weighting and Assumptions*	Rationale	Products Included	NDB No.
	Infants 0–3 months: Composite powder formula weighted by type and brand	Powder form is recommended for partially breastfed infants 0–3 months in the Final Rule	Liquid concentrate, routine:	
			Enfamil Premium Infant	33865
	All other infants: Composite formula weighted by type, brand, and form		Liquid concentrate, soy:	
			Enfamil ProSobee	03854
			Isomil Advance Soy	03952
			Gerber Good Start Soy	03966
			Liquid concentrate, milk-based lactose-free	
			Similac Sensitive	03947
	Estimates used the specified maximum monthly allowance (MMA) ounces in the Final Rule	In alignment with foods across other WIC food packages, the maximum monthly allowance multiplied by redemption was assumed in the absence of data on issuance		
	Powder scoop to liquid conversion: 1 scoop + 2 oz water = 2.2 fl oz prepared formula	Mead Johnson website		
	Liquid concentrate to prepared form conversion: 1-to-1 dilution at 20 kcal/fl oz (standard dilution)	Mead Johnson and Abbott Nutrition websites		
Infant food cereal	Oatmeal: 38% Rice: 39% Whole wheat/multigrain: 23%	Wyoming and Massachusetts redemption data, 2015	Infant food cereal, oatmeal, dry, fortified	03189
			Infant food cereal, brown rice, dry, instant	42285
			Infant food whole wheat/ multigrain, dry, fortified	03996

Infant food, fruits	Applesauce: 28% Banana: 27% Peach: 18% Pear: 18% Prunes: 9%	Wyoming and Massachusetts redemption data, 2015	Applesauce Banana Peach Pear Prunes	03116 43546 03130 03132 03139
Infant food, vegetables	Carrots: 23% Green beans: 8% Peas: 15% Squash: 23% Sweet potatoes: 31%	Wyoming and Massachusetts redemption data, 2015	Carrots Green beans Peas Squash Sweet potatoes	03099 03091 03121 03104 03108
Infant food, fruit and vegetable composite	Vegetable: 44.3% Fruit: 55.7%	Wyoming and Massachusetts redemption data, 2015		
Infant food, meats	Beef: 27% Chicken: 34% Turkey: 24% Ham: 15%	Wyoming, Chickasaw Nation, and Massachusetts redemption data, 2015	Beef Chicken Turkey Ham	03002 03012 03015 03008

NOTES: FNB = full nutrition benefit; NDB = National Nutrient Database for Standard Reference, Release 28 (USDA/ARS, 2016); PC = WIC Participant and Program Characteristics Report.

* State data were incorporated into weighting only when the committee judged the data to be reasonable and complete.

TABLE R-4 Assumptions Used in Nutrient Analyses of Current and Revised Food Packages for Women and Children

Food Category	Weighting and Assumptions[a]	Rationale	Products Included	NDB No.
Juice	Apple juice: 59% Orange juice: 11% Grape juice: 30%	Wyoming and Massachusetts redemption data, 2015	Apple juice, prepared from frozen concentrate, added vitamin C	09411
			Orange juice, prepared from frozen concentrate	09215
	Assumes women and children consume the same types of juice		Grape juice, canned or bottled, added vitamin C	09130
Milk and milk alternatives[b]	Mozzarella: 24% Natural cheddar: 34% Colby: 18% American: 24%	Average of Texas, Wyoming, and Massachusetts redemption data, 2015	Nonfat milk	01086
			1% milk	01083
			Whole milk	01077
			Soy milk	16139
			Lactose-free milk, 1%	N/A*
	Weighted low-fat yogurt: Vanilla: 70% Plain: 30%	Average of Texas and Massachusetts redemption data, 2015	Tofu	16426
			Yogurt, plain, low fat	01117
			Yogurt, vanilla, low fat	01119
			Yogurt, plain, whole milk	01116
	Weighted whole milk yogurt: Fruit: 70% Plain: 30%	Average of Texas and Massachusetts redemption data, 2015	Yogurt, fruit, whole milk	N/A*
			Cheese, mozzarella	01028
			Cheese, natural cheddar	01009
			Cheese, Colby	01011
	Weighted whole milk: Whole milk: 98% Lactose-free milk: 1%	Average of Texas redemption data July–August 2015 and Wyoming redemption data May 2015	*Used Supertracker for items not found in the NDB (lactose-free milk, fruited whole milk yogurt)	
	Soymilk: 1% weighted low-fat milk: 1% milk: 93% Nonfat milk: 4%	Average of Texas redemption data July–August 2015 and Wyoming redemption data May 2015		

Soymilk: 1% Lactose-free milk: 1% Children receiving IV-A: 30.4% Children receiving IV-B: 69.6%	Calculated from WIC PC 2014 Food Package Report (USDA/FNS, 2016) and FY2015 Monthly Data—State Level Participation by Category and Program Costs (FNS website)
Current FP IV-A (children 1 to <2 years receiving whole milk), per 16 qt: 12 qt weighted whole milk 1 lb cheese 1 qt whole milk yogurt Revised FP IV-A, per 12 qt: 8 qt weighted whole milk 1 lb cheese 1 qt whole milk yogurt	Current food packages: Assumed max substitution of yogurt and cheese (1 qt of yogurt for 1 qt of milk; 1 lb of cheese for 3 qt of milk or 2 lb of cheese for 6 qt of milk in baseline FP VII). This is a conservative estimate; no data are available on substitution rate
Current FP IV-B (children 2 to <5 years receiving low-fat milk), per 16 qt: 12 qt weighted low-fat milk 1 lb cheese 1 qt low-fat yogurt	Revised food packages: Assumed max substitution of yogurt and cheese. In the revised package, an additional quart of yogurt may substitute for 1 qt of milk while maintaining the milk substitution limit, presenting additional max substitution scenarios. All scenarios and weighting are described
Revised FP IV-B, per 14 qt (50%): 10 qt weighted low-fat milk	Revised FP IV-A: Given the high redemption rate and public

continued

TABLE R-4 Continued

Food Category	Weighting and Assumptions[a]	Rationale	Products Included	NDB No.
	1 lb cheese 1 qt low-fat yogurt OR (50%): 12 qt weighted low-fat milk 0 lb cheese 2 qt low-fat yogurt	feedback received about whole milk, the committee made the assumption that substitution of 2 qt of yogurt may not be a likely scenario for food package IV-A. The substitution scheme used in the weighting, therefore, only represents the cheese and yogurt pattern. This is the higher price substitution scenario, so cost differences for this food package are most likely conservative		
	Current FP V, per 22 qt: 18 qt weighted low-fat milk 1 lb cheese 1 qt low-fat yogurt			
	Revised FP V and VI, per 16 qt (50%): 12 qt weighted low-fat milk 1 lb cheese 1 qt low-fat yogurt OR (50%): 14 qt weighted low-fat milk 0 lb cheese 2 qt low-fat yogurt			
	Current FP VI, per 16 qt: 12 qt weighted low-fat milk 1 lb cheese 1 qt low-fat yogurt			

	Current FP VII, per 24 qt: 17 qt weighted low-fat milk 2 lbs cheese 1 qt low-fat yogurt Revised FP VII, per 16 qt (33.33%): 12 qt weighted low-fat milk 1 lb cheese 1 qt low-fat yogurt OR (33.33%): 14 qt weighted low-fat milk 0 lb cheese 2 qt low-fat yogurt OR (33.33%): 10 qt weighted low-fat milk 2 lb cheese 0 qt low-fat yogurt			
Breakfast cereal	Current: Honey Bunches of Oats, Almonds: 34% Cheerios (whole grain): 13% Corn Flakes: 10% Frosted Mini-Wheats (whole grain): 13% Kix: 8% Life (whole grain): 8% Rice Krispies: 9% Dora the Explorer: 6% Revised packages include whole grain cereals only	Average of Texas redemption data July–August 2015 and Wyoming redemption data May 2015 Cereals chosen for the profile represent the top five most redeemed cereals in Texas and Wyoming	Honey Bunches of Oats, Almonds Cheerios Corn Flakes Frosted Mini-Wheats Kix Life Rice Krispies Dora the Explorer	42240 08013 08020 08319 08048 08049 08065 08582

continued

TABLE R-4 Continued

Food Category	Weighting and Assumptions[a]	Rationale	Products Included	NDB No.
	Naturally occurring sugars per 18 oz subtracted from cereals to obtain added sugars: Oats: 7.65 g Wheat: 2.05 g Corn: 7.71 g Rice: 0.61 g			
Cheese	Mozzarella: 24% Natural cheddar: 34% Colby: 18% American: 24%	Average of Massachusetts, Texas, and Wyoming redemption data, 2015	Mozzarella Natural cheddar Colby American	01028 01009 01011 01042
Eggs	Large eggs		Large eggs	01123
Whole wheat bread and alternatives	Whole wheat bread: 76% Corn tortillas: 19% Instant oatmeal: 6% Note on folic acid in corn tortillas: A new federal rule (21 C.F.R. part 172) established on April 15, 2016, allows folic acid to be added to corn masa flour at a level not to exceed 0.7 milligrams of folic acid per pound of corn masa flour. The folic acid content in the nutrient profile for corn masa flour was thus recalculated from the value in the standard reference database assuming a corn tortilla recipe of	Average of Chickasaw Nation, Texas, and Wyoming redemption data, 2015	Whole wheat bread Corn tortillas Instant oatmeal, fortified	18075 18363 08122

	2 cups of masa per 1.5 cups of water. Assumes no loss of folic acid during cooking			
Canned fish	Tuna: 85% Salmon: 15%	Average of Massachusetts, Texas, and Wyoming redemption data, 2015	Tuna, light in water Salmon, pink	15121 15084
Legumes and peanut butter	Current: legumes and peanut butter weighting: Legumes: 50% Peanut butter: 50%	Specifically for FP IV and VI in which legumes OR peanut butter may be prescribed	Pinto beans, dry Black beans, dry Pinto beans, canned Black beans, canned Peanut butter	16042 16014 16146 16316 16098
	Revised: legumes and peanut butter weighting: Legumes: 67% Peanut butter: 33%	Weighted mean of peanut butter and legumes used for FP V, VI, and VII (participants receive a 3-month rotation of legumes, legumes, peanut butter) Unweighted mean of peanut butter and legumes used for FP IV (participants receive a 3-month rotation of legumes, peanut butter, nothing)		
	Current: canned versus dry beans weighting: Canned: 37% Dry: 63% Revised: canned versus dry weighting: Canned: 42% Dry: 58%	FNS redemption data		

continued

TABLE R-4 Continued

Food Category	Weighting and Assumptions[a]	Rationale	Products Included	NDB No.
	5% shift of dry to canned due to recommendation that states allow more canned options Bean type weighting: Pinto beans: 75% Black beans: 25%			
	Naturally occurring sugars per 18 oz peanuts subtracted from peanut butter to obtain added sugars: 21.3 g			
Fruits	Apples: 16% Bananas: 25% Watermelon: 8% Oranges: 9% Strawberries: 23% Grapes: 19%	Average of Texas redemption data July–August 2015, Wyoming redemption data May 2015, and Massachusetts redemption data June 2016. Assumes all fresh (no data available to determine percent of processed fruits redeemed).	Apples Bananas Watermelon Oranges Strawberries Grapes	09003 09040 09326 09200 09316 09131

Vegetables	Tomatoes: 31% Potatoes: 18% Avocados: 19% Peppers: 20% Lettuce: 12% No potato data in Wyoming; assumed to equal Texas % potato redemption	Average of Texas redemption data July–August 2015, Wyoming redemption data May 2015, and Massachusetts redemption data June 2016. Assumes all fresh (no data available to determine percent of processed vegetables redeemed)	Tomatoes Potatoes Avocados Peppers Lettuce	11529 11354 09037 11333 11253
Fruit and vegetable composite (CVV)	Vegetable: 33% Fruit: 67%	Texas WIC redemption, January 2016, Wyoming redemption data May 2015		

NOTES: CVV = cash value voucher; FP = food package; NDB = National Nutrient Database for Standard Reference, Release 28 (USDA/ARS, 2016); PC = WIC Participant and Program Characteristics Report.

[a] State data were incorporated into weighting only when the committee judged the data to be reasonable and complete.

[b] Weighting for milk and milk alternatives for each food package do not total to 1 due to the 1:3 substitution of cheese for milk.

DESCRIPTION OF METHOD FOR CALCULATING REDEMPTION RATES

Two sets of redemption rates were applied in the cost analysis: rates for the current set of food packages and rates for the revised set of food packages. The primary data source for the current package redemption rates was data provided to the committee by USDA-FNS (herein referenced as the FNS redemption data) (personal communication, K. Castellanos-Brown, USDA-FNS, April 7, 2016 and June 30, 2016). The FNS redemption data included 12 months (August 2013 through July 2014) of price and redemption data from a convenience sample of six WIC state agencies, representing five of the seven regions of the country. The identity of the agencies was not known to the committee.[1] Redemption rates were available for the following WIC foods: juice, breakfast cereal, whole grains, CVV, eggs, legumes/peanut butter, and fish. For foods for which redemption data were not available in the FNS redemption dataset, redemption rates were calculated as the average (unweighted) from several states that provided the committee with information (see Chapter 2, Table 2-14). Together, these sources resulted in a consensus list of redemption rates that were applied to develop the current food package nutrient and cost profiles.

Redemption rates for milk were a special case. The FNS redemption dataset did not include a separate redemption rate for whole milk. Considering that redemption might be different for milk in food package IV-A (because of the different fat level of the product, and the different age group of children), the average redemption rate from three states of 75 percent was applied to the current food package IV-A. For low-fat milk, the average redemption rate from the FNS redemption data was 65 percent. This represented average redemption of low-fat milk for women and children, combined. The difference in redemption rates for whole milk and low-fat milk, in combination with the committee's data on dairy intake of children and women, suggested that redemption rates may be higher for children ages 2 to less than 5 years, compared to women. The group average rate of 65 percent redemption for low-fat milk was decomposed into values of 71 percent for children ages 2 to less than 5 and 56 percent for women, rates that were consistent with the observed 65 percent redemption when

[1] To keep maintain anonymity of the state agencies, USDA-FNS inputted average monthly participation by participant category for each state into a spreadsheet containing the redemption equations created by the committee, and returned the overall unweighted average redemption across the state agencies per food package item. Through this process, USDA-FNS identified one of the six states as a clear outlier, and removed it from the averages (personal communication, K. Castellanos-Brown, USDA-FNS, June 22, 2016). As such, redemption estimates represent five of the six state agencies included in the FNS redemption dataset. Sensitivity analysis (see Chapter 8) explores the effect of shifting specific redemption rates up or down.

weighted by the population proportion of WIC-participating children and women.

Accounting for the Distribution of Redemption Rates

The redemption rates for WIC foods in the revised set of food packages are based on a distribution of redemption practices among WIC participants that ranged from no redemption of a food to partial redemption to full redemption of the package allotment. In 2012, Altarum conducted a study of redemption rates in three states (Kentucky, Michigan, and Nevada) (USDA/ERS, 2014) that provided basic information on the redemption distribution. All three states had implemented EBT issuance systems. The study classified redemption practices in three groups: *full redemption*, *partial redemption* and *nonredemption*. As stated in the Altarum report:

> The amount redeemed in a given month was subtracted from the amount issued to all participants in the family for that benefit month; if the remaining amount was zero or less than an approved minimum size food item, then the redemption was considered a *full redemption*. (USDA/ERS, 2014)

If the amount remaining was greater than the approved minimum amount but less than the amount issued, this was considered *partial redemption*. If none of the amount issued was redeemed, this was *nonredemption*. The redemption amounts were calculated for more than 14 individual food categories, for each of the food categories, and over all of the categories. Overall, 12.6 percent of the families receiving WIC benefits redeemed all of their benefits.

The information on redemption rates by product category from Altarum's report can also be used to develop data-based assumptions for redemption behaviors, specifically those used to guide committee choices of redemption rates to apply for the revised packages. The committee used a combination of the Altarum and FNS data to develop a range of revised redemption rates, and the final rates used were close to the implied new FNS-based rates with some adjustments.

WIC-participating families that did not redeem a food category in the current food package (the nonredemption group) were assumed not to redeem under the revised package if there was no change to the food category or if the only change was to change the amount offered. This seems like a plausible assumption given that there was relatively little change in the type of foods offered for each food group. If WIC-participating families fully redeemed foods in the category (the full redemption group), the families were assumed to continue to fully redeem the benefits in the food category with the revised packages as long as the amount offered was less than in the current package. This was also the case if the amount of the food provided increased, as in the case of the CVV, the full redemption rate was assumed to stay approximately unchanged. The CVV is the main category with a large increase in the amount of food provided. If there were partial redemption in the food category, the committee compared the revised amount offered in the package with the average partial redemption amount of the food before the change. (The average partial redemption amount redeemed can be derived from the redemption rates, the full amount offered, and the total average amount redeemed.) If the revised package amount was less than the average partial redemption amount, the partial redeemers were treated as were the full redeemers and assumed to fully redeem the revised package. If the revised amount was more than the average partial redemption amount, then a new implied average redemption rate consistent with the other numbers was calculated. The degree to which partial redemption affects the projected redemption rates can be derived from the available information.

Application of the Altarum Redemption Distributions (None, Partial, Full): Assumptions

To apply the Altarum redemption distribution information to estimate the revised redemption rates, several assumptions were applied, as listed below:

- The redemption rate patterns follow the distributions—full, partial, and none—observed in the Altarum study.
- The redemption patterns are constant and independent of the overall percentage redemption observed. That is, the Altarum distribution of rates of no, partial, and full redemption was applied to all redemption rates assumed for each food item, including the redemption rates based on the FNS redemption data provided to the committee as well as the observed state average rates included in the current food package consensus rates.[2]

[2] Note that the ideal data for this task would be nationally-representative redemption distributions across food items by package type. These data were not available. Although the Altarum redemption data and distribution of full, partial, and no-redemption are the best available, there are several limitations that should be noted. First, the Altarum report indicates the share of full, partial, and nonredeemers, but these percentages are not adequate to back-calculate anything other than the average amount redeemed by the partial redeemers without further more complex assumptions. Second, although there may be differences in the redemption shares (full, partial, and nonredeemers) by group across locations (e.g., states), the committee assumes that the shares are constant across locations. Finally, the committee assumes that the partial redemption average amount calculated from the Altarum study is consistent with the overall partial redemption mean and can be applied to overall redemption rates based on the FNS average redemption rates and state average rates.

- Implied adjustments occur because of changes in quantities only; adjustment for changes attributable to new products or available substitutions are made separately from the adjustments to the quantities.

The committee was interested in obtaining estimates for the implied new redemption rate (*Redemption%New*) for each food item.
The relationship observed from Altarum is:

Redemption%Alt = (*Partial%Alt* × *PartialAmtAlt* + *Full%Alt* × *FullAmt*) / *FullAmt*

Where:

Redemption%Alt = the overall redemption rate observed in Altarum
PartialAmtAlt = the implied average partial redemption amount in Altarum
FullAmt = the full amount issued
Partial%Alt = the % (share) with partial redemption from Altarum
Full%Altarum = the % (share) with full redemption from Altarum.

In this equation, all of the numbers are known from the data except *PartialAmtAlt*. Solving for *PartialAmtAlt* (the implied average partial redemption amount in Altarum):

Redemption%Alt = (*Partial%Alt* × *PartialAmtAlt* + *Full%Altarum* × *FullAmt*) / *FullAmt*
Redemption%Alt × *FullAmt* = (*Partial%Alt* × *PartialAmtAlt* + *Full%Altarum* × *FullAmt*)

Rearranging terms:

Partial%Alt × *PartialAmtAlt* = [(*Redemption%Alt* – *Full%Altarum*) × *FullAmt*]
PartialAmtAlt = [(*Redemption%Alt* – *Full%Altarum*) × *FullAmt*] / *Partial%Alt*

Similarly, the committee knows the overall average redemption rates in the FNS (or state average) data and can combine it with the no, full, and partial rates from the Altarum data to calculate the implied average partial redemption amounts assumed for the FNS data as well (*PartialAmtAssumed*). As the same redemption shares are assumed to hold for different overall redemption levels across all locations, the value

Redemption%Assumed can be substituted in the below calculation for the overall redemption rate observed in the Altarum study (*Redemption%Alt*) to solve for *PartialAmtAssumed* if this leads to nonnegative amounts. In this case, replacing *Redemption%Alt*, the reported overall Altarum redemption rate, with *Redemption%Assumed*, the FNS reported (consensus) redemption rate, yields:

$$PartialAmtAssumed = [(Redemption\%Assumed - Full\%Altarum) \times FullAmt] / Partial\%Alt$$

As long as the *PartialAmtAssumed*, our calculated assumed partial redemption amount on average is positive, this calculation is not inconsistent with observed patterns and yet incorporates the distribution of redemptions rates across full, no, and partial rates.

Now when the implied partial amount assumed is nonnegative, we use this calculation of the assumed Partial Amount (*PartialAmtAssumed*) to adjust our overall redemption rate for the revised package. Then we consider a further adjustment to our revised rates to account for whether the distribution of full and partial redeemers (based on the mean) is above the newly projected amount in the new package. If the revised amount is below the current amount and the current average redeemed partial amount, we assume the new redemption rate is 1 minus the share that has no redemption (that is, all participants except the nonredemption group will redeem the revised full amount). However, if the revised full amount is more than the current amount redeemed by partial redeemers, then the redemption amount is down-weighted to incorporate their lower levels.

Following this procedure generates implied new redemption rates based on the changes between the current and revised food packages (see Table R-5). These implied rates do not account for behavioral changes, such as those resulting from the offering of new substitutions. Slight adjustments were made (see the "Revised" column, Table R-5) to account for these changes.

TABLE R-5 Redemption Rates Applied to Generate the Set of Cost-Neutral Food Packages

Food Package and Food	Change to the Current Food Package	Redemption Rates Applied to the Food Package Cost and Nutrient Profiles			Rationale for Revised Package Redemption Rate
		Current[a]	Implied[b]	Revised[c]	
All packages for women and children					
CVV	Mandate fresh + 1 processed form; allow flexibility wherever vegetable and fruits are mentioned (fresh, frozen, or canned)	77[d]	77	75	Reduced rate of redemption because the additional CVV amount may not be redeemed at the same rate; accounts for time costs of preparation
Legumes	Mandate provision of canned beans; provide once (children) or twice (women) every 3 months	51[d]	51	53	Increased rate of redemption (approximately a 5% increase from the Altarum implied redemption that accounts for bimodal[e] distributions) due to additional options and reduced amounts
Peanut butter	Reduce to a rotation of 16–18 oz every 3 months	51[d]	51	53	Increased rate of redemption (approximately a 5% increase from the Altarum implied redemption that accounts for bimodal distributions) due to additional options and reduced amounts
RTE cereals	All adhere to whole grain-rich criteria	60[d]	60	54	Decreased rate by 10% (6 percentage points) below current redemption because state-level redemption data indicate that whole grain cereals are less preferred in some states and the number of options are reduced
Whole grains	Expand to allow 16–24 oz	53[d]	52	60	Slight increase in rate of redemption (set to the current redemption rate for RTE cereals) with increased options and package size range

continued

TABLE R-5 Continued

Food Package and Food	Change to the Current Food Package	Redemption Rates Applied to the Food Package Cost and Nutrient Profiles			Rationale for Revised Package Redemption Rate
		Current[a]	Implied[b]	Revised[c]	
Eggs	Allow a 1 lb substitution of legumes	80[d]	80	80	No change
Cheese	No change	70	70	70	No change
Infants–all relevant packages					
Jarred veg/fr, formula fed, and partially breastfed	Allow CVV in place of 1/2 or all of jarred veg/fr	51	51	65	Increased rate of redemption with the CVV substitution option; the revised redemption rate is approximately the average of the implied redemption rate (Altarum) and the revised redemption rate for the CVV; it is also the average redemption rate from Altarum so represents a reasonable redemption rate
Jarred veg/fr, fully breastfed	Allow CVV in place of 1/2 or all of jarred veg/fr	51	53	65	Increased rate of redemption with the CVV substitution option; the revised redemption rate is approximately the average of the implied redemption rate (Altarum) and the revised redemption rate for the CVV; it is also the actual average redemption rate from Altarum so represents a reasonable redemption rate
Infant formula	No change	94	94	94	There are no available data to suggest that the redemption rate should be adjusted; no changes were made to formula amounts
Infant meat/fish	Reduce to half; allow some portion as fish	31	39	43	Increase rate of redemption due to decreased amounts and fish option; used Altarum average to account for bimodal distribution; value is average redemption from the Altarum study so represents a feasible increase

Infant cereal, formula fed, and partially breastfed	Reduce by 66% for formula-fed and partially breastfed	47	45	57	Increased rate of redemption with reduction in amounts; used the Altarum report average to account for bimodal distribution; average may increase because the amount of infant cereal was excessive; value is average redemption from the Altarum study so represents a feasible increase
Infant cereal, fully breastfed	Reduce by 30% for fully breastfed	47	41	57	Increased rate of redemption with reduction in amounts; used the Altarum report average to account for bimodal distribution; average may increase because the amount of infant cereal was excessive; value is average redemption from the Altarum study so represents a feasible increase
FP IV: Children					
Juice	Reduce to 64 oz	70[d]	75	78	Increased rate of redemption due to reduced amount (approximately a 5% increase from the Altarum implied redemption that accounts for bimodal distributions), and shift of individuals that prefer the CVV to that option (individuals that prefer juice will be issued and redeem juice)
Milk (applies to composite of milk, cheese, and yogurt)	IV-A: Reduce to 3 gallons	75	87	87	Uses the implied new redemption rate based on Altarum distributions; public comments and redemption indicate that whole milk is a preferred food, so do not anticipate full yogurt substitution
Milk (applies to composite of milk, cheese, and yogurt)	IV-B: Reduce to 3.5 gallons	71[d,f]	76	80	Uses the implied new redemption rate based on Altarum distributions; increased rate of redemption 4 percentage points (a 5% increase from the Altarum implied redemption) due to additional yogurt option

continued

TABLE R-5 Continued

Food Package and Food	Change to the Current Food Package	Redemption Rates Applied to the Food Package Cost and Nutrient Profiles			Rationale for Revised Package Redemption Rate
		Current[a]	Implied[b]	Revised[c]	
Fish	Include 10 oz every 3 months	NA	68	68	Uses the implied new redemption rate based on Altarum distributions
FP V: P and partially BF women					
Juice	Reduce to 64 oz	70[d]	76	79	Increased rate of redemption due to reduced amount (approximately a 5% increase from the Altarum implied redemption that accounts for bimodal distributions), and shift of individuals that prefer the CVV to that option (individuals that prefer juice will be issued and redeem juice)
Milk (applies to composite of milk, cheese, and yogurt)	Reduce to 4 gallons	56[d,f]	62	66	Uses the implied new redemption rate based on Altarum distributions; increased rate of redemption 4 percentage points (a 5% increase from the Altarum implied redemption) due to additional yogurt option
Fish	Include 10 oz every 3 months (V-A); 20 oz per month (V-B)	NA	68	68	Uses the implied new redemption rate based on Altarum distributions
FP VI: PP (non-BF) women					
Juice	Remove juice	70[d]	NA	NA	NA

Milk (applies to composite of milk, cheese, and yogurt)	No change	56[d,f]	56	59	Uses the implied new redemption rate based on Altarum distributions; increased rate of redemption 3 percentage points (a 5% increase from the Altarum implied redemption) due to additional yogurt option
Fish	Include 10 oz every 3 months	NA	68	68	Uses the implied new redemption rate based on Altarum distributions
FP VII: Fully BF women					
Juice	Reduce to 64 oz	70[d]	76	79	Increased rate of redemption due to reduced amount (approximately a 5% increase from the Altarum implied redemption that accounts for bimodal distributions), and shift of individuals that prefer the CVV to that option (individuals that prefer juice will be issued and redeem juice)
Milk (applies to composite of milk, cheese, and yogurt)	Reduce to 4 gallons	56[d,f]	65	68	Uses the implied new redemption rate based on Altarum distributions; increased rate of redemption 3 percentage points (a 5% increase from the Altarum implied redemption) due to additional yogurt option
Fish	Reduce to 20 oz	69[d]	68	68	Uses the implied new redemption rate based on Altarum distributions

NOTES: BF = breastfeeding; CVV = cash value voucher; FP = food package; veg/fr = vegetables and fruits; NA = not applicable; P = pregnant; PP = postpartum; RTE = ready-to-eat.

[a] These values were applied to estimate the costs of the current set of food packages. Values represent the unweighted mean values from five states provided by FNS, except for whole milk, cheese, and infant foods and formula. For these foods, the unweighted average of available state data was used.

[b] These values were generated using the method described in this appendix, and account for the redemption distributions reported in USDA/ERS, 2014. These values account for changes in amounts, but they do not account for changes in composition or substitution options.

continued

TABLE R-5 Continued

[c] These values include upward adjustments to account for changes in composition or substitution options. Values represent the anticipated mean redemption over the course of the revised program.

[d] USDA-FNS provided the committee with 12 months (August 2013 through July 2014) of price and redemption data from a convenience sample of six WIC state agencies, representing five of the seven regions of the country (herein referenced as the FNS redemption data). The identity of the agencies was not known to the committee. The states were diverse in terms of size and did not include Indian Tribal Organizations or territories. Redemption values from the five states may be slightly underestimated: The PC2014 report indicates that 17.7 percent of minimally breastfeeding women are included in reported participants, but do not receive a food package. FNS indicated that these women are included in administrative data for participation. Because these women are not issued and, therefore, do not redeem WIC foods, the redemption rates may be slightly deflated.

[e] Bimodal distribution refers to cases where the tails of the distribution (none and full redemption) had a relatively large share of the redemptions and the "partial redemptions" were a small share (USDA/ERS, 2014).

[f] The group average rate of 65 percent redemption for low-fat milk (women and children, combined) was decomposed into values of 71 percent for children ages 2 to less than 5 and 56 percent for women, rates that were consistent with the observed 65 percent redemption when weighted by the population proportion of WIC-participating children and women.

SOURCES: Personal communication, USDA/FNS, June 30, 2016; USDA/ERS, 2014; redemption data provided to the committee by individual states, available in the public access file for the study (Email: paro@nas.edu).

REFERENCES

USDA/ARS (U.S. Department of Agriculture/Agricultural Research Service). 2016. *USDA National Nutrient Database for Standard Reference, release 28*. https://www.ars.usda.gov/northeast-area/beltsville-md/beltsville-human-nutrition-research-center/nutrient-data-laboratory/docs/usda-national-nutrient-database-for-standard-reference (accessed December 22, 2016).

USDA/ERS (U.S. Department of Agriculture/Economic Research Service). 2014. *Transition to EBT in WIC: Review of impact and examination of participant redemption patterns: Final report*. http://altarum.org/sites/default/files/uploaded-publication-files/Altarum_Transition%20to%20WIC%20EBT_Final%20Report_071614.pdf (accessed December 22, 2016).

USDA/FNS (U.S. Department of Agriculture/Food and Nutrition Service). 2013. Fiscal year 2010: WIC food cost report. http://www.fns.usda.gov/sites/default/files/WICFoodCost2010_0.pdf (accessed December 22, 2016).

USDA/FNS. 2015. *WIC food packages policy options II*. Final report. Alexandria, VA: USDA/FNS. http://www.fns.usda.gov/wic-food-package-policy-options-ii (accessed December 21, 2016).

USDA/FNS. 2016. *WIC participant and program characteristics 2014 food package report*. Alexandria, VA: USDA/FNS. http://www.fns.usda.gov/wic-participant-and-program-characteristics-2014-food-package-report (accessed August 30, 2016).

Appendix S

Sensitivity Tests and Results

TABLES

TABLE S-1 List of Sensitivity Tests Conducted for Food Packages IV-B (Children Ages 2 to Less Than 5 Years), V-A (Pregnant Women), and VII (Fully Breastfeeding Women)

Food Package	Food Category	Current Package (Applies the Current Package Redemption Rate)[a]	Revised Food Package (Applies the Revised Package Redemption Rate Only for the Tested Food Category)[a]	Tests[b]		
				1	2	3
IV-B	Milk	16 qt + additional substitutions, 71% redemption	–2 qt + additional substitutions, 80% redemption	–4 qt + additional substitutions, 86% redemption	–2 qt, no substitutions (only fluid milk), 76% redemption	—
V-A	Milk	22 qt + additional substitutions, 56% redemption	–6 qt + additional substitutions, 66% redemption	–10 qt + additional substitutions, 74% redemption	—	—
VII	Milk	24 qt + additional substitutions, 56% redemption	–8 qt + additional substitutions, 68% redemption	–12 qt + additional substitutions, 77% redemption	–8 qt, no substitutions (only fluid milk), 65% redemption	—
IV-B	Breakfast cereal	36 oz, 50/50 WG/non-WG, 60% redemption	36 oz, all WG, 54% redemption	36 oz, all WG, 60% (current redemption)	36 oz, all WG, 69% redemption (highest of available rates)	—
V-A	Breakfast cereal	36 oz, 50/50 WG/non-WG, 60% redemption	36 oz, all WG, 54% redemption	36 oz, all WG, 60% (current redemption)	—	—
VII	Breakfast cereal	36 oz, 50/50 WG/non-WG, 60% redemption	36 oz, all WG, 54% redemption	36 oz, all WG, 60% (current redemption)	—	—
IV-B	CVV	$8	+$4; 75% redemption	+$4; 65% redemption	+$4; 80% redemption	+$4; 85% redemption

continued

TABLE S-1 Continued

Food Package	Food Category	Current Package (Applies the Current Package Redemption Rate)[a]	Revised Food Package (Applies the Revised Package Redemption Rate Only for the Tested Food Category)[a]	Tests[b] 1	2	3
V-A	CVV	$11	+$4, 75% redemption	+$4, 65% redemption	+$4, 80% redemption	+$4, 85% redemption
VII	CVV	$11	+$24, 75% redemption	+$24, 85% redemption	+$9, 75% redemption	+$34, 75% redemption
IV-B	CVV	$8	+$4, 75% redemption, 33/67 vegetable/fruit	+$4, 50/50 vegetable/fruit	—	—
V-A	CVV	$11	+$4, 75% redemption, 33/67 vegetable/fruit	+$4, 50/50 vegetable/fruit	—	—
VII	CVV	$11	+$24, 75% redemption, 33/67 vegetable/fruit	+$24, 50/50 vegetable/fruit		
IV-B	Juice/CVV	128 oz juice, $8 CVV	–64 oz juice, 78% redemption; +$4 CVV, 75% redemption	–64 oz juice, 75% redemption, +$4 CVV	–128 oz juice, +$18 CVV	—
V-A	Juice/CVV	144 oz juice, $11 CVV	–80 oz juice, 79% redemption, +$4 CVV, 75% redemption	–144 oz juice, +$10 CVV	—	—
VII	Juice/CVV	144 oz juice, $11 CVV	–80 oz juice, 79% redemption, +$24 CVV, 75% redemption	–144 oz juice, +$41 CVV	—	—
IV-B	Fish	No fish	+10 oz every 3 mo, 68% redemption	+10 oz every 3 mo, 59% redemption	+10 oz every 3 mo, 79% redemption	—

V-A	Fish	No fish	+10 oz every 3 mo, 68% redemption	Revised fish, 59% redemption	Revised fish, 79% redemption	—
VII	Fish	30 ounces per month	−10 oz per mo, 68% redemption	−10 oz per mo, 59% redemption	−10 oz per mo, 79% redemption	—
IV-B	Peanut butter/ legumes/fish	1 lb choice legumes or peanut butter, no fish	−2.7 oz legumes/mo, 53% redemption; −3 oz peanut butter/mo; +3.3 oz fish/mo	−2.7 oz legumes/ mo; −3 oz peanut butter/mo; no fish	−2.7 oz legumes/mo, 38% redemption; −3 oz peanut butter/mo; +3.3 oz fish/mo	−2.7 oz legumes/ mo, 69%; −3 oz peanut butter/mo; +3.3 oz fish/mo
V-A	Peanut butter/ legumes/fish	1 lb legumes, and 18 oz peanut butter, no fish	−5.3 oz legumes/mo, 53% redemption; −12 oz peanut butter/mo; no fish	−5.3 oz legumes/ mo, 38% redemption; −12 oz peanut butter/mo; +3.3 oz fish/mo	−5.3 oz legumes/mo, 69% redemption; −12 oz peanut butter/mo; +3.3 oz fish/mo	—
II	Infant vegetables and fruits	128 oz	128 oz, 65% redemption	128 oz, 50% of infant food as CVV	—	—
I/II/V-B (cost only)[c]		Current participation	Shift of 5% from FF to partial	Shift of 8% from FF to partial	—	—

NOTES: — = No test 2 and/or test 3 was conducted; CVV = cash value voucher; FF = formula-fed; WG = whole grain. Results were based on the food package nutrient and cost profiles and calculated redemption rates developed using the method outlined in Appendix R.

[a] To test the effect of the changes that were made to the revised package, the current food package amounts and redemption rates were held constant, changing only the food amounts and redemption rates of the food or foods in the category being tested.

[b] The revised food package redemption rate is applied in each test, unless otherwise indicated.

[c] Results are presented in Chapter 8.

TABLE S-2 Food Package IV-B Sensitivity Results: Impact of Changes to Milk Amounts and Substitutions

FP Nutrients, Food Groups, HEI–2010 Components, and Cost	EAR/AI,* 1–3y/4–8y	Current Amount: 16 qt (71% Redemption), Additional Substitutions	Change from Current (Redemption Rate)					
			Revised: –2 qt (80%), Additional Substitutions		Test 1: –4 qt (86%), Additional Substitutions		Test 2: –2 qt (76%), No Yogurt or Cheese Substitutes for Milk (Only Fluid Milk)	
			Absolute Change	%	Absolute Change	%	Absolute Change	%
Energy (kcal)	1300	423	+2.9	+0.7	–12.9	-3.1	–17.4	–4.1
Protein (g)	13 (RDA)	21	+0.2	+1.0	–1.2	-5.9	–0.7	–3.3
Total fat (g)	ND	11	–0.7	-6.2	+0.0	+0.3	–1.9	–16.8
Carbohydrate (g)	130 (RDA)	61	+2.1	+3.5	–2.0	-3.4	+0.5	+0.8
Fiber (g)	19/25*	4.3	+0.0	+0.0	–0.0	-0.0	+0.0	+0.0
Added sugar (g)	NA/32.5	4.3	+0.7	+17.6	+0.2	+5.5	–1.1	-25.8
Calcium (mg)	500/800	543	+11.1	+2.0	–47.5	-8.7	–11.0	-2.0
Iron (mg)	3/4.1	8.2	+0.0	+0.1	–0.0	-0.2	–0.0	-0.1
Magnesium (mg)	65/110	98.9	+2.7	+2.7	–6.3	-6.3	+3.8	+3.9
Phosphorus (mg)	380/405	513	+12.8	+2.5	–38.7	-7.5	–0.3	-0.1
Potassium (mg)	3000/3800*	927	+44.1	+4.8	–74.2	-8.0	+52.9	+5.7
Sodium (mg)	1000/1200*	412	–8.1	-2.0	–13.7	-3.3	–30.9	-7.5
Zinc (mg)	2.5/4	3.7	+0.0	+1.3	–0.1	-3.2	–0.2	-5.0
Copper (mg)	0.26/0.34	0.22	+0.0	+0.8	–0.0	-2.4	+0.0	+1.2
Selenium (μg)	17/23	21	+0.1	+0.6	–0.7	-3.1	–1.1	-5.3
Vitamin C (mg)	13/22	43	+0.2	+0.5	–0.5	-1.1	+0.5	+1.2

Thiamin (mg)	0.4/0.5	0.51	+0.0	+1.7	−0.0	−3.7	+0.0	+3.1
Riboflavin (mg)	0.4/0.5	0.95	+0.0	+3.3	−0.1	−8.0	+0.0	+4.4
Niacin (mg)	5/6	5.3	+0.0	+0.4	−0.0	−0.8	+0.0	+0.6
Vitamin B6 (mg)	0.4/0.5	0.71	+0.0	+1.1	−0.0	−2.9	+0.0	+2.1
Folate (μg DFE)	120/160	263	+1.4	+0.5	−1.8	−0.7	−0.6	−0.2
Choline (mg)	200/250*	58	0	0	0	0	0	0
Vitamin B12 (μg)	0.7/1	2.4	+0.1	+3.3	−0.2	−6.9	+0.1	+2.7
Vitamin A (μg RAE)	210/275	357	−2.5	−0.7	−26.7	−7.5	+17.6	+4.9
Vitamin E (mg)	5/6	1.78	−0.0	−0.6	+0.0	+0.4	−0.0	−2.2
Vitamin D (IU)	400	148	+2.4	+1.6	−21.1	−14.2	+25.9	+17.5
Saturated fat (g)	NA/14	4.49	−0.4	−9.1	+0.0	+0.3	−1.1	−25.2
Total dairy (c-eq)		1.5	−0.03	−2.0	−0.1	−9.2	−0.1	−6.3
HEI dairy (0 to 10)		9.95	−0.15	−1.6	−0.7	−7.1	−0.49	−4.9
HEI overall (0 to 100)		66.26	+0.06	+0.1	−0.8	−1.2	+0.76	+1.1
FP cost		$33.88	+$0.08	+0.2	−$0.89	−2.6	−$4.29	−12.7
Average per-participant FP cost		$37.27	+$0.03	+0.1	−$0.27	−0.7	−$2.18	−5.9

NOTES: Tests of decreases in the amount of milk and milk substitutions may result in increases or decreases of nutrients due to changes in redemption rates and allowable substitutions. For example, revised and alternative packages allow an additional quart of yogurt compared to the current packages; 1 qt of fat-free milk contains 363 kcal and no added sugars, whereas 1 qt of low-fat vanilla yogurt contains 833 kcal 66 g of added sugars. See additional notes following Table S-22.

TABLE S-3 Food Package V-A Sensitivity Results: Impact of Changes to Milk Amounts and Substitutions

			Change from Current (Redemption Rate)			
			Revised: –6 qt (66%), Additional Substitutions		Test 1: –10 qt (74%), Additional Substitutions	
FP Nutrients, Food Groups, and Cost	EAR/AI,* 19–30y/31–50y	Current Amount (56% Redemption): 22 qt, Additional Substitutions	Absolute Change	%	Absolute Change	%
Energy (kcal)	2,625	468	–19.4	–4.1	–49.1	–10.5
Protein (g)	71 (RDA)	22.5	–1.6	–7.2	–3.8	–16.9
Total fat (g)	ND	13.4	–1.0	–7.5	–1.5	–11.1
Carbohydrate (g)	175 (RDA)	65.2	–0.9	–1.4	–5.1	–7.8
Fiber (g)	28*	4.9	–0.0	–0.0	–0.0	–0.0
Added sugar (g)	65.0	4.3	+0.7	+15.4	–0.3	–6.8
Calcium (mg)	800	581.5	–57.7	–9.9	–136.4	–23.5
Iron (mg)	22	8.2	–0.0	–0.3	–0.1	–0.7
Magnesium (mg)	290/300	114	–5.3	–4.6	–13.6	–11.9
Phosphorus (mg)	580	559	–41.8	–7.5	–103.9	–18.6
Potassium (mg)	4,700*	1,096	–50.9	–4.6	–154.9	–14.1
Sodium (mg)	1,500*	416	–32.7	–7.9	–62.3	–15.0
Zinc (mg)	9.5	3.8	–0.2	–4.2	–0.5	–12.1
Copper (mg)	0.8	0.26	–0.0	–1.9	–0.0	–4.5
Selenium (μg)	49	19.3	–1.1	–5.5	–2.7	–14.0

Vitamin C (mg)	70	50.8	–0.4	–0.7	–0.9	–1.7
Thiamin (mg)	1.2	0.54	–0.0	–2.6	–0.0	–6.9
Riboflavin (mg)	1.2	1.04	–0.1	–6.4	–0.2	–16.4
Niacin (mg)	14	5.8	–0.0	–0.6	–0.1	–1.5
Vitamin B6 (mg)	1.6	0.77	–0.0	–2.3	–0.0	–5.6
Folate (µg DFE)	520	283	–1.4	–0.5	–5.4	–1.9
Choline (mg)	450*	57.4	0	0	0	0
Vitamin B12 (µg)	2.2	2.54	–0.1	–5.5	–0.4	–15.2
Vitamin A (µg RAE)	550	381	–33.8	–8.9	–56.9	–14.9
Vitamin E (mg)	12	2.08	–0.0	–0.4	–0.0	–0.6
Vitamin D (IU)	400	167.9	–20.1	–12.0	–35.1	–20.9
Saturated fat (g)	29	6	–1.2	–20.4	–1.8	–30.4
Total dairy (c-eq)	3	1.6	–0.24	–14.4	–0.45	–27.6
FP cost		$36.68	–$1.11	–3.0	–$2.97	–8.1
Average per-participant FP cost		$37.27	–$0.11	–0.3	–$0.28	–0.9

NOTES: Tests of decreases in the amount of milk and milk substitutions may result in increases or decreases of nutrients due to changes in redemption rates and allowable substitutions. For example revised and test packages allow an additional quart of yogurt compared to the current packages; 1 qt of fat-free milk contains 363 kcal and no added sugars, whereas 1 qt of low-fat vanilla yogurt contains 833 kcal 66 g of added sugars. See additional notes following Table S-22.

TABLE S-4 Food Package VII Sensitivity Results: Impact of Changes to Milk Amounts and Substitutions

FP Nutrients, Food Groups, and Cost	EAR/AI* 19–30y/31–50y	Current Amount (56% Redemption): 24 qt, Additional Substitutions	Change from Current (Redemption Rate)					
			Revised: –8 qt (68%), Additional Substitutions		Test 1: –12 qt (77%), Additional Substitutions		Test 2: –8 qt (65%), No Yogurt or Cheese Substitutes for Milk (Only Fluid Milk)	
			Absolute Change	%	Absolute Change	%	Absolute Change	%
Energy (kcal)	2,492	559	–30.1	–5.4	–51.9	–9.3	–43.7	–7.8
Protein (g)	71 (RDA)	32	–2.5	–8.0	–4.4	–13.9	–2.9	–9.2
Total Fat (g)	ND	19	–1.1	–5.6	–1.4	–7.1	–2.8	–14.7
Carbohydrate (g)	210 (RDA)	66	–2.5	–3.8	–5.3	–8.1	–1.7	–2.5
Fiber (g)	29*	4.9	–0.0	–0.0	–0.0	–0.1	–0.0	–0.0
Added sugar (g)	65.0	3.9	+0.6	+16.1	+0.8	+19.7	–0.4	–11.2
Calcium (mg)	800	717	-92.0	–12.8	-162.7	–22.7	-93.5	–13.0
Iron (mg)	6.5	8.8	–0.0	–0.4	–0.1	–0.8	–0.0	–0.5
Magnesium (mg)	255/265	125	–9.5	–7.6	–17.8	–14.3	–4.8	–3.8
Phosphorus (mg)	580	698	-69.4	–9.9	-125.4	–18.0	-62.6	–9.0
Potassium (mg)	5,100*	1,181	-101.2	–8.6	-199.1	–16.9	-39.2	–3.3
Sodium (mg)	1,500*	608	-43.8	–7.2	-69.2	–11.4	-69.7	–11.5
Zinc (mg)	10.4	4.6	–0.3	–5.7	–0.5	–10.1	–0.4	–8.9
Copper (mg)	1	0.29	–0.0	–2.9	–0.0	–5.3	–0.0	–1.7

Selenium (µg)	59	41.4	–1.6	–3.9	–2.8	–6.7	–2.5	-6.1
Vitamin C (mg)	100	50.9	-0.7	-1.3	-1.3	-2.5	-0.1	-0.3
Thiamin (mg)	1.2	0.56	-0.0	-4.7	-0.1	-9.1	-0.0	-1.5
Riboflavin (mg)	1.3	1.2	-0.1	-9.9	-0.2	-18.5	-0.1	-5.5
Niacin (mg)	13	7.8	-0.1	-0.8	-0.1	-1.5	-0.0	-0.3
Vitamin B6 (mg)	1.7	0.87	-0.0	-3.6	-0.1	-6.7	-0.0	-1.6
Folate (µg DFE)	450	293	-2.9	-1.0	-5.7	-1.9	-3.2	-1.1
Choline (mg)	550*	113	0	0	0	0	0	0
Vitamin B12 (µg)	2.4	3.4	-0.3	-7.4	-0.5	-14.0	-0.2	-4.8
Vitamin A (µg RAE)	900	456	-49.8	-10.9	-85.3	-18.7	-28.8	-6.3
Vitamin E (mg)	16	2.4	-0.0	-0.2	-0.0	-0.1	-0.0	-1.8
Vitamin D (IU)	400	223	-32.2	-14.4	-58.1	-26.1	-4.5	-2.0
Saturated fat (g)	29	7.8	-0.6	-8.3	-0.8	-10.6	-1.7	-21.7
Total dairy (c-eq)	3	2.0	-0.6	-28.7	-0.8	-39.4	-0.6	-42.7
FP Cost		$47.41	–$1.59	–3.4	–$2.49	–5.3	–$5.51	–11.6
Average per-participant FP cost		$37.27	–$0.06	–0.2	–$0.12	–0.3	–$0.19	–0.5

NOTES: Tests of decreases in the amount of milk and milk substitutions may result in increases or decreases of nutrients due to changes in redemption rates and allowable substitutions. For example, revised and test packages allow an additional quart of yogurt compared to the current packages; 1 qt of fat-free milk contains 363 kcal and no added sugars, whereas 1 qt of low-fat vanilla yogurt contains 833 kcal 66 g of added sugars. See additional notes following Table S-22.

TABLE S-5 Food Package IV-B Sensitivity Results: Impact of Changes to Cereal Form and Redemption

FP Nutrients, Food Groups, HEI Components, and Cost	EAR/AI,* 1–3y/4–8y	Current Cereal (60% Redemption)	Change from Current (Redemption Rate)					
			Revised: All WG Cereal (54%)		Test 1: All WG (60%)		Test 2: All WG (69%)[a]	
			Absolute Change	%	Absolute Change	%	Absolute Change	%
Energy (kcal)	1,300	423	–9.4	–2.2	–1.7	–0.4	+9.2	+2.2
Protein (g)	13 (RDA)	20.5	+0.2	+0.8	+0.4	+1.8	+0.7	+3.3
Total fat (g)	ND	11.2	–0.1	–0.8	+0.0	+0.0	+0.1	+1.3
Carbohydrate (g)	130 (RDA)	60.6	–2.1	–3.5	–0.5	–0.8	+1.8	+3.0
Fiber (g)	19/25*	4.3	+0.3	+6.0	+0.4	+10.2	+0.7	+16.3
Added sugar (g)	NA/32.5	4.3	–0.5	–10.9	–0.2	–4.6	+0.2	+4.5
Calcium (mg)	500/800	543	+8.7	+1.6	+13.4	+2.5	+20.1	+3.7
Iron (mg)	3/4.1	8.2	–0.7	–8.7	–0.1	–0.8	+0.9	+10.5
Magnesium (mg)	65/110	98.9	+4.1	+4.2	+6.1	+6.1	+8.9	+9.0
Phosphorus (mg)	380/405	513	+23.9	+4.7	+32.0	+6.2	+43.7	+8.5
Potassium (mg)	3,000/3,800*	927	+22.2	+2.4	+31.0	+3.3	+43.7	+4.7
Sodium (mg)	1,000/1,200*	412	–29.8	–7.3	–23.0	–5.6	–13.2	–3.2
Zinc (mg)	2.5/4	3.7	+0.5	+14.0	+0.7	+19.5	+1.0	+27.4
Copper (mg)	0.26/0.34	0.22	+0.0	+0.5	+0.0	+2.6	+0.0	+5.6
Selenium (μg)	17/23	21.1	+0.2	+0.9	+0.5	+2.4	+0.9	+4.5
Vitamin C (mg)	13/22	42.5	–1.4	–3.2	–1.2	–2.8	–1.0	–2.3

Thiamin (mg)	0.4/0.5	0.51	–0.1	–12.2	–0.0	–7.8	–0.0	–1.4
Riboflavin (mg)	0.4/0.5	0.95	–0.1	–11.4	–0.1	–9.8	–0.1	–7.5
Niacin (mg)	5/6	5.3	–0.5	–10.0	–0.2	–3.9	+0.3	+4.9
Vitamin B6 (mg)	0.4/0.5	0.71	–0.0	–6.9	–0.0	–2.0	+0.0	+5.2
Folate (μg DFE)	120/160	263	–14.8	–5.6	+6.1	+2.3	+36.2	+13.8
Choline (mg)	200/250*	58.0	–0.1	–0.2	+0.3	+0.4	+0.8	+1.3
Vitamin B12 (μg)	0.7/1	2.4	–0.2	–10.0	–0.2	–6.6	–0.0	–1.7
Vitamin A (μg RAE)	210/275	357	–42.1	–11.8	–33.0	–9.2	–19.8	–5.6
Vitamin E (mg)	5/6	1.78	–0.5	–29.8	–0.5	–29.1	–0.5	–28.2
Vitamin D (IU)	400	148	–9.8	–6.6	–8.5	–5.7	–6.6	–4.4
Saturated fat (g)	NA/14	4.5	+0.0	+0.5	+0.0	+0.9	+0.1	+1.5
Total grains (c-eq)	4.5	1.3	–0.07	–5.6	0.00	0	0.10	8.1
Whole grains (c-eq)	2.3	0.7	+0.19	+26.9	+0.22	+32.0	0.28	+39.4
HEI whole grains	0 to 10	2.6	+0.84	+32.4	+1.00	+38.6	+1.23	+47.5
HEI overall	0 to 100	66	+0.84	+1.3	+1.00	+1.5	+1.23	+1.9
FP cost		$33.88	–$0.08	–0.2	+$0.43	+1.3	+$1.16	+3.4
Average per-participant FP cost		$37.27	–$0.03	–0.1	+$0.15	+0.4	+$0.42	+1.1

NOTES: See additional notes following Table S-22.
[a] Represents the highest redemption rate for breakfast cereals among those made available to the committee.

TABLE S-6 Food Package V-A Sensitivity Results: Impact of Changes to Cereal Form and Redemption

FP Nutrients, Food Groups, and Cost	EAR/AI,* 19–30y/ 31–50y	Current Amount (60% Redemption)	Change from Current (Redemption Rate) Revised: All WG Cereal (54%) Absolute Change	%	Test 1: All WG (60%) Absolute Change	%
Energy (kcal)	2,625	468	-9.4	-2.0	-1.7	-0.4
Protein (g)	71 (RDA)	23	+0.2	+0.7	+0.4	+1.7
Total Fat (g)	ND	13	-0.1	-0.7	+0.0	+0.0
Carbohydrate (g)	175 (RDA)	65	-2.1	-3.2	-0.5	-0.8
Fiber (g)	28*	4.9	+0.3	+5.3	+0.4	+9.0
Added sugar (g)	65.0	4.3	-0.5	-10.8	-0.2	-4.5
Calcium (mg)	800	581	+8.7	+1.5	+13.4	+2.3
Iron (mg)	22	8.2	-0.7	-8.7	-0.1	-0.8
Magnesium (mg)	290/300	114	+4.1	+3.6	+6.1	+5.3
Phosphorus (mg)	580	559	+23.9	+4.3	+32.0	+5.7
Potassium (mg)	4,700*	1,096	+22.2	+2.0	+31.0	+2.8
Sodium (mg)	1,500*	416	-29.8	-7.2	-23.0	-5.5
Zinc (mg)	9.5	3.8	+0.5	+13.4	+0.7	+18.6
Copper (mg)	0.8	0.26	+0.0	+0.4	+0.0	+2.2
Selenium (μg)	49	19.3	+0.2	+1.0	+0.5	+2.6
Vitamin C (mg)	70	50.8	-1.4	-2.7	-1.2	-2.3
Thiamin (mg)	1.2	0.54	-0.1	-11.6	-0.0	-7.4
Riboflavin (mg)	1.2	1.04	-0.1	-10.5	-0.1	-9.0
Niacin (mg)	14	5.8	-0.5	-9.2	-0.2	-3.6
Vitamin B6 (mg)	1.6	0.77	-0.0	-6.4	-0.0	-1.8
Folate (μg DFE)	520	283	-14.8	-5.2	+6.1	+2.2
Choline (mg)	450*	57.4	-0.1	-0.2	+0.3	+0.4
Vitamin B12 (μg)	2.2	2.5	-0.2	-9.4	-0.2	-6.2
Vitamin A (μg RAE)	550	381	-42.1	-11.0	-33.0	-8.7
Vitamin E (mg)	12	2.08	-0.5	-25.5	-0.5	-25.0
Vitamin D (IU)	400	168	-9.8	-5.8	-8.5	-5.1
Saturated fat (g)	29	6.0	+0.0	+0.8	+0.0	+0.8
Total grains (c-eq)	9	1.01	-0.1	-7.2	0	0
Whole grains (c-eq)	4.5	0.42	+0.2	+44.9	+0.2	+53.5
FP cost		$36.68	-$0.08	-0.2	+$0.43	+1.2
Average per-participant FP cost		$37.27	-$0.01	-0.0	+$0.04	+0.1

NOTES: See notes following Table S-22.

TABLE S-7 Food Package VII Sensitivity Results: Impact of Changes to Cereal Form and Redemption

FP Nutrients, Food Groups, and Cost	EAR/AI,* 19–30y/ 31–50y	Current Amount (60% Redemption)	Change from Current (Redemption Rate)			
			Revised: All WG (54%)		Test 1: All WG (60%)	
			Absolute Change	%	Absolute Change	%
Energy (kcal)	2,492	559	-9.4	-1.7	-1.7	-0.3
Protein (g)	71 (RDA)	31.7	+0.2	+0.5	+0.4	+1.2
Total fat (g)	ND	19.1	-0.1	-0.5	+0.0	+0.0
Carbohydrate (g)	210 (RDA)	65.6	-2.1	-3.2	-0.5	-0.8
Fiber (g)	29*	4.9	+0.3	+5.3	+0.4	+9.0
Added sugar (g)	65.0	3.9	-0.5	-12.0	-0.2	-5.0
Calcium (mg)	800	717	+8.7	+1.2	+13.4	+1.9
Iron (mg)	6.5	8.8	-0.7	-8.1	-0.1	-0.8
Magnesium (mg)	255/265	125	+4.1	+3.3	+6.1	+4.9
Phosphorus (mg)	580	698	+23.9	+3.4	+32.0	+4.6
Potassium (mg)	5,100*	1,181	+22.2	+1.9	+31.0	+2.6
Sodium (mg)	1,500*	608	-29.8	-4.9	-23.0	-3.8
Zinc (mg)	10.4	4.6	+0.5	+11.1	+0.7	+15.5
Copper (mg)	1	0.29	+0.0	+0.4	+0.0	+1.9
Selenium (μg)	59	41.4	+0.2	+0.5	+0.5	+1.2
Vitamin C (mg)	100	50.9	-1.4	-2.7	-1.2	-2.3
Thiamin (mg)	1.2	0.56	-0.1	-11.2	-0.0	-7.2
Riboflavin (mg)	1.3	1.2	-0.1	-9.1	-0.1	-7.9
Niacin (mg)	13	7.8	-0.5	-6.9	-0.2	-2.7
Vitamin B6 (mg)	1.7	0.87	-0.0	-5.6	-0.0	-1.6
Folate (μg DFE)	450	293	-14.8	-5.0	+6.1	+2.1
Choline (mg)	550*	113	-0.1	-0.1	+0.3	+0.2
Vitamin B12 (μg)	2.4	3.42	-0.2	-7.0	-0.2	-4.6
Vitamin A (μg RAE)	900	456	-42.1	-9.2	-33.0	-7.2
Vitamin E (mg)	16	2.41	-0.5	-22.1	-0.5	-21.6
Vitamin D (IU)	400	223	-9.8	-4.4	-8.5	-3.8
Saturated fat (g)	29	7.8	+0.0	+0.3	+0.0	+0.5
Total grains (c-eq)	9	1.01	-0.1	-7.2	0	0
Whole grains (c-eq)	4.5	0.42	+0.2	+44.9	+0.2	+53.5
FP cost		$47.41	-$0.08	-0.2	+$0.43	+0.9
Average per-participant FP cost		$37.27	-$0.01	-0.0	+$0.01	+0.0

NOTES: See notes following Table S-22.

TABLE S-8 Food Package IV-B Sensitivity Results: Impact of Changes to CVV Redemption

FP Nutrients, Food Groups, HEI Components, and Cost	EAR/AI,* 1–3y/4–8y	Current Amount (77% Redemption): $8	Change from Current (Redemption Rate)							
			Revised: +$4 (75%)		Test 1: +$4 (65%)		Test 2: +$4 (80%)		Test 3: +$4 (85%)	
			Absolute Change	%	Absolute Change	%	Absolute Change	%	Absolute Change	%
Energy (kcal)	1,300	423	+16.1	+3.8	+9.2	+2.2	+19.5	+4.6	+22.9	+5.4
Protein (g)	13 (RDA)	20.5	+0.2	+1.1	+0.1	+0.6	+0.3	+1.3	+0.3	+1.5
Total fat (g)	ND	11.2	+0.3	+2.6	+0.2	+1.5	+0.3	+3.1	+0.4	+3.6
Carbohydrate (g)	130 (RDA)	60.6	+2.8	+4.6	+1.6	+2.7	+3.4	+5.6	+4.0	+6.6
Fiber (g)	19/25*	4.3	+0.5	+12.0	+0.3	+6.9	+0.6	+14.5	+0.7	+17.1
Added sugar (g)	NA/32.5	4.3	0	0	0	0	0	0	0	0
Calcium (mg)	500/800	543	+3.1	+0.6	+1.8	+0.3	+3.8	+0.7	+4.5	+0.8
Iron (mg)	3/4.1	8.2	+0.1	+0.9	+0.0	+0.5	+0.1	+1.1	+0.1	+1.3
Magnesium (mg)	65/110	99	+3.5	+3.6	+2.0	+2.1	+4.3	+4.3	+5.0	+5.1
Phosphorus (mg)	380/405	513	+5.7	+1.1	+3.3	+0.6	+6.9	+1.3	+8.1	+1.6
Potassium (mg)	3,000/3,800*	927	+57.1	+6.2	+32.8	+3.5	+69.2	+7.5	+81.4	+8.8
Sodium (mg)	1,000/1,200*	412	+0.9	+0.2	+0.5	+0.1	+1.1	+0.3	+1.3	+0.3
Zinc (mg)	2.5/4	3.7	+0.0	+1.1	+0.0	+0.6	+0.0	+1.3	+0.1	+1.5
Copper (mg)	0.26/0.34	0.22	+0.0	+7.3	+0.0	+4.2	+0.0	+8.8	+0.0	+10.4
Selenium (μg)	17/23	21.1	+0.1	+0.4	+0.1	+0.2	+0.1	+0.5	+0.1	+0.6
Vitamin C (mg)	13/22	42.5	+5.8	+13.7	+3.3	+7.9	+7.0	+16.6	+8.3	+19.5
Thiamin (mg)	0.4/0.5	0.51	+0.0	+2.2	+0.0	+1.2	+0.0	+2.6	+0.0	+3.1

Riboflavin (mg)	0.4/0.5	0.95	+0.0	+1.1	+0.0	+0.6	+0.0	+1.4	+0.0	+1.6
Niacin (mg)	5/6	5.3	+0.1	+2.4	+0.1	+1.4	+0.2	+3.0	+0.2	+3.5
Vitamin B6 (mg)	0.4/0.5	0.71	+0.0	+5.0	+0.0	+2.9	+0.0	+6.1	+0.1	+7.2
Folate (μg DFE)	120/160	263	+5.0	+1.9	+2.9	+1.1	+6.0	+2.3	+7.1	+2.7
Choline (mg)	200/250*	58.0	+1.8	+3.1	+1.0	+1.8	+2.2	+3.8	+2.6	+4.4
Vitamin B12 (μg)	0.7/1	2.40	0	0	0	0	0	0	0	0
Vitamin A (μg RAE)	210/275	357	+5.2	+1.4	+3.0	+0.8	+6.3	+1.8	+7.4	+2.1
Vitamin E (mg)	5/6	1.8	+0.1	+4.7	+0.0	+2.7	+0.1	+5.7	+0.1	+6.6
Vitamin D (IU)	400	148	0	0	0	0	0	0	0	0
Saturated fat (g)	NA/14	4.5	+0.0	+1.0	+0.0	+0.6	+0.1	+1.2	+0.1	+1.4
Total fruit (c-eq)	1.25	0.63	+0.11	+18.4	0.07	+10.6	0.14	+22.2	0.16	+26.1
Fruit, whole (c-eq)	0.8	0.25	+0.11	+45.7	0.07	+26.3	0.14	+55.5	0.16	+65.2
Total vegetables (c-eq)	1.5	0.19	+0.06	+30.1	0.03	+17.3	0.07	+36.5	0.08	+42.8
HEI fruit, total	0 to 5	5.0	0	0	0	0	0	0	0	0
HEI fruit, whole	0 to 5	5.0	0	0	0	0	0	0	0	0
HEI vegetables, total	0 to 5	1.8	+0.17	+9.3	+0.10	+5.3	0.21	+11.3	+0.24	+13.2
HEI overall	0 to 100	66.3	+0.17	+0.3	+0.10	+0.1	0.21	+0.3	+0.24	+0.4
FP cost		$33.88	+$2.82	+8.3	+$1.62	+4.8	+$3.42	+10.1	+$4.02	+11.9
Average per-participant FP cost		$37.27	+$1.03	+2.8	+$0.59	+1.6	+$1.25	+3.4	+$1.47	+3.9

NOTES: See notes following Table S-22.

TABLE S-9 Food Package V-A Sensitivity Results: Impact of Changes to CVV Redemption

			Change from Current (Redemption Rate)							
			Revised: +$4 (75%)		Test 1: +$4 (65%)		Test 2: +$4 (80%)		Test 3: +$4 (85%)	
FP Nutrients, Food Groups, and Cost	EAR/AI,* 19–30y/ 31–50y	Current Amount (77% Redemption): $11	Absolute Change	%	Absolute Change	%	Absolute Change	%	Absolute Change	%
Energy (kcal)	2,625	468	+15.7	+3.4	+7.2	+1.5	+19.9	+4.3	+24.2	+5.2
Protein (g)	71 (RDA)	22.5	+0.2	+1.0	+0.1	+0.4	+0.3	+1.2	+0.3	+1.5
Total fat (g)	ND	13.4	+0.3	+2.1	+0.1	+1.0	+0.4	+2.7	+0.4	+3.2
Carbohydrate (g)	175 (RDA)	65.2	+2.7	+4.2	+1.2	+1.9	+3.5	+5.3	+4.2	+6.5
Fiber (g)	28*	4.9	+0.5	+10.3	+0.2	+4.7	+0.6	+13.1	+0.8	+15.9
Added sugar (g)	65.0	4.3	0	0	0	0	0	0	0	0
Calcium (mg)	800	581	+3.1	+0.5	+1.4	+0.2	+3.9	+0.7	+4.7	+0.8
Iron (mg)	22	8.2	+0.1	+0.9	+0.0	+0.4	+0.1	+1.2	+0.1	+1.4
Magnesium (mg)	290/300	114	+3.4	+3.0	+1.6	+1.4	+4.4	+3.9	+5.3	+4.7
Phosphorus (mg)	580	559	+5.6	+1.0	+2.5	+0.5	+7.1	+1.3	+8.6	+1.5
Potassium (mg)	4,700*	1,096	+55.8	+5.1	+25.4	+2.3	+70.9	+6.5	+86.1	+7.9
Sodium (mg)	1,500*	416	+0.9	+0.2	+0.4	+0.1	+1.1	+0.3	+1.4	+0.3
Zinc (mg)	9.5	3.8	+0.0	+1.0	+0.0	+0.5	+0.0	+1.3	+0.1	+1.5
Copper (mg)	0.8	0.26	+0.0	+5.9	+0.0	+2.7	+0.0	+7.5	+0.0	+9.1
Selenium (μg)	49	19.3	+0.1	+0.5	+0.0	+0.2	+0.1	+0.6	+0.1	+0.7
Vitamin C (mg)	70	50.8	+5.7	+11.2	+2.6	+5.1	+7.2	+14.2	+8.8	+17.2
Thiamin (mg)	1.2	0.54	+0.0	+2.0	+0.0	+0.9	+0.0	+2.6	+0.0	+3.1

Riboflavin (mg)	1.2	1.04	+0.0	+1.0	+0.0	+0.5	+0.0	+1.3	+0.0	+1.6
Niacin (mg)	14	5.80	+0.1	+2.2	+0.1	+1.0	+0.2	+2.8	+0.2	+3.4
Vitamin B6 (mg)	1.6	0.77	+0.0	+4.5	+0.0	+2.1	+0.0	+5.7	+0.1	+6.9
Folate (μg DFE)	520	283	+4.9	+1.7	+2.2	+0.8	+6.2	+2.2	+7.5	+2.7
Choline (mg)	450*	57.44	+1.8	+3.1	+0.8	+1.4	+2.2	+3.9	+2.7	+4.7
Vitamin B12 (μg)	2.2	2.54	0	0	0	0	0	0	0	0
Vitamin A (μg RAE)	550	381	+5.1	+1.3	+2.3	+0.6	+6.4	+1.7	+7.8	+2.0
Vitamin E (mg)	12	2.08	+0.1	+3.9	+0.0	+1.8	+0.1	+5.0	+0.1	+6.0
Vitamin D (IU)	400	168	0	0	0	0	0	0	0	0
Saturated fat (g)	29	6.0	+0.0	+0.7	+0.0	+0.7	+0.0	+0.7	+0.0	+0.7
Fruit, total (c-eq)	2.0	0.77	+0.11	+14.6	+0.1	+6.7	0.14	+18.6	+0.2	+22.6
Fruit, whole (c-eq)	1.0	0.34	+0.11	+32.5	+0.1	+14.8	0.14	+41.3	+0.2	+50.2
Vegetables, total (c-eq)	3.5	0.30	+0.06	+18.5	+0.03	+8.4	0.07	+23.5	+0.1	+28.5
FP cost		$36.68	+$2.76	+7.5	+$1.26	+3.4	+$3.51	+9.6	+$4.26	+11.6
Average per-participant FP cost		$37.27	+$0.26	+0.7	+$0.12	+0.3	+$0.34	+.09	+$0.41	+1.1

NOTES: See notes following Table S-22.

TABLE S-10 Food Package VII Sensitivity Results: Impact of Changes to CVV Amount and Redemption

FP Nutrients, Food Groups, and Cost	EAR/AI,* 19–30y/ 31–50y	Current Amount (77% Redemption): $11	Change from Current (Redemption Rate)							
			Revised: +$24 (75%)		Test 1: +$24 (85%)		Test 2: +$9 (75%)		Test 3: +$34 (75%)	
			Absolute Change	%	Absolute Change	%	Absolute Change	%	Absolute Change	%
Energy (kcal)	2,492	559	+101.0	+18.1	+120.9	+21.6	+37.0	+6.6	+143.6	+25.7
Protein (g)	71 (RDA)	32	+1.4	+4.4	+1.7	+5.3	+0.5	+1.6	+2.0	+6.3
Total fat (g)	ND	19	+1.8	+9.4	+2.2	+11.3	+0.7	+3.5	+2.6	+13.4
Carbohydrate (g)	210 (RDA)	66	+17.6	+26.8	+21.1	+32.1	+6.5	+9.8	+25.0	+38.2
Fiber (g)	29*	4.9	+3.3	+66.5	+3.9	+79.6	+1.2	+24.4	+4.6	+94.6
Added sugar (g)	65.0	3.9	0	0	0	0	0	0	0	0
Calcium (mg)	800	717	+19.7	+2.7	+23.5	+3.3	+7.2	+1.0	+28.0	+3.9
Iron (mg)	6.5	8.8	+0.5	+5.4	+0.6	+6.5	+0.2	+2.0	+0.7	+7.7
Magnesium (mg)	255/265	125	+22.2	+17.8	+26.6	+21.3	+8.1	+6.5	+31.6	+25.3
Phosphorus (mg)	580	698	+35.9	+5.1	+43.0	+6.2	+13.2	+1.9	+51.1	+7.3
Potassium (mg)	5,100*	1,181	+359.0	+30.4	+429.7	+36.4	+131.6	+11.1	+510.6	+43.2
Sodium (mg)	1,500*	608	+5.8	+0.9	+6.9	+1.1	+2.1	+0.3	+8.2	+1.3
Zinc (mg)	10.4	4.6	+0.2	+5.3	+0.3	+6.4	+0.1	+2.0	+0.3	+7.6
Copper (mg)	1	0.29	+0.1	+34.4	+0.1	+41.2	+0.0	+12.6	+0.1	+48.9
Selenium (μg)	59	41.4	+0.6	+1.4	+0.7	+1.7	+0.2	+0.5	+0.8	+2.0

Vitamin C (mg)	100	50.9	+36.5	+71.7	+43.7	+85.8	+13.4	+26.3	+51.9	+101.9
Thiamin (mg)	1.2	0.56	+0.1	+12.5	+0.1	+15.0	+0.0	+4.6	+0.1	+17.8
Riboflavin (mg)	1.3	1.19	+0.1	+5.7	+0.1	+6.8	+0.0	+2.1	+0.1	+8.1
Niacin (mg)	13	7.75	+0.8	+10.6	+1.0	+12.7	+0.3	+3.9	+1.2	+15.1
Vitamin B6 (mg)	1.7	0.87	+0.2	+25.7	+0.3	+30.8	+0.1	+9.4	+0.3	+36.6
Folate (µg DFE)	450	293	+31.3	+10.7	+37.5	+12.8	+11.5	+3.9	+44.5	+15.2
Choline (mg)	550*	113	+11.3	+10.0	+13.6	+12.0	+4.2	+3.7	+16.1	+14.2
Vitamin B12 (µg)	2.4	3.42	0	0	0	0	0	0	0	0
Vitamin A (µg RAE)	900	456	+32.5	+7.1	+38.9	+8.5	+11.9	+2.6	+46.3	+10.1
Vitamin E (mg)	16	2.41	+0.5	+21.7	+0.6	+26.0	+0.2	+8.0	+0.7	+30.9
Vitamin D (IU)	400	223	0	0	0	0	0	0	0	0
Saturated fat (g)	29	7.8	+0.3	+3.6	+0.3	+4.4	+0.1	+1.3	+0.4	+5.2
Fruit, total (c-eq)	2.0	0.77	+0.7	+94.2	+0.9	+112.7	+0.3	+34.5	+1.0	+133.9
Fruit, whole (c-eq)	1.0	0.34	+0.7	+209.1	+0.9	+250.4	+0.3	+76.7	+1.0	+297.5
Vegetables, total (c-eq)	3.5	0.30	+0.4	+119.0	+0.4	+142.4	0.13	+43.6	0.51	+169.2
FP cost		$47.41	+$17.76	+37.5	+$21.26	+44.8	+$6.51	+13.7	+$25.26	+53.3
Average per-participant FP cost		$37.27	+$0.58	+1.6	+$0.70	+1.9	+$0.21	+0.6	+$0.83	+2.2

NOTES: See notes following Table S-22.

TABLE S-11 Food Package IV-B Sensitivity Results: Impact of Changes to Proportions of Vegetables and Fruits Redeemed with the CVV

			Change from Current (Redemption Rate)			
			Revised: +$4 (75%), 33/67 Vegetable/Fruit		Test 1: +$4 (75%), 50/50 Vegetable/Fruit	
FP Nutrients, Food Groups, HEI Components, and Cost	EAR/AI,* 1–3y/4–8y	Current Amount (77% Redemption): $8	Absolute Change	%	Absolute Change	%
Energy (kcal)	1,300	423	+16.1	+3.8	+14.5	+3.4
Protein (g)	13 (RDA)	20.5	+0.2	+1.1	+0.3	+1.5
Total fat (g)	ND	11.2	+0.3	+2.6	+0.7	+5.9
Carbohydrate (g)	130 (RDA)	60.6	+2.8	+4.6	+2.0	+3.3
Fiber (g)	19/25*	4.3	+0.5	+12.0	+0.6	+14.5
Added sugar (g)	NA/32.5	4.3	0	0	0	0
Calcium (mg)	500/800	543	+3.1	+0.6	+3.2	+0.6
Iron (mg)	3/4.1	8.2	+0.1	+0.9	+0.1	+1.3
Magnesium (mg)	65/110	99	+3.5	+3.6	+4.1	+4.1
Phosphorus (mg)	380/405	513	+5.7	+1.1	+8.6	+1.7
Potassium (mg)	3,000/3,800*	927	+57.1	+6.2	+73.2	+7.9
Sodium (mg)	1,000/1,200*	412	+0.9	+0.2	+2.0	+0.5
Zinc (mg)	2.5/4	3.7	+0.0	+1.1	+0.1	+1.8
Copper (mg)	0.26/0.34	0.22	+0.0	+7.3	+0.0	+10.3
Selenium (μg)	17/23	21.1	+0.1	+0.4	+0.1	+0.3
Vitamin C (mg)	13/22	42.5	+5.8	+13.7	+5.8	+13.6

Thiamin (mg)	0.4/0.5	0.51	+0.0	+2.2	+0.0	+2.6
Riboflavin (mg)	0.4/0.5	0.95	+0.0	+1.1	+0.0	+1.3
Niacin (mg)	5/6	5.34	+0.1	+2.4	+0.2	+3.8
Vitamin B6 (mg)	0.4/0.5	0.71	+0.0	+5.0	+0.0	+5.7
Folate (μg DFE)	120/160	263	+5.0	+1.9	+7.0	+2.7
Choline (mg)	200/250*	58.0	+1.8	+3.1	+2.3	+3.9
Vitamin B12 (μg)	0.7/1	2.4	0	0	0	0
Vitamin A (μg RAE)	210/275	357	+5.2	+1.4	+11.6	+3.3
Vitamin E (mg)	5/6	1.8	+0.1	+4.7	+0.2	+8.7
Vitamin D (IU)	400	148	0	0	0	0
Saturated fat (g)	NA/14	4.5	+0.0	+1.0	+0.1	+2.2
Fruit, total (c-eq)	1.25	0.63	+0.11	+18.4	+0.02	+3.5
Fruit, whole (c-eq)	0.8	0.25	+0.11	+45.7	+0.02	+8.8
Vegetables, total (c-eq)	1.5	0.19	+0.06	+30.1	+0.15	+79.4
HEI fruit, total	0 to 5	5.00	0	0	0	0
HEI fruit, whole	0 to 5	5.00	0	0	0	0
HEI vegetables, total	0 to 5	1.84	+0.57	+30.9	+0.45	+24.6
HEI overall	0 to 100	66.26	+0.57	+0.9	+0.45	+0.7
FP cost		$33.88	+$2.82	+8.3	+$2.82	+8.3
Average per-participant FP cost		$37.27	+$1.03	+2.8	+$1.03	+2.8

NOTES: See notes following Table S-22.

TABLE S-12 Food Package V-A Sensitivity Results: Impact of Changes to Proportions of Vegetables and Fruits Redeemed with the CVV

			Change from Current (Redemption Rate)			
			Revised: +$4 (75%), 33/67 Vegetable/Fruit		Test 1: +$4 (75%), 50/50 Vegetable/Fruit	
FP Nutrients, Food Groups, and Cost	EAR/AI,* 19–30y/31–50y	Current Amount (77% Redemption): $11	Absolute Change	%	Absolute Change	%
Energy (kcal)	2,625	468	+15.7	+3.4	+13.8	+2.9
Protein (g)	71 (RDA)	22.5	+0.2	+1.0	+0.3	+1.4
Total fat (g)	ND	13.4	+0.3	+2.1	+0.8	+5.6
Carbohydrate (g)	175 (RDA)	65.2	+2.7	+4.2	+1.7	+2.7
Fiber (g)	28*	4.9	+0.5	+10.3	+0.6	+13.1
Added sugar (g)	65.0	4.3	0	0	0	0
Calcium (mg)	800	581	+3.1	+0.5	+3.1	+0.5
Iron (mg)	22	8.2	+0.1	+0.9	+0.1	+1.3
Magnesium (mg)	290/300	114	+3.4	+3.0	+4.1	+3.6
Phosphorus (mg)	580	559	+5.6	+1.0	+9.1	+1.6
Potassium (mg)	4,700*	1,096	+55.8	+5.1	+75.8	+6.9
Sodium (mg)	1,500*	416	+0.9	+0.2	+2.3	+0.6
Zinc (mg)	9.5	3.8	+0.0	+1.0	+0.1	+1.8
Copper (mg)	0.8	0.26	+0.0	+5.9	+0.0	+9.1

Selenium (μg)	49	19.3	+0.1	+0.5	+0.0	+0.2
Vitamin C (mg)	70	50.8	+5.7	+11.2	+5.6	+11.1
Thiamin (mg)	1.2	0.54	+0.0	+2.0	+0.0	+2.6
Riboflavin (mg)	1.2	1.04	+0.0	+1.0	+0.0	+1.2
Niacin (mg)	14	5.80	+0.1	+2.2	+0.2	+3.7
Vitamin B6 (mg)	1.6	0.77	+0.0	+4.5	+0.0	+5.2
Folate (μg DFE)	520	283	+4.9	+1.7	+7.4	+2.6
Choline (mg)	450*	57.4	+1.8	+3.1	+2.3	+4.1
Vitamin B12 (μg)	2.2	2.5	0	0	0	0
Vitamin A (μg RAE)	550	381	+5.1	+1.3	+13.1	+3.4
Vitamin E (mg)	12	2.08	+0.1	+3.9	+0.2	+8.2
Vitamin D (IU)	400	168	0	0	0	0
Saturated fat (g)	29	6.0	+0.0	+0.7	+0.1	+1.8
Fruit, total (c-eq)	2.0	0.77	+0.11	+14.6	−0.004	−0.5
Fruit, whole (c-eq)	1.0	0.34	+0.11	+32.5	−0.004	−1.1
Vegetables, total (c-eq)	3.5	0.30	+0.06	+18.5	+0.2	+57.3
FP cost		$36.68	+$2.76	+7.5	+$2.76	+7.5
Average per-participant FP cost		$37.27	+$0.26	+0.7	+$0.26	+0.7

NOTES: See notes following Table S-22.

TABLE S-13 Food Package VII Sensitivity Results: Impact of Changes to Proportions of Vegetables and Fruits Redeemed with the CVV

			Change from Current (Redemption Rate)			
			Revised: +$24, (75%), 33/67 Vegetable/Fruit		Test 1: +$24 (75%), 50/50 Vegetable/Fruit	
FP Nutrients, Food Groups, and Cost	EAR/AI,* 19–30y/31–50y	Current Amount (77% Redemption): $11	Absolute Change	%	Absolute Change	%
Energy (kcal)	2,492	559	+101.0	+18.1	+96.5	+17.3
Protein (g)	71 (RDA)	31.7	+1.4	+4.4	+1.6	+5.2
Total fat (g)	ND	19.1	+1.8	+9.4	+2.9	+15.2
Carbohydrate (g)	210 (RDA)	65.6	+17.6	+26.8	+15.3	+23.3
Fiber (g)	29*	4.9	+3.3	+66.5	+3.6	+73.1
Added sugar (g)	65.0	3.8	0	0	0	0
Calcium (mg)	800	717	+19.7	+2.7	+19.8	+2.8
Iron (mg)	6.5	8.8	+0.5	+5.4	+0.6	+6.4
Magnesium (mg)	255/265	125	+22.2	+17.8	+23.8	+19.0
Phosphorus (mg)	580	698	+35.9	+5.1	+44.2	+6.3
Potassium (mg)	5,100*	1,181	+359.0	+30.4	+405.8	+34.4
Sodium (mg)	1,500*	608	+5.8	+0.9	+9.0	+1.5
Zinc (mg)	10.4	4.6	+0.2	+5.3	+0.3	+6.9
Copper (mg)	1	0.29	+0.1	+34.4	+0.1	+41.0
Selenium (µg)	59	41.4	+0.6	+1.4	+0.5	+1.1

Vitamin C (mg)	100	50.9	+36.5	+71.7	+36.4	+71.5
Thiamin (mg)	1.2	0.56	+0.1	+12.5	+0.1	+13.8
Riboflavin (mg)	1.3	1.19	+0.1	+5.7	+0.1	+6.1
Niacin (mg)	13	7.8	+0.8	+10.6	+1.0	+13.3
Vitamin B6 (mg)	1.7	0.87	+0.2	+25.7	+0.2	+27.3
Folate (µg DFE)	450	293	+31.3	+10.7	+37.3	+12.7
Choline (mg)	550*	113	+11.3	+10.0	+12.7	+11.2
Vitamin B12 (µg)	2.4	3.42	0	0	0	0
Vitamin A (µg RAE)	900	456	+32.5	+7.1	+51.4	+11.3
Vitamin E (mg)	16	2.41	+0.5	+21.7	+0.7	+30.4
Vitamin D (IU)	400	223	0	0	0	0
Saturated fat (g)	29	7.8	+0.3	+3.6	+0.4	+5.7
Fruit, total (c-eq)	2.0	0.77	+0.7	+94.2	+0.5	+58.8
Fruit, whole (c-eq)	1.0	0.34	+0.7	+209.1	+0.5	+130.7
Vegetables, total (c-eq)	3.5	0.30	+0.4	+119.0	+0.6	+209.5
FP cost		$47.41	+$17.76	+37.5	+$17.76	+37.5
Average per-participant FP cost		$37.27	+$0.58	+1.6	+$0.58	+1.6

NOTES: See notes following Table S-22.

TABLE S-14 Food Package IV-B Sensitivity Results: Impact of Changes to Juice/CVV Amounts

			Change from Current (Redemption Rate)					
			Revised: –64 oz (78%), +$4 CVV		Test 1: –64 oz (75%), +$4 CVV		Test 2: –128 oz (no juice), +$18 CVV	
FP Nutrients, Food Groups, HEI Components, and Cost	EAR/AI,* 1–3y/4–8y	Current Amount: 128 oz Juice (70%), $8 CVV	Absolute Change	%	Absolute Change	%	Absolute Change	%
Energy (kcal)	1,300	423	–4.1	–1.0	–5.2	–1.2	–3.9	–0.9
Protein (g)	13 (RDA)	20.5	+0.1	+0.6	+0.1	+0.5	+0.3	+1.6
Total fat (g)	ND	11.2	+0.2	+2.2	+0.2	+2.2	+0.6	+5.8
Carbohydrate (g)	130 (RDA)	60.6	–2.1	–3.5	–2.4	–4.0	–3.9	–6.5
Fiber (g)	19/25*	4.3	+0.5	+10.6	+0.5	+10.5	+1.2	+27.9
Added sugar (g)	NA/32.5	4.3	0	0	0	0	0	0
Calcium (mg)	500/800	543	–0.2	–0.0	–0.4	–0.1	+0.5	+0.1
Iron (mg)	3/4.1	8.2	–0.0	–0.2	–0.0	–0.3	–0.0	–0.2
Magnesium (mg)	65/110	99	+0.6	+0.7	+0.5	+0.5	+2.6	+2.7
Phosphorus (mg)	380/405	513	+1.6	+0.3	+1.3	+0.3	+5.4	+1.1
Potassium (mg)	3,000/3,800*	927	+7.5	+0.8	+4.9	+0.5	+35.9	+3.9
Sodium (mg)	1,000/1,200*	412	–1.5	–0.4	–1.7	–0.4	–3.2	–0.8
Zinc (mg)	2.5/4	3.7	+0.0	+0.5	+0.0	+0.5	+0.1	+1.6
Copper (mg)	0.26/0.34	0.22	+0.0	+4.3	+0.0	+4.1	+0.0	+12.1
Selenium (μg)	17/23	21.1	+0.1	+0.3	+0.1	+0.3	+0.2	+0.8
Vitamin C (mg)	13/22	42.5	–4.8	–11.3	–5.4	–12.6	–8.9	–21.0
Thiamin (mg)	0.4/0.5	0.51	+0.0	+1.0	+0.0	+1.0	+0.0	+3.0

Riboflavin (mg)	0.4/0.5	0.95	+0.0	+0.4	+0.0	+0.3	+0.0	+1.2
Niacin (mg)	5/6	5.34	+0.1	+1.7	+0.1	+1.7	+0.3	+4.7
Vitamin B6 (mg)	0.4/0.5	0.71	+0.0	+3.0	+0.0	+2.8	+0.1	+8.3
Folate (µg DFE)	120/160	263	+4.1	+1.6	+4.1	+1.6	+11.0	+4.2
Choline (mg)	200/250*	58.0	+1.8	+3.1	+1.8	+3.1	+4.7	+8.1
Vitamin B12 (µg)	0.7/1	2.4	0	0	0	0	0	0
Vitamin A (µg RAE)	210/275	357	+5.0	+1.4	+5.0	+1.4	+13.1	+3.7
Vitamin E (mg)	5/6	1.8	+0.1	+4.3	+0.1	+4.3	+0.2	+11.2
Vitamin D (IU)	400	148	0	0	0	0	0	0
Saturated fat (g)	NA/14	4.5	+0.04	+0.8	+0.04	+0.8	+0.1	+2.2
Total fruit (c-eq)	1.25	0.63	–0.05	–8.1	–0.06	–9.5	–0.08	–12.3
Fruit, whole (c-eq)	0.8	0.25	+0.11	+45.7	+0.11	+45.7	+0.30	+119
Total vegetables (c-eq)	1.5	0.19	+0.06	+30.1	+0.06	+30.1	+0.15	+78.0
HEI fruit, total	0 to 5	5.0	0	0	0	0	0	0
HEI fruit, whole	0 to 5	5.0	0	0	0	0	0	0
HEI vegetables, total	0 to 5	1.8	+0.2	+9.3	+0.2	+9.3	+0.44	+24.1
HEI overall	0 to 100	66.3	+0.2	+0.3	+0.2	+0.3	+0.44	+0.7
FP cost		$33.88	+$0.87	+2.6	+$0.77	+2.3	$2.91	+8.6
Average per-participant FP cost		$37.27	+$0.32	+0.8	+$0.28	+0.7	$0.32	+0.8

NOTES: See notes following Table S-22.

TABLE S-15 Food Package V-A Sensitivity Results: Impact of Changes to Juice/CVV Amounts

FP Nutrients, Food Groups, and Cost	EAR/AI,* 19–30y/31–50y	Current Amount: 144 oz Juice (70%), $11 CVV	Change from Current (Redemption Rate)			
			Revised: –80 oz (79%), +$4 CVV		Test 1: –144 oz (no juice), +$10 CVV	
			Absolute Change	%	Absolute Change	%
Energy (kcal)	2,625	468	–9.8	–2.1	–10.0	–2.1
Protein (g)	71 (RDA)	22.5	+0.1	+0.4	+0.3	+1.4
Total fat (g)	ND	13.4	+0.2	+1.7	+0.6	+4.7
Carbohydrate (g)	175 (RDA)	65.2	–3.5	–5.4	–5.4	–8.3
Fiber (g)	28*	4.9	+0.4	+8.7	+1.2	+23.9
Added sugar (g)	65.0	4.3	0	0	0	0
Calcium (mg)	800	581	–1.2	–0.2	–0.5	–0.1
Iron (mg)	22	8.2	–0.0	–0.6	–0.0	–0.6
Magnesium (mg)	290/300	114	–0.2	–0.2	+1.7	+1.5
Phosphorus (mg)	580	559	+0.3	+0.1	+4.1	+0.7
Potassium (mg)	4,700*	1,096	–7.0	–0.6	+20.5	+1.9
Sodium (mg)	1,500*	416	–2.2	–0.5	–3.9	–0.9
Zinc (mg)	9.5	3.8	+0.0	+0.4	+0.1	+1.3
Copper (mg)	0.8	0.26	+0.0	+2.8	+0.0	+9.2
Selenium (μg)	49	19.3	+0.0	+0.3	+0.2	+0.8

Vitamin C (mg)	70	50.8	−7.7	−15.2	−12.1	−23.7
Thiamin (mg)	1.2	0.54	+0.0	+0.6	+0.0	+2.5
Riboflavin (mg)	1.2	1.04	+0.0	+0.1	+0.0	+0.9
Niacin (mg)	14	5.80	+0.1	+1.4	+0.2	+4.1
Vitamin B6 (mg)	1.6	0.77	+0.0	+2.1	+0.1	+7.0
Folate (µg DFE)	520	283	+3.8	+1.3	+10.7	+3.8
Choline (mg)	450*	57.4	+1.8	+3.1	+4.6	+8.1
Vitamin B12 (µg)	2.2	2.5	0	0	0	0
Vitamin A (µg RAE)	550	381	+4.9	+1.3	+12.9	+3.4
Vitamin E (mg)	12	2.08	+0.1	+3.5	+0.2	+9.4
Vitamin D (IU)	400	168	0	0	0	0
Saturated fat (g)	29	6.0	+0.8	+13.8	+0.9	+14.9
Fruit, total (c-eq)	2.0	0.77	−0.10	−12.7	−0.13	−16.5
Fruit, whole (c-eq)	1.0	0.34	+0.11	+32.5	+0.29	+85.5
Vegetables, total (c-eq)	3.5	0.30	+0.06	+18.5	+0.15	+48.6
FP cost		$36.68	+$0.29	+0.8	+$2.29	+6.2
Average per-participant FP cost		$37.27	+$0.03	+0.1	+$0.22	+0.6

NOTES: See notes following Table S-22.

TABLE S-16 Food Package VII Sensitivity Results: Impact of Changes to Juice/CVV Amounts

FP Nutrients, Food Groups, and Cost	EAR/AI,* 19–30y/31–50y	Current Amount: 144 oz Juice (70%), $11 CVV	Change from Current (Redemption Rate)			
			Revised: –80 oz (79%), +$24 CVV		Test 1: –144 oz (no juice), +$41 CVV	
			Absolute Change	%	Absolute Change	%
Energy (kcal)	2,492	559	+75.5	+13.5	+75.3	+13.5
Protein (g)	71 (RDA)	31.7	+1.3	+4.0	+1.5	+4.7
Total fat (g)	ND	19.1	+1.8	+9.2	+2.2	+11.3
Carbohydrate (g)	210 (RDA)	65.6	+11.4	+17.3	+9.5	+14.5
Fiber (g)	29*	4.9	+3.2	+64.9	+3.9	+80.1
Added sugar (g)	65.0	3.8	0	0	0	0
Calcium (mg)	800	717	+15.4	+2.2	+16.1	+2.2
Iron (mg)	6.5	8.8	+0.4	+4.1	+0.4	+4.0
Magnesium (mg)	255/265	125	+18.6	+14.8	+20.5	+16.4
Phosphorus (mg)	580	698	+30.7	+4.4	+34.4	+4.9
Potassium (mg)	5,100*	1,181	+296.2	+25.1	+323.7	+27.4
Sodium (mg)	1,500*	608	+2.7	+0.4	+1.0	+0.2
Zinc (mg)	10.4	4.6	+0.2	+4.8	+0.3	+5.6
Copper (mg)	1	0.29	+0.1	+31.6	+0.1	+37.4

Selenium (µg)	59	41.4	+0.5	+1.3	+0.6	+1.5
Vitamin C (mg)	100	50.9	+23.1	+45.4	+18.8	+36.9
Thiamin (mg)	1.2	0.56	+0.1	+11.2	+0.1	+13.0
Riboflavin (mg)	1.3	1.19	+0.1	+4.9	+0.1	+5.6
Niacin (mg)	13	7.8	+0.8	+10.0	+0.9	+12.0
Vitamin B6 (mg)	1.7	0.87	+0.2	+23.6	+0.2	+27.9
Folate (µg DFE)	450	293	+30.2	+10.3	+37.1	+12.6
Choline (mg)	550*	113	+11.3	+10.0	+14.2	+12.5
Vitamin B12 (µg)	2.4	3.42	0	0	0	0
Vitamin A (µg RAE)	900	456	+32.3	+7.1	+40.4	+8.9
Vitamin E (mg)	16	2.41	+0.5	+21.4	+0.6	+26.5
Vitamin D (IU)	400	223	0	0	0	0
Saturated fat (g)	29	7.8	+0.3	+3.5	+0.3	+4.3
Fruit, total (c-eq)	2.0	0.77	+0.5	+66.8	+0.5	+63.0
Fruit, whole (c-eq)	1.0	0.34	+0.7	+209	+0.9	+262.1
Vegetables, total (c-eq)	3.5	0.30	+0.4	+119	+0.4	+149.1
FP cost		$47.41	+$15.29	+32.2	+$17.29	+36.5
Average per-participant FP cost		$37.27	+$0.50	+1.3	+$0.57	+1.5

NOTES: See notes following Table S-22.

TABLE S-17 Food Package IV-B Sensitivity Results: Impact of Changes to Fish Amounts and Redemption

			Change from Current (Redemption Rate)					
			Revised: +10 oz every 3 mo (68%)		Test 1: +10 oz every 3 mo (59%)		Test 2: +10 oz every 3 mo (79%)	
FP Nutrients, Food Groups, HEI Components, and Cost	EAR/AI,* 1–3y/4–8y	Current Amount: No Fish	Absolute Change	%	Absolute Change	%	Absolute Change	%
Energy (kcal)	1,300	423	+2.0	+0.5	+1.7	+0.4	+2.3	+0.6
Protein (g)	13 (RDA)	20.5	+0.4	+2.1	+0.4	+1.8	+0.5	+2.4
Total fat (g)	ND	11.2	+0.0	+0.3	+0.0	+0.3	+0.0	+0.3
Carbohydrate (g)	130 (RDA)	60.6	0	0	0	0	0	0
Fiber (g)	19/25*	4.3	0	0	0	0	0	0
Added sugar (g)	NA/32.5	4.3	0	0	0	0	0	0
Calcium (mg)	500/800	543	+1.2	+0.2	+1.0	+0.2	+1.4	+0.3
Iron (mg)	3/4.1	8.2	+0.0	+0.4	+0.0	+0.3	+0.0	+0.5
Magnesium (mg)	65/110	99	+0.5	+0.5	+0.5	+0.5	+0.6	+0.6
Phosphorus (mg)	380/405	513	+3.7	+0.7	+3.2	+0.6	+4.3	+0.8
Potassium (mg)	3,000/3,800*	927	+4.3	+0.5	+3.7	+0.4	+5.0	+0.5
Sodium (mg)	1,000/1,200*	412	+5.7	+1.4	+5.0	+1.2	+6.6	+1.6
Zinc (mg)	2.5/4	3.7	+0.0	+0.4	+0.0	+0.4	+0.0	+0.5
Copper (mg)	0.26/0.34	0.22	+0.0	+0.5	+0.0	+0.5	+0.0	+0.6
Selenium (μg)	17/23	21.1	+1.4	+6.7	+1.2	+5.8	+1.6	+7.8
Vitamin C (mg)	13/22	42.5	0	0	0	0	0	0

Thiamin (mg)	0.4/0.5	0.51	+0.0	+0.1	+0.0	+0.1	+0.0	+0.1
Riboflavin (mg)	0.4/0.5	0.95	+0.0	+0.2	+0.0	+0.2	+0.0	+0.3
Niacin (mg)	5/6	5.34	+0.2	+3.9	+0.2	+3.4	+0.2	+4.5
Vitamin B6 (mg)	0.4/0.5	0.71	+0.0	+0.9	+0.0	+0.8	+0.0	+1.0
Folate (μg DFE)	120/160	263	+0.1	+0.0	+0.1	+0.0	+0.1	+0.0
Choline (mg)	200/250*	58.0	+0.8	+1.4	+0.7	+1.2	+0.9	+1.6
Vitamin B12 (μg)	0.7/1	2.4	+0.1	+2.6	+0.1	+2.3	+0.1	+3.0
Vitamin A (μg RAE)	210/275	357	+0.4	+0.1	+0.3	+0.1	+0.4	+0.1
Vitamin E (mg)	5/6	1.8	+0.0	+0.6	+0.0	+0.5	+0.0	+0.7
Vitamin D (IU)	400	148	+2.7	+1.8	+2.3	+1.6	+3.1	+2.1
Saturated fat (g)	NA/14	4.5	+0.0	+0.1	+0.0	+0.1	+0.0	+0.2
Total protein (oz-eq)	3.5	0.62	+0.08	+12.1	+0.07	+10.5	+0.09	+14.0
Seafood (oz-eq)	0.57	0	+0.08	NA	+0.07	NA	+0.09	NA
HEI seafood and plant proteins	0 to 5	1.25	+0.31	+25.1	+0.27	+21.8	+0.37	+29.3
HEI total protein foods	0 to 5	3.90	+0.10	+2.6	+0.09	+2.2	+0.12	+3.0
HEI overall	0 to 100	66.26	+0.41	+0.6	+0.36	+0.5	+0.48	+0.7
FP cost		$33.88	+$0.46	+1.4	+$0.40	+1.2	+$0.53	+1.6
Average per-participant FP cost		$37.27	+$0.16	+0.4	+$0.14	+0.4	+$0.19	+0.5

NOTES: See notes following Table S-22.

TABLE S-18 Food Package V-A Sensitivity Results: Impact of Changes to Fish Amounts and Redemption

FP Nutrients, Food Groups, and Cost	EAR/AI,* 19–30y/31–50y	Current Amount: No Fish	Change from Current (Redemption Rate)					
			Revised: +10 oz every 3 mo (68%)		Test 1: +10 oz every 3 mo (59%)		Test 2: +10 oz every 3 mo (79%)	
			Absolute Change	%	Absolute Change	%	Absolute Change	%
Energy (kcal)	2,625	468	+2.0	+0.4	+1.7	+0.4	+2.3	+0.5
Protein (g)	71 (RDA)	22.5	+0.4	+1.9	+0.4	+1.7	+0.5	+2.2
Total fat (g)	ND	13.4	+0.0	+0.2	+0.0	+0.2	+0.0	+0.3
Carbohydrate (g)	175 (RDA)	65.2	0	0	0	0	0	0
Fiber (g)	28*	4.9	0	0	0	0	0	0
Added sugar (g)	65.0	4.3	0	0	0	0	0	0
Calcium (mg)	800	581	+1.2	+0.2	+1.0	+0.2	+1.4	+0.2
Iron (mg)	22	8.2	+0.0	+0.4	+0.0	+0.3	+0.0	+0.5
Magnesium (mg)	290/300	114	+0.5	+0.5	+0.5	+0.4	+0.6	+0.5
Phosphorus (mg)	580	559	+3.7	+0.7	+3.2	+0.6	+4.3	+0.8
Potassium (mg)	4,700*	1,096	+4.3	+0.4	+3.7	+0.3	+5.0	+0.5
Sodium (mg)	1,500*	416	+5.7	+1.4	+5.0	+1.2	+6.6	+1.6
Zinc (mg)	9.5	3.8	+0.0	+0.4	+0.0	+0.4	+0.0	+0.5
Copper (mg)	0.8	0.26	+0.0	+0.5	+0.0	+0.4	+0.0	+0.5

Selenium (μg)	49	19.3	+1.4	+7.3	+1.2	+6.4	+1.6	+8.5
Vitamin C (mg)	70	50.8	0	0	0	0	0	0
Thiamin (mg)	1.2	0.54	+0.0	+0.1	+0.0	+0.1	+0.0	+0.1
Riboflavin (mg)	1.2	1.04	+0.0	+0.2	+0.0	+0.2	+0.0	+0.2
Niacin (mg)	14	5.80	+0.2	+3.6	+0.2	+3.1	+0.2	+4.2
Vitamin B6 (mg)	1.6	0.77	+0.0	+0.8	+0.0	+0.7	+0.0	+0.9
Folate (μg DFE)	520	283	+0.1	+0.0	+0.1	+0.0	+0.1	+0.0
Choline (mg)	450*	57.4	+0.8	+1.4	+0.7	+1.2	+0.9	+1.6
Vitamin B12 (μg)	2.2	2.5	+0.1	+2.4	+0.1	+2.1	+0.1	+2.8
Vitamin A (μg RAE)	550	381	+0.4	+0.1	+0.3	+0.1	+0.4	+0.1
Vitamin E (mg)	12	2.08	+0.0	+0.5	+0.0	+0.4	+0.0	+0.6
Vitamin D (IU)	400	168	+2.7	+1.6	+2.3	+1.4	+3.1	+1.9
Saturated fat (g)	29	6.0	+0.0	+0.1	+0.0	+0.1	+0.0	+0.1
Total protein (oz-eq)	6.5	0.93	+0.1	+8.1	+0.1	+7.0	+0.1	+9.4
Seafood (oz-eq)	1.4	0	+0.1	NA	+0.1	NA	+0.1	NA
FP cost		$36.68	+$0.46	+1.2	+$0.40	+1.1	+$0.53	+1.5
Average per-participant FP cost		$37.27	+$0.04	+0.1	+$0.04	+0.1	+$0.05	+0.1

NOTES: See notes following Table S-22.

TABLE S-19 Food Package VII Sensitivity Results: Impact of Changes to Fish Amounts and Redemption

			Change from Current (Redemption Rate)					
			Revised: –10 oz per mo (68%)		Test 1: –10 oz per mo (59%)		Test 2: –10 oz per mo (79%)	
FP Nutrients, Food Groups, and Cost	EAR/AI,* 19–30y/31–50y	Current Amount: 30 oz per mo (69% Redemption)	Absolute Change	%	Absolute Change	%	Absolute Change	%
Energy (kcal)	2,492	559	–6.4	–1.1	–8.0	–1.4	–4.4	–0.8
Protein (g)	71 (RDA)	31.7	–1.4	–4.3	–1.7	–5.4	–0.9	–3.0
Total fat (g)	ND	19.1	–0.1	–0.6	–0.1	–0.7	–0.1	–0.4
Carbohydrate (g)	210 (RDA)	65.6	0	0	0	0	0	0
Fiber (g)	29*	4.9	0	0	0	0	0	0
Added sugar (g)	65.0	3.8	0	0	0	0	0	0
Calcium (mg)	800	717	–3.9	–0.5	–4.8	–0.7	–2.7	–0.4
Iron (mg)	6.5	8.8	–0.1	–1.2	–0.1	–1.5	–0.1	–0.8
Magnesium (mg)	255/265	125	–1.7	–1.3	–2.1	–1.7	–1.2	–0.9
Phosphorus (mg)	580	698	–11.9	–1.7	–14.9	–2.1	–8.3	–1.2
Potassium (mg)	5,100*	1,181	–13.8	–1.2	–17.2	–1.5	–9.6	–0.8
Sodium (mg)	1,500*	608	–18.3	–3.0	–22.7	–3.7	–12.7	–2.1
Zinc (mg)	10.4	4.6	–0.0	–1.1	–0.1	–1.3	–0.0	–0.8
Copper (mg)	1	0.29	–0.0	–1.3	–0.0	–1.6	–0.0	–0.9

Selenium (μg)	59	41.4	–4.5	–10.9	–5.6	–13.6	–3.1	–7.6
Vitamin C (mg)	100	50.9	0	0	0	0	0	0
Thiamin (mg)	1.2	0.56	–0.0	–0.4	–0.0	–0.5	–0.0	–0.3
Riboflavin (mg)	1.3	1.19	–0.0	–0.6	–0.0	–0.7	–0.0	–0.4
Niacin (mg)	13	7.8	–0.7	–8.6	–0.8	–10.7	–0.5	–6.0
Vitamin B6 (mg)	1.7	0.87	–0.0	–2.3	–0.0	–2.8	–0.0	–1.6
Folate (μg DFE)	450	293	–0.3	–0.1	–0.3	–0.1	–0.2	–0.1
Choline (mg)	550*	113	–2.6	–2.3	–3.2	–2.8	–1.8	–1.6
Vitamin B12 (μg)	2.4	3.42	–0.2	–5.8	–0.2	–7.2	–0.1	–4.0
Vitamin A (μg RAE)	900	456	–1.2	–0.3	–1.5	–0.3	–0.8	–0.2
Vitamin E (mg)	16	2.41	–0.0	–1.3	–0.0	–1.7	–0.0	–0.9
Vitamin D (IU)	400	223	–8.6	–3.9	–10.7	–4.8	–6.0	–2.7
Saturated fat (g)	29	7.8	–0.0	–0.3	–0.0	–0.3	–0.0	–0.2
Total protein (oz-eq)	6.5	1.94	–0.2	–12.4	–0.3	–15.5	–0.2	–8.6
Seafood (oz-eq)	1.4	0.69	–0.2	–34.8	–0.3	–43.3	–0.2	–24.1
FP cost		$47.41	–$1.47	–3.1	–$1.83	–3.9	–$1.02	–2.1
Average per-participant FP cost		$37.27	–$0.05	–0.1	–$0.06	–0.2	–$0.04	–0.1

NOTES: See notes following Table S-22.

TABLE S-20 Food Package IV-B Sensitivity Results: Impact of Changes to Peanut Butter/Legumes/Fish Rotation

FP Nutrients, Food Groups, HEI Components, and Cost	EAR/AI,* 1–3y/4–8y	Current Amount: 1 lb Choice Legumes or Peanut Butter (51% Redemption), No Fish	Change from Current (Redemption Rate)							
			Revised: –2.7 oz Legumes/mo (53%); –3 oz Peanut Butter/mo (53%); +3.3 oz Fish/mo (68%)		Test 1: –2.7 oz Legumes/mo (53%); –3 oz Peanut Butter/mo (53%); No Fish		Test 2: –2.7 oz Legumes/mo (38%); –3 oz Peanut Butter/mo (53%); +3.3 oz Fish/mo (68%)		Test 3: –2.7 oz Legumes/mo (69%); –3 oz Peanut Butter/mo (53%); +3.3 oz Fish/mo (68%)	
			Absolute Change	%	Absolute Change	%	Absolute Change	%	Absolute Change	%
Energy (kcal)	1,300	423	–13.1	–3.1	–15.1	–3.6	–18.9	–4.5	–7.1	–1.7
Protein (g)	13 (RDA)	20.5	–0.2	–0.8	–0.6	–2.9	–0.4	–2.1	+0.1	+0.6
Total fat (g)	ND	11.2	–1.2	–10.4	–1.2	–10.7	–1.5	–13.1	–0.9	–7.6
Carbohydrate (g)	130 (RDA)	60.6	–0.7	–1.2	–0.7	–1.2	–1.3	–2.1	–0.2	–0.3
Fiber (g)	19/25*	4.3	–0.2	–3.9	–0.2	–3.9	–0.3	–7.1	–0.0	–0.6
Added sugar (g)	NA/32.5	4.3	–0.1	–3.4	–0.1	–3.4	–0.2	–4.3	–0.1	–2.6
Calcium (mg)	500/800	543	–0.3	–0.1	–1.5	–0.3	–1.4	–0.3	+0.8	+0.2
Iron (mg)	3/4.1	8.2	–0.0	–0.3	–0.1	–0.7	–0.1	–0.9	+0.0	+0.2
Magnesium (mg)	65/110	99	–4.0	–4.0	–4.5	–4.6	–6.1	–6.2	–1.8	–1.9
Phosphorus (mg)	380/405	513	–5.4	–1.1	–9.1	–1.8	–10.0	–1.9	–0.7	–0.1
Potassium (mg)	3,000/3,800*	927	–13.5	–1.5	–17.8	–1.9	–25.9	–2.8	–0.8	–0.1
Sodium (mg)	1,000/1,200*	412	–4.1	–1.0	–9.8	–2.4	–7.2	–1.7	–1.0	–0.2
Zinc (mg)	2.5/4	3.7	–0.1	–1.4	–0.1	–1.8	–0.1	–2.3	–0.0	–0.5
Copper (mg)	0.26/0.34	0.22	–0.0	–5.4	–0.0	–5.9	–0.0	–9.2	–0.0	–1.5
Selenium (µg)	17/23	21.1	+1.2	+5.9	–0.2	–0.8	+1.1	+5.1	+1.4	+6.6
Vitamin C (mg)	13/22	42.5	0	0	0	0	–0.0	–0.1	0	0
Thiamin (mg)	0.4/0.5	0.51	–0.0	–1.1	–0.0	–1.2	–0.0	–2.2	+0.0	+0.1
Riboflavin (mg)	0.4/0.5	0.95	–0.0	–0.3	–0.0	–0.5	–0.0	–0.6	0	0

Niacin (mg)	5/6	5.34	−0.1	−1.9	−0.3	−5.8	−0.2	−3.5	−0.0	−0.3
Vitamin B6 (mg)	0.4/0.5	0.71	−0.0	−0.8	−0.0	−1.7	−0.0	−1.5	0	0
Folate (µg DFE)	120/160	263	−3.7	−1.4	−3.8	−1.4	−7.3	−2.8	0	0
Choline (mg)	200/250*	58.0	+0.8	+1.4	0	0	+0.8	+1.4	+0.8	+1.4
Vitamin B12 (µg)	0.7/1	2.4	+0.1	+2.6	0	0	+0.1	+2.6	+0.1	+2.6
Vitamin A (µg RAE)	210/275	357	+0.4	+0.1	0	0	+0.4	+0.1	+0.4	+0.1
Vitamin E (mg)	5/6	1.8	−0.2	−11.3	−0.2	−11.9	−0.3	−14.4	−0.1	−8.2
Vitamin D (IU)	400	148	+2.7	+1.8	0	0	+2.7	+1.8	+2.7	+1.8
Saturated fat (g)	NA/14	4.5	−0.2	−5.2	−0.2	−5.4	−0.3	−6.6	−0.2	−3.8
Total vegetables (c-eq)	1.5	0.19	−0.02	−9.9	−0.02	−9.9	−0.03	−17.3	−0.01	−3.4
Beans (oz-eq)	0.1	0.06	−0.02	−28.8	−0.02	−28.8	−0.03	−50.4	−0.01	−9.9
Total protein (oz-eq)	3.5	0.62	−0.02	−2.8	−0.09	−14.9	−0.02	−2.8	−0.12	−19.9
Nuts, seeds, and soy (oz-eq)	0.36	0.31	−0.09	−30.3	−0.09	−30.3	−0.09	−30.3	−0.09	−30.3
Seafood (oz-eq)	0.57	0	0.08	NA	0.00	NA	0.08	NA	0.08	NA
HEI greens and beans	0 to 5	1.10	−0.31	−28.1	−0.31	−28.1	−0.54	−49.1	−0.11	−9.6
HEI seafood and plant proteins	0 to 5	1.25	−0.07	−5.8	−0.39	−30.9	−0.07	−5.8	−0.07	−5.8
HEI total protein foods	0 to 5	3.90	−0.02	−0.6	−0.12	−3.2	−0.02	−0.6	−0.17	−4.2
HEI overall	0 to 100	66.26	−0.46	−0.7	−0.88	−1.3	−0.73	−1.1	−0.36	−0.5
FP cost		$33.88	+$0.11	+0.3	−$0.34	−1.0	−$0.13	−0.4	+$0.37	+1.1
Average per-participant FP cost		$37.27	+$0.04	+0.1	−$0.13	−0.3	−$0.05	−0.1	+$0.13	+0.4

NOTES: See notes following Table S-22.

TABLE S-21 Food Package V-A Sensitivity Results: Impact of Changes to Peanut Butter/Legumes/Fish Rotation

			Change from Current (Redemption Rate)							
		Current Amount: 1 lb Legumes and 18 oz Peanut Butter (53% Redemption), No Fish	Revised: –5.3 oz Legumes/mo (53%); –12 oz Peanut Butter/mo (53%); +3.3 oz Fish/mo (68%)		Test 1: –5.3 oz Legumes/mo (53%); –12 oz Peanut Butter/mo (53%); No Fish		Test 2: –5.3 oz Legumes/mo (38%); –12 oz Peanut Butter/mo (53%); +3.3 oz Fish/mo (68%)		Test 3: –5.3 oz Legumes/mo (69%); –12 oz Peanut Butter/mo (53%); +3.3 oz Fish/mo (68%)	
FP Nutrients, Food Groups, and Cost	EAR/AI,* 19–30y/31–50y		Absolute Change	%	Absolute Change	%	Absolute Change	%	Absolute Change	%
Energy (kcal)	2,625	468	–38.2	–8.2	–40.2	–8.6	–46.9	–10.0	–29.3	–6.3
Protein (g)	71 (RDA)	22.5	–1.2	–5.5	–1.7	–7.4	–1.6	–7.3	–0.8	–3.6
Total fat (g)	ND	13.4	–2.9	–21.7	–2.9	–21.9	–3.4	–25.1	–2.4	–18.1
Carbohydrate (g)	175(RDA)	65.2	–2.4	–3.7	–2.4	–3.7	–3.2	–5.0	–1.6	–2.4
Fiber (g)	28*	4.9	–0.6	–11.7	–0.6	–11.7	–0.8	–16.0	–0.4	–7.4
Added sugar (g)	65.0	4.3	–0.4	–8.3	–0.4	–8.3	–0.4	–9.6	–0.3	–7.0
Calcium (mg)	800	581	–3.8	–0.6	–5.0	–0.9	–5.4	–0.9	–2.1	–0.4
Iron (mg)	22	8.2	–0.2	–2.0	–0.2	–2.3	–0.2	–2.8	–0.1	–1.1
Magnesium (mg)	290/300	114	–12.1	–10.7	–12.7	–11.1	–15.3	–13.4	–8.9	–7.8
Phosphorus (mg)	580	559	–22.5	–4.0	–26.2	–4.7	–29.4	–5.3	–15.5	–2.8
Potassium (mg)	4,700*	1,096	–52.9	–4.8	–57.2	–5.2	–71.6	–6.5	–33.9	–3.1
Sodium (mg)	1,500*	416	–19.3	–4.6	–25.0	–6.0	–23.9	–5.8	–14.6	–3.5
Zinc (mg)	9.5	3.8	–0.2	–4.5	–0.2	–4.9	–0.2	–5.8	–0.1	–3.3
Copper (mg)	0.8	0.26	–0.0	–15.0	–0.0	–15.5	–0.1	–19.8	–0.0	–10.1
Selenium (µg)	49	19.3	+1.4	+7.3	0	0	+1.4	+7.3	+1.4	+7.3

Vitamin C (mg)	70	50.8	–0.1	–0.2	–0.1	–0.2	–0.1	–0.3	–0.0	–0.1
Thiamin (mg)	1.2	0.54	–0.0	–4.0	–0.0	–4.1	–0.0	–5.5	–0.0	–2.4
Riboflavin (mg)	1.2	1.04	–0.0	–1.2	–0.0	–1.4	–0.0	–1.6	–0.0	–0.8
Niacin (mg)	14	5.80	–0.6	–9.6	–0.8	–13.2	–0.7	–11.8	–0.4	–7.4
Vitamin B6 (mg)	1.6	0.77	–0.0	–3.4	–0.0	–4.2	–0.0	–4.4	–0.0	–2.4
Folate (µg DFE)	520	283	–13.7	–4.9	–13.8	–4.9	–19.2	–6.8	–8.2	–2.9
Choline (mg)	450*	57.4	+0.8	+1.4	0	0	+0.8	+1.4	+0.8	+1.4
Vitamin B12 (µg)	2.2	2.5	+0.1	+2.4	0	0	+0.1	+2.4	+0.1	+2.4
Vitamin A (µg RAE)	550	381	+0.4	+0.1	0	0	+0.4	+0.1	+0.4	+0.1
Vitamin E (mg)	12	2.08	–0.5	–24.5	–0.5	–25.0	–0.6	–28.4	–0.4	–20.5
Vitamin D (IU)	400	168	+2.7	+1.6	0	0	+2.7	+1.6	+2.7	+1.6
Saturated fat (g)	29	6.0	–0.8	–13.7	–0.8	–13.8	–0.8	–13.7	–0.8	–13.7
Total vegetables (c-eq)	3.5	0.30	–0.04	–12.4	–0.04	–12.4	–0.06	–21.7	–0.01	–4.3
Beans (oz-eq)	0.4	0.13	–0.04	–28.8	–0.04	–28.8	–0.06	–50.4	–0.01	–9.9
Total protein (oz-eq)	6.5	0.93	–0.32	–34.8	–0.40	–42.9	–0.32	–34.8	–0.32	–34.8
Nuts, seeds, and soy (oz-eq)	0.7	0.61	–0.40	–65.2	–0.40	–65.2	–0.40	–65.2	–0.40	–65.2
Seafood (oz-eq)	1.4	0.00	+0.08	NA	0.00	NA	+0.08	NA	+0.08	NA
FP cost		$36.68	–$0.64	–1.7	–$1.09	–3.0	–$1.02	–2.8	–$0.25	–0.7
Average per-participant FP cost		$37.27	–$0.06	–0.2	–$0.10	+0.3	–$0.10	+0.3	–$0.02	+0.1

NOTES: See notes following Table S-22.

TABLE S-22 Food Package II Sensitivity Results: Impact of the Infant Food Vegetable and Fruit CVV Substitute

			Change from Current (Redemption Rate)			
			Revised (65%)		Test 1: 50% of Infant Food as CVV (65%)	
FP Nutrients and Cost	AI, 6–11 mo	Current Amount	Absolute Change	%	Absolute Change	%
Energy (kcal)		443	+2.2	+0.5	+2.2	+0.5
Protein (g)		9.9	+0.0	+0.4	+0.0	+0.4
Total fat (g)	30	20.3	0	0	0	0
Carbohydrate (g)	95	56.3	+0.5	+0.9	+0.5	+0.9
Fiber (g)	ND	1.97	+0.1	+3.6	+0.1	+3.6
Added sugar (g)	NA	0.36	0	0	0	0
Calcium (mg)	260	420	+0.6	+0.1	+0.6	+0.1
Iron (mg)	6.9 (EAR)	12.5	+0.0	+0.2	+0.0	+0.2
Magnesium (mg)	75	45.0	+0.5	+1.2	+0.5	+1.2
Phosphorus (mg)	275	269	+0.9	+0.3	+0.9	+0.3
Potassium (mg)	700	572	+7.6	+1.3	+7.6	+1.3
Sodium (mg)	370	119	+0.5	+0.4	+0.5	+0.4
Zinc (mg)	2.5 (EAR)	4.07	+0.0	+0.1	+0.0	+0.1
Copper (mg)	0.22	0.37	+0.0	+0.6	+0.0	+0.6
Selenium (μg)	20	12.2	+0.0	+0.1	+0.0	+0.1
Vitamin C (mg)	50	50.8	+0.7	+1.5	+0.7	+1.5
Thiamin (mg)	0.3	0.46	+0.0	+0.2	+0.0	+0.2
Riboflavin (mg)	0.4	0.63	+0.0	+0.4	+0.0	+0.4
Niacin (mg)	4	6.2	+0.0	+0.4	+0.0	+0.4
Vitamin B6 (mg)	0.3	0.22	0	0	0	0
Folate (μg DFE)	80	111	+0.5	+0.4	+0.5	+0.4
Choline (mg)	150	74.0	+0.4	+0.5	+0.4	+0.5
Vitamin B12 (μg)	0.5	1.41	0	0	0	0
Vitamin A (μg RAE)	500	400	+4.4	+1.1	+4.4	+1.1
Vitamin E (mg)	5	5.05	+0.0	+0.4	+0.0	+0.4
Vitamin D (IU)	400	229	0	0	0	0
Saturated fat (g)	NA	8.3	0	0	0	0
FP cost		$51.37	+$3.25	+6.3	–$0.31	–0.6
Average per-participant FP cost		$37.27	+$0.38	+1.0	–$0.04	–0.1

TABLE S-22 Continued

NOTES for Tables S-2 through S-22: * = AI value; AI = Adequate Intake; c-eq = cup-equivalents; DFE = dietary folate equivalents; EAR = Estimated Average Requirement; FP = food package; HEI = Healthy Eating Index–2010; IU = international units; oz-eq = oz equivalents; NA = not applicable; ND = not determined; RAE = retinol activity equivalents; WG = whole grain.

Current amounts reflect the foods as currently redeemed. Revised amounts reflect calculated revised redemption rates. Tests apply the calculated revised redemption rates to the changed food category unless noted otherwise. Details on methods used to develop the food package nutrient and cost profiles and to generate redemption rates are available in Appendix R.

Appendix T

Amounts of Food Groups and Nutrients Provided by the Current, Compared to the Revised WIC Food Packages

FIGURES

TABLES

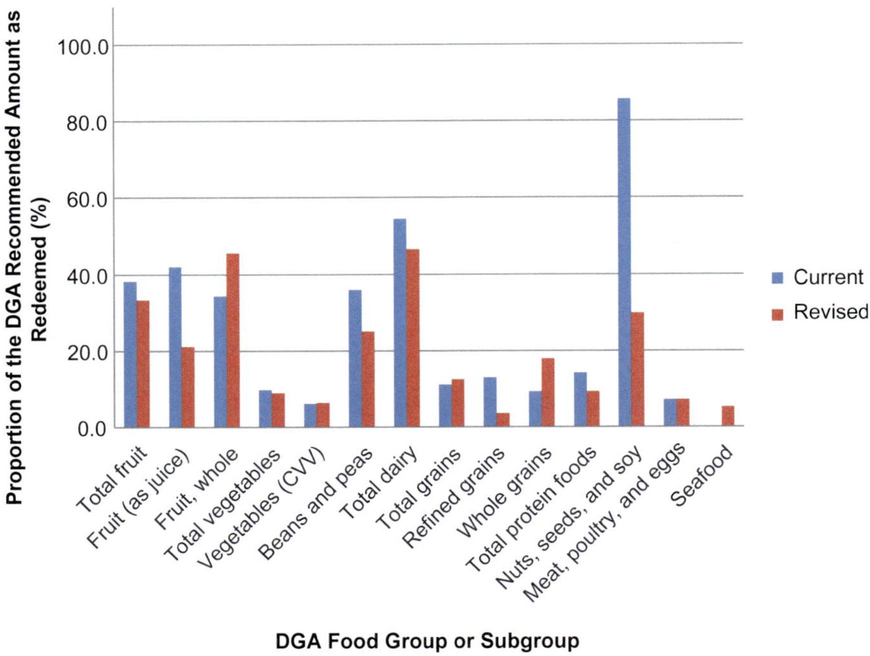

FIGURE T-1 Current compared to the revised food package V-A: Redeemed amounts as the proportion of the DGA recommended amounts.
NOTES: CVV = cash value voucher; DGA = *Dietary Guidelines for Americans*.

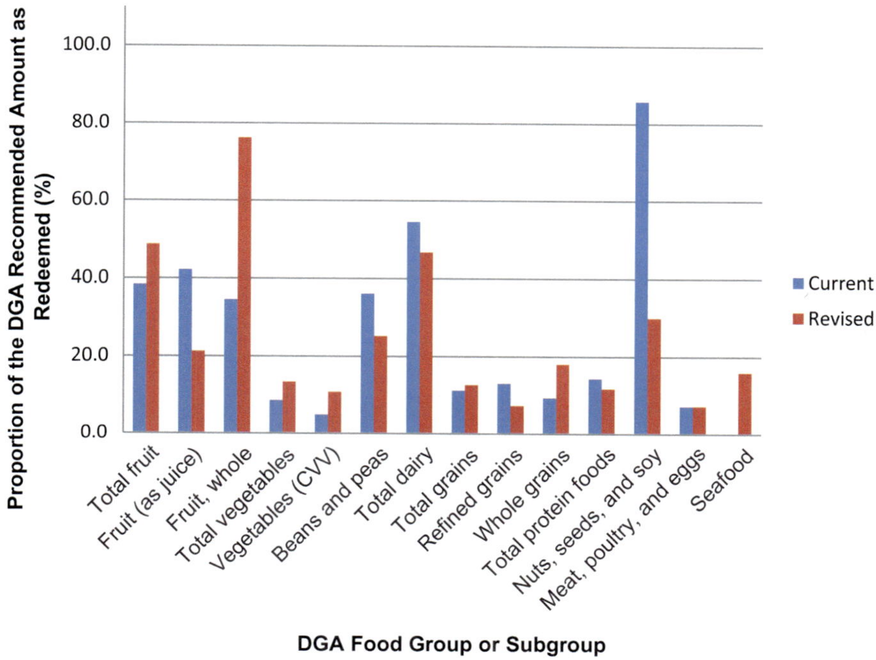

FIGURE T-2 Current compared to the revised food package V-B: Redeemed amounts as the proportion of the DGA recommended amounts.
NOTES: CVV = cash value voucher; DGA = *Dietary Guidelines for Americans.*

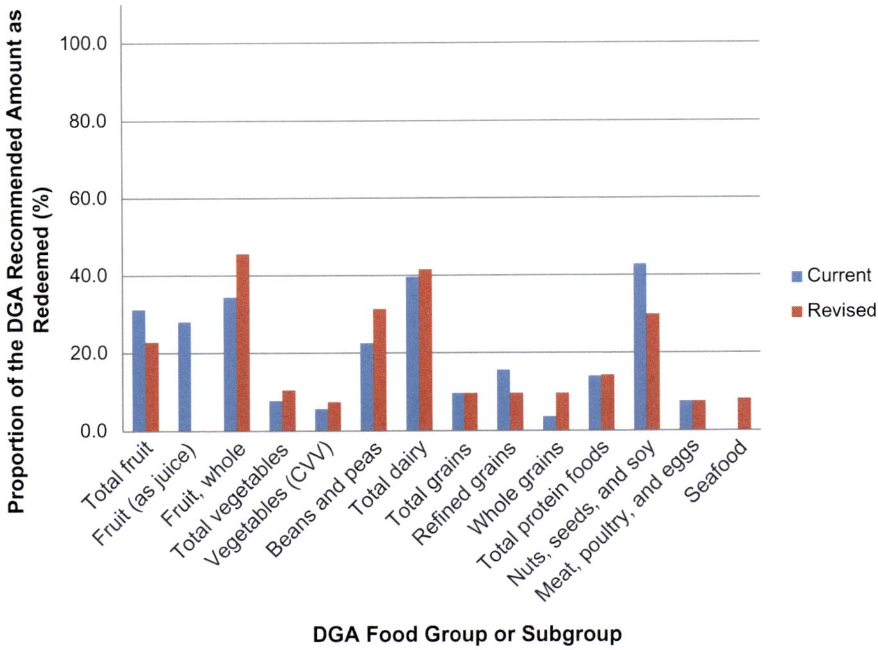

FIGURE T-3 Current compared to the revised food package VI: Redeemed amounts as the proportion of the DGA recommended amounts. This figure is corrected from the original prepublication version.
NOTES: CVV = cash value voucher; DGA = *Dietary Guidelines for Americans.*

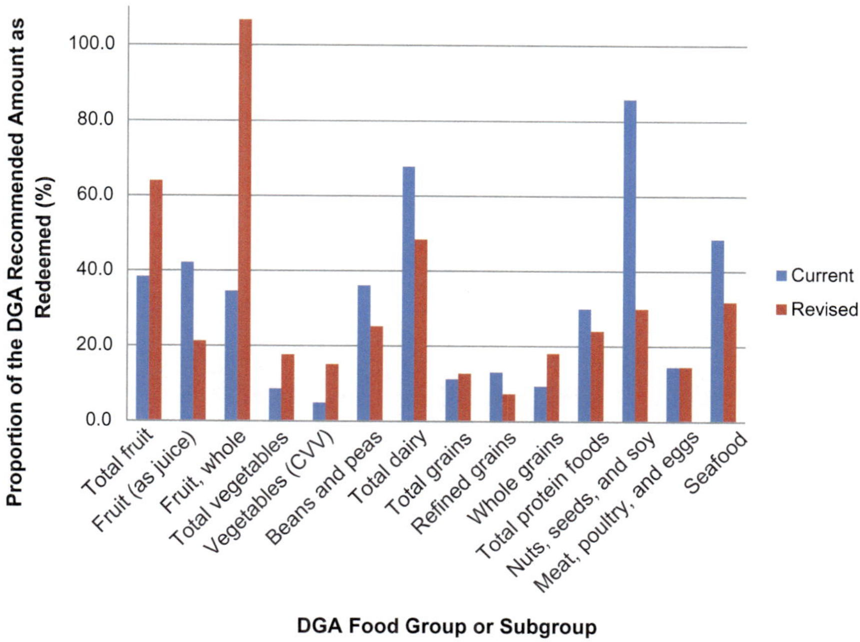

FIGURE T-4 Current compared to the revised food package VII: Redeemed amounts as the proportion of the DGA recommended amounts.
NOTES: CVV = cash value voucher; DGA = *Dietary Guidelines for Americans*.

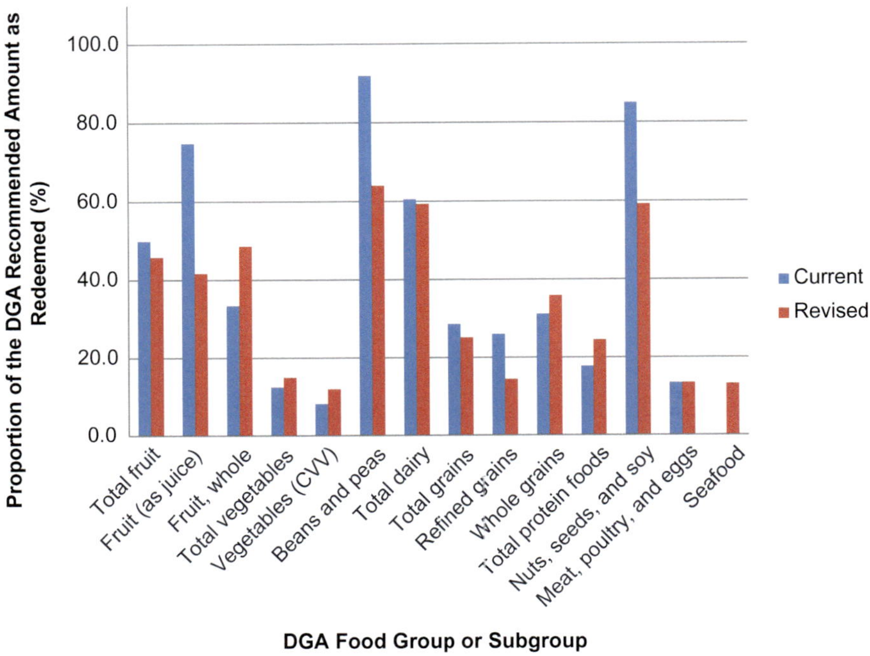

FIGURE T-5 Current compared to the revised food package IV-B: Redeemed amounts as the proportion of the DGA recommended amounts.
NOTES: CVV = cash value voucher; DGA = *Dietary Guidelines for Americans.*

TABLE T-1a Proportion of 2015–2020 DGA Recommended Amounts of Food Groups in the Current and Revised Food Packages for Pregnant Women Assuming Full Redemption: Food Package V-A

			Current		Revised			
WIC Food Category	DGA Food Group	Units/d	WIC Maximum Allowance	Proportion of the DGA Recom-mendation (%)[a]	WIC Maximum Allowance	Proportion of the DGA Recom-mendation (%)[a]	Change in Proportion of DGA Recom-mendation (%)[a]	DGA 2,600 Kcal Food Pattern[b]
Total fruit	*Total fruit*	*c-eq*	1.0	52	0.9	44	–9	2.0
Juice, 100%	Fruit, as juice	c-eq	0.6	60	0.3	27	–33	1.0
Fruit, 67% of CVV[c]	Fruit, whole	c-eq	0.4	45	0.6	61	16	1.0
Total vegetables	*Total vegetables*	*c-eq*	0.5	13	0.5	13	0	3.5
Vegetables, 43% of CVV[d]		c-eq	0.2	6	0.3	9	2	3.5
Legumes (as vegetable)[e]	Legumes (beans and peas)	c-eq	0.3	71	0.2	47	–24	0.4
Total dairy	*Total dairy*	*c-eq*	2.9	98	2.1	71	–27	3.0
Milk		c-eq	2.9	98	2.1	71	–27	3.0
Total grains	*Total grains*	*oz-eq*	1.7	19	2.0	22	3	9.0
Breakfast cereal[f]	Refined grains	oz-eq	1.0	22	0.6	13	–8	4.5
Breakfast cereal	Whole grains	oz-eq	0.2	17[g]	0.6	31[g]	14	4.5
Whole wheat bread	Whole grains	oz-eq	0.5		0.8			
Total protein foods	*Total protein foods*	*oz-eq*	1.6	25	0.9	14	–11	6.5
Peanut butter	Nuts, seeds, and soy	oz-eq	1.2	168	0.4	56	–112	0.7
Eggs	Meat, poultry, and eggs	oz-eq	0.4	9	0.4	9	0	4.4
Fish	Seafood	oz-eq	0.0	0	0.1	8	8	1.4

continued

TABLE T-1a Continued

NOTES: c-eq = cup-equivalent; CVV = cash value voucher; DGA = *Dietary Guidelines for Americans*; oz-eq = ounce-equivalent.

[a] Percentages represent the proportion of the recommended food pattern amount in the corresponding row of the DGA food pattern column. Values may not be replicable from the table due to rounding.

[b] The 2,600-kcal food pattern was applied to evaluate this package. This kcal level most closely matched the calculated Estimated Energy Requirement (EER) for pregnant WIC-participating women in National Health and Nutrition Examination Survey (NHANES) 2005–2012. In the current WIC food packages, pregnant women and partially breastfeeding women receive the same benefits.

[c] Assumes that 67 percent of the CVV is used to purchase fruits, based on redemption data from Texas and Wyoming. A weighted composite cost of fruit ($0.55/c-eq) was developed, based on the most commonly consumed fruits (bananas, apples, oranges, berries, grapes, melon [watermelon was used in this case]) from an average of Massachusetts, Texas, and Wyoming redemption data. Only fresh fruit was included as all states allow fresh forms; Economic Research Service (ERS) 2013 price data were updated with a Consumer Price Index to 2015 values.

[d] Assumes that 33 percent of the CVV is used to purchase vegetables, based on redemption data from Texas and Wyoming. A weighted composite cost of vegetables ($0.55/c-eq) was developed, based on the most commonly consumed vegetables (tomatoes, avocados, potatoes, peppers, lettuce) from an average of Massachusetts, Texas, and Wyoming redemption data. Only fresh vegetables were included as all states allow fresh forms; ERS 2013 price data were updated with a Consumer Price Index to 2015 values. Because potatoes were not yet available in Wyoming, the same proportion of potatoes was assumed for this state as for Texas.

[e] Legumes can also be assessed as a protein, but they were placed in the vegetable group because a higher proportion of individuals had low intakes of vegetables across WIC-participating subgroups compared to protein.

[f] In the current food packages, a ratio of 81 percent refined grains and 19 percent whole grains was applied, based on redemption data; in the revised packages, a ratio of 50 percent refined grains and 50 percent whole grains was applied to account for the requirement that all cereals meet the whole grain-rich criteria.

[g] To compare the food package contribution to the DGA recommended amounts of whole grains, the whole grain portion of breakfast cereal was added to the whole grain contribution of bread.

SOURCES: USDA/ARS, 2014; USDA/FNS, 2014; USDA/HHS, 2016.

TABLE T-1b Proportion of 2015–2020 DGA Recommended Amounts of Food Groups in the Current and Revised Food Packages for Pregnant Women as Redeemed[a]: Food Package V-A

			Current		Revised			
WIC Food Category	DGA Food Group	Units/d	WIC Redeemed Amounts of the Maximum Allowance	Proportion of the DGA Recom-mendation (%)[b]	WIC Redeemed Amounts of the Maximum Allowance	Proportion of the DGA Recom-mendation (%)[b]	Change in Proportion of DGA Recom-mendation (%)[b]	DGA 2,600 Kcal Food Pattern[c]
Total fruit	*Total fruit*	*c-eq*	*0.8*	*38*	*0.7*	*33*	*–5*	*2.0*
Juice, 100%	Fruit, as juice	c-eq	0.4	42	0.2	21	–21	1.0
Fruit, 67% of CVV[d]	Fruit, whole	c-eq	0.3	34	0.5	46	11	1.0
Total vegetables	*Total vegetables*	*c-eq*	*0.3*	*9*	*0.3*	*9*	*–1*	*3.5*
Vegetables, 33% of CVV[e]		c-eq	0.2	5	0.2	6	2	3.5
Legumes (as vegetable)[f]	Legumes (beans and peas)	c-eq	0.1	36	0.1	25	–11	0.4
Total dairy	*Total dairy*	*c-eq*	*1.6*	*55*	*1.4*	*47*	*–8*	*3.0*
Milk		c-eq	1.6	55	1.4	47	–8	3.0
Total grains	*Total grains*	*oz-eq*	*1.0*	*11*	*1.1*	*13*	*1*	*9.0*
Breakfast cereal[g]	Refined grains	oz-eq	0.6	13	0.3	4	–9	4.5
Breakfast cereal	Whole grains	oz-eq	0.1	9.3[h]	0.3	18[h]	15	4.5
Whole wheat bread	Whole grains	oz-eq	0.3		0.5			
Total protein foods	*Total protein foods*	*oz-eq*	*0.9*	*14*	*0.6*	*9*	*–5*	*6.5*
Peanut butter	Nuts, seeds, and soy	oz-eq	0.6	86	0.2	30	–56	0.7
Eggs	Meat, poultry, and eggs	oz-eq	0.3	7	0.3	7	0	4.4
Fish	Seafood	oz-eq	0.0	0	0.1	5	5	1.4

continued

TABLE T-1b Continued

NOTES: c-eq = cup-equivalent; CVV = cash value voucher; DGA = *Dietary Guidelines for Americans*; oz-eq = ounce-equivalent.

[a] Applies redemption factors presented in Appendix R, Table R-5.

[b] Percentages represent the proportion of the recommended food pattern amount in the corresponding row of the DGA food pattern column. Values may not be replicable from the table due to rounding.

[c] The 2,600-kcal food pattern was applied to evaluate this package. This kcal level most closely matched the calculated Estimated Energy Requirement (EER) for pregnant WIC-participating women in National Health and Nutrition Examination Survey (NHANES) 2005–2012. In the current WIC food packages, pregnant women and partially breastfeeding women receive the same benefits.

[d] Assumes that 67 percent of the CVV is used to purchase fruits, based on redemption data from Texas and Wyoming. A weighted composite cost of fruit ($0.55/c-eq) was developed, based on the most commonly consumed fruits (bananas, apples, oranges, berries, grapes, melon [watermelon was used in this case]) from an average of Massachusetts, Texas, and Wyoming redemption data. Only fresh fruit was included as all states allow fresh forms; Economic Research Service (ERS) 2013 price data were updated with a Consumer Price Index to 2015 values.

[e] Assumes that 33 percent of the CVV is used to purchase vegetables, based on redemption data from Texas and Wyoming. A weighted composite cost of vegetables ($0.55/c-eq) was developed, based on the most commonly consumed vegetables (tomatoes, avocados, potatoes, peppers, lettuce) from an average of Massachusetts, Texas, and Wyoming redemption data. Only fresh vegetables were included as all states allow fresh forms; ERS 2013 price data were updated with a Consumer Price Index to 2015 values. Because potatoes were not yet available in Wyoming, the same proportion of potatoes was assumed for this state as for Texas.

[f] Legumes can also be assessed as a protein, but they were placed in the vegetable group because a higher proportion of individuals had low intakes of vegetables across WIC-participating subgroups compared to protein.

[g] In the current food packages, a ratio of 81 percent refined grains and 19 percent whole grains was applied, based on redemption data; in the revised packages, a ratio of 50 percent refined grains and 50 percent whole grains was applied to account for the requirement that all cereals meet the whole grain-rich criteria.

[h] To compare the food package contribution to the DGA recommended amounts of whole grains, the whole grain portion of breakfast cereal was added to the whole grain contribution of bread.

SOURCES: USDA/ARS, 2014; USDA/FNS, 2014; USDA/HHS, 2016.

TABLE T-2a Proportion of 2015–2020 DGA Recommended Amounts of Food Groups in the Current and Revised Food Packages for Partially Breastfeeding Women Assuming Full Redemption: Food Package V-B[a]

			Current		Revised			
WIC Food Category	DGA Food Group	Units/d	WIC Maximum Allowance	Proportion of the DGA Recommendation (%)[b]	WIC Maximum Allowance	Proportion of the DGA Recommendation (%)[b]	Change in Proportion of DGA Recommendation (%)[b]	DGA 2,600-Kcal Food Pattern[c]
Total fruit	*Total fruit*	*c-eq*	*1.0*	*52*	*1.3*	*64*	*12*	*2.0*
Juice, 100%	Fruit, as juice	c-eq	0.6	60	0.3	27	–33	1.0
Fruit, 67% of CVV[d]	Fruit, whole	c-eq	0.4	45	1.0	102	57	1.0
Total vegetables	*Total vegetables*	*c-eq*	*0.5*	*13*	*0.7*	*19*	*6*	*3.5*
Vegetables, 33% of CVV[e]		c-eq	0.2	0.2	0.4	14	5	3.5
Legumes (as vegetable)[f]	Legumes (beans and peas)	c-eq	0.3	71	0.2	47	–24	0.4
Total dairy	*Total dairy*	*c-eq*	*2.9*	*98*	*2.1*	*71*	*–27*	*3.0*
Milk		c-eq	2.9	98	2.1	71	–27	3.0
Total grains	*Total grains*	*oz-eq*	*1.7*	*19*	*2.0*	*22*	*3*	*9.0*
Breakfast cereal[g]	Refined grains	oz-eq	1.0	22	0.6	13	–8	4.5
Breakfast cereal	Whole grains	oz-eq	0.2	17[h]	0.6	31[h]	14	4.5
Whole wheat bread	Whole grains	oz-eq	0.5		0.8			
Total protein foods	*Total protein foods*	*oz-eq*	*1.6*	*25*	*1.1*	*17*	*–7*	*6.5*
Peanut butter	Nuts, seeds, and soy	oz-eq	1.2	168	0.4	56	–112	0.7
Eggs	Meat, poultry, and eggs	oz-eq	0.4	9	0.4	9	0	4.4
Fish	Seafood	oz-eq	0.0	0	0.3	23	23	1.4

continued

TABLE T-2a Continued

NOTES: c-eq = cup-equivalent; CVV = cash value voucher; DGA = *Dietary Guidelines for Americans*; oz-eq = ounce-equivalent.

[a] This table compares the current food package V (provided to both pregnant and partially breastfeeding women) to the revised food package V-B for partially breastfeeding women only.

[b] Percentages represent the proportion of the recommended food pattern amount in the corresponding row of the DGA food pattern column. Values may not be replicable from the table due to rounding.

[c] The 2,600 kcal food pattern was applied to evaluate this package. This kcal level most closely matched the calculated Estimated Energy Requirement (EER) for breastfeeding WIC-participating women in National Health and Nutrition Examination Survey (NHANES) 2005–2012.

[d] Assumes that 67 percent of the CVV is used to purchase fruits, based on redemption data from Texas and Wyoming. A weighted composite cost of fruit ($0.55/c-eq) was developed, based on the most commonly consumed fruits (bananas, apples, oranges, berries, grapes, melon [watermelon was used in this case]) from an average of Massachusetts, Texas, and Wyoming redemption data. Only fresh fruit was included as all states allow fresh forms; Economic Research Service (ERS) 2013 price data were updated with a Consumer Price Index to 2015 values.

[e] Assumes that 33 percent of the CVV is used to purchase vegetables, based on redemption data from Texas and Wyoming. A weighted composite cost of vegetables ($0.55/c-eq) was developed, based on the most commonly consumed vegetables (tomatoes, avocados, potatoes, peppers, lettuce) from an average of Massachusetts, Texas, and Wyoming redemption data. Only fresh vegetables were included as all states allow fresh forms; ERS 2013 price data were updated with a Consumer Price Index to 2015 values. Because potatoes were not yet available in Wyoming, the same proportion of potatoes was assumed for this state as for Texas.

[f] Legumes can also be assessed as a protein, but were placed in the vegetable group because a higher proportion of individuals had low intakes of vegetables across WIC-participating subgroups compared to protein.

[g] In the current food packages, a ratio of 81 percent refined grains and 19 percent whole grains was applied, based on redemption data; in the revised packages, a ratio of 50 percent refined grains and 50 percent whole grains was applied to account for the requirement that all cereals meet the whole grain-rich criteria.

[h] To compare the food package contribution to the DGA recommended amounts of whole grains, the whole grain portion of breakfast cereal was added to the whole grain contribution of bread.

SOURCES: USDA/ARS, 2014; USDA/FNS, 2014; USDA/HHS, 2016.

TABLE T-2b Proportion of 2015–2020 DGA Recommended Amounts of Food Groups in the Current and Revised Food Packages for Partially Breastfeeding[a] Women as Redeemed[b]: Food Package V-B

WIC Food Category	DGA Food Group	Units/d	Current: WIC Redeemed Amounts of the Maximum Allowance	Current: Proportion of the DGA Recommendation (%)[c]	Revised: WIC Redeemed Amounts of the Maximum Allowance	Revised: Proportion of the DGA Recommendation (%)[c]	Change in Proportion of DGA Recommendation (%)[c]	DGA 2,600-Kcal Food Pattern[d]
Total fruit	*Total fruit*	*c-eq*	*0.8*	*38*	*1.0*	*49*	*10*	*2.0*
Juice, 100%	Fruit, as juice	c-eq	0.4	42	0.2	21	−21	1.0
Fruit, 67% of CVV[e]	Fruit, whole	c-eq	0.3	34	0.8	76	42	1.0
Total vegetables	*Total vegetables*	*c-eq*	*0.3*	*9*	*0.5*	*13*	*5*	*3.5*
Vegetables, 33% of CVV[f]		c-eq	0.2	5	0.4	11	6	3.5
Legumes (as vegetable)[g]	Legumes (beans and peas)	c-eq	0.1	36	0.1	25	−11	0.4
Total dairy	*Total dairy*	*c-eq*	*1.6*	*55*	*1.4*	*47*	*−8*	*3.0*
Milk		c-eq	1.6	55	1.4	47	−8	3.0
Total grains	*Total grains*	*oz-eq*	*1.0*	*11*	*1.1*	*13*	*1*	*9.0*
Breakfast cereal[h]	Refined grains	oz-eq	0.6	13	0.3	7	−6	4.5
Breakfast cereal	Whole grains	oz-eq	0.1	9[i]	0.3	18[i]	9	4.5
Whole wheat bread	Whole grains	oz-eq	0.3		0.5			
Total protein foods	*Total protein foods*	*oz-eq*	*0.9*	*14*	*0.8*	*12*	*−3*	*6.5*
Peanut butter	Nuts, seeds, and soy	oz-eq	0.6	86	0.2	30	−56	0.7
Eggs	Meat, poultry, and eggs	oz-eq	0.3	7	0.3	7	0	4.4
Fish	Seafood	oz-eq	0.0	0	0.2	16	16	1.4

continued

TABLE T-2b Continued

NOTES: c-eq = cup-equivalent; CVV = cash value voucher; DGA = *Dietary Guidelines for Americans*; oz-eq = ounce-equivalent.

[a] This table compares the current food package V (provided to both pregnant and partially breastfeeding women) to the revised food package V-B for partially breastfeeding women only.

[b] Applies redemption factors presented in Appendix R, Table R-5.

[c] Percentages represent the proportion of the recommended food pattern amount in the corresponding row of the DGA food pattern column. Values may not be replicable from the table due to rounding.

[d] The 2,600 kcal food pattern was applied to evaluate this package. This kcal level most closely matched the calculated Estimated Energy Requirement (EER) for breastfeeding WIC-participating women in National Health and Nutrition Examination Survey (NHANES) 2005–2012.

[e] Assumes that 67 percent of the CVV is used to purchase fruits, based on redemption data from Texas and Wyoming. A weighted composite cost of fruit ($0.55/c-eq) was developed, based on the most commonly consumed fruits (bananas, apples, oranges, berries, grapes, melon [watermelon was used in this case]) from an average of Massachusetts, Texas, and Wyoming redemption data. Only fresh fruit was included as all states allow fresh forms; Economic Research Service (ERS) 2013 price data were updated with a Consumer Price Index to 2015 values.

[f] Assumes that 33 percent of the CVV is used to purchase vegetables, based on redemption data from Texas and Wyoming. A weighted composite cost of vegetables ($0.55/c-eq) was developed, based on the most commonly consumed vegetables (tomatoes, avocados, potatoes, peppers, lettuce) from an average of Massachusetts, Texas, and Wyoming redemption data. Only fresh vegetables were included as all states allow fresh forms; ERS 2013 price data were updated with a Consumer Price Index to 2015 values. Because potatoes were not yet available in Wyoming, the same proportion of potatoes was assumed for this state as for Texas.

[g] Legumes can also be assessed as a protein, but were placed in the vegetable group because a higher proportion of individuals had low intakes of vegetables across WIC-participating subgroups compared to protein.

[h] In the current food packages, a ratio of 81 percent refined grains and 19 percent whole grains was applied, based on redemption data; in the revised packages, a ratio of 50 percent refined grains and 50 percent whole grains was applied to account for the requirement that all cereals meet the whole grain-rich criteria.

[i] To compare the food package contribution to the DGA recommended amounts of whole grains, the whole grain portion of breakfast cereal was added to the whole grain contribution of bread.

SOURCES: USDA/ARS, 2014; USDA/FNS, 2014; USDA/HHS, 2016.

TABLE T-3a Proportion of 2015–2020 DGA Recommended Amounts of Food Groups in the Current and Revised Food Packages for Postpartum Women Assuming Full Redemption: Food Package VI

			Current		Revised			
WIC Food Category	DGA Food Group	Units/d	WIC Maximum Allowance	Proportion of the DGA Recom-mendation (%)[a]	WIC Maximum Allowance	Proportion of the DGA Recom-mendation (%)[a]	Change in Proportion of DGA Recom-mendation (%)[a]	DGA 2,300 Kcal Food Pattern[b]
Total fruit	*Total fruit*	*c-eq*	*0.8*	*42*	*0.6*	*30*	*–14*	*2.0*
Juice, 100%	Fruit, as juice	c-eq	0.4	40	0.0	0	–40	1.0
Fruit, 67% of CVV[c]	Fruit, whole	c-eq	0.4	45	0.6	61	12	1.0
Total vegetables	*Total vegetables*	*c-eq*	*0.3*	*12*	*0.5*	*16*	*4*	*3.0*
Vegetable, 33% of CVV[d]		c-eq	0.2	7	0.3	10	3	3.0
Legumes (as vegetable)[e,f]	Legumes (beans and peas)	c-eq	0.1	44	0.2	59	15	0.3
Total dairy	*Total dairy*	*c-eq*	*2.1*	*71*	*2.1*	*71*	*0*	*3.0*
Milk		c-eq	2.1	71	2.1	71	0	3.0
Total grains	*Total grains*	*oz-eq*	*1.2*	*16*	*1.2*	*16*	*0*	*7.5*
Breakfast cereal[g]	Refined grains	oz-eq	1.0	26	0.6	16	–10	3.8
Breakfast cereal	Whole grains	oz-eq	0.2	6	0.6	16	10	3.8
Total protein foods	*Total protein foods*	*oz-eq*	*1.3*	*20*	*1.2*	*19*	*–1*	*6.3*
Peanut butter[f]	Nuts, seeds, and soy	oz-eq	0.6	84	0.4	56	–28	0.7
Eggs	Meat, poultry, and eggs	oz-eq	0.4	9.5	0.4	9.5	0	4.2
Fish	Seafood	oz-eq	0.0	0	0.1	8	8	1.4

continued

TABLE T-3a Continued

NOTES: c-eq = cup-equivalent; CVV = cash value voucher; DGA = *Dietary Guidelines for Americans*; oz-eq = ounce-equivalent.

[a] Percentages represent the proportion of the recommended food pattern amount in the corresponding row of the DGA food pattern column. Values may not be replicable from the table due to rounding.

[b] The 2,300 kcal food pattern was applied to evaluate this package. This kcal level most closely matched the calculated Estimated Energy Requirement (EER) for nonbreastfeeding postpartum WIC-participating women in National Health and Nutrition Examination Survey (NHANES) 2005–2012.

[c] Assumes that 67 percent of the CVV is used to purchase fruits, based on redemption data from Texas and Wyoming. A weighted composite cost of fruit ($0.55/c-eq) was developed, based on the most commonly consumed fruits (bananas, apples, oranges, berries, grapes, melon [watermelon was used in this case]) from an average of Massachusetts, Texas, and Wyoming redemption data. Only fresh fruit was included as all states allow fresh forms; Economic Research Service (ERS) 2013 price data were updated with a Consumer Price Index to 2015 values.

[d] Assumes that 33 percent of the CVV is used to purchase vegetables, based on redemption data from Texas and Wyoming. A weighted composite cost of vegetables ($0.55/c-eq) was developed, based on the most commonly consumed vegetables (tomatoes, avocados, potatoes, peppers, lettuce) from an average of Massachusetts, Texas, and Wyoming redemption data. Only fresh vegetables were included as all states allow fresh forms; ERS 2013 price data were updated with a Consumer Price Index to 2015 values. Because potatoes were not yet available in Wyoming, the same proportion of potatoes was assumed for this state as for Texas.

[e] Legumes can also be assessed as a protein, but they were placed in the vegetable group because a higher proportion of individuals had low intakes of vegetables across WIC-participating subgroups compared to protein.

[f] For the current food package, assumes 50 percent legumes and 50 percent peanut butter; for the revised package, the proportion provided on a monthly basis was calculated.

[g] In the current food packages, a ratio of 81 percent refined grains and 19 percent whole grains was applied, based on redemption data; in the revised packages, a ratio of 50 percent refined grains and 50 percent whole grains was applied to account for the requirement that all cereals meet the whole grain-rich criteria.

SOURCES: USDA/ARS, 2014; USDA/FNS, 2014; USDA/HHS, 2016.

TABLE T-3b Proportion of 2015–2020 DGA Recommended Amounts of Food Groups in the Current and Revised Food Packages for Postpartum Women as Redeemed[a]: Food Package VI*

			Current		Revised			
WIC Food Category	DGA Food Group	Units/d	WIC Redeemed Amounts of the Maximum Allowance	Proportion of the DGA Recommendation (%)[b]	WIC Redeemed Amounts of the Maximum Allowance	Proportion of the DGA Recommendation (%)[b]	Change in Proportion of DGA Recommendation (%)[b]	DGA 2,300-Kcal Food Pattern[c]
Total fruit	*Total fruit*	*c-eq*	*0.6*	*31*	*0.5*	*23*	*-8*	*2.0*
Juice, 100%	Fruit, as juice	c-eq	0.3	28	0	0	–28	1.0
Fruit, 67% of CVV[d]	Fruit, whole	c-eq	0.3	34	0.5	46	11	1.0
Total vegetables	*Total vegetables*	*c-eq*	*0.2*	*8*	*0.3*	*10*	*3*	*3.0*
Vegetables, 33% of CVV[e]		c-eq	0.2	6	0.2	8	2	3.0
Legumes (as vegetable)[f,g]	Legumes (beans and peas)	c-eq	0.1	23	0.1	31	9	0.3
Total dairy	*Total dairy*	*c-eq*	*1.2*	*40*	*1.2*	*42*	*2*	*3.0*
Milk		c-eq	1.2	40	1.2	42	2	3.0
Total grains	*Total grains*	*oz-eq*	*0.7*	*10*	*0.7*	*9*	*–1*	*7.5*
Breakfast cereal[h]	Refined grains	oz-eq	0.6	16	0.3	9	–7	3.8
Breakfast cereal	Whole grains	oz-eq	0.1	4	0.3	9	5	3.8
Total protein foods	*Total protein foods*	*oz-eq*	*0.9*	*14*	*0.9*	*14*	*0*	*6.3*
Peanut butter[g]	Nuts, seeds, and soy	oz-eq	0.3	43	0.2	30	–13	0.7
Eggs	Meat, poultry, and eggs	oz-eq	0.3	8	0.3	8	0	4.2
Fish	Seafood	oz-eq	0.0	0	0.1	8	8	1.4

continued

TABLE T-3b Continued

NOTES: c-eq = cup-equivalent; CVV = cash value voucher; DGA = *Dietary Guidelines for Americans*; oz-eq = ounce-equivalent.

* Some values in this table are corrected from the original prepublication.

[a] Applies redemption factors presented in Appendix R, Table R-5.

[b] Percentages represent the proportion of the recommended food pattern amount in the corresponding row of the DGA food pattern column. Values may not be replicable from the table due to rounding.

[c] The 2,300 kcal food pattern was applied to evaluate this package. This kcal level most closely matched the calculated Estimated Energy Requirement (EER) for nonbreastfeeding postpartum WIC-participating women in National Health and Nutrition Examination Survey (NHANES) 2005–2012.

[d] Assumes that 67 percent of the CVV is used to purchase fruits, based on redemption data from Texas and Wyoming. A weighted composite cost of fruit ($0.55/c-eq) was developed, based on the most commonly consumed fruits (bananas, apples, oranges, berries, grapes, melon [watermelon was used in this case]) from an average of Massachusetts, Texas, and Wyoming redemption data. Only fresh fruit was included as all states allow fresh forms; Economic Research Service (ERS) 2013 price data were updated with a Consumer Price Index to 2015 values.

[e] Assumes that 33 percent of the CVV is used to purchase vegetables, based on redemption data from Texas and Wyoming. A weighted composite cost of vegetables ($0.55/c-eq) was developed, based on the most commonly consumed vegetables (tomatoes, avocados, potatoes, peppers, lettuce) from an average of Massachusetts, Texas, and Wyoming redemption data. Only fresh vegetables were included as all states allow fresh forms; ERS 2013 price data were updated with a Consumer Price Index to 2015 values. Because potatoes were not yet available in Wyoming, the same proportion of potatoes was assumed for this state as for Texas.

[f] Legumes can also be assessed as a protein, but were placed in the vegetable group because a higher proportion of individuals had low intakes of vegetables across WIC-participating subgroups compared to protein.

[g] For the current food package, assumes 43 percent legumes and 57 percent peanut butter, based on prescription data from the PC 2014 Food Package Report (USDA/FNS, 2016).

[h] In the current food packages, a ratio of 81 percent refined grains and 19 percent whole grains was applied, based on redemption data; in the revised packages, a ratio of 50 percent refined grains and 50 percent whole grains was applied to account for the requirement that all cereals meet the whole grain-rich criteria.

SOURCES: USDA/ARS, 2014; USDA/FNS, 2014; USDA/HHS, 2016.

TABLE T-4a Proportion of 2015–2020 DGA Recommended Amounts of Food Groups in the Current and Revised Food Packages for Fully Breastfeeding Women Assuming Full Redemption: Food Package VII

			Current		Revised			
WIC Food Category	DGA Food Group	Units/d	WIC Maximum Allowance	Proportion of the DGA Recom-mendation (%)[a]	WIC Maximum Allowance	Proportion of the DGA Recom-mendation (%)[a]	Change in Proportion of DGA Recom-mendation (%)[a]	DGA 2,600-Kcal Food Pattern[b]
Total fruit	*Total fruit*	*c-eq*	*1.0*	*52*	*1.7*	*84*	*32*	*2.0*
Juice, 100%	Fruit, as juice	c-eq	0.6	60	0.3	27	–33	1.0
Fruit, 67% of CVV[c]	Fruit, whole	c-eq	0.4	45	1.4	142	97	1.0
Total vegetables	*Total vegetables*	*c-eq*	*0.5*	*13*	*0.9*	*25*	*11*	*3.5*
Vegetables, 33% of CVV[d]		c-eq	0.2	6	0.7	20	14	3.5
Legumes (as vegetable)[e]	Legumes (beans and peas)	c-eq	0.3	71	0.2	47	–24	0.4
Total dairy	*Total dairy*	*c-eq*	*3.6*	*119*	*2.1*	*71*	*–47*	*3.0*
Milk		c-eq	3.2	107	2.1	71	–36	3.0
Cheese		c-eq	0.4	12	0.0	0	–12	3.0
Total grains	*Total grains*	*oz-eq*	*1.7*	*19*	*2.0*	*22*	*3*	*9.0*
Breakfast cereal[f]	Refined grains	oz-eq	1.0	22	0.6	13	–8	4.5
Breakfast cereal	Whole grains	oz-eq	0.2	17[g]	0.6	31[g]	14	4.5
Whole wheat bread	Whole grains	oz-eq	0.5		0.8			
Total protein foods	*Total protein foods*	*oz-eq*	*3.3*	*50*	*2.1*	*33*	*–17*	*6.5*
Peanut butter	Nuts, seeds, and soy	oz-eq	1.2	168	0.4	56	–112	0.7
Eggs	Meat, poultry, and eggs	oz-eq	0.8	18	0.8	18	0	4.4
Fish	Seafood	oz-eq	1.0	70	0.7	47	–23	1.4

continued

TABLE T-4a Continued

NOTES: c-eq = cup-equivalent; CVV = cash value voucher; DGA = *Dietary Guidelines for Americans*; oz-eq = ounce-equivalent.

[a] Percentages represent the proportion of the recommended food pattern amount in the corresponding row of the DGA food pattern column. Values may not be replicable from the table due to rounding.

[b] The 2,600-kcal food pattern was applied to evaluate this package. This kcal level most closely matched the calculated Estimated Energy Requirement (EER) for WIC-participating women coded as breastfeeding in National Health and Nutrition Examination Survey (NHANES) 2005–2012.

[c] Assumes that 67 percent of the CVV is used to purchase fruits, based on redemption data from Texas and Wyoming. A weighted composite cost of fruit ($0.55/c-eq) was developed, based on the most commonly consumed fruits (bananas, apples, oranges, berries, grapes, melon [watermelon was used in this case]) from an average of Massachusetts, Texas, and Wyoming redemption data. Only fresh fruit was included as all states allow fresh forms; Economic Research Service (ERS) 2013 price data were updated with a Consumer Price Index to 2015 values.

[d] Assumes that 33 percent of the CVV is used to purchase vegetables, based on redemption data from Texas and Wyoming. A weighted composite cost of vegetables ($0.55/c-eq) was developed, based on the most commonly consumed vegetables (tomatoes, avocados, potatoes, peppers, lettuce) from an average of Massachusetts, Texas, and Wyoming redemption data. Only fresh vegetables were included as all states allow fresh forms; ERS 2013 price data were updated with a Consumer Price Index to 2015 values. Because potatoes were not yet available in Wyoming, the same proportion of potatoes was assumed for this state as for Texas.

[e] Legumes can also be assessed as a protein, but they were placed in the vegetable group because a higher proportion of individuals had low intakes of vegetables across WIC-participating subgroups compared to protein.

[f] In the current food packages, a ratio of 81 percent refined grains and 19 percent whole grains was applied, based on redemption data; in the revised packages, a ratio of 50 percent refined grains and 50 percent whole grains was applied to account for the requirement that all cereals meet the whole grain-rich criteria.

[g] To compare the food package contribution to the DGA recommended amounts of whole grains, the whole grain portion of breakfast cereal was added to the whole grain contribution of bread.

SOURCES: USDA/ARS, 2014; USDA/FNS, 2014; USDA/HHS, 2016.

TABLE T-4b Proportion of 2015–2020 DGA Recommended Amounts of Food Groups in the Current and Revised Food Packages for Postpartum Women as Redeemed[a]: Food Package VII

			Current		Revised			
WIC Food Category	DGA Food Group	Units/d	WIC Redeemed Amounts of the Maximum Allowance	Proportion of the DGA Recom-mendation (%)[b]	WIC Redeemed Amounts of the Maximum Allowance	Proportion of the DGA Recom-mendation (%)[b]	Change in Proportion of DGA Recom-mendation (%)[b]	DGA 2,600-Kcal Food Pattern[c]
Total fruit	*Total fruit*	*c-eq*	*0.8*	*38*	*1.3*	*64*	*26*	*2.0*
Juice, 100%	Fruit, as juice	c-eq	0.4	42	0.2	21	–21	1.0
Fruit, 67% of CVV[d]	Fruit, whole	c-eq	0.3	34	1.1	107	72	1.0
Total vegetables	*Total vegetables*	*c-eq*	*0.3*	*9*	*0.6*	*18*	*9*	*3.5*
Vegetables, 33% of CVV[e]		c-eq	0.2	5	0.5	15	10	3.5
Legumes (as vegetable)[f]	Legumes (beans and peas)	c-eq	0.1	36	0.1	25	–11	0.4
Total dairy	*Total dairy*	*c-eq*	*2.0*	*68*	*1.4*	*48*	*–19*	*3.0*
Milk		c-eq	1.8	59	1.4	48	–11	3.0
Cheese		c-eq	0.2	8	0.0	0	–8	3.0
Total grains	*Total grains*	*oz-eq*	*1.0*	*11*	*1.1*	*13*	*1*	*9.0*
Breakfast cereal[g]	Refined grains	oz-eq	0.6	13	0.3	7	–5.8	4.5
Breakfast cereal	Whole grains	oz-eq	0.1	9[h]	0.3	18[h]	8.6	4.5
Whole wheat bread	Whole grains	oz-eq	0.3		0.5			
Total protein foods	*Total protein foods*	*oz-eq*	*1.9*	*30*	*1.6*	*24*	*–6*	*6.5*
Peanut butter	Nuts, seeds, and soy	oz-eq	0.6	86	0.2	30	–56	0.7
Eggs	Meat, poultry, and eggs	oz-eq	0.6	14	0.6	14	0	4.4
Fish	Seafood	oz-eq	0.7	49	0.5	32	–17	1.4

continued

TABLE T-4b Continued

NOTES: c-eq = cup-equivalent; CVV = cash value voucher; DGA = *Dietary Guidelines for Americans*; oz-eq = ounce-equivalent.

[a] Applies redemption factors presented in Appendix R, Table R-5.

[b] Percentages represent the proportion of the recommended food pattern amount in the corresponding row of the DGA food pattern column. Values may not be replicable from the table due to rounding.

[c] The 2,600-kcal food pattern was applied to evaluate this package. This kcal level most closely matched the calculated Estimated Energy Requirement (EER) for WIC-participating women coded as breastfeeding in National Health and Nutrition Examination Survey (NHANES) 2005–2012.

[d] Assumes that 67 percent of the CVV is used to purchase fruits, based on redemption data from Texas and Wyoming. A weighted composite cost of fruit ($0.55/c-eq) was developed, based on the most commonly consumed fruits (bananas, apples, oranges, berries, grapes, melon [watermelon was used in this case]) from an average of Massachusetts, Texas, and Wyoming redemption data. Only fresh fruit was included as all states allow fresh forms; Economic Research Service (ERS) 2013 price data were updated with a Consumer Price Index to 2015 values.

[e] Assumes that 33 percent of the CVV is used to purchase vegetables, based on redemption data from Texas and Wyoming. A weighted composite cost of vegetables ($0.55/c-eq) was developed, based on the most commonly consumed vegetables (tomatoes, avocados, potatoes, peppers, lettuce) from an average of Massachusetts, Texas, and Wyoming redemption data. Only fresh vegetables were included as all states allow fresh forms; ERS 2013 price data were updated with a Consumer Price Index to 2015 values. Because potatoes were not yet available in Wyoming, the same proportion of potatoes was assumed for this state as for Texas.

[f] Legumes can also be assessed as a protein, but they were placed in the vegetable group because a higher proportion of individuals had low intakes of vegetables across WIC-participating subgroups compared to protein.

[g] In the current food packages, a ratio of 81 percent refined grains and 19 percent whole grains was applied, based on redemption data; in the revised packages, a ratio of 50 percent refined grains and 50 percent whole grains was applied to account for the requirement that all cereals meet the whole grain-rich criteria.

[h] To compare the food package contribution to the DGA recommended amounts of whole grains, the whole grain portion of breakfast cereal was added to the whole grain contribution of bread.

SOURCES: USDA/ARS, 2014; USDA/FNS, 2014; USDA/HHS, 2016.

TABLE T-5a Proportion of 2015–2020 DGA Recommended Amounts of Food Groups in the Current and Revised Food Packages for Children Ages 2 to Less Than 5 Years Assuming Full Redemption: Food Package IV-B[a]

			Current		Revised			
WIC Food Category	DGA Food Group	Units/d	WIC Redeemed Amounts of the Maximum Allowance	Proportion of the DGA Recom-mendation (%)[b]	WIC Redeemed Amounts of the Maximum Allowance	Proportion of the DGA Recom-mendation (%)[b]	Change in % of DGA Recom-mendation[b]	DGA 1,300-Kcal Food Pattern[c]
Total fruit	*Total fruit*	*c-eq*	*0.9*	*69*	*0.8*	*60*	*–8*	*1.3*
Juice, 100%	Fruit, as juice	c-eq	0.5	107	0.3	53	–53	0.5[j]
Fruit, 67% of CVV[d]	Fruit, whole	c-eq	0.3	43	0.5	65	22	0.8
Total vegetables	*Total vegetables*	*c-eq*	*0.3*	*19*	*0.3*	*22*	*3*	*1.5*
Vegetables, 33% of CVV[e]		c-eq	0.2	11	0.2	16	5	1.5
Legumes (as vegetable)[f,g]	Legumes (beans and peas)	c-eq	0.13	177	0.08	120	–56	0.1
Total dairy	*Total dairy*	*c-eq*	*2.1*	*85*	*1.9*	*75*	*–11*	*2.5*
Milk		c-eq	2.1	85	1.9	75	–11	2.5
Total grains	*Total grains*	*oz-eq*	*2.3*	*50*	*2.0*	*44*	*–6*	*4.5*
Breakfast cereal[h]	Refined grains	oz-eq	1.0	43	0.6	27	–17	2.3
Breakfast cereal	Whole grains	oz-eq	0.2	58[i]	0.6	61[i]	3	2.3
Whole wheat bread	Whole grains	oz-eq	1.1		0.8			
Total protein foods	*Total protein foods*	*oz-eq*	*1.0*	*29*	*1.2*	*33*	*5*	*3.5*
Peanut butter[g]	Nuts, seeds, and soy	oz-eq	0.6	167	0.4	111	–56	0.4
Eggs	Meat, poultry, and eggs	oz-eq	0.4	17	0.4	17	0	2.4
Fish	Seafood	oz-eq	0.0	0	0.1	19	19	0.6

continued

TABLE T-5a Continued

NOTES: c-eq = cup-equivalent; CVV = cash value voucher; DGA = *Dietary Guidelines for Americans*; oz-eq = ounce-equivalent.

[a] The DGA apply to individuals ages 2 years and older; therefore, although food package IV-A is also issued to younger children, food groups can only be evaluated for food package IV-B.

[b] Percentages represent the proportion of the recommended food pattern amount in the corresponding row of the DGA food pattern column. Values may not be replicable from the table due to rounding.

[c] A pattern of 1,300 kcal was selected for this age group because (1) the latter level reflects increases in body weights for young children and was considered too high for normal weight children in this age group, particularly in light of efforts to reduce and/or contain the prevalence of childhood obesity, and (2) the 1,300-kcal pattern was applied in both the previous WIC food package review (IOM, 2006) and the Child and Adult Food Care Program (CACFP) report (IOM, 2011) and should similarly be appropriate for current WIC-participating children of the same ages.

[d] Assumes that 67 percent of the CVV is used to purchase fruits, based on redemption data from Texas and Wyoming. A weighted composite cost of fruit ($0.55/c-eq) was developed, based on the most commonly consumed fruits (bananas, apples, oranges, berries, grapes, melon [watermelon was used in this case]) from an average of Massachusetts, Texas, and Wyoming redemption data. Only fresh fruit was included as all states allow fresh forms; Economic Research Service (ERS) 2013 price data were updated with a Consumer Price Index to 2015 values.

[e] Assumes that 33 percent of the CVV is used to purchase vegetables, based on redemption data from Texas and Wyoming. A weighted composite cost of vegetables ($0.55/c-eq) was developed, based on the most commonly consumed vegetables (tomatoes, avocados, potatoes, peppers, lettuce) from an average of Massachusetts, Texas, and Wyoming redemption data. Only fresh vegetables were included as all states allow fresh forms; ERS 2013 price data were updated with a Consumer Price Index to 2015 values. Because potatoes were not yet available in Wyoming, the same proportion of potatoes was assumed for this state as for Texas.

[f] Legumes can also be assessed as a protein, but they were placed in the vegetable group because a higher proportion of individuals had low intakes of vegetables across WIC-participating subgroups compared to protein.

[g] For the current food package, assumes 50 percent legumes and 50 percent peanut butter; for the revised package, the proportions of each provided per month were calculated.

[h] In the current food packages, a ratio of 81 percent refined grains and 19 percent whole grains was applied, based on redemption data; in the revised packages, a ratio of 50 percent refined grains and 50 percent whole grains was applied to account for the requirement that all cereals meet the whole grain-rich criteria.

[i] To compare the food package contribution to the DGA recommended amounts of whole grains, the whole grain portion of breakfast cereal was added to the whole grain contribution of bread.

[j] Equivalent to 4 oz per day, the lower end of AAP guideline of not more than 4–6 ounces per day.

SOURCES: IOM, 2006, 2011; USDA/ARS, 2014; USDA/FNS, 2014, 2016; USDA/HHS, 2016.

TABLE T-5b Proportion of 2015–2020 DGA Recommended Amounts of Food Groups in the Current and Revised Food Packages for Children Ages 2 to Less Than 5 Years as Redeemed[a]: Food Package IV-B[b]

			Current		Revised			
WIC Food Category	DGA Food Group	Units/d	WIC Redeemed Amounts of the Maximum Allowance	Proportion of the DGA Recom-mendation (%)[c]	WIC Redeemed Amounts of the Maximum Allowance	Proportion of the DGA Recom-mendation (%)[c]	Change in % of DGA Recom-mendation[c]	DGA 1,300-Kcal Food Pattern[d]
Total fruit	*Total fruit*	*c-eq*	*0.6*	*50*	*0.6*	*46*	*–4*	*1.3*
Juice, 100%	Fruit, as juice	c-eq	0.4	75	0.2	42	–33	0.5[k]
Fruit, 67% of CVV[e]	Fruit, whole	c-eq	0.3	33	0.4	49	15	0.8
Total vegetables	*Total vegetables*	*c-eq*	*0.2*	*13*	*0.2*	*15*	*2*	*1.5*
Vegetables, 33% of CVV[f]		c-eq	0.1	8	0.2	12	4	1.5
Legumes (as vegetable)[g,h]	Legumes (beans and peas)	c-eq	0.06	92	0.04	64	–28	0.1
Total dairy	*Total dairy*	*c-eq*	*1.5*	*61*	*1.5*	*59*	*–1*	*2.5*
Milk		c-eq	1.5	61	1.5	59	–1	2.5
Total grains	*Total grains*	*oz-eq*	*1.3*	*29*	*1.1*	*25*	*–3*	*4.5*
Breakfast cereal[i]	Refined grains	oz-eq	0.6	26	0.3	14	–12	2.3
Breakfast cereal	Whole grains	oz-eq	0.1	31[j]	0.3	36[j]	30	2.3
Whole wheat bread	Whole grains	oz-eq	0.6		0.5			
Total protein foods	*Total protein foods*	*oz-eq*	*0.6*	*18*	*0.9*	*25*	*7*	*3.5*
Peanut butter[h]	Nuts, seeds and soy	oz-eq	0.3	85	0.2	59	–26	0.4
Eggs	Meat, poultry, eggs	oz-eq	0.3	14	0.3	14	0	2.4
Fish	Seafood	oz-eq	0.0	0	0.1	13	13	0.6

continued

TABLE T-5b Continued

NOTES: c-eq = cup-equivalent; CVV = cash value voucher; DGA = *Dietary Guidelines for Americans*; oz-eq = ounce-equivalent.

[a] Applies redemption factors presented in Appendix R, Table R-5.

[b] The DGA apply to individuals ages 2 years and older; therefore, although food package IV-A is also issued to younger children, food groups can only be evaluated for food package IV-B.

[c] Percentages represent the proportion of the recommended food pattern amount in the corresponding row of the DGA food pattern column. Values may not be replicable from the table due to rounding.

[d] A pattern of 1,300 kcal was selected for this age group because (1) the latter level reflects increases in body weights for young children and was considered too high for normal weight children in this age group, particularly in light of efforts to reduce and/or contain the prevalence of childhood obesity, and (2) the 1,300-kcal pattern was applied in both the previous WIC food package review (IOM, 2006) and the CACFP report (IOM, 2011) and should similarly be appropriate for current WIC participating children of the same ages.

[e] Assumes that 67 percent of the CVV is used to purchase fruits, based on redemption data from Texas and Wyoming. A weighted composite cost of fruit ($0.55/c-eq) was developed, based on the most commonly consumed fruits (bananas, apples, oranges, berries, grapes, melon [watermelon was used in this case]) from an average of Massachusetts, Texas, and Wyoming redemption data. Only fresh fruit was included as all states allow fresh forms; Economic Research Service (ERS) 2013 price data were updated with a Consumer Price Index to 2015 values.

[f] Assumes that 33 percent of the CVV is used to purchase vegetables, based on redemption data from Texas and Wyoming. A weighted composite cost of vegetables ($0.55/c-eq) was developed, based on the most commonly consumed vegetables (tomatoes, avocados, potatoes, peppers, lettuce) from an average of Massachusetts, Texas, and Wyoming redemption data. Only fresh vegetables were included as all states allow fresh forms; ERS 2013 price data were updated with a Consumer Price Index to 2015 values. Because potatoes were not yet available in Wyoming, the same proportion of potatoes was assumed for this state as for Texas.

[g] Legumes can also be assessed as a protein, but they were placed in the vegetable group because a higher proportion of individuals had low intakes of vegetables across WIC-participating subgroups compared to protein.

[h] For the current food package, assumes 43 percent legumes and 57 percent peanut butter, based on prescription data from the PC 2014 Food Package Report (USDA/FNS, 2016).

[i] In the current food packages, a ratio of 81 percent refined grains and 19 percent whole grains was applied, based on redemption data; in the revised packages, a ratio of 50 percent refined grains and 50 percent whole grains was applied to account for the requirement that all cereals meet the whole grain-rich criteria.

[j] To compare the food package contribution to the DGA recommended amounts of whole grains, the whole grain portion of breakfast cereal was added to the whole grain contribution of bread.

[k] Equivalent to 4 oz per day, the lower end of the AAP guideline of not more than 4–6 ounces per day.

SOURCES: IOM, 2006, 2011; USDA/ARS, 2014; USDA/FNS, 2014, 2016; USDA/HHS, 2016.

TABLE T-6a Proportion of Dietary Reference Intakes or DGA Limits Provided by the Current and Revised Food Packages for Pregnant and Partially Breastfeeding Women Assuming Full Redemption: Food Packages V-A and V-B*

Nutrient	EAR/AI[a] (19–30y/31–50y)	Current		Revised				
		Amount	% DRI	Amount, Pregnant	Amount, Partial BF	% DRI, Pregnant	% Change, Pregnant	% Change, Partial BF
Higher Priority								
Iron (mg)	22	14	62	13.0	13	59	–4	–1
Choline (mg)	450[b]	74.9	17	78.6	87	17	+5	+17
Potassium (mg)	4,700[b]	1,837	39	1,473	1,688	31	–20	–8
Fiber (g)	28[b]	8.0	29	7.4	9.3	27	–7	+16
Sodium (mg)	1,500[b]	727	48	572	592	38	–21	–19
Saturated fat (g)	29	8.5	29	5.7	5.9	19	–34	–31
Added sugars (g)	65.6	7.4	11	7.5	7.5	11	+1	+1
Middle Priority								
Folate (µg DFE)	520	473	91	442	460	85	–7	–3
Lower Priority								
Magnesium (mg)	290/300	198	68/68	150.3	164	52/50	–24	–17
Vitamin A (µg RAE)	550	646	117	544.7	564	99	–16	–13
Zinc (mg)	9.5	6.6	69	5.5	5.7	58	–16	–13
Vitamin C (mg)	70	72.2	103	57.4	78.0	82	–20	+8
Vitamin B6 (mg)	1.6	1.3	79	1.2	1.3	73	–8	+3
Vitamin D (IU)	400	291	73	229	237	57	–21	–19
Calcium (mg)	800	1,029	129	796	811	100	–23	–21

continued

TABLE T-6a Continued

Nutrient	EAR/AI[a] (19–30y/31–50y)	Current		Revised				
		Amount	% DRI	Amount, Pregnant	Amount, Partial BF	% DRI, Pregnant	% Change, Pregnant	% Change, Partial BF
Other								
Energy (kcal)	2,625[c]	787	30	614	677	23	–22	–14
Protein (g)	71 (RDA)[d]	39	55	30.3	32	43	–23	–17
Phosphorus (mg)	580	976	168	762	793	131	–22	–19
Copper (mg)	0.8	0.4	55	0.3	0.4	44	–21	–7
Selenium (µg)	49	31.6	65	31.0	36	63	–2	+12
Thiamin (mg)	1.2	0.9	76	0.8	0.9	68	–11	–6
Riboflavin (mg)	1.2	1.8	148	1.5	1.5	123	–17	–14
Niacin (mg)	14	9.9	71	8.7	9.7	62	–13	–2
Vitamin B12 (µg)	2.2	4.4	198	3.8	4.0	175	–12	–7
Vitamin E (mg)	12	3.6	30	2.6	3.0	22	–26	–17

NOTES: BF = breastfeeding; DFE = dietary folate equivalents; DGA = *Dietary Guidelines for Americans*; DRI = Dietary Reference Intake; EAR/AI = Estimated Average Requirement/Adequate Intake; RAE = retinol activity equivalents; RDA = Recommended Dietary Allowance. Shading indicates nutrients to limit. See Chapter 5 for description of nutrient priorities.

*Some values in this table are corrected from the original prepublication version.

[a] Values represent the EAR/AI for pregnant women.

[b] Indicates AI.

[c] Value is the median estimated energy requirement (EER) calculated by the committee. Values differ slightly from those in Chapter 4 because EER values for that chapter were re-calculated in a different statistical program to generate percentiles. The means are equivalent for the two analyses.

[d] The RDA (provided in units of g/d) was used for evaluation of the food package content because the EAR is provided in units of g/kg/d.

SOURCE: USDA National Nutrient Database for Standard Reference, Release 28 (USDA/ARS, 2016).

TABLE T-6b Proportion of Dietary Reference Intakes or DGA Limits Provided by the Current and Revised Food Packages for Pregnant and Partially Breastfeeding Women as Redeemed[a]: Food Packages V-A and V-B*

		Current		Revised				
Nutrient	EAR/AI[b] (19–30y/31–50y)	Amount	% DRI	Amount, Pregnant	Amount, Partial BF	% DRI, Pregnant	% Change, Pregnant	% Change, Partial BF
Higher Priority								
Iron (mg)	22	8.2	37	7.3	7.6	33	–10	–7
Choline (mg)	450[c]	57.4	13	60	66	13	+4	+16
Potassium (mg)	4,700[c]	1,096	23	983	1,143	21	–10	+4
Fiber (g)	28[c]	4.9	17	4.7	6.0	17	–4	24
Sodium (mg)	1,500[c]	416	28	356	370	24	–14	–11
Added sugars (g)	66	4.3	6.6	4.3	4.3	7	0	0
Saturated fat (g)	29	6.0	21	3.7	3.9	13	–38	–36
Middle Priority								
Folate (μg DFE)	520	283	54	251	265	48	–11	–6
Lower Priority								
Magnesium (mg)	290/300	114	39/38	96	106	33/32	–16	–7
Vitamin A (μg RAE)	550	381	69	341	355	62	–11	–7
Zinc (mg)	9.5	3.8	40	3.4	3.5	36	–11	–8
Vitamin C (mg)	70	50.8	73	42	58	61	–17	–14
Vitamin B6 (mg)	1.6	0.8	48	0.7	0.8	44	–8	+6

continued

TABLE T-6b Continued

Nutrient	EAR/AI[b] (19–30y/31–50y)	Current		Revised				
		Amount	% DRI	Amount, Pregnant	Amount, Partial BF	% DRI, Pregnant	% Change, Pregnant	% Change, Partial BF
Vitamin D (IU)	400	168	42	148	154	37	–12	–8
Calcium (mg)	800	581	73	517	528	65	–11	–9
Other								
Energy (kcal)	2,625[d]	468	18	396	442	15	–15	–5
Protein (g)	71 (RDA)[e]	22.4	32	19.6	21.1	28	–13	–6
Phosphorus (mg)	580	559	96	493	515	85	–12	–8
Copper (mg)	0.8	0.3	32	0.2	0.3	28	–15	–2
Selenium (μg)	49	19	39	21	24	42	6	+22
Thiamin (mg)	1.2	0.5	45	0.5	0.5	40	–10	–4
Riboflavin (mg)	1.2	1.0	86	0.9	1.0	78	–10	–7
Niacin (mg)	14	5.8	41	5.0	5.7	36	–14	–1
Vitamin B12 (μg)	2.2	2.5	116	2.4	2.5	108	–7	–2
Vitamin E (mg)	12	2.1	17	1.6	1.8	13	–23	–12

NOTES: BF = breastfeeding; DFE = dietary folate equivalents; DGA = *Dietary Guidelines for Americans*; DRI = Dietary Reference Intake; EAR/AI = Estimated Average Requirement/Adequate Intake; IU = international units; RAE = retinol activity equivalents; RDA = Recommended Dietary Allowance. Shading indicates nutrients to limit. See Chapter 5 for description of nutrient priorities.

*Some values in this table are corrected from the original prepublication version.

[a] Applies redemption factors presented in Appendix R, Table R-5.

[b] Values represent the EAR/AI for pregnant women.

[c] Indicates an AI.

[d] Value is the median estimated energy requirement (EER) calculated by the committee. Values differ slightly from those in Chapter 4 because EER values for that chapter were re-calculated in a different statistical program to generate percentiles. The means are equivalent for the two analyses.

[e] The RDA (provided in units of g/d) was used for evaluation of the food package content because the EAR is provided in units of g/kg/d.

SOURCE: USDA National Nutrient Database for Standard Reference, Release 28 (USDA/ARS, 2016).

TABLE T-7a Proportion of Dietary Reference Intakes or DGA Limits Provided by the Current and Revised Food Packages for Postpartum Women Assuming Full Redemption: Food Package VI*

Nutrient	EAR/AI (19–30y/31–50y)	Current Amount	Current % DRI	Revised Amount	Revised % DRI	% Change
Higher Priority						
Calcium (mg)	800	739	92	766	96	+4
Potassium (mg)	4,700[a]	1,302	28	1,356	29	+4
Fiber (g)	25[a]	5.7	23	6.4	25	+12
Sodium (mg)	1,500[a]	527	35	512	34	–3
Added sugars (g)	59	6.9	12	7.5	13	+9
Middle Priority						
Folate (μg DFE)	320	425	133	436	136	+3
Vitamin D (IU)	400	213	53	229	57	+8
Iron (mg)	8.1	12	152	12.3	152	0
Saturated fat (g)	26	6.4	25	5.6	21	–13
Lower Priority						
Magnesium (mg)	255/265	132	52/50	134	52/50	+2
Vitamin A (μg RAE)	500	522	104	537	107	+3
Vitamin C (mg)	60	57	95	40.3	67	–30
Copper (mg)	0.7	0.3	42	0.3	43	+4
Zinc (mg)	6.8	5.2	76	5.2	77	+2
Thiamin (mg)	0.9	0.7	81	0.8	84	+4

continued

TABLE T-7a Continued

Nutrient	EAR/AI (19–30y/31–50y)	Current		Revised		
		Amount	% DRI	Amount	% DRI	% Change
Vitamin B6 (mg)	1.1	1.1	97	1.1	101	+3
Vitamin B12 (μg)	2	3.6	180	3.8	192	+7
Riboflavin (mg)	0.9	1.4	153	1.4	160	+5
Niacin (mg)	11	8.0	72	8.0	73	+1
Other						
Energy (kcal)	2,350[b]	572	24	543	23	–5
Protein (g)	46 (RDA)[c]	28	60	28.4	62	+3
Phosphorus (mg)	580	690	119	718	124	+4
Selenium (μg)	45	25	56	28	61	+10
Choline (mg)	425[a]	71	17	75	18	+5
Vitamin E (mg)	12	2.5	20	2.3	19	–6

NOTES: DFE = dietary folate equivalents; DGA = *Dietary Guidelines for Americans*; DRI = Dietary Reference Intake; EAR/AI = Estimated Average Requirement/Adequate Intake; RAE = retinol activity equivalents; RDA = Recommended Dietary Allowance. Shading indicates nutrients to limit. See Chapter 5 for description of nutrient priorities.

*Some values in this table are corrected from the original prepublication version.

[a] Indicates AI.

[b] Value is the median estimated energy requirement (EER) calculated by the committee. Values differ slightly from those in Chapter 4 because EER values for that chapter were re-calculated in a different statistical program to generate percentiles. The means are equivalent for the two analyses.

[c] The RDA (provided in units of g/d) was used for evaluation of the food package content because the EAR is provided in units of g/kg/d.

SOURCE: USDA National Nutrient Database for Standard Reference, Release 28 (USDA/ARS, 2016).

TABLE T-7b Proportion of Dietary Reference Intakes or DGA Limits Provided by the Current and Revised Food Packages for Postpartum Women as Redeemed[a]: Food Package VI*

		Current		Revised		
Nutrient	EAR/AI (19–30y/31–50y)	Amount	% DRI	Amount	% DRI	% Change
Higher Priority						
Calcium (mg)	800	421	53	451	56	+7
Potassium (mg)	4,700[b]	796	17	839	18	+5
Fiber (g)	25[b]	3.7	15	4.0	16	+9
Sodium (mg)	1,500[b]	307	24	299	20	–2
Added sugars (g)	58.7	4.0	7	4.1	7	+3
Middle Priority						
Folate (μg DFE)	320	257	80	245	77	–5
Vitamin D (IU)	400	124	31	136	34	+10
Iron (mg)	8.1	7.5	93	6.9	85	–9
Saturated fat (g)	26	3.7	15	3.4	13	–9
Lower Priority						
Magnesium (mg)	255/265	78	31/29	80	31/30	+3
Vitamin A (μg RAE)	500	312	62	317	63	1
Vitamin C (mg)	60	40.7	68	29	47	–30
Copper (mg)	0.7	0.2	26	0.2	27	+4
Zinc (mg)	6.8	3.1	45	3.1	45	0
Thiamin (mg)	0.9	0.4	48	0.4	48	–1

continued

TABLE T-7b Continued

Nutrient	EAR/AI (19–30y/31–50y)	Current		Revised		
		Amount	% DRI	Amount	% DRI	% Change
Vitamin B6 (mg)	1.1	0.7	60	0.7	60	–1
Vitamin B12 (μg)	2	2.1	106	2.2	111	+5
Riboflavin (mg)	0.9	0.8	91	0.9	95	+5
Niacin (mg)	11	4.8	43	4.6	42	–4
Other						
Energy (kcal)	2,350[c]	349	15	330	14	–5
Protein (g)	46 (RDA)[d]	16	35	17	37	+6
Phosphorus (mg)	580	402	69	428	74	+7
Selenium (μg)	45	16	35	18	39	+12
Choline (mg)	425[b]	56	13	58	14	+4
Vitamin E (mg)	12	1.5	13	1.4	12	–7

NOTES: DFE = dietary folate equivalents; DGA = *Dietary Guidelines for Americans*; DRI = Dietary Reference Intake; EAR/AI = Estimated Average Requirement/Adequate Intake; RAE = retinol activity equivalents; RDA = Recommended Dietary Allowance. Shading indicates nutrients to limit. See Chapter 5 for description of nutrient priorities.

*Some values in this table are corrected from the original prepublication version.

[a] Indicates AI.

[b] Applies redemption factors presented in Appendix R, Table R-5.

[c] Value is the median estimated energy requirement (EER) calculated by the committee. Values differ slightly from those in Chapter 4 because EER values for that chapter were re-calculated in a different statistical program to generate percentiles. The means are equivalent for the two analyses.

[d] The RDA (provided in units of g/d) was used for evaluation of the food package content because the EAR is provided in units of g/kg/d.

SOURCE: USDA National Nutrient Database for Standard Reference, Release 28 (USDA/ARS, 2016).

TABLE T-8a Proportion of Dietary Reference Intakes or DGA Limits Provided by the Current and Revised Food Packages for Fully Breastfeeding Women Assuming Full Redemption: Food Package VII*

Nutrient	EAR/AI (19–30y/31–50y)	Current		Revised		
		Amount	% DRI	Amount	% DRI	% Change
Higher Priority						
Potassium (mg)	5,100[a]	1,958	38	1,853	36	–5
Fiber (g)	29[a]	8.0	28	11.1	38	38
Sodium (mg)	1,500[a]	1,007	67	657	44	–35
Saturated fat (g)	28	12.8	44	7.3	26	–43
Added sugars (g)	62.3	6.6	10	6.7	11	+1
Middle Priority						
Folate (μg DFE)	450	487	108	485	108	0
Vitamin D (IU)	400	371	93	253	63	–32
Calcium (mg)	800	1,232	154	810	101	–34
Lower Priority						
Vitamin A (μg RAE)	900	754	84	609	68	–19
Magnesium (mg)	255/265	214	84/81	176	69/66	–18
Zinc (mg)	10.4	7.7	74	6.1	59	–21
Vitamin C (mg)	100	72	72	98	98	+36
Vitamin B6 (mg)	1.7	1.4	83	1.5	87	+5
Copper (mg)	1	0.5	48	0.5	48	0
Thiamin (mg)	1.2	0.9	78	0.9	74	–6

continued

TABLE T-8a Continued

Nutrient	EAR/AI (19–30y/31–50y)	Current		Revised		
		Amount	% DRI	Amount	% DRI	% Change
Other						
Energy (kcal)	2,492[b]	918	37	764	31	–17
Protein (g)	71 (RDA)[c]	52.3	74	36.9	52	–29
Iron (mg)	6.5	14.4	221	14.1	217	–2
Phosphorus (mg)	580	1,178	203	841	145	–29
Selenium (μg)	59	63.5	108	47.9	81	–25
Riboflavin (mg)	1.3	2.0	153	1.6	122	–20
Niacin (mg)	13	12.7	98	11.1	85	–13
Choline (mg)	550[a]	147	27	156	28	+6
Vitamin B12 (μg)	2.4	5.6	234	4.3	180	–23
Vitamin E (mg)	16	4.0	25	2.9	18	–27

NOTES: DFE = dietary folate equivalents; DGA = *Dietary Guidelines for Americans*; DRI = Dietary Reference Intake; EAR/AI = Estimated Average Requirement/Adequate Intake; RAE = retinol activity equivalents; RDA = Recommended Dietary Allowance. Shading indicates nutrients to limit. See Chapter 5 for description of nutrient priorities.

* Some values in this table are corrected from the original prepublication version.

[a] Indicates AI.

[b] Value is the median estimated energy requirement (EER) calculated by the committee. Values differ slightly from those in Chapter 4 because EER values for that chapter were re-calculated in a different statistical program to generate percentiles. The means are equivalent for the two analyses.

[c] The RDA (provided in units of g/d) was used for evaluation of the food package content because the EAR is provided in units of g/kg/d.

SOURCE: USDA National Nutrient Database for Standard Reference, Release 28 (USDA/ARS, 2016).

TABLE T-8b Proportion of Dietary Reference Intakes or DGA Limits Provided by the Current and Revised Food Packages for Fully Breastfeeding Women as Redeemed[a]: Food Package VII*

Nutrient	EAR/AI (19–30y/31–50y)	Current		Revised		
		Amount	% DRI	Amount	% DRI	% Change
Higher Priority						
Potassium (mg)	5,100[b]	1,181	23	1,291	25	+9
Fiber (g)	29[b]	4.9	17	7.4	26	+52
Sodium (mg)	1,500[b]	608	41	425	28	–30
Saturated fat (g)	28	7.8	27	5.0	18	–36
Added sugars (g)	62.3	3.9	6	3.8	6	–1
Middle Priority						
Folate (μg DFE)	450	293	65	285	63	–3
Vitamin D (IU)	400	223	56	171	43	–23
Calcium (mg)	800	717	90	545	68	–24
Lower Priority						
Vitamin A (μg RAE)	900	456	51	397	44	–13
Magnesium (mg)	255/265	125	49/47	117	46/44	–7
Zinc (mg)	10.4	4.6	44	3.9	37	–16
Vitamin C (mg)	100	51	51	73	73	+43
Vitamin B6 (mg)	1.7	0.9	51	1.0	56	+9
Copper (mg)	1	0.3	29	0.3	32	+12
Thiamin (mg)	1.2	0.6	46	0.5	45	–2

continued

TABLE T-8b Continued

Nutrient	EAR/AI (19–30y/31–50y)	Current Amount	Current % DRI	Revised Amount	Revised % DRI	% Change
Other						
Energy (kcal)	2,492[c]	559	22	515	21	–8
Protein (g)	71 (RDA)[d]	31.7	45	25.0	35	–21
Iron (mg)	6.5	8.8	136	8.2	126	–7
Phosphorus (mg)	580	698	120	566	98	–19
Selenium (μg)	59	41.4	70	33.0	56	–20
Riboflavin (mg)	1.3	1.2	92	1.1	81	–12
Niacin (mg)	13	7.7	60	6.7	52	–13
Choline (mg)	550[b]	114	21	120	22	+6
Vitamin B12 (μg)	2.4	3.4	143	2.8	115	–19
Vitamin E (mg)	16	2.4	15	1.9	12	–19

NOTES: DFE = dietary folate equivalents; DGA = *Dietary Guidelines for Americans*; DRI = Dietary Reference Intake; EAR/AI = Estimated Average Requirement/Adequate Intake; RAE = retinol activity equivalents; RDA = Recommended Dietary Allowance. Shading indicates nutrients to limit. See Chapter 5 for description of nutrient priorities.

*Some values in this table are corrected from the original prepublication version.

[a] Applies redemption factors presented in Appendix R, Table R-5.

[b] Indicates AI.

[c] Value is the median estimated energy requirement (EER) calculated by the committee. Values differ slightly from those in Chapter 4 because EER values for that chapter were re-calculated in a different statistical program to generate percentiles. The means are equivalent for the two analyses.

[d] The RDA (provided in units of g/d) was used for evaluation of the food package content because the EAR is provided in units of g/kg/d.

SOURCE: USDA National Nutrient Database for Standard Reference, Release 28 (USDA/ARS, 2016).

TABLE T-9a Proportion of Dietary Reference Intakes or DGA Limits Provided by the Current and Revised Food Packages for Infants Ages 6 to Less Than 12 Months Assuming Full Redemption: Food Package II*

		Current Amount			Revised Amount			% Change		
Nutrient	EAR/AI	FF 6–11 mo	BF/FF 6–11 mo	BF 6–11 mo	FF 6–11 mo	BF/FF 6–11 mo	BF 6–11 mo	FF 6–11 mo	BF/FF 6–11 mo	BF 6–11 mo
Priority										
Iron (mg)	6.9[a]	20.9	17.0	14.1	13.2	9.3	8.9	–37	–45	–37
Zinc (mg)	2.5[a]	5.9	4.1	3.3	4.8	2.9	1.8	–19	–28	–46
Other										
Energy (kcal)	727[b]	621	409	300	559	347	156	–10	–15	–48
Protein (g)	11 (RDA)[c]	13.5	8.8	13.4	12.1	7.4	6.0	–10	–16	–55
Fiber (g)	ND	3.7	3.7	5.9	2.7	2.7	3.2	–29	–29	–45
Calcium (mg)	260	604	404	208	504	304	126	–17	–25	–39
Magnesium (mg)	75	69	52	58	57	41	31	–17	–22	–47
Phosphorus (mg)	275	388	266	220	324	202	118	–17	–24	–46
Potassium (mg)	700	830	599	669	765	534	338	–8	–11	–50
Copper (mg)	0.22	0.52	0.35	0.28	0.46	0.29	0.15	–11	–16	–48
Selenium (μg)	20	18	13	14	14	8.7	7.1	–22	–31	–49
Vitamin C (mg)	50	71	49	46	71	49	23	0	0	–50
Thiamin (mg)	0.30	0.70	0.52	0.35	0.52	0.34	0.22	–26	–35	–38
Riboflavin (mg)	0.40	0.92	0.63	0.47	0.77	0.48	0.26	–16	–24	–45
Niacin (mg)	4	9.7	7.4	7.5	7.0	4.7	4.2	–28	–37	–44

continued

TABLE T-9a Continued

Nutrient	EAR/AI	Current Amount FF 6–11 mo	BF/FF 6–11 mo	BF 6–11 mo	Revised Amount FF 6–11 mo	BF/FF 6–11 mo	BF 6–11 mo	% Change FF 6–11 mo	BF/FF 6–11 mo	BF 6–11 mo
Vitamin B6 (mg)	0.30	0.29	0.16	0.09	0.29	0.16	0.04	0	0	-61
Folate (μg DFE)	80	158	105	62	139	86	35	-12	-18	-43
Choline (mg)	150	100	63	60	95	58	28	-5	-8	-54
Vitamin B12 (μg)	0.5	2.1	1.4	1.2	1.6	1.0	0.7	-22	-31	-46
Vitamin A (μg RAE)	500	550	358	262	550	358	131	0	0	-50
Vitamin E (mg)	5	7.0	4.4	2.2	6.5	3.9	1.2	-7	-11	-45
Vitamin D (IU)	400	313	192	58	282	160	36	-10	-16	-39
Added sugars (g)	NA	0.5	0.3	0.0	0.5	0.3	0.0	0	0	0
Saturated fat (g)	NA	11	5.9	1.4	11	5.8	0.6	-1	-2	-57
Sodium (mg)	370	157	93	64	155	91	29	-1	-2	-55

NOTES: BF = breastfeeding; DFE = dietary folate equivalents; DGA = *Dietary Guidelines for Americans*; DRI = Dietary Reference Intake; EAR/AI = Estimated Average Requirement/Adequate Intake; FF = formula-feeding; RAE = retinol activity equivalents; RDA = Recommended Dietary Allowance. Shading indicates nutrients to limit. See Chapter 5 for description of nutrient priorities.

*Some values in this table are corrected from the original prepublication version.

[a] Indicates EAR.

[b] Value is the median estimated energy requirement (EER) calculated by the committee.

[c] The RDA (provided in units of g/d) was used for evaluation of the food package content because the EAR is provided in units of g/kg/d.

SOURCE: USDA National Nutrient Database for Standard Reference, Release 28 (USDA/ARS, 2016).

TABLE T-9b Proportion of Dietary Reference Intakes or DGA Limits Provided by the Current and Revised Food Packages for Infants Ages 6 to Less Than 12 Months as Redeemed[a]: Food Package II*

		Current Amount			Revised Amount			% Change		
Nutrient	EAR/AI	FF 6–11 mo	BF/FF 6–11 mo	BF 6–11 mo	FF 6–11 mo	BF/FF 6–11 mo	BF 6–11 mo	FF 6–11 mo	BF/FF 6–11 mo	BF 6–11 mo
Priority										
Iron (mg)	6.9[b]	13.8	10.2	6.6	10.7	7.1	5.1	–22	–30	–22
Zinc (mg)	2.5[b]	4.7	2.9	1.4	4.2	2.5	1.0	–9	–15	–29
Other										
Energy (kcal)	727[c]	513	313	134	496	296	90	–3	–5	–33
Protein (g)	11 (RDA)[d]	11	6.8	4.9	11	6.4	3.0	–4	–6	–39
Fiber (g)	ND	1.8	1.8	2.9	1.7	1.7	2.0	–8	–8	–32
Calcium (mg)	260	490	302	95	451	263	72	–8	–13	–24
Magnesium (mg)	75	50	34	27	47	32	18	–6	–8	–32
Phosphorus (mg)	275	308	194	94	285	171	65	–8	–12	–30
Potassium (mg)	700	637	420	315	641	424	204	1	1	–35
Copper (mg)	0.22	0.42	0.26	0.13	0.41	0.25	0.08	–3	–5	–33
Selenium (μg)	20	13.8	8.9	5.4	12.3	7.3	3.7	–11	–18	–31
Vitamin C (mg)	50	58	36	23	61	39	15	–5	–8	–37
Thiamin (mg)	0.30	0.52	0.35	0.16	0.45	0.28	0.13	–14	–20	–23
Riboflavin (mg)	0.40	0.73	0.46	0.21	0.67	0.41	0.15	–7	–12	–29
Niacin (mg)	4	6.9	4.8	3.2	5.9	3.7	2.3	–15	–22	–28

continued

TABLE T-9b Continued

Nutrient	EAR/AI	Current Amount FF 6–11 mo	Current Amount BF/FF 6–11 mo	Current Amount BF 6–11 mo	Revised Amount FF 6–11 mo	Revised Amount BF/FF 6–11 mo	Revised Amount BF 6–11 mo	% Change FF 6–11 mo	% Change BF/FF 6–11 mo	% Change BF 6–11 mo
Vitamin B6 (mg)	0.30	0.27	0.15	0.03	0.27	0.15	0.02	0	0	–46
Folate (μg DFE)	80	129	79	30	123	74	21	–5	–7	–29
Choline (mg)	150	86	51	24	85	50	15	–1	–1	–38
Vitamin B12 (μg)	0.5	1.6	1.0	0.5	1.4	0.8	0.3	–11	–18	–29
Vitamin A (μg RAE)	500	461	281	134	479	299	85	–4	–6	–37
Vitamin E (mg)	5	5.9	3.5	1.1	5.8	3.4	0.7	–2	–3	–31
Vitamin D (IU)	400	272	158	25	259	145	20	–5	–8	–22
Added sugars (g)	NA	0.4	0.2	0.0	0.4	0.2	0.0	0	0	0
Saturated fat (g)	NA	10.0	5.5	0.5	9.9	5.4	0.3	0	–1	–41
Sodium (mg)	370	140	80	26	141	89	16	–1	–1	–40

NOTES: AI = adequate intake; BF = breastfeeding; DFE = dietary folate equivalents; DGA = *Dietary Guidelines for Americans*; DRI = Dietary Reference Intake; EAR/AI = Estimated Average Requirement/Adequate Intake; FF = formula-feeding; RAE = retinol activity equivalents; RDA = Recommended Dietary Allowance. Shading indicates nutrients to limit. See Chapter 5 for description of nutrient priorities.

*Some values in this table are corrected from the original prepublication version.

[a] Applies redemption factors presented in Appendix R, Table R-5.

[b] Indicates EAR.

[c] Value is the median estimated energy requirement (EER) calculated by the committee.

[d] The RDA (provided in units of g/d) was used for evaluation of the food package content because the EAR is provided in units of g/kg/d.

SOURCE: USDA National Nutrient Database for Standard Reference, Release 28 (USDA/ARS, 2016).

TABLE T-10a Proportion of Dietary Reference Intakes or DGA Limits Provided by the Current and Revised Food Packages for Children Ages 1 to Less Than 2 Years Assuming Full Redemption: Food Package IV-A*

		Current		Revised		
Nutrient	EAR/AI	Amount	% DRI	Amount	% DRI	% Change
Priority						
Fiber (g)	19[a]	7.1	38	6.3	33	-11
Potassium (mg)	3,000[a]	1,267	42	1,007	34	-20
Added sugars (g)	NA	8.4	NA	7.1	NA	-16
Saturated fat (g)	NA	11.9	NA	9.1	NA	-23
Sodium (mg)	1,000[a]	587	59	472	47	-20
Other						
Energy (kcal)	917[b]	725	79	577	63	-20
Protein (g)	13 (RDA)[c]	29	224	23	177	-21
Calcium (mg)	500	717	143	542	108	-24
Iron (mg)	3	13	445	13	420	-6
Magnesium (mg)	65	138	212	106	163	-23
Phosphorus (mg)	380	690	182	534	140	-23
Zinc (mg)	2.5	5.5	221	4.7	188	-15
Copper (mg)	0.26	0.4	161	0.3	129	-20
Selenium (µg)	17	35	207	30	177	-15
Vitamin C (mg)	13	56	429	47	360	-16
Thiamin (mg)	0.4	0.8	211	0.7	181	-15
Riboflavin (mg)	0.4	1.4	345	1.1	284	-18
Niacin (mg)	5	8.9	179	8.3	166	-7
Vitamin B6 (mg)	0.4	1.1	268	1.0	252	-6
Folate (µg DFE)	120	430	358	412	343	-4
Choline (mg)	200[a]	71.4	36	127	64	78
Vitamin B12 (µg)	0.7	3.8	546	3.3	474	-13
Vitamin A (µg RAE)	210	417	199	380	181	-9
Vitamin E (mg)	5	1.1	22	2.7	55	+148
Vitamin D (IU)	400	254	63	192	48	-25

NOTES: DFE = dietary folate equivalents; DGA = *Dietary Guidelines for Americans*; DRI = Dietary Reference Intake; EAR/AI = Estimated Average Requirement/Adequate Intake; RAE = retinol activity equivalents; RDA = Recommended Dietary Allowance. Shading indicates nutrients to limit. See Chapter 5 for description of nutrient priorities.

*Some values in this table are corrected from the original prepublication version.

[a] Indicates AI.

[b] Value is the median estimated energy requirement (EER) calculated by the committee.

[c] The RDA (provided in units of g/d) was used for evaluation of the food package content because the EAR is provided in units of g/kg/d.

SOURCE: USDA National Nutrient Database for Standard Reference, Release 28 (USDA/ARS, 2016).

TABLE T-10b Proportion of Dietary Reference Intakes or DGA Limits Provided by the Current and Revised Food Packages for Children Ages 1 to Less Than 2 Years as Redeemed[a]: Food Package IV-A*

		Current		Revised		
Nutrient	EAR/AI	Amount	% DRI	Amount	% DRI	% Change
Priority						
Fiber (g)	19[b]	4.3	23	4.0	21	-8
Potassium (mg)	3,000[b]	888	30	770	26	-13
Added sugars (g)	NA	5.4	NA	4.5	NA	-18
Saturated fat (g)	NA	8.6	NA	7.6	NA	-12
Sodium (mg)	1,000[b]	385	38	333	33	-14
Other						
Energy (kcal)	917[c]	491	54	421	46	-14
Protein (g)	13 (RDA)[d]	20	154	18	135	-12
Calcium (mg)	500	516	103	441	88	-14
Iron (mg)	3	8.1	270	7.1	237	-12
Magnesium (mg)	65	88.9	137	74	114	-17
Phosphorus (mg)	380	479	126	409	108	-15
Zinc (mg)	2.5	3.6	145	3.2	128	-12
Copper (mg)	0.26	0.3	104	0.2	90	-14
Selenium (μg)	17	25	144	23	133	-8
Vitamin C (mg)	13	40	306	35	267	-13
Thiamin (mg)	0.4	0.5	134	0.5	113	-15
Riboflavin (mg)	0.4	1.0	241	0.8	208	-14
Niacin (mg)	5	5.3	107	4.8	96	-10
Vitamin B6 (mg)	0.4	0.7	172	0.6	158	-8
Folate (μg DFE)	120	264	220	237	197	-10
Choline (mg)	200[b]	55	27	101	50	84
Vitamin B12 (μg)	0.7	2.6	376	2.3	333	-12
Vitamin A (μg RAE)	210	281	134	256	122	-9
Vitamin E (mg)	5	0.7	14	1.7	34	+143
Vitamin D (IU)	400	186	46	153	38	-18

NOTES: DFE = dietary folate equivalents; DGA = *Dietary Guidelines for Americans*; DRI = Dietary Reference Intake; EAR/AI = Estimated Average Requirement/Adequate Intake; RAE = retinol activity equivalents; RDA = Recommended Dietary Allowance. Shading indicates nutrients to limit. See Chapter 5 for description of nutrient priorities.

*Some values in this table are corrected from the original prepublication version.

[a] Applies redemption factors presented in Appendix R, Table R-5.

[b] Indicates AI (used when EAR could not be determined).

[c] Value is the median estimated energy requirement (EER) calculated by the committee.

[d] The RDA (provided in units of g/d) was used for evaluation of the food package content because the EAR is provided in units of g/kg/d.

SOURCE: USDA National Nutrient Database for Standard Reference, Release 28 (USDA/ARS, 2016).

TABLE T-11a Proportion of Dietary Reference Intakes or DGA Limits Provided by the Current and Revised Food Packages for Children Ages 2 to Less Than 5 Years Assuming Full Redemption: Food Package IV-B*

			Current			Revised			
Nutrient	EAR/AI children 1–3 y	EAR/AI children 4–8 y	Amount	% DRI children 1–3 y	% DRI children 4–5 y	Amount	% DRI children 1–3 y	% DRI children 4–5 y	% Change
Priority									
Fiber (g)	19[a]	25[a]	7.1	38	29	6.3	33	25	–11
Potassium (mg)	3,000[a]	3,800[a]	1,357	45	36	1,262	42	33	–7
Added sugars (g)	32.5	32.5	6.9	21	21	7.5	23	23	+9
Saturated fat (g)	14	14	6.6	47	47	5.2	37	37	–20
Sodium (mg)	1,000[a]	1,200[a]	639	64	53	534	53	44	–16
Other									
Energy (kcal)	917[b]	1,517[b]	648	71	43	557	61	37	–14
Protein (g)	13 (RDA)[c]	19 (RDA)[c]	31	236	162	27.1	208	143	–12
Calcium (mg)	500	800	787	157	98	705	141	88	–10
Iron (mg)	3	4.1	14	449	328	13	424	310	–5
Magnesium (mg)	65	110	154	237	140	132	203	120	–14
Phosphorus (mg)	380	405	762	201	188	678	178	167	–11
Zinc (mg)	2.5	4	5.7	227	142	5.2	206	129	–9
Copper (mg)	0.26	0.34	0.3	134	102	0.3	114	87	–15
Selenium (μg)	17	23	32	187	138	29	169	125	–9

continued

TABLE T-11a Continued

Nutrient	EAR/AI children 1–3 y	EAR/AI children 4–8 y	Current			Revised			% Change
			Amount	% DRI children 1–3 y	% DRI children 4–5 y	Amount	% DRI children 1–3 y	% DRI children 4–5 y	
Vitamin C (mg)	13	22	60	458	271	51	388	229	–15
Thiamin (mg)	0.4	0.5	0.8	206	165	0.8	188	151	–9
Riboflavin (mg)	0.4	0.5	1.4	353	282	1.3	336	268	–5
Niacin (mg)	5	6	9.0	179	150	8.4	169	140	–6
Vitamin B6 (mg)	0.4	0.5	1.1	277	222	1.1	270	216	–2
Folate (µg DFE)	120	160	431	359	269	418	349	261	–3
Choline (mg)	200[a]	250[a]	77	38	31	77	38	31	0
Vitamin B12 (µg)	0.7	1	3.6	514	360	3.6	514	360	0
Vitamin A (µg RAE)	210	275	532	253	194	501	238	182	–6
Vitamin E (mg)	5	6	3.0	60	50	2.5	51	42	–16
Vitamin D (IU)	400	400	213	53	53	202	51	51	–5

NOTES: DFE = dietary folate equivalents; DGA = *Dietary Guidelines for Americans*; DRI = Dietary Reference Intake; EAR/AI = Estimated Average Requirement/Adequate Intake; RAE = retinol activity equivalents; RDA = Recommended Dietary Allowance. Shading indicates nutrients to limit. See Chapter 5 for description of nutrient priorities.

*Some values in this table are corrected from the original prepublication version.

[a] Indicates AI.

[b] Value is the median estimated energy requirement (EER) calculated by the committee.

[c] The RDA (provided in units of g/d) was used for evaluation of the food package content because the EAR is provided in units of g/kg/d.

SOURCE: USDA National Nutrient Database for Standard Reference, Release 28 (USDA/ARS, 2016).

TABLE T-11b Proportion of Dietary Reference Intakes or DGA Limits Provided by the Current and Revised Food Packages for Children Ages 2 to Less Than 5 Years as Redeemed[a]: Food Package IV-B*

			Current			Revised			
Nutrient	EAR/AI children 1–3 y	EAR/AI children 4–8 y	Amount	% DRI children 1–3 y	% DRI children 4–5 y	Amount	% DRI children 1–3 y	% DRI children 4–5 y	% Change
Priority									
Fiber (g)	19[b]	25[b]	4.3	23	17	4.0	21	16	–8
Potassium (mg)	3,000[b]	3,800[b]	927	31	24	940	31	25	+1
Added sugars (g)	32.5	32.5	4.3	13	13	4.6	14	14	+9
Saturated fat (g)	14	14	4.5	32	32	3.9	27	27	–13
Sodium (mg)	1,000[b]	1,200[b]	412	41	34	367	37	31	–11
Other									
Energy (kcal)	917[c]	1,517[c]	423	46	28	388	42	26	–8
Protein (g)	13 (RDA)[d]	19 (RDA)[d]	21	158	108	20	153	104	–3
Calcium (mg)	500	800	543	109	68	539	108	67	–1
Iron (mg)	3	4.1	8.2	272	199	7.2	240	176	–12
Magnesium (mg)	65	110	99	152	90	92	142	84	–7
Phosphorus (mg)	380	405	513	135	127	501	132	124	–2
Zinc (mg)	2.5	4	3.7	146	92	3.4	137	86	–6
Copper (mg)	0.26	0.34	0.21	83	63	0.2	75	57	–10
Selenium (μg)	17	23	21	124	92	21	122	90	–2

continued

TABLE T-11b Continued

Nutrient	EAR/AI Children 1–3 y	EAR/AI Children 4–8 y	Current Amount	Current % DRI Children 1–3 y	Current % DRI Children 4–5 y	Revised Amount	Revised % DRI Children 1–3 y	Revised % DRI Children 4–5 y	% Change
Vitamin C (mg)	13	22	43	327	193	38	289	171	–12
Thiamin (mg)	0.4	0.5	0.5	128	102	0.5	117	94	–9
Riboflavin (mg)	0.4	0.5	1.0	239	191	1.0	238	191	0
Niacin (mg)	5	6	5.3	107	89	4.9	97	81	–9
Vitamin B6 (mg)	0.4	0.5	0.7	177	142	0.7	171	137	–4
Folate (μg DFE)	120	160	263	219	164	241	200	150	–9
Choline (mg)	200[b]	250[b]	58	29	23	59	29	23	+1
Vitamin B12 (μg)	0.7	1	2.4	342	240	2.4	349	244	+2
Vitamin A (μg RAE)	210	275	357	170	130	344	164	125	–4
Vitamin E (mg)	5	6	1.8	36	30	1.5	31	25	–14
Vitamin D (IU)	400	400	148	37	37	151	38	38	+2

NOTES: DFE = dietary folate equivalents; DGA = *Dietary Guidelines for Americans*; DRI = Dietary Reference Intake; EAR/AI = Estimated Average Requirement/Adequate Intake; RAE = retinol activity equivalents; RDA = Recommended Dietary Allowance. Shading indicates nutrients to limit. See Chapter 5 for description of nutrient priorities.

*Some values in this table are corrected from the original prepublication version.

[a] Applies redemption factors presented in Appendix R, Table R-5.

[b] Indicates AI.

[c] Value is the median estimated energy requirement (EER) calculated by the committee.

[d] The RDA (provided in units of g/d) was used for evaluation of the food package content because the EAR is provided in units of g/kg/d.

SOURCE: USDA National Nutrient Database for Standard Reference, Release 28 (USDA/ARS, 2016).

TABLE T-12 Vegetables Provided in Food Packages IV, V-B, and VII Considering 33% or 100% Redemption of the CVV for Vegetables (c-eq/d)

			Amount in Food Package				
Food Package	Recommended Intake	Current Intake (Mean)	Current	Revised, 33% Veg	Difference from Current	Revised, 100% Veg	Difference from Current
IV	1.5	0.65	0.19	0.22	+0.04	0.59	+0.40
V-B	3.5	0.94	0.30	0.46	+0.17	1.23	+0.93
VII	3.5	0.94	0.30	0.61	+0.32	1.68	+1.38

NOTES: Food group amounts based on the food package food group profiles, as presented in Chapter 3, Tables 3-1, 3-3, and 3-4.

TABLE T-13 Fiber Provided in Food Packages IV, V-B, and VII Considering 33% or 100% Redemption of the CVV for Vegetables (g/d)

			Amount in Food Package				
Food Package	AI	Current Intake (Mean)	Current	Revised, 33% Veg	Difference from Current in FP	Revised, 100% Veg	Difference from Current
IV	19	8.5,12*	4.31	3.98	−0.33	4.42	+0.11
V-B	29	16	4.89	6.05	+1.16	6.96	+2.07
VII	29	16	4.89	7.42	+2.53	8.70	+3.81

NOTES: Nutrient data based on the food package nutrient profiles developed using the method described in Appendix R.

* Values represent mean intake for children ages 1 to less than 2 years, ages 2 to less than 5 years.

REFERENCES

IOM (Institute of Medicine). 2006. *WIC food packages: Time for a change*. Washington, DC: The National Academies Press.

IOM. 2011. *Child and Adult Care Food Program: Aligning dietary guidance for all*. Washington, DC: The National Academies Press.

USDA/ARS (U.S. Department of Agriculture/Agricultural Research Service). 2005–2012. *What we eat in America, NHANES 2005–2012*. Beltsville, MD: USDA/ARS. http://www.ars.usda.gov/services/docs.htm?docid=13793 (accessed December 15, 2016).

USDA/ARS. 2014. *Food patterns equivalents database 2011–12: Methodology and user guide*. Beltsville, MD: USDA/ARS. http://www.ars.usda.gov/SP2UserFiles/Place/80400530/pdf/fped/FPED_1112.pdf (accessed August 31, 2016).

USDA/ARS. 2016. *USDA National Nutrient Database for Standard Reference*. Release 28. Beltsville, MD: USDA/ARS. https://www.ars.usda.gov/northeast-area/beltsville-md/beltsville-human-nutrition-research-center/nutrient-data-laboratory/docs/usda-national-nutrient-database-for-standard-reference/ (accessed November 11, 2016).

USDA/FNS (U.S. Department of Agriculture/Food and Nutrition Service). 2014. *Special Supplemental Nutrition Program for Women, Infants and Children (WIC): Revisions in the WIC food packages*; final rule, 7 C.F.R. § 246.

USDA/FNS. 2016. *WIC participant and program characteristics 2014: Food package report.* Alexandria, VA: USDA/FNS. http://www.fns.usda.gov/wic-participant-and-program-characteristics-2014-food-package-report (accessed August 30, 2016).

USDA/HHS (U.S. Department of Agriculture/U.S. Department of Health and Human Development). 2016. *2015–2020 Dietary Guidelines for Americans*. Washington, DC: U.S. Government Printing Office. https://health.gov/dietaryguidelines/2015 (accessed August 29, 2016).

Appendix U

The Regulatory Impact Analysis (Complete)

This appendix presents a regulatory impact analysis (RIA) for the proposed revisions to the Special Supplemental Nutrition Program for Women, Infants, and Children (WIC) food packages. This RIA was guided by the overall structure and analytic approach presented in the 2007 Revisions to the WIC Food Package Interim Rule and associated appendix (USDA/FNS, 2007a,b), along with those prepared for the Proposed Rule and Final Rule (USDA/FNS, 2006, 2014a). Unlike WIC RIAs found in the *Federal Register*, this analysis is not part of the federal rulemaking process nor has it been reviewed by the U.S. Department of Agriculture (USDA), the Office of Budget and Program Analysis, the Office of Management and Budget, or any other federal entity. Accordingly, all estimates should be considered provisional.

An overview of the types of estimates in this RIA is presented in Box U-1. Throughout this appendix, the committee compares the projected costs of the proposed revised food packages (assuming all recommendations are fully implemented) to the projected costs of the current set of food packages (assuming the current regulations remain intact). Estimated costs are based on the forecasted program participation levels, calculated redemption of each food package item, and inflated prices of each food package item. Unless otherwise noted, cost differences describe how much more the revised food packages would save or cost program-wide, as compared to the current food package.

BOX U-1

Overview of the Types of Estimates Presented in This Regulatory Impact Analysis

Current Food Costs

- Costs to the WIC program if the current food package regulations are left intact.

Revised Food Costs

- Costs to the WIC program if all proposed revisions are fully implemented.

Total Food Costs

- The sum of food costs from fiscal year (FY) 2018 through FY2022.

Cost Differences

- Current food costs subtracted from the revised food costs
  - Negative values (–) indicate that the revised food packages costs less than the current food packages.
  - Positive values (+) indicate that the revised food packages costs more than the current food packages.

Total Cost Differences (Total Cost Savings, Total Cost Increases)

- The sum of the cost differences.
- Describe how much more the revised food packages will cost or save compared to the current food packages or another food package scenario.

Unadjusted

- Assumes all state agencies fully implement the revisions as of April 1, 2018.

Phased-In

- Assumes one-third of participants will be served by an agency that implements the revised food packages on April 1, 2018. The remaining state agencies are assumed to implement the food package revisions on October 1, 2019.

KEY CONSIDERATIONS

Assumptions underlie this analysis. Some—such as how program participation and prices are projected to change through fiscal year (FY) 2022—pertain to one specific component of the analysis and are described in detail later in this appendix (see "Cost Estimate Methodology" section). Other assumptions affect the interpretation of the estimated costs and cost differences. Three such broad considerations are the representativeness of the available data, timing of implementation, and food package nomenclature.

Representativeness of the Available Data

A number of factors affect the total food costs to the WIC program, including interstate variation in food prices, caseload composition, and cost-containment practices (USDA/ERS, 2005). Accurate estimates of total food costs, therefore, need to be based on data that capture this variability. To project the cost effects associated with specific changes to the food packages, data need to provide insight into how each individual food item within each specific food package contributes to the total food costs. At the present, this level of granularity does not exist in data sources representative of the entire WIC program.

The data and assumptions used throughout this analysis are primarily based on WIC agency and administrative data sources. These include the participation data from the *WIC Participant and Program Characteristics 2014: Food Package Report* (USDA/FNS, 2016a), national participation levels presented on the USDA's Food and Nutrition Services (USDA-FNS) website (USDA/FNS, 2016b), redemption data from six de-identified state agencies provided to the committee by USDA-FNS, redemption data provided to the committee from six individual state agencies, and a 2014 report detailing redemption in three states as they transitioned to the electronic benefit transfer (EBT) food benefit issuance method (USDA/ERS, 2014).

The committee estimated total food costs and cost differences by integrating the available WIC data sources, some of which were from a relatively small number of state agencies. This analysis assumes the data are representative of the WIC population at large. The committee, however, recognizes that the cost estimates calculated are not identical to costs derived from FNS administrative data. For FY2015, the committee estimated the per-participant food cost to be $37.09[1] per month, based on assumptions about prices per unit, substitutions of allowable options, and redemption of each food package item. USDA-FNS, however, reported the FY2015 per-participant food costs to be $43.37 per month. The committee was unable to discern what component(s) of its analysis led to this difference, because some of the data available to the committee were de-identified and the majority of the data represented only a small portion of states and territories. The estimates presented in this RIA should be interpreted in context of these limitations.

[1] A per participant cost of $37.27 per month was presented previously in this report. This higher estimate reflects the $1 increase in women's cash value voucher, which was implemented in FY2016 (from $10 to $11). The committee used this monthly per participant cost to assess the cost neutrality of the revised food packages, because it reflects current regulations. The $37.09 estimate, in contrast, reflects the regulations existed in FY2015.

Timing of Implementation

The magnitude of the cost effects and stability of the projections in this analysis are largely defined by the timeframe evaluated. The exact timing of when the revised food packages will be implemented, however, depends on a number of factors, including when the federal regulations are put forth and how quickly state agencies can operationalize the changes. For the purposes of this analysis, the committee assumes that the earliest implementation of the revised food packages could occur would be April 1, 2018, approximately 15 months after the release of this consensus report. Food cost estimates for both the current and revised food packages are projected through FY2022. This RIA, therefore, encompasses a 54-month period.[2]

The committee assumes within each state agency all proposed food package changes will be fully implemented at one time, but that across the WIC program, state agencies may begin offering the revised food packages at different times. As such, two sets of cost projections were generated: unadjusted and phased in. Unadjusted estimates assume that all agencies fully implement the revised food packages on April 1, 2018. Phased-in estimates, in contrast, account for states implementing the revised food packages at different times. The phased-in scenario assumes that states with EBT systems operational as of the August 2016 EBT Detail Status Report (USDA/FNS, 2016c) would be early implementers of the proposed food package changes (i.e., those implementing the changes on April 1, 2018).[3] The remaining state agencies would have up to 18 additional months to implement the proposed food package changes (i.e., implemented by October 1, 2019). As evidenced by the final implementation dates from the previous food package revision (USDA/FNS, 2012), most state agencies instituted changes on the regulatory deadline, rather than before or after. This analysis assumes the same will occur for these proposed revisions. Accordingly, the phased-in cost differences between the current food packages and proposed revised food packages are 33.3 percent of the unadjusted cost differences for FY2018 (6 months) and FY2019 (12 months), and 100 percent of the unadjusted differences thereafter. The dates and rates of implementation used in this RIA are not intended to be prescriptive or to be the committee's recommended timeline for implementation, but rather are the committee's informed assumptions necessary for this analysis.

---

[2] The fiscal year starts October 1. April 1, 2018, is halfway through FY2018.

[3] This estimate was calculated by identifying agencies that have implemented EBT statewide as of August 2016 (USDA/FNS, 2016c) and determining what proportion of participants are served by those agencies from total participation administrative data (USDA/FNS, 2016b). For FY2015, EBT states serve 34.3 percent of WIC participants. Given this, the assumption for the phased-in estimate is that one-third of participants would be served by an "early implementer" state agency. This assumption only affects the phased-in estimates, not the unadjusted estimates.

Food Package Nomenclature

The WIC food packages are specific to the age, life stage, physiological state, and, if applicable, breastfeeding status of the participant. Several of the broad food package categories (both current and revised) are actually composed of two or more specific food package types. Both the quantity of foods and the food items prescribed in each specific food package can differ within a broad food package category. Infants ages 6 to less than 12 months receiving food package II, for example, may be prescribed food package II-BF, fully breastfed; II-BF/FF partially (mostly) breastfed; or II-FF, fully formula fed. Currently, food package II-BF recipients are prescribed infant food meat (77.5 ounces), infant cereal (24 ounces), and jarred infant food vegetables and fruits (256 ounces). In contrast, food package II-BF/FF recipients are currently prescribed infant formula, infant cereal (24 ounces), and jarred infant food vegetables and fruits (128 ounces). Food package II-FF recipients are prescribed the same quantity of complementary foods as II-BF/FF recipients, but they are prescribed more infant formula. These types of differences exist across all specific food packages and must be accounted for when estimating food package costs.

As Table U-1 highlights, the proposed revisions largely leave the current structure of the food packages unchanged. There are, however, three important considerations:

- Food package V is currently a single food package prescribed to both pregnant women and partially (mostly) breastfeeding women, up to 1 year postpartum. Under the proposed revisions, it would be split into two distinct food packages, V-A for pregnant women and V-B for partially (mostly) breastfeeding women.
- Revised food package I-BF/FF-A for a partially (mostly) breastfed infant, age 0 to less than 1 month, may not ultimately be operationalized as separate from food package I-BF/FF-B for a partially (mostly) breastfed infant, age 1 to less than 4 months. Under the proposed revisions, infants issued food package I-BF/FF-A could potentially be prescribed the same amount of formula as food package I-BF/FF-B, on a case-by-case basis. In implementing the proposed revisions, it may be decided to consolidate the two food packages and align the naming structure across the infant food packages (i.e., I-BF/FF-A for infants ages 0 to less than 4 months, I-BF/FF-B for infants ages 4 to less than 6 months). The committee chose to keep the revised food package I-BF/FF-A separate in this analysis because the proposed revision maintains the provision that issuing infant formula to breastfed infants in the first month of life should not be standard. The committee expects that infants

TABLE U-1 Current and Revised Food Packages and Corresponding Participant Categories

Food Package	Abbreviation of Specific Food Package	Applicable Version of the Food Packages	Participant Category
I	I-BF-A	Current, revised	Fully breastfed infants, ages 0 to less than 4 months
	I-BF-B	Current, revised	Fully breastfed infants, ages 4 to less than 6 months
	I-BF/FF-A	Current, revised[a]	Partially (mostly) breastfed infants,[b] ages 0 to less than 1 month
	I-BF/FF-B	Current, revised	Partially (mostly) breastfed infants,[b] ages 1 to less than 4 months
	I-BF/FF-C	Current, revised	Partially (mostly) breastfed infants,[b] ages 4 to less than 6 months
	I-FF-A	Current, revised	Fully formula-fed infants, ages 0 to less than 4 months
	I-FF-B	Current, revised	Fully formula-fed infants, ages 4 to less than 6 months
II	II-BF	Current, revised	Fully breastfed infants, ages 6 to less than 12 months
	II-BF/FF	Current, revised	Partially breastfed infants, ages 6 to less than 12 months
	II-FF	Current, revised	Fully formula-fed infants, ages 6 to less than 12 months
III	III[c]	Current, revised	Infants, children, and women with a qualifying condition[d]
IV	IV-A	Current, revised	Children, ages 1 to less than 2 years
	IV-B	Current, revised	Children, ages 2 to less than 5 years
V	V	Current	Pregnant women Partially (mostly) breastfeeding women,[b] up to 1-year postpartum
V-A	V-A	Revised	Pregnant women

V-B	V-B	Revised	Partially (mostly) breastfeeding women,[b] up to 1-year postpartum
VI	VI	Current, revised	Nonbreastfeeding postpartum women, up to 6-months postpartum Partially (minimally) breastfeeding women,[e] up to 6-months postpartum
VII	VII	Current, revised	Fully breastfeeding women, up to 1-year postpartum
N/A	N/A	Current, revised	Partially (minimally) breastfeeding women, more than 6-months postpartum[e]

[a] Despite revised food packages I-BF/FF-A and I-BF/FF-B having the same maximum ("up to") amount for infant formula, the two food packages remain separate in this analysis. The committee supports issuance of infant formula to food package I-FF/BF-A recipients only on a case-by-case basis after a breastfeeding assessment. Accordingly, the committee assumes the average quantity of infant formula prescribed in food package I-BF/FF-A to be less than the average amount prescribed to I-BF/FF-B recipients. Food package I-BF/FF-A may not ultimately be operationalized as separate from food package I-BF/FF-B for partially (mostly) breastfed infants, ages 1 to less than 4 months.

[b] The parenthetical "mostly" is determined by the amount of formula provided to the infant through the WIC program. Women and their infants are classified as partially (mostly) breastfeeding if the infant's formula prescription does not exceed the monthly maximum allowance for the age-specific BF/FF food packages.

[c] Food package III recipients are prescribed food packages appropriate to their age and physiological state. There are specific food packages for women, infants, and children within food package III that correspond to specific food packages I, II, IV, V, VI, and VII.

[d] Participants prescribed food package III have one or more medically documented qualifying conditions that require use of a WIC formula. Recipients are eligible to receive WIC formula (i.e., infant formula, exempt infant formula, and WIC-eligible nutritionals) and supplementary foods.

[e] The parenthetical "minimally" is determined by the amount of formula provided to the infant through the WIC program. Women and infants are classified as partially (minimally) breastfeeding if the infant's formula prescription exceeds the monthly maximum allowance for the age-specific BF/FF food packages but does not exceed the full amount allowed in the age-specific fully formula-fed food packages. Women who are minimally breastfeeding less than 6 months postpartum receive food package VI, along with breastfeeding support. Women who are minimally breastfeeding and with infants more than 6 months of age that receive more formula than is allowed for a partially breastfed infant do not receive a food benefit. These women, however, are eligible to continue to receive other benefits through WIC, such as breastfeeding support, nutrition education, and health and social services referrals (USDA/FNS, 2013). This group of participants is included in one of the committee's assumption regarding the revised food package cost estimates, and is therefore included in the above table.

issued the revised food package I-BF/FF-A would continue to be prescribed only small quantities of infant formula, markedly less than what is prescribed to food package I-BF/FF-B recipients.

- Food package "N/A" is listed as a food package because it is included in an assumption about how participation is expected to change with the revised food packages. Women who are minimally breastfeeding more than 6-months postpartum do not receive a food benefit (referred to herein as "food package N/A"), but are still eligible to continue to receive breastfeeding support, nutrition education, health and social services referrals, and other program benefits (USDA/FNS, 2013a). These program participants do not contribute to the total food costs of the program. The committee assumes that preventing premature classification of mother–infant dyads as fully formula fed is likely to shift dyads toward the partially (mostly) breastfeeding food packages. This projected participant shift includes women more than 6-months postpartum.

ACTION

Nature

This RIA was conducted by the Committee to Review WIC Food Packages as part of a National Academies of Sciences, Engineering, and Medicine (the National Academies) consensus study.

Need

The WIC program serves low-income, nutritionally at-risk pregnant women, breastfeeding and nonbreastfeeding postpartum women, and children younger than 5 years of age. The program provides participants with nutritious supplemental foods, breastfeeding support, nutrition education, and referrals to health and social services. Supplemental foods are intended to be appropriate for the participants' life stage and are designed to provide specific nutrients that current nutrition research indicates are lacking in the diets of WIC's target population groups (7 C.F.R. § 246). Given the nature and funding of the program, the supplemental foods must provide these specific nutrients to participants in a manner that is both effective and economical. To ensure this, regulatory language explicitly defines the specifications and amount of each authorized food item.

In 2006, an Institute of Medicine (IOM) committee offered its first set of recommended changes to the quantity and types of foods included in the WIC food packages (IOM, 2006). The recommended revisions aligned the food benefit with the 2005 *Dietary Guidelines for Americans* (DGA) and the American Academy of Pediatrics' (AAP's) infant feeding guidelines, and led to the first major revisions to the WIC food packages since the inception of the program. A decade has passed since the IOM's first set of recommendations and with it has come advances in nutrition research and insight into the effects of WIC generally and the food package changes specifically. Congress asked the USDA, which administers the WIC program, to review and update the food packages to be consistent with the current (2015–2020) DGA.[4] To accomplish this, USDA-FNS asked the National Academies to recommend revisions to the food packages to align with current research and dietary guidance, be culturally suitable to the increasingly diverse WIC population, be relatively cost-neutral compared to current food packages, be efficient for nationwide distribution, and be nonburdensome to state and local agencies that administer the program.

Affected Parties

The proposed changes to the food packages affect a broad range of individuals and entities associated with the WIC program, including, but not limited to, USDA-FNS; the 90 agencies that administer WIC and their associated staff; authorized vendors; food producers, manufacturers, and distributors; and program participants.

EFFECT

The proposed changes to the food packages are consistent with the DGA, current recommendations of the AAP, and other recently-available scientific evidence. Revisions also consider the Dietary Reference Intakes (DRIs). The proposed changes take into account the nutrient and food group intake, health status, and cultural needs of the program participant population, while simultaneously considering the efficiency and efficacy of program operations and administration. The analyses and sections that follow describe the potential economic impact of the proposed revisions.

Background

Piloted by the USDA-FNS in 1972, WIC was established as a permanent program in 1975 (P.L. 94-105, 1975). While its mission has remained the same—to "safeguard the health of low-income women, infants, and children up to age 5 who are at nutritional risk"—WIC's goals have evolved over time. Goals currently include promoting and supporting successful long-term breastfeeding; providing WIC participants with a wider variety

[4] References to the DGA in this appendix are specific to 2015-2020 unless otherwise noted.

of foods, including vegetables, fruits, and whole grains; and providing WIC state agencies greater flexibility in prescribing food packages to accommodate cultural food preferences of WIC participants (USDA/FNS, 2014b). WIC supports the national health goals of *Healthy People 2020*, specifically those related to birth weight, childhood and adult weight, and breastfeeding prevalence (NWA, 2013; HHS, 2015).

WIC is funded through discretionary grants that are appropriated by Congress on an annual basis. Grants are administered to 90 WIC state agencies, which include agencies in each of the 50 states, the District of Columbia, 5 territories, and 34 Indian Tribal Organizations (USDA/FNS, 2015a). WIC is not an entitlement program and is not guaranteed unlimited funds. The maximum number of eligible women, infants, and children who can be served has the potential to be limited by the amount of funding appropriated in a given year. In 2014, the WIC program served an average of approximately 8.2 million women, infants, and children on a monthly basis through its 1,900 local agencies in 10,000 clinic sites (USDA/FNS, 2015a). Approximately 50 percent of infants and 40 percent of pregnant women in the United States benefit from WIC services (USDA/FNS, 2015a; personal communication, J. Hirschman, USDA-FNS, October 15, 2014).

Participants in the WIC program must meet eligibility criteria for life stage, income, and nutritional risk in order to receive benefits. Specifically, applicants must be: (1) women who are pregnant and up to 6-months postpartum, or, if breastfeeding, 1-year postpartum; infants or children up to 5 years of age; (2) at or below 185 percent of federal poverty guidelines or enrolled in Temporary Assistance for Needy Families, Supplemental Nutrition Assistance Program, or Medicaid; and (3) at nutritional risk (e.g., anemia, obesity, underweight, high-risk pregnancy). WIC participants receive a range of benefits, including nutrition education, breastfeeding support, health and social services referrals, and nutritious supplemental foods. The supplemental foods provided in the WIC food packages are designed to provide specific nutrients determined to be lacking in the diets of the WIC target population (7 C.F.R. § 246).

The composition of the food packages offered to participants remained relatively unchanged throughout the first 30 years of the program, aside from enhancing the breastfeeding food package in 1992. In 2006, an IOM committee proposed the first significant revisions to the WIC food packages, at the request of USDA-FNS (IOM, 2006). Most, but not all, of the 2006 IOM report recommendations were fully implemented, which dramatically changed the food benefit offerings. While most were instituted by fall of 2009 in accordance with the Interim Rule (USDA/FNS, 2007c), some changes have taken up to 6 years to be implemented.

A decade has passed since the first set of recommended changes to the WIC food packages. In that time, the WIC population has changed in ways that reflect demographic changes across the United States, which have included declining birthrates (CDC, 2015) and population growth coming from immigration, temporary and permanent residency, and other population shifts (DHS, 2014). Shifts have also occurred in the public's attention to food production, sustainability, and food systems. Since 2006, the DGA, which serve as a foundation for the WIC food packages, have undergone two revisions. Changes have also been seen in the administration of the WIC program. During this period, many state agencies have made significant updates to their Management Information Systems, moving toward more efficient, Web-based technologies. Some states have migrated to an EBT card to issue food benefits, which is required of all state agencies by 2020. Research has been conducted that provides insight into the effect of WIC generally and the food package changes specifically. Given the changing landscape of participants, advances in science, and lessons learned from the previous revision to the food packages, an opportunity exists to further refine and enhance the WIC food packages.

The USDA-FNS charged the National Academies' current Committee to Review WIC Food Packages to conduct a two-phase evaluation of the WIC food packages and develop recommendations for revising the packages to be consistent with the current DGA and to consider the health and cultural needs of a diverse WIC population while remaining cost neutral, efficient for nationwide distribution, and nonburdensome to administration in national, state, and local agencies.

Summary of Proposed Changes and Benefits

In 2014, USDA-FNS contracted with the National Academies to conduct a comprehensive examination of the WIC food packages in relation to the best science available on food and nutrient intake relative to needs, food security and operational factors, and make recommendations for future improvements in the types and quantities of foods provided. The food package revisions recommended in this report reflect the consensus of an expert committee. Compared to the current food packages, the proposed revisions do the following:

- *Provide supplemental quantities of foods across food packages.* The committee's concept of the word *supplemental*, as described in Chapter 6 of this report, is that the amounts of nutrients and food groups in the WIC packages should provide a moderate proportion of an individual's requirement for a particular nutrient or recommended amount of a food group. The current food packages provide widely varying proportions of required nutrients (5 to 400 percent of DRIs) and DGA food groups (0 to 190 percent of recommended intake). In developing the revised food packages, the committee sought to balance the food package offerings. While it did not create or apply a strict definition of "*supplemental*," the committee considered that a supplemental amount was less than 100 percent of recommended amounts of nutrients and food groups. Therefore, adjustments were made to the extent permitted by marketplace options.[5] The primary exception to this is for fully formula-fed infants less than 6 months of age (food packages I-FF-A and I-FF-B), as no other household food is appropriate for substitution in instances of formula insufficiency. For these food packages, the committee emphasizes the need to tailor the food package to meet the specific needs of the infant.

- *Align the food packages with the DGA.* Analyses presented in the DGA indicate that vegetable consumption across all age groups (ages 2 years and older) and fruit consumption among adolescents and adults do not currently meet the recommended intake ranges. To support the recommended dietary shift toward more vegetables and (mainly whole) fruits put forth in the DGA, the proposed food package revisions provide larger cash value vouchers (CVVs) to children and women and allow for additional CVV value to be substituted for juice.[6] The DGA also report that average seafood intake falls well below what is recommended for all age groups. To support the DGA's recommendation to increase seafood intake, the revised food packages include fish in all children's and women's food packages. Furthermore, DGA analyses also indicate that while most age groups' consumption of total grains is within the recommended intake ranges, average refined grain consumptions exceeds

[5] One of the challenges the committee faced in developing revised food packages that provided supplemental quantities of foods was the standard container sizes of products currently available on the market. Infant cereal, as will be discussed later in this appendix, serves as an illustrative example. The committee aimed to provide more infant cereal to fully breastfed infants in food package II than to their partially breastfed and fully formula-fed counterparts, because of greater need for certain micronutrients from complementary foods. Infant cereal, however, is typically available in 8- and 16-ounce containers, which would provide infants with 50 and 100 percent of recommended infant cereal intake, respectively. As such, either all food package II recipients would receive the same amount of infant cereal at a supplemental quantity (i.e., 8 ounces per month = 50 percent of recommended intake), or fully breastfed infants would receive 100 percent of the recommended amount of infant cereal. While the revisions better align with the concept of supplemental, it was not always possible to provide all nutrients and food groups in quantities less than 100 percent of the recommended amounts across all food packages.

[6] The DGA currently apply to individuals ages 2 years and older. The revised food package IV-A for children ages 1 to less than 2 years, was modeled after the revisions to food package IV-B for children ages 2 to less than 5 years. Proposed revisions to the infant food package are discussed in the next section.

recommend intake limits and average whole grain consumption falls well below recommended intake ranges for nearly every age group. The revised food packages support the DGA's recommendation of daily intake of whole grains being at least half of total grain intake by recommending that all ready-to-eat (RTE) breakfast cereal provided by WIC meet the "whole grain-rich" criteria and by recommending that additional whole grain substitutes (e.g., cornmeal, buckwheat, teff) be added as state options.

- *Align the food packages with current dietary guidance for infants.* To better align food package II (infants ages 6 to less than 12 months) with current complementary feeding recommendations from the AAP, the quantity of infant cereal, jarred infant food vegetables and fruits (for fully breastfed infants only), and jarred infant food meat (for fully breastfed infants only) prescribed in food package II are revised. Additional options for substitutions (CVV for some or all of the jarred infant food vegetables and fruits; canned fish for infant food meat) are also provided to encourage redemption and consumption.
- *Enhance food packages for any level of breastfeeding.* The proposed revisions to the food packages are intended to encourage breastfeeding. Revised food packages V-B and VII are enhanced to support and incentivize both partial (mostly) and full breastfeeding to the extent possible within the cost-containment parameters. The proposed revisions also clarify the maximum amount of formula that may be prescribed to a partially breastfed infant in the first 30 days of life through individual nutrition tailoring. The proposed revision would create an opportunity for mother–infant dyads that would otherwise be categorized as fully formula-fed to achieve and maintain a partially breastfeeding status within the program.

The committee is proposing changes to each of the food packages, along with changes to the specifications of select authorized food items. The proposed food package revisions, and the corresponding rationale and anticipated benefits, are outlined in the sections that follow.

Food Package I—Infants Under 6 Months

Proposed revision *Modify/clarify what constitutes partial (mostly) breastfeeding in the first 30 days.*

- After a breastfeeding assessment by a competent professional authority, an infant can be prescribed up to 364 fluid ounces of

infant formula and still be classified as a partially (mostly) breastfed infant (food package I-BF/FF-A).
- The infant's mother is eligible to be prescribed food package V-B (partially [mostly] breastfeeding woman).

Rationale and benefit The current rule was intended to encourage women who initiated breastfeeding to do so exclusively, while allowing a small amount of infant formula as a supplement. Under this provision, infants receiving more than 104 fluid ounces of reconstituted infant formula in the first month of life are considered fully formula fed, even if the provision of infant formula is substantially less than the amount that can be prescribed in food package I-FF-A (full nutrition benefit = 806 fluid ounces). The proposed revision is intended to support partial breastfeeding and to prevent premature categorization of the dyad as fully formula-fed. This recommendation is not intended to undermine the success of states or local agencies that have identified the resources needed to support breastfeeding. Rather, it is meant to bolster the importance of the support and counseling needed to establish and sustain breastfeeding in the immediate postpartum period. The proposed revision maintains the federal requirement that routine issuance of infant formula in the first month is not standard; it would give state agencies and WIC staff greater flexibility to tailor food package I-BF/FF-A and to support women who choose to partially (mostly) breastfeed their infants.

Proposed revision *Allow tailoring of all prescribed infant formula quantities.*

- Across all infant food packages, the maximum formula quantities should be considered "up to" amounts. All formula prescribed to infants should be tailored to the individual needs of the infant.
- The amount of formula that can be prescribed in food package I-BF/FF-A and I-BF/FF-B is up to 364 fluid ounces (monthly maximum allowances of 388 fluid ounces reconstituted liquid concentrate, 384 fluid ounces ready-to-feed, or 435 fluid ounces reconstituted powder).
- The amount of formula that can be provided in food package I-BF/FF-C is up to 442 fluid ounces (monthly maximum allowances of 460 fluid ounces, reconstituted liquid concentrate, 474 fluid ounces ready-to-feed or 522 fluid ounces reconstituted powder).
- The amount of formula that can be prescribed in food package I-FF-A is up to 806 fluid ounces (monthly maximum allowances of 823 fluid ounces, reconstituted liquid concentrate, 832 fluid ounces ready-to-feed, or 870 fluid ounces reconstituted powder).

- The amount of formula that can be prescribed in food package I-FF-B is up to 884 fluid ounces (monthly maximum allowances of 896 fluid ounces reconstituted liquid concentrate, 913 fluid ounces ready-to-feed or 960 fluid ounces reconstituted powder).

Rationale and benefit The current WIC policy guidelines state that the maximum monthly allowance of infant formula should not be used as the standard for issuance unless the mother is not breastfeeding the infant at all (USDA/FNS, 2016d). The committee, however, recommends formula prescriptions be tailored to the individual needs of the infant. This proposed revision would give clinics greater flexibility to tailor the infant formula quantities prescribed to all infants who are not fully breastfed. Aside from food package I-BF/FF-A (previously described), the maximum quantities are unchanged.

Food Package II—Infants Ages 6 to Less Than 12 Months

Proposed revision *Allow tailoring of all prescribed infant formula quantities.*

- Similar to food package I, across all infant food packages, the maximum formula quantities should be considered "up to" amounts. All formula prescribed to infants should be tailored to the individual needs of the infant.
- The amount of formula that can be provided in food package II-BF/FF is up to 312 fluid ounces (monthly maximum allowances of 315 fluid ounces reconstituted liquid concentrate, 338 fluid ounces ready-to-feed, or 384 fluid ounces reconstituted powder).
- The amount of formula that can be provided in food package II-FF is up to 624 fluid ounces (monthly maximum allowances of 630 fluid ounces reconstituted liquid concentrate, 643 fluid ounces ready-to-feed, or 696 fluid ounces reconstituted powder).

Rationale and benefit Rationale and benefits of allowing tailoring of the prescribed infant formula quantities are the same as for younger infants. See "Food Package I—Infants Under 6 Months" for details.

Proposed revision *Reduce the quantity of infant cereal prescribed in food package II.*

- Food package II-BF recipients are prescribed 16 ounces of infant cereal per month.
- Food packages II-BF/FF and II-FF recipients are prescribed 8 ounces infant cereal per month.

Rationale and benefit

- The amount of infant cereal currently prescribed in food package II provides approximately 150 percent of the amount recommended by the AAP (AAP, 2014). Reducing the amount of infant cereal prescribed in food package II aligns with the concept of supplemental.
- Infant cereals are a favored first food and are good sources of zinc and iron. Because fully breastfed infants are not likely to receive zinc and iron from infant formula, food package II-BF recipients are prescribed more infant cereal per month compared to their partially (mostly) breastfed and fully formula-fed counterparts.

Proposed revision *Reduce the quantity of jarred infant food vegetables and fruits provided to fully breastfed infants; offer CVV substitution option to all food package II recipients.*

- Food package II-BF recipients are prescribed 128 ounces jarred infant food vegetables and fruits per month.
- All food package II recipients can substitute a $10 or $20 CVV for half or all of the jarred infant food vegetables and fruits, respectively.
- The CVV can be used to purchased vegetables and fruits in all forms allowed by the state agency (i.e., fresh, frozen, canned) except dried.

Rationale and benefit

- The IOM committee (2006) that put forth the first set of recommended food package changes did not provide nutrient-based rationale for the selected quantity of jarred infant food vegetables and fruits for food package II-BF recipients. Rather, it stated, "to encourage or promote full breastfeeding, the recommended amounts of [infant] food fruits and vegetables are more generous for fully breastfed infants than other infants" (page 103).
- The AAP does not provide specific intake recommendations for infant food vegetables and fruits, but it does acknowledge they are useful for transitioning infants to solid foods (AAP, 2014).
- Public comments indicated that 256 ounces of jarred infant food vegetables and fruits per month can exceed the need of the infant.
- The reduction of jarred infant food vegetables and fruits brings the fully breastfed infant's food package in better alignment with the concept of supplemental. Other incentives for full breastfeeding have been included in other aspects of the mother–infant dyad's

food packages. For example, the quantity and variety of foods available to the breastfeeding mother during the infant's first 6 months are greater compared to the postpartum (nonbreastfeeding) package (increasing proximal incentives) and extend for 12 as opposed to 6 months (increasing distal incentives).

- Jarred infant food is retained in food package II as a convenient, shelf-stable form of vegetables and fruits for infants. The options for partial or complete substitution of jarred infant food vegetables and fruits with CVVs are intended to help participants meet their cultural needs and personal preferences. Caregivers can use the vegetables and fruits purchased with the CVV to prepare infant foods of varying textures that are suitable to the infant's developmental stage.
- Participants may be able to buy more servings of fruits or vegetables using the CVV compared to the jarred varieties.

Proposed revision *Reduce the quantity of jarred infant food meat prescribed; offer canned fish substitution option.*

- Food package II-BF recipients are prescribed 40 ounces of jarred infant food meat per month.
- Food package II-BF recipients have the option of substituting four jars (10 ounces) of infant food meat with 10 ounces of canned fish per month.

Rationale and benefit

- The AAP (2014) recommends provision of 1 to 2 ounces of meat per day, which corresponds to 30 to 60 ounces per month. Currently, food package II-BF provides 130 percent of the maximum of this recommended range.
- Redemption of jarred infant food meat is particularly low; published data and public comments indicate that it is not a preferred infant food.
- The committee considered, but could not identify nutritionally equivalent but preferred alternatives to jarred infant food meat suitable for inclusion in the WIC food packages. For these reasons, jarred infant food meat is retained in food package II-BF, at a reduced quantity.
- The option of substituting canned fish for some of the jarred infant food meat provides participants with a choice that better meets their cultural needs and personal preferences, while still providing key nutrients and within cost-containment parameters. Canned fish

provides slightly more iron and some (but less) zinc per ounce and costs approximately half as much per ounce compared to jarred infant food meat. Because the nutrient profiles of jarred infant food meat and canned fish are not equivalent, the proposed revision does not allow for full substitution.

Food Package III—Participants with Qualifying Conditions

Proposed revision *Clarify the role of WIC formula in food package III.*

- Food package III recipients are permitted access to foods in the package that are appropriate for their age, physiological state, and medical condition without the requirement of a WIC formula (i.e., infant formula, exempt formula, WIC-eligible nutritionals).

Rationale and benefit

- The proposed revision is intended to facilitate the issuance of a food package appropriate for participants with qualifying conditions, without the provision of unnecessary items.
- Public comments indicated that a WIC formula in addition to supplemental foods for food package III recipients may not be necessary in all cases. The proposed revision would allow participants to be prescribed supplemental food(s) that qualifies them for food package III with medical documentation (e.g., whole milk for older children and women) without being required to be prescribed a WIC formula.
- The proposed revision upholds the provision in the current rule that states' health care providers providing oversight of the medical management of the participant may refer to the WIC registered dietitian and/or qualified nutritionist for identifying appropriate supplemental foods (excluding WIC formula) and their prescribed amounts, as well as the length of time the supplemental foods are required by the participant.

Food Package IV—Children Ages 1 to Less Than 5 Years

Proposed revision *Reduce the amount of juice prescribed; offer a CVV substitution option.*

- Children are prescribed 64 fluid ounces of juice per month.
- A $3 CVV can be substituted for the 64 ounces of juice.

Rationale and benefit

- The role of juice in the food package has historically been to provide a source of vitamin C (which overlaps with one of the roles of the CVV) and is a convenient means of providing fruit to children.
- The amount of juice in the current packages for children provides more than 100 percent of the lower end of the AAP recommended limit of 4 ounces per day (AAP, 2014). The reduction of juice, therefore, better aligns with the concept of supplemental.
- The AAP (2014) recommends that most fruit intake should be from whole fruit because whole fruit also contributes fiber and other plant-based compounds that are removed during processing. The DGA include a recommendation that at least half of fruit intake should be from whole fruit, and state that most individuals in the United States "would benefit from increasing intakes of fruit, mostly whole fruit" (USDA/HHS, 2016). The option for CVV substitution aligns with both the AAP and DGA recommendations and allows recipients to select from options that may better meet their cultural needs and personal preferences.
- All juice offered through the WIC program (across food packages) would be 64 fluid ounces, decreasing vendor burden and streamlining options across food packages.
- The cost savings from the reduction of juice allows for other revisions across the food packages.

Proposed revision *Reduce the amount of milk prescribed to children; specify substitution options.*

- Food package IV-A recipients are prescribed 12 quarts of milk per month. Food package IV-B recipients are prescribed 14 quarts of milk per month.
- Children can substitute up to 4 quarts of milk per month, choosing either to substitute 2 quarts of yogurt for 2 quarts for milk or to substitute 1 pound of cheese and 1 quart of yogurt for 4 quarts of milk.
- Soy-based yogurt substitute and soy-based cheese substitute are allowable yogurt and cheese substitution options, respectively, for individuals with lactose intolerance, a milk allergy, or who consume a vegan diet. Soy-based yogurt and cheese substitutes must meet calcium and protein specifications (described later).

Rationale and benefit

- Milk in the current food packages provides what the committee considered a greater than supplemental amount of dairy (e.g.,

85 percent of the recommended dairy amount for children ages 2 to less than 5 years). At the same time, intakes of dairy foods, were below recommended amounts. These data suggest that redemption of milk and/or consumption of redeemed amounts of milk are less than optimal.

- The committee received public comments requesting a reduction in the amount of milk prescribed. Comments requesting reductions indicated that participants are unable to use the amount of milk provided and that milk is not always compatible with cultural needs or personal preferences.
- The revised food package IV-B provides 75 percent of the recommended amounts of dairy for children ages 2 to less than 5 years. Because the DGA food patterns do not apply to children ages 1 to less than 2 years, the committee considered that the dairy needs for this group are likely lower than those for children ages 2 to less than 5 years. Milk prescribed in food package IV-A, therefore, is 2 quarts less than the amount provided in food package IV-B.
- The two substitution options are structured to allow full redemption of fluid milk in gallon and half gallon sizes, and eliminate the single quart ("dangling quart") of milk, which public comments indicated was difficult to find and is often more expensive.
- The option for substitution of two quarts of yogurt in place of two quarts of milk may improve intakes for participants who prefer dairy in this form. Soy options are allowable for participants with lactose intolerance, a milk allergy, and those who consume a vegan diet. The options are intended to provide participants with flexibility to select substitutions that better meet cultural needs and personal preferences.

Proposed revision *Limit the whole grain bread option to 100% whole wheat bread; expand list of whole grain options that states may choose to allow; provide a range of allowable sizes; reduce the maximum amount of bread prescribed.*

- Food packages IV recipients are prescribed 16 to 24 ounces of 100% whole wheat bread or other allowable whole grain options per month.
- In addition to current whole grain options, states may authorize corn masa flour (nonwhole grain), cornmeal, teff, and buckwheat (specifications described later). States should authorize as many options as cost constraints allow.

Rationale and benefit

- Very few states offer whole grain bread options other than 100% whole wheat. Identification of suitable whole grain breads (greater than 50% whole grain) can be challenging for participants. Restricting authorized breads to 100% whole-wheat aligns with the current practices of most state agencies and reduces state agency burden to identify allowable whole grain options.
- When the current food packages were first introduced, the 16-ounce size of bread was uncommon in the marketplace. Manufacturers had to create this size of bread specifically for WIC participants and vendors had to stock it. This created vendor, manufacturer, and participant burden. The allowable bread size range allows for the purchase of more commonly available sizes of products, including bread ranging in size from 22- to 24-ounce. The range would also eliminate the need for manufacturers to create WIC-specific product sizes. Decreasing participant burden and expanding options may also increase availability and promote intake of whole grains, for which intake is below recommended amounts across most WIC participant groups.
- The proposed revisions would slightly reduce the amount of whole wheat bread and allowable options provided to children, from a maximum 32 ounces per month in the current package to a maximum of 24 ounces in the revised food package. This slight reduction helps to offset the cost of offering the range of bread sizes across food packages.
- Additional whole wheat bread substitutions are added as state options (corn masa flour [nonwhole grain], cornmeal, teff, and buckwheat) to provide culturally appropriate alternatives, which in turn, may help to promote intake.

Proposed revision *Create a quarterly rotation of legumes, peanut butter, and fish; clarify authorized types of legumes and canned fished.*

- Food package IV recipients are prescribed legumes, peanut butter, and fish in a rotation over the course of 3 months.
- The rotation consists of 1 pound (16 ounces of dry or 64 ounces canned [four 15- to 16-ounce cans]) of legumes, 16–18 ounces of peanut butter, and 10 ounces of canned fish.
- State agencies must authorize both dried and canned legumes.
- Authorized canned fish may be packed in water or currently authorized sauces and flavorings. Oil-packed is no longer authorized.

Rationale and benefit

- The amount of peanut butter prescribed in the current food packages provides 167 percent of recommend amounts of the protein food subgroup of nuts, seeds, and soy, and the amount of legumes provides approximately 177 percent of recommended amounts of beans and peas for children. Both items exceed what the committee considers to be a supplemental amount.
- The proposed revision specifies that state agencies must authorize both canned and dried legumes. According to the 2015 Food Policy Options report, 85 percent of WIC state agencies have already authorized canned legumes (USDA/FNS, 2015b). Therefore, the committee considered this change an administratively feasible strategy with the potential to promote redemption and consumption.
- Authoritative groups recommend consumption of 1.0 to 1.7 ounces of lower-mercury fish per day by children ages 1 to 4 years (AAP, 2014; FDA/EPA, 2014; USDA/HHS, 2016). Intake of seafood was either low or uncommon across subgroups of WIC participants. As such, the committee considered it important to include fish in additional food packages as costs allowed.
- In the revised food package IV, legumes, peanut butter, and fish are rotated on a quarterly basis in order to provide supplemental amounts and amounts that better align with participant preferences. Although the amount of fish offered in the food packages is small compared to DGA recommended amounts of seafood (19 percent for children), it is a significant improvement over the current packages that offer no fish. It also introduces this food into participants' diets.
- In the revised food packages, canned fish may be water packed, and may include the same sauces and flavorings that are currently allowed as a state option. Oil packed is no longer authorized. Water-packed varieties are more nutrient dense because water-packed fish is lower in energy but contains the same amounts of key nutrients per serving.

Proposed revision *Increase the CVV. Food package IV recipients are prescribed a $12 vegetable and fruit CVV per month.*

Rationale and benefit

- The CVV offers participants the most flexibility to meet their cultural food preferences and provides them with access to two food groups (vegetables and fruits) and nutrients (potassium and fiber) for which intakes were inadequate.

- The current amount of the CVV permits participants to purchase less than one serving of fruits or vegetables per day. Based on the committee's composite cost for vegetables and fruits most commonly purchased among WIC participants,[7] $23 would be required for individuals who consumed a 1,300-kcal diet to meet half of the recommended intakes of vegetables and fruits.
- The committee increased the CVV across food packages to the extent possible within cost-neutral restrictions.

Food Package V-A—Pregnant Women

Proposed revision *Create separate food packages for pregnant and partially (mostly) breastfeeding women.*

- Pregnant women are issued food package V-A, which is different from food package V-B for partially (mostly) breastfeeding women, up to 1-year postpartum.

Rationale and benefit One of the committee's objectives with the revised food packages was to promote and incentivize any level of breastfeeding. To do this within cost-neutral parameters, food package V was divided into two distinct food packages.

Proposed revision *Reduce the amount of juice prescribed; offer a CVV substitution option.*

- Pregnant women are prescribed 64 fluid ounces of juice per month.
- A $3 CVV can be substituted for the 64 ounces of juice.

Rationale and benefit The rationale and benefits are comparable to those presented for the children's food package. See "Food Package IV—Children Ages 1 to Less Than 5 Years" for details.

Proposed revision *Reduce the amount of milk prescribed; specify substitution options.*

- All women are prescribed 16 quarts of milk per month.

---

[7] Based on the vegetable and fruit composite ($0.55 per cup-equivalent) applied in this report, which considered the vegetables and fruits most commonly purchased by WIC participants in Massachusetts, Texas, and Wyoming.

- Food package V-A recipients can substitute up to 4 quarts of milk per month, choosing either to substitute 2 quarts of yogurt for 2 quarts for milk or to substitute 1 pound of cheese and 1 quart of yogurt for 4 quarts of milk.
- Soy-based yogurt substitute and soy-based cheese are authorized yogurt and cheese substitution options, respectively, for individuals with lactose intolerance, a milk allergy, or who consume a vegan diet. Authorized soy-based yogurt and cheese must meet calcium and protein specifications (described later).

Rationale and benefit

- For women who are pregnant, postpartum, or breastfeeding, the Estimated Average Requirement (EAR) for calcium is 800 mg, and the corresponding DGA recommendation for the intake of dairy, which is the major dietary source of calcium, is 3 cup-equivalents per day. Therefore, it is reasonable to provide the same quantity of the key food group for this nutrient (dairy) across food packages for women. As revised, the food packages for women provide 71 percent of the recommended amounts of dairy. The revised food packages for women provide approximately 100 percent of the calcium EAR for women.
- Rationale and benefits of the milk substitution options are the same as for children. See "Food Package IV—Children Ages 1 to Less Than 5 Years" for details.

Proposed revision *Limit the whole grain bread option to 100% whole wheat bread; expand the list of whole grain options states may choose to authorize; provide a range of authorized sizes.*

- Food packages V-A recipients are prescribed 16 to 24 ounces of 100% whole wheat bread or authorized whole grain options per month.
- In addition to current whole grain options, states may authorize corn masa flour (nonwhole grain), cornmeal, teff, and buckwheat (specifications described later). States should authorize as many options as cost constraints allow.

Rationale and benefit Rationale and benefits of the revisions to the whole grain bread and associated substitution options are the same as for children. See "Food Package IV—Children Ages 1 to Less Than 5 Years" for details.

Proposed revision *Create a quarterly rotation of legumes, peanut butter, and fish; clarify authorized types of legumes and canned fish.*

- Food package V-A recipients are prescribed legumes, peanut butter, and fish in a rotation over the course of 3 months.
- Food package V-A recipients are prescribed 2 pounds (32 ounces of dry or 128 ounces canned [eight 15- to 16-ounce cans]) of legumes, 16 to 18 ounces of peanut butter, and 10 ounces canned fish on a quarterly basis. States may decide to issue 2 pounds of legumes in 1 month (to create a quarterly rotation with tuna) or spread the legumes over 2 months. Peanut butter may only be issued once per quarter. State agencies must authorize both dried and canned legumes.
- Authorized canned fish may be packed in water or currently authorized sauces and flavorings. Oil packed is no longer authorized.

Rationale and benefit

- Legumes are key sources of many nutrients (potassium, fiber, and folate) for which intakes below recommended amounts were prevalent across participant subgroups. Therefore, legumes are a valuable component of the WIC food packages. Provision of 2 pounds of dry legumes (or eight 15- to 16-ounce cans) every 3 months brings the amount prescribed closer to what is considered supplemental for women: between 47 and 59 percent of the DGA recommended amount.
- The amount of peanut butter in the current food packages for women provides up to 168 percent of recommended amounts. In the proposed revisions to the food packages, the same quantities of peanut butter currently provided every month will still be provided but only once every 3 months, which brings the prescription in better alignment with the concept of supplemental.
- Authoritative groups recommend consumption of 1.0 to 1.7 ounces of lower-mercury fish per day by pregnant and breastfeeding women (FDA/EPA, 2014; AHA, 2015; USDA/HHS, 2016).
- Inasmuch as intake of seafood was either low or uncommon across subgroups of WIC participants, the committee considered it important to include fish in additional food packages as costs allowed. Although the amount of fish offered in the food packages is small compared to DGA recommended amounts of seafood, it is a significant improvement over the current packages that offer no fish.
- Canned fish may be packed in water and may include the same sauces and flavorings that are currently allowed as a state option.

Oil-packed is no longer authorized. Water-packed varieties are more nutrient dense because water-packed fish is lower in energy but contains the same levels of key nutrients per serving.
- In the revised food package V-A, legumes, peanut butter, and fish are rotated on a quarterly basis in order to provide supplemental amounts, and amounts that better align with participant preferences. Although the amount of fish offered in the food packages is small compared to DGA recommended amounts of seafood, it is a significant improvement over the current packages that offer no fish.

Proposed revision *Increase the CVV. Food package V-A recipients are prescribed a $15 vegetable and fruit CVV per month.*

Rationale and benefit Rationale and benefits of the increase in CVV are the same as for children. See "Food Package IV—Children Ages 1 to Less Than 5 Years" for details. In addition:

- The CVV provides access to vitamins A and C, folate, and other nutrients for which intakes were inadequate.
- Based on the committee's composite cost for vegetables and fruits most commonly purchased among WIC participants, $45 would be required for individuals who consumed a 2,600-kcal diet to meet half of the recommended intakes of vegetables and fruits.

Food Package V-B—Partially (Mostly) Breastfeeding Women Up to 1-Year Postpartum

Proposed revision *Create separate food packages for pregnant and partially (mostly) breastfeeding women.*

- Pregnant women are issued food package V-A, which is different from food package V-B for partially (mostly) breastfeeding women, up to 1-year postpartum.

Rationale and benefit

- One of the committee's objectives with the revised food packages was to promote and incentivize any level of breastfeeding. To do this within cost-neutral parameters, food package V was divided into two distinct food packages.

Proposed revision *Reduce the amount of juice prescribed; offer a CVV substitution option.*

- Partially (mostly) breastfeeding women are prescribed 64 fluid ounces of juice per month. A $3 CVV can be substituted for the 64 ounces of juice.

Rationale and benefit The rationale and benefits are comparable to those presented for the children's food package. See "Food Package IV—Children Ages 1 to Less Than 5 Years" for details.

Proposed revision *Prescribe legumes and peanut butter on a quarterly rotation; clarify authorized types of legumes.*

- Food package V-B recipients are prescribed 2 pounds (32 ounces of dry or 128 ounces canned [eight 15- to 16-ounce cans]) of legumes and 16 to 18 ounces of peanut butter on a quarterly basis. States may decide to issue 2 pounds of legumes in 1 month or spread the legumes over 2 months. Peanut butter may only be issued once per quarter.
- State agencies must authorize both dried and canned legumes.

Rationale and benefit The rationale and benefits are comparable to those presented for the pregnant women's food package. See "Food Package V-A—Pregnant Women" for details.

Proposed revision *Add fish to the food package.*

- Women receiving food package V-B are prescribed 10 ounces of canned fish per month.
- Authorized canned fish may be packed in water or currently authorized sauces and flavorings. Oil packed is no longer authorized.

Rationale and benefit

- Provision of canned fish on a monthly basis, rather than on a quarterly rotating basis, is intended to incentivize the partial (mostly) breastfeeding food package.
- Rationale and benefits for inclusion of fish in food package V-B are comparable to those presented for the pregnant women's food package. See "Food Package V-A—Pregnant Women" for details.

Proposed revision *Reduce the amount of milk prescribed; specify substitution options.*

- All women are prescribed 16 quarts of milk per month.
- Food package V-B recipients can substitute up to 4 quarts of milk per month, choosing either to substitute 2 quarts of yogurt for 2 quarts for milk or to substitute 1 pound of cheese and 1 quart of yogurt for 4 quarts of milk.
- Soy-based yogurt substitute and soy-based cheese are authorized yogurt and cheese substitution options, respectively, for individuals with lactose intolerance, a milk allergy, or who consume a vegan diet. Authorized soy-based yogurt and cheese must meet calcium and protein specifications (described later).

Rationale and benefit The rationale and benefits are comparable to those presented for the pregnant women's food package. See "Food Package V-A—Pregnant Women" for details.

Proposed revision *Limit the whole grain bread option to 100% whole wheat bread; expand list of whole grain options that states may choose to authorize; provide a range of authorized sizes.*

- Food packages V-B recipients are prescribed 16 to 24 ounces of 100% whole wheat bread or authorized grain options per month.
- In addition to current whole grain options, states may authorize corn masa flour (nonwhole grain), cornmeal, teff, and buckwheat (specifications described later). States should authorize as many options as cost constraints allow.

Rationale and benefit Rationale and benefits of the revisions to the whole grain bread and associated substitution options are the same as for children. See "Food Package IV—Children Ages 1 to Less Than 5 Years" for details.

Proposed revision *Increase the CVV.* Food package V-B recipients are prescribed a $25 vegetable and fruit CVV per month.

Rationale and benefit

- Provision of a larger CVV compared to the postpartum and partially (minimally) breastfeeding food package (food package VI) is intended to incentivize the partial (mostly) breastfeeding food package.

- Rationale and benefits of the increase in CVV are the same as for pregnant women. See "Food Package V-A—Pregnant Women" for details.

Food Package VI—Nonbreastfeeding Postpartum Women, Up to 6-Months Postpartum and Partially (Minimally) Breastfeeding Women, Up to 6-Months Postpartum

Proposed revision *Eliminate juice.*

- Postpartum and partially (minimally) breastfeeding women, up to 6-months postpartum, are no longer prescribed juice through food package VI.

Rationale and benefit Juice was removed from food package VI to achieve cost-neutrality and to increase the relative value of the partially (V-B) and fully (VII) breastfeeding packages. To compensate for the reduced juice, the CVV for food package VI was increased (described later).

Proposed revision *Align milk prescription across women's food packages; specify substitution options.*

- All women are prescribed 16 quarts of milk per month.
- Food package VI recipients can substitute up to 4 quarts of milk per month, choosing either to substitute 2 quarts of yogurt for 2 quarts for milk or to substitute 1 pound of cheese and 1 quart of yogurt for 4 quarts of milk.
- Soy-based yogurt substitute and soy-based cheese are authorized yogurt and cheese substitution options, respectively, for individuals with lactose intolerance, a milk allergy, or who consume a vegan diet. Authorized soy-based yogurt and cheese must meet calcium and protein specifications (described later).

Rationale and benefit The rationale and benefits are comparable to those presented for pregnant women. See "Food Package V-A—Pregnant Women" for details.

Proposed revision *Create a quarterly rotation of legumes, peanut butter, and fish; clarify authorized types of legumes and canned fished.*

- Food package V-A recipients are prescribed legumes, peanut butter, and fish in a rotation over the course of 3 months.

- Food package VI recipients are prescribed 2 pounds (32 ounces of dry or 128 ounces canned [eight 15- to 16-ounce cans]) of legumes, 16 to 18 ounces of peanut butter, and 10 ounces of canned fish on a quarterly basis. States may decide to issue 2 pounds of legumes in 1 month (to create a quarterly rotation with peanut butter and canned fish) or spread the legumes over 2 months. Peanut butter may only be issued once per quarter.
- State agencies must authorize both dried and canned legumes.
- Authorized canned fish may be packed in water or currently authorized sauces and flavorings. Oil packed is no longer authorized.

Rationale and benefit The rationale and benefits are comparable to those presented for the pregnant women's food package. See "Food Package V-A—Pregnant Women" for details.

Proposed revision *Increase the CVV.* Food package VI recipients are prescribed a $15 vegetable and fruit CVV per month.

Rationale and benefit Rationale and benefits of the increase in CVV are the same as for pregnant women. See "Food Package V-A—Pregnant Women" for details.

Food Package VII—Fully Breastfeeding Women, Up to 1-Year Postpartum

Proposed revision *Reduce the amount of juice prescribed; offer a CVV substitution option.* Fully breastfeeding women are prescribed 64 fluid ounces of juice per month. A $3 CVV can be substituted for the 64 ounces of juice.

Rationale and benefit The rationale and benefits are comparable to those presented for the children's food package. See "Food Package IV—Children Ages 1 to Less Than 5 Years" for details.

Proposed revision *Reduce the amount of milk prescribed; specify substitution options.*

- All women are prescribed 16 quarts of milk per month.
- Food package VII recipients can substitute up to 6 quarts of milk per month, choosing either to substitute 2 quarts of yogurt for 2 quarts of milk or to substitute 1 pound of cheese and 1 quart of yogurt for 4 quarts of milk or to substitute 2 pounds of cheese for 6 quarts of milk.
- Soy-based yogurt substitute and soy-based cheese are authorized yogurt and cheese substitution options, respectively, for individuals

with lactose intolerance, a milk allergy or who consume a vegan diet. Authorized soy-based yogurt and cheese must meet calcium and protein specifications (described later).

Rationale and benefit

- The retention of additional substitution options is intended to incentivize the fully breastfeeding food package.
- The rationale and benefits are comparable to those presented for the pregnant women's food package. See "Food Package V-A—Pregnant Women" for details.

Proposed revision *Limit the whole grain bread option to 100% whole wheat bread; expand list of whole grain options that states may choose to authorize; provide a range of authorized sizes.*

- Food packages VII recipients are prescribed 16–24 ounces of 100% whole wheat bread or authorized whole grain options per month.
- In addition to current whole grain options, states may authorize corn masa flour (nonwhole grain), cornmeal, teff, and buckwheat (specifications described later). States should authorize as many options as cost constraints allow.

Rationale and benefit Rationale and benefits of the revisions to the whole grain bread and associated substitution options are the same as for children. See "Food Package IV—Children Ages 1 to Less Than 5 Years" for details.

Proposed revision *Prescribe legumes and peanut butter on a quarterly rotation; clarify authorized types of legumes.*

- Food package VII recipients are prescribed 2 pounds (32 ounces of dry or 128 ounces canned [eight 15- to 16-ounce cans]) of legumes and 16 to 18 ounces of peanut butter on a quarterly basis. States may decide to issue 2 pounds of legumes in 1 month or spread the legumes over 2 months. Peanut butter may only be issued once per quarter.
- State agencies must authorize both dried and canned legumes.

Rationale and benefit The rationale and benefits are comparable to those presented for the pregnant women's food package. See "Food Package V-A—Pregnant Women" for details.

Proposed revision *Reduce fish in the food package; modify specifications.*

- Women receiving food package VII are prescribed 20 ounces of canned fish per month.
- Authorized canned fish may be packed in water or currently authorized sauces and flavorings. Oil packed is no longer authorized.

Rationale and benefit

- Fully breastfeeding women are prescribed the greatest quantity of fish on a monthly basis in order to incentivize the food package.
- The fish provision was slightly reduced from 30 ounces per month in the current food package to 20 ounces per month in the revised food package in order to achieve cost neutrality and allow for a monthly provision of fish in the partially breastfeeding package.
- Rationale and benefits for maintaining fish in food package VII are comparable to those presented for the pregnant women's food package. See "Food Package V-A—Pregnant Women" for details.

Proposed revision *Increase the CVV.* Food package VII recipients are prescribed a $35 vegetable and fruit CVV per month.

Rationale and benefit

- Provision of the largest monthly CVV compared to all other food packages is intended to incentivize the fully breastfeeding food package.
- Rationale and benefits of the increase in CVV are the same as for pregnant women. See "Food Package V-A—Pregnant Women" for details.

Other Provisions (Not Specific to a Single Food Package)

Proposed revision *Modify specifications for milk. Only unflavored milk is permitted. All other specifications remain unchanged.*

Rationale and benefit

- The proposed revision aligns the milk offering with Child and Adult Care Food Program (CACFP) provision of milks to children less than 5 years of age. The specification reduces the amount of added sugars that can be provided through the WIC food packages.

- At present, flavored milk is offered in 6 percent of states and 40 percent of Indian Tribal Organizations (ITOs), which together cover 3 percent of WIC participants (USDA/FNS, 2015b). At least one ITO is removing flavored milk from its food list to align with CACFP policy (personal communication, D. Tipton, Chickasaw Nation WIC, July 2016). Therefore, the recommendation is not expected to cause a significant disruption in administration of food packages nationally.

Proposed revision *Increase federal minimum vegetable stocking requirement; increase number of vegetable and fruit forms states must authorize.*

- Require WIC vendors to stock a minimum of three varieties of vegetables and two varieties of fruits.
- States must authorize fresh and at least one additional form (frozen, canned, and/or dried) of vegetables and fruits.

Rationale and benefit

- The committee foresees the need to provide participants with a greater variety of options, given the larger CVVs and opportunities to substitute juice and jarred infant food vegetables and fruits with CVVs.
- The proposed revision seeks to enhance the amount and forms of vegetables and fruits available in WIC authorized stores, while minimizing burden on small vendors.
- The increased vegetable requirement is intended to encourage participants to prioritize the use of the CVV for vegetables.

Proposed revision *Increase soy substitution options; specify nutrient profiles of soy options.*

- Soy-based yogurt and cheese are authorized yogurt and cheese substitution options, respectively, for individuals with lactose intolerance, a milk allergy, or who consume a vegan diet.
- Soy-based yogurt must contain at least 250 mg of calcium and 6.5 grams of protein per 8 ounce serving.
- Soy-based cheese must contain at least 250 mg of calcium and 6.5 grams of protein per 1.5-ounce serving.
- In addition to current standards for authorized soy-based beverages, the total sugars content should be as low as possible, not to exceed 12 grams per 8-ounce serving.

- Authorized tofu must contain a minimum of 200 milligram of calcium per 100 grams of tofu. Calcium-set is no longer part of the specification. Authorized tofu may not contain added fats, sugars, oils, or sodium.

Rationale and benefit

- The soy substitutions for yogurt or cheese are intended to meet the needs of individuals with lactose intolerance, a milk allergy, or who consume a vegan diet. The soy-based options in the food packages serve as milk substitutions. As such, the revised specification ensures that items in the food packages provide an amount of calcium as close to the amount in a serving of milk as reasonable, considering marketplace options.
- Sugars in soy-based beverages are 100 percent added; added sugars intakes are excessive in the WIC population, therefore the committee considered it important to apply a limit that considers nationwide availability of these products.

Proposed revision *Create a range of authorized yogurt sizes; reduce the total sugars limit.*

- At the discretion of the state agency, the yogurt quart substitution may range from 30 to 32 ounces to accommodate the smaller container sizes (approximately 5 ounces).
- In addition to the current specifications, authorized yogurts must contain no more than 30 grams total sugars per 8-ounce serving (≤3.75 grams total sugars per ounce).

Rationale and benefit

- The yogurt container sizes commonly available in the marketplace vary in total ounces, especially the single serving sizes. The proposed range of ounces of yogurt that substitutes for 1 quart of milk would allow for smaller container sizes to be authorized as a state option. State agencies would need to determine if provision of the smaller containers is within cost-containment parameters.
- The availability of yogurts that contain 30 grams or less of total sugars per 8-ounce serving has expanded substantially in recent years. The reduced total sugar limits for yogurt is more closely aligned with the DGA.

Proposed revision *Modify the bread specifications; expand the list of state options for substitutions; specify specific nutrient parameters.*

- Whole grain bread is no longer permitted; only 100% whole wheat bread is permitted.
- In addition to current whole grain options, states may authorize corn masa flour (nonwhole grain), teff, and buckwheat (specifications described later). States should authorize as many options as cost constraints allow.
- Cornmeal (including blue) meeting the FDA standard of identity (21 C.F.R. 137.260) and that is in alignment with USDA specifications for cornmeal in School Meal Programs (USDA-CNP-01-2008) may also be added as an option.
- Once available in the marketplace, states are encouraged to offer folic acid fortified corn masa flour and tortillas made with folic acid-fortified corn masa flour.

Rationale and benefit

- Very few states offer whole grain bread options other than 100% whole wheat. From the participant's perspective, identification of suitable whole grain breads (more than 50 percent whole grain) is challenging. As such, restricting to 100% whole wheat bread aligns with most current state WIC authorized food lists.
- Culturally appropriate alternatives are provided as state options. The selected options correspond to nutritionally appropriate items that participants and WIC staff expressed an interest in adding to the food packages. The expanded list allows state agencies to tailor their offerings to better accommodate the cultural needs and personal preferences of WIC clientele.

Proposed revision *Changing whole grain specification of authorized breakfast cereals.*

- In addition to meeting current nutrient specifications, all ready-to-eat cereals on a state agency's authorized food list must adhere to the "whole grain-rich" criteria as outlined by USDA-FNS for the School Lunch Program (USDA/FNS, 2014c).

Rationale and benefit

- The committee's analysis of NHANES data indicated that intakes of whole grains continue to be poor and intakes of refined-grains excessive across the WIC subgroups studied. Focusing on whole grains in the WIC food packages may also improve acceptability of whole grains for the longer term. This change increases the amount of whole grains in the food packages. This change also aligns WIC specifications with those of CACFP (USDA/FNS, 2014c).

- Whole grain cereal options have expanded substantially since the last review of the WIC food packages, removing marketplace availability as a barrier to access. Launches of whole grain products including cereal (wheat and other grains) doubled between 2006 and 2011 (Oldways, 2015).
- Two large national manufacturers of RTE breakfast cereals produce at least 14 different types of RTE cereals that meet the current WIC whole grain criteria (which is similar to the whole grain rich criteria), including 4 gluten-free whole grain varieties.
- The previous committee to review WIC food packages (IOM, 2006) recommended that all breakfast cereals provided through WIC be whole grain (that is, the grain component is at least 50 percent whole grain) to align with the 2005 DGA. Since 2005, the DGA have consistently specified that at least half of grain intake should be from whole grains. The DGA specifically state that intake of refined grains should be limited, although individuals (particularly women capable of becoming pregnant) who consume all grains as whole should include some sources fortified with folic acid as a means of preventing neural tube defects. RTE, fortified whole grain cereals are an example such a source (USDA/HHS, 2016).

Proposed revision *Modify the specifications for canned fish.*

- Authorized canned fish may be packed in water. Pack may include bones or skin. Added sauces and flavorings, such as tomato sauce, mustard, lemon, are authorized at the state agency's option. May be regular or lower in sodium content. Oil-packed is no longer authorized.

Rationale and benefit

- Water-packed varieties are more nutrient dense because water-packed fish is lower in energy but contains the same levels of key nutrients per serving.
- Few states currently offer oil-packed fish. The effect of this specification, therefore, is expected to have little effect on participant choice.

Summary of Key Provisions

The anticipated effects of the proposed food package revisions on four broad stakeholder groups—the USDA/federal government, state and local agencies, vendors and industry, and WIC participants—are summarized in Table U-2. The overall projected net cost difference are also noted; a detailed evaluation of the cost effects is presented in the section that follows Table U-2. The direction and magnitude of the presented cost differences are dependent on the committee's assumptions. The cost effects of alternative assumptions are evaluated in the "Uncertainties" section of this appendix.

COST

Proposed Revisions to the Benefit

Unadjusted Estimates of Food Costs and Total Cost Differences

Table U-3 presents unadjusted food cost estimates for the current and revised food packages. The total unadjusted food costs from FY2018 through FY2022 are estimated to be $17.7 billion (averaging $3.93 billion per year) for the current food packages and $17.4 billion (averaging $3.87 billion per year) for the revised food packages. Over the course of FY2018 through FY2022, the proposed revisions are projected to lead to a total unadjusted cost savings of $263 million, as compared to the current food packages.

Phased-in Cost Differences

Table U-4 presents the phased-in cost differences between the current and revised food packages, from FY2018 through FY2022. Assuming phased-in implementation across the WIC program inherently decreases the projected total cost savings. The total phased-in cost savings for FY2018 through FY2022 are approximately $42 million less than the total unadjusted cost savings ($220.4 million versus $262.8 million). The estimated cost differences not only reflect changes to the type and quantity of items in the specific food packages, but also the proportion of participants who are prescribed each food package. The cost savings in food package I in FY2021 and FY2022, for example, is driven by the anticipated 5 percent shift of fully formula-fed mother–infant dyads to the partially (mostly) breastfeeding participant categories, due to the incentives incorporated in to the revised food packages (see the "Participation" subsection in the section "Cost Estimate Methodology" for additional details about this assumption).

TABLE U-2 Summary of Key Revisions

Current Rules, Proposed Revisions, and Projected Net Cost Differences*	Effect of the Proposed Revision			
	USDA/Federal Government	State/Local Agencies	Vendors/Industry	WIC Participants
Current rule: State agencies have the option to prescribe breastfed infants up to 104 fl oz of infant formula (not more than one can of powdered infant formula) during the first 30 days of life, on a case-by-case basis. *Proposed revision:* Breastfed infants can be prescribed up to 364 fl oz of infant formula during the first 30 days of life, on a case-by-case basis after a breastfeeding assessment by a competent professional authority, and remain categorically classified as a partially breastfed infant. (*Net cost effect: savings*)	The cost of food package I-BF/FF-A itself may slightly increase, depending on how frequently competent professional authorities identify need for issuance of formula beyond 104 fl oz. The anticipated shift in fully formula-fed dyads toward the partial (mostly) breastfeeding food packages is expected to largely offset additional costs of the infant formula.	At the staff and clinic level, the proposed revision is expected to provide greater flexibility in tailoring the partially (mostly) breastfed infant's food package and create opportunities to support partial breastfeeding in dyads who would otherwise be considered fully formula-fed. Management Information Systems will need to be updated. State and local agencies will encounter a short-term burden of retraining staff.	The effect on vendors or industry is anticipated to be minimal. The anticipated shift in fully formula-fed dyads to the partial (mostly) breastfeeding food packages may reduce the amount of infant formula purchased by WIC participants with their food benefit.	The revision is intended to allow more flexibility for women and infants in the first month, as opposed to the current situation in which only two options are available (fully breastfeeding or fully formula-feeding). The proposed revision is intended to provide security for women who may try to breastfeed in the immediate postpartum period but are not yet certain they can succeed.

Current rule: The maximum monthly allowance of formula should not be used as the standard for issuance unless the mother is not breastfeeding the infant at all. *Proposed revision:* The quantity of infant formula prescribed to infants should be tailored based on needs. All maximum monthly allowances for infant formula should be considered "up to" amounts. (*Net cost effect: minimal*)	The cost effect of the proposed revision will depend on the extent to which infant formula tailoring occurs. If minimal tailoring occurs, the cost effects would be minimal. If it is fully executed, the proposed revision would result in a cost savings.	At the staff and clinic level, the proposed revision is expected to provide greater flexibility in tailoring the amount of formula provided to infants. Management Information Systems will need to be updated. State and local agencies will encounter a short-term burden of retraining staff.	The effect on the vendors will depend on the amount of infant formula tailoring that occurs. If minimal tailoring occurs, the effect on infant formula sales would be minimal. Full execution is likely to result in a decrease of infant formula sales to WIC participants using their food benefit.	Participants would still have access to the quantities of infant formula currently being offered by WIC. The proposed revision, however, would help participants receive the amount of infant formula needed to meet their infants' needs.
Current rule: All food package II recipients are prescribed 24 oz of infant cereal per month *Proposed revision:* Food package II-BF recipients are prescribed 16 oz of infant cereal per month; II-FF and II-BF/FF	The proposed revision would reduce the cost of food package II. This reduction helps offset costs elsewhere in the food packages.	Administrative burden is expected to be minimal. State agencies currently authorize 8 oz infant cereal containers; some state agencies also authorize 16 oz containers. Management Information Systems will need to be updated. State and local agencies will	The proposed revision may result in reduced infant cereal sales to WIC participants. It is not anticipated to affect stocking requirements.	Although infants will receive less infant cereal under the revised food package, the amount provided is more consistent with current complementary feeding recommendations.

continued

TABLE U-2 Continued

Current Rules, Proposed Revisions, and Projected Net Cost Differences*	Effect of the Proposed Revision			
	USDA/Federal Government	State/Local Agencies	Vendors/Industry	WIC Participants
recipients are prescribed 8 oz per month (*Net cost effect: savings*)		encounter a short-term burden of retraining staff and communicating the change to participants when the revisions are initially implemented.		
Current rule: Food package II-BF recipients are prescribed 256 oz of jarred infant food vegetables and fruits per month. All other food package II recipients receive 128 oz of jarred infant food vegetables and fruits. Up to 16 oz of jarred infant food fruits can be substituted with fresh bananas, one banana per 4 oz jar. *Proposed revision:* All infants receiving food package II are prescribed 128 oz of jarred infant food vegetables and fruits.	Despite the decrease in jarred infant vegetable and fruit issuance to fully breastfed infants, the option for CVV substitution is expected to lead to an increase in redemption, thereby increasing costs to the program.	Administrative burden is expected to be minimal. Management Information Systems will need to be updated, but overall it will improve Management Information Systems efficiency by authorizing the same vegetable and fruit varieties for all CVVs. State and local agencies will encounter a short-term burden of retraining staff and communicating the change to participants when the revisions are initially implemented. State and local agencies will also face an	The proposed revision may result in slight reductions in jarred infant food vegetable and fruit sales to WIC participants, but it may increase fresh, frozen, and/or canned vegetables and fruits via the CVV. This is not anticipated to affect stocking requirements.	The proposed revision is intended to provide fully breastfed infants with a supplemental quantity of infant food vegetables and fruits, in the absence of definitive guidance on recommended intake. The CVV substitution option provides participants the opportunity to prepare their own infant food vegetables and fruits, which can be used to better meet diverse cultural needs, personal preferences, and the infant's developmental stage. Participants may be able to buy more servings

A CVV can be prescribed for partial substitution ($10 for 64 oz jarred infant food vegetables and fruits) or complete substitution ($20 for the 128 oz). The CVV can be used to purchased vegetables and fruits in all forms authorized by the state agency (i.e., fresh, frozen, canned) except dried. (*Net cost effect: increase*)		administrative burden developing educational messages and materials related to selecting and preparing vegetables and fruits appropriate for complementary feeding.		of vegetables or fruit using the CVV compared to the jarred varieties.
Current rule: Food package II-BF recipients are prescribed 77.5 oz of infant food meat per month. *Proposed revision:* Food package II-BF recipients are prescribed 40 oz of infant food meat per month. Ten oz of canned fish can be substituted for 4 jars (10 oz) of infant food meat per month. (*Net cost effect: savings*)	Because redemption of infant food meat is low, reducing the amount prescribed is expected to result in slight cost savings. The option for substitution of canned fish may slightly increase redemption in this category. Given that canned fish is currently less expensive per oz than jarred infant food meat, increase in redemption may be offset by the slightly lower price.	Implementation of the proposed revision will require training WIC staff and participants of the change and new substitution option. Management Information Systems will need to be updated.	The revision may reduce the amount of infant food meat purchased by WIC participants. The substitution option may slightly increase the amount of canned fish purchased by WIC participants.	The proposed revision addresses participants' feedback about the quantity and preference in the infant food meat category, while still providing key nutrients to fully breastfed infants. The substitution option provides participants with greater flexibility in this food category.

continued

TABLE U-2 Continued

Current Rules, Proposed Revisions, and Projected Net Cost Differences*	Effect of the Proposed Revision			
	USDA/Federal Government	State/Local Agencies	Vendors/Industry	WIC Participants
Current rule: Food package III is reserved for participants who have one or more qualifying conditions that require an exempt infant formula or WIC-eligible nutritional (formerly WIC-eligible medical food) to supplement their nutrition needs, as determined by the participant's health care professional. *Proposed revision:* Participants with a qualifying condition in which a WIC formula is not medically necessary are still eligible to receive appropriate supplementary foods through food package III. (*Net cost effect: minimal*)	Clarifies that WIC formula is not an absolute requirement of food package III. The cost effects of the proposed revision will be minimal, as the number of applicable participants is expected to be extremely small.	Administrative burden increases in the short term. Management Information Systems will need to be updated.	No impact.	Some participants receiving food package III may be prescribed a package that is more appropriate for their needs.

Current rule: Children are prescribed 128 fl oz of juice per month; pregnant, partially (mostly) breastfeeding, and fully breastfeeding women are prescribed 144 fl oz of juice per month; postpartum and partially (minimally) breastfeeding women are prescribed 96 fl oz of juice per month. *Proposed revision:* Children, pregnant women, partially (mostly) breastfeeding women, and fully breastfeeding women are prescribed 64 fl oz of juice per month. Recipients may opt to substitute a $3 CVV for the 64 fl oz of juice. Postpartum and partially (minimally) breastfeeding women no longer receive juice. (*Net cost effect: savings*)	The reduction in juice prescribed would reduce the costs of the food packages. This reduction helps offset costs elsewhere in the food packages.	Implementation of the proposed revision will require training WIC staff and participants of the change and new substitution option. Management Information Systems will need to be updated.	Less juice would be purchased with the WIC food benefits. The minimum stocking requirements for juice would be simplified, as all participants prescribed juice would receive 64 fl oz (or frozen equivalent).	The proposed revision provides a supplemental amount of juice, which can help participants meet their daily fruit intake goals. The CVV substitution option allows participants greater flexibility to tailor their food package for personal preferences. The reduction and eliminations (food package VI) of juice from the food packages also allowed for larger CVVs across all food packages provided to children and women.

continued

TABLE U-2 Continued

Current Rules, Proposed Revisions, and Projected Net Cost Differences*	Effect of the Proposed Revision: USDA/Federal Government	State/Local Agencies	Vendors/Industry	WIC Participants
Current rule: Food package IV and VI recipients are prescribed 16 qt of milk per month. Food package V recipients are prescribed 22 qt of milk per month. Food package VII recipients are prescribed 24 qt of milk per month. Three qt of milk can be substituted for 1 lb of cheese, with the maximum amount of cheese being 1 lb for food packages IV, V, and VI and 2 lb for food package VII. Food package VII recipients are also prescribed 1 lb of cheese as a separate food package category. At state agency option, 1 qt of yogurt may be substituted for 1 qt of milk for women and children in food packages III–VII.	The proposed revisions would reduce the costs of the food packages. This reduction helps offset costs elsewhere in the food packages.	The administrative burden is expected to be short term, as the revision changes quantities rather than adding new items. It will require training WIC staff and participants of the changes and revised substitution options. Management Information Systems will need to be updated.	The total amount of milk purchased by WIC participants with their food benefit is expected to decrease. The revised quantities and substitution options eliminate participants' need for milk in a quart-sized container. More yogurt may be purchased by WIC participants under the revised substitution options, as 1 and 2 qt substitution options are allowed. The state agency option of a range of yogurt container sizes (30 to 32 oz) may also lead to increased redemption. Stocking requirements are not expected to substantially expand or change.	The proposed revisions provide supplemental quantities of milk across the food packages. The substitution structure eliminates the possibility of a dangling quart and may be more compatible with cultural needs or preferences.

No more than 1 qt of yogurt is authorized per participant. No more than a total of 4 qt of milk may be substituted for a combination of cheese, yogurt, or tofu for children and women in food packages IV–VI. No more than a total of 6 qt of milk may be substituted for a combination of cheese, yogurt, or tofu for women in food package VII.

Proposed revision:
Food package IV-A recipients are prescribed 12 qt of milk per month. Food package IV-B recipients are prescribed 14 qt of milk per month. All women are prescribed 16 qt of milk per month. Cheese is no longer offered as a separate food package item. Children and women can substitute up to 4 qt of milk per month, choosing either

continued

TABLE U-2 Continued

Current Rules, Proposed Revisions, and Projected Net Cost Differences*	Effect of the Proposed Revision			
	USDA/Federal Government	State/Local Agencies	Vendors/Industry	WIC Participants
to substitute 2 qt of yogurt for 2 qt for milk or to substitute 1 lb of cheese and 1 qt of yogurt for 4 qt of milk. Fully breastfeeding women can choose from a third substitution option of 2 lb of cheese for 6 qt of milk. Only one substitution option can be selected per month. At the discretion of the state agency, yogurt may be prescribed as a range of 30 to 32 oz, to accommodate different container sizes available on the market.				
(*Net cost effect: savings*)				
Current rule: Food packages V and VII recipients are prescribed 1 lb of whole wheat	The proposed revisions are expected to decrease food package costs. The expanded list of whole	The expanded list of whole grain options that states can authorize are intended to better meet	The range of whole wheat bread sizes may lead to the elimination of the 16 oz bread size	WIC participants will benefit by allowing whole wheat breads that are readily available in the

bread or other authorized options. Food package IV recipients are prescribed 2 lb of whole wheat bread or other authorized options. Authorized whole grain options include brown rice, bulgur, oats, whole grain barley, tortillas, and pastas. *Proposed revision:* Food packages IV, V, and VII recipients are prescribed one 16 to 24 oz 100% whole wheat bread or other authorized whole grain option. Allowable whole grain options include brown rice, bulgur, oats, whole grain barley, tortillas, pastas, corn masa flour (nonwhole grain), cornmeal, teff, and buckwheat. (*Net cost effect: savings*)	grain options is available at the discretion of state agencies, within cost-containment parameters.	the cultural and personal preferences of the participants they serve, within cost containment parameters. The expansion of whole grain sizes will require the Management Information Systems to be updated. WIC staff, vendors, and participants will need to be trained on new sizes and options.	in the market, which was principally created for the WIC population. The proposed revision is likely to lead to stocking requirements that better reflect widely available sizes. Vendors will need to train personnel to identify WIC-eligible breads and grains.	market. The expanded state options for substitutions may allow options that better meet diverse cultural needs and personal preferences.

continued

TABLE U-2 Continued

Current Rules, Proposed Revisions, and Projected Net Cost Differences*	Effect of the Proposed Revision			
	USDA/Federal Government	State/Local Agencies	Vendors/Industry	WIC Participants
Current rule: Food package VII recipients are prescribed 30 oz of canned fish per month. May be packed in water or oil. Pack may include bones or skin. May be regular or lower in sodium content. At the state agency's option, added sauces and flavorings are allowable. *Proposed revision:* Food packages IV, V-A, and VI recipients are prescribed 10 oz of fish once every 3 months. Food package V-B recipients are prescribed 10 oz of fish every month and food package VII recipients are prescribed 20 oz per month. May be packed in water, but may not be packed in oil.	Addition of fish across the food packages will increase food packages costs. The additional costs are offset by other changes across food packages.	Implementing the proposed change will increase the short-term administrative burden. Management Information Systems will need to be revised. WIC staff, vendors, and participants will need to be trained on new quantities and rotation pattern for food packages IV, V-A, and VI. The burden is expected to be relatively minor, as all food packages would be authorized the same canned fish.	The proposed revision is expected to increase the amount of water-packed canned fish purchased by WIC participants with their food benefit. The revision may increase minimum stocking requirements for small vendors. Vendors will need to train personnel to identify authorized canned fish products.	Provision of water-packed canned fish provides a high nutrient-density source of nonperishable seafood, and better aligns the food packages with DGA recommendations.

All other specifications remain the same. (*Net cost effect: increase*)				
Current rule: Food packages IV and VI recipients have the option of being prescribed 1 lb dried legumes (or 64 oz of canned legumes) or 16 to 18 oz of peanut butter per month. Food packages V and VII are prescribed 1 lb legumes (or 64 oz of canned legumes) and 16 to 18 oz of peanut butter per month. *Proposed revision:* Food package IV recipients receive peanut butter, legumes, and canned fish in rotation over 3 months. All women receive legumes and peanut butter once each in a quarter. Both canned and dried legumes must be allowed by all state agencies. (*Net cost effect: savings*)	Reduction of the amount of legumes and peanut butter prescribed in food packages IV through VII will result in a cost savings.	States and local agencies will need to educate participants about the legume and peanut butter rotation patterns for children and women. States that do not currently authorize canned legumes will incur a short-term administrative burden of expanding to include the canned option. Management Information Systems will need to be revised.	Sales of legumes and peanut butter to WIC participants using their food instrument will decrease. Market effect is expected to be minimal.	This change brings children's and women's food packages in better alignment with the concept of supplemental and the recommendations of the DGA. Cost savings help offset costs of revisions throughout the food packages.

continued

TABLE U-2 Continued

Current Rules, Proposed Revisions, and Projected Net Cost Differences*	Effect of the Proposed Revision			
	USDA/Federal Government	State/Local Agencies	Vendors/Industry	WIC Participants
Current rule: Children are prescribed an $8 CVV per month. Women are prescribed an $11 CVV per month. *Proposed revision:* The monthly CVVs for food packages IV, V-A, V-B, VI, and VII are $12, $15, $25, $15, and $35, respectively. (*Net cost effect: increase*)	Increasing the CVV across the food packages will increase food package costs. The additional costs are offset by other changes across food packages.	The infrastructure already exists to provide the CVV through the program, which greatly reduces the administrative burden associated with the proposed changes. Management Information Systems will need to be updated. States and local agencies will need to develop ways to communicate the change in the short term, and encourage use of the CVV for vegetables, to align use with the DGA.	Sales of vegetables and fruits will increase through WIC participants using their food benefit. Minimum stocking requirements will slightly increase for vendors that meet the current federal minimum stocking requirement for vegetables. Vendors in states that currently only allow fresh fruits may experience additional stocking requirements, as frozen, canned, and/or dried options are authorized.	Increasing the CVV expands the amount of vegetables and fruits participants are able to buy with their food instrument. Provision of a dollar amount allows participants flexibility and choice to meet cultural needs and personal preferences. Larger CVV values in food packages V-B and VII are intended as incentives to partial (mostly) and full breastfeeding.

NOTES: CVV = cash value voucher; DGA = *Dietary Guidelines for Americans*; fl oz = fluid ounce(s); lb = pound(s); oz = ounce(s); qt = quart(s).

* The projected net cost differences described in this table are contingent on the committee's assumptions, which are detailed in the "Cost" section of this appendix. The magnitude and even the direction of some of the cost differences can change with different assumptions that would still be considered reasonable. The cost effects of various different assumptions are evaluated in the "Uncertainties" section of this appendix.

TABLE U-3 Estimated Unadjusted Food Costs of the Current and Proposed Food Packages, FY2018 Through FY2022

Food Package Version	Food Package	Unadjusted Food Costs ($, millions)					
		FY2018[a]	FY2019	FY2020	FY2021[b]	FY2022	Total, FY2018 Through FY2022
Current	I	213.5	441.3	451.0	461.8	472.9	2,040.6
	II	300.3	620.5	634.2	649.4	665.0	2,869.4
	III[c]	45.2	93.4	95.3	97.5	99.7	431.2
	IV-A	277.7	571.7	582.1	593.7	605.5	2,630.7
	IV-B	616.5	1,268.9	1,291.9	1,317.4	1,343.6	5,838.3
	V	202.4	416.3	423.5	431.6	448.1	1,922.0
	VI	128.2	263.5	267.8	272.7	284.0	1,216.3
	VII	76.9	158.3	161.2	164.5	170.2	731.1
Total food costs		1,860.7	3,833.9	3,907.1	3,988.7	4,089.2	17,679.6
Revised	I	213.5	441.3	451.0	450.7	461.5	2,018.1
	II	297.5	614.7	628.3	634.0	649.2	2,823.7
	III[c]	45.4	93.7	95.7	97.8	100.0	432.6
	IV-A	264.8	544.5	553.7	563.9	574.3	2,501.2
	IV-B	602.2	1,237.9	1,258.7	1,281.9	1,305.6	5,686.4
	V-A	166.0	340.9	346.3	352.3	358.4	1,563.9
	V-B	35.4	72.4	73.4	97.6	99.1	377.9
	VI	129.0	264.5	268.4	259.0	263.2	1,184.1
	VII	87.6	179.4	184.0	186.5	191.3	828.8
Total food costs		1,841.4	3,789.5	3,859.4	3,923.7	4,002.7	17,416.7
Total unadjusted cost differences[d]		*–19.2*	*–44.4*	*–47.7*	*–65.0*	*–86.6*	*–262.8*

NOTES: Unadjusted costs and cost differences assume full implementation of the proposed revisions in all state agencies as of April 1, 2018. Column and row totals may not be exact owing to independent rounding.

[a] This analysis assumes the earliest date of implementation of the proposed changes would be April 1, 2018. Accordingly all estimates for FY2018 only encompass a 6-month period.

[b] This analysis assumes the proposed revisions will incentivize partially (mostly) breastfeeding food packages for mother–infant dyads The cost estimates for the revised food package anticipates a 5 percent shift of fully formula-fed dyads to the partially (mostly) breastfed participant categories in the year after full implementation of the food package revisions under the phased-in implementation assumption. Difference in food package costs in FY2021 and FY2022 are due, in part, to this anticipated shift in participants.

[c] Estimated costs for food package III only include standard issuance food package items, and do not account for exempt infant formula or WIC-eligible nutritionals.

[d] Calculated by subtracting the current food package costs from the revised food package costs. Negative values (–) indicate that the revised food packages result in cost savings as compared to the current food packages. Positive values (+) indicate that the revised food packages result in cost increases as compared to the current food packages.

TABLE U-4 Estimated Phased-in Cost Differences of the Proposed Revised Food Packages as Compared to the Current Food Packages, FY2018 Through FY2022

	Phased-in Cost Differences of the Revised Food Packages Compared to Current Food Packages ($, millions)[a]					
Food Package	FY2018[b,c]	FY2019[c]	FY2020	FY2021[d]	FY2022[d]	Total, FY2018 Through FY2022
I	0.0	0.0	0.0	−11.1	−11.4	−22.5
II	−0.9	−1.9	−5.9	−15.4	−5.8	−40.0
III[e]	+0.1	+0.1	+0.3	+0.3	+0.3	+1.1
IV-A	−4.3	−9.1	−28.4	−29.8	−31.2	−102.8
IV-B	−4.8	−10.3	−33.1	−35.6	−38.0	−121.8
V-A[f]	−2.1	−4.6	−14.7	−15.6	−23.5	−60.5
V-B[f]	+1.8	+3.6	+10.8	+33.9	+32.9	+83.0
VI	+0.2	+0.3	+0.5	−13.6	−20.8	−33.4
VII	+3.6	+7.0	+22.8	+22.0	+21.1	+76.5
Total phased-in cost differences	−6.4	−14.8	−47.7	−65.0	−86.6	−220.4

NOTES: Phased-in estimates assume full implementation of the proposed revisions in state agencies serving one-third of all WIC participants as of April 1, 2018. All other state agencies are assumed to implement the proposed revisions as of FY2020.

[a] Cost differences were calculated by subtracting the estimated food costs for the current food packages from the estimated food costs for the revised food packages. Negative values (−) indicate that the revised food packages result in cost savings as compared to the current food packages. Positive values (+) indicate that the revised food packages result in cost increases as compared to the current food packages. Column and row totals may not be exact owing to independent rounding.

[b] This analysis assumes the earliest date of implementation of the proposed changes would be April 1, 2018. Accordingly all estimates for FY2018 only encompass 6 months.

[c] Phased-in cost differences in FY2018 and FY2019 are 33.3 percent of the unadjusted cost differences.

[d] This analysis assumes the proposed revisions will incentivize partially (mostly) breastfeeding food packages for mother–infant dyads. Accordingly, the cost estimates for the revised food package anticipates a 5 percent shift of fully formula-fed dyads to the partially (mostly) breastfed participant categories in the year after full implementation of the food package revisions. The participant shift is assumed to take place in FY2021. The shift is expected to be sustained, but to not recur in FY2022. The difference in food package costs for both FY2021 and FY2022 is due, in part, to the participant shift assumptions.

[e] Estimates for food package III only include standard issuance food package items for both the current and revised food packages. Costs and cost differences do not account for exempt infant formula or WIC-eligible nutritionals.

[f] Currently, food package V is issued to both pregnant and partially (mostly) breastfeeding women. To arrive at cost differences, the proportion of food package V recipients categorized as pregnant and partially (mostly) breastfeeding were applied to the estimated costs of food package V for the current food packages to create estimates that could be compared to revised food package V-A and V-B, respectively.

Sources of Cost Differences

Cost Difference of Each Food Package Item

To determine the source(s) of the projected cost savings of the revised food package, the committee evaluated the total costs of each food package item category within the current and revised food packages. The total costs of each of the food items presented in Table U-5 include assumptions about substitutions and allowable options within each category and assumptions about changes in redemption rates (see "Cost Estimate Methodology" for additional details). Across the food package items, the total cost savings are larger than the total added costs, resulting in estimated total cost savings of the revised food packages as compared to the current food packages. Two major sources of cost differences between the current and revised food packages are juice and the CVV. In the current food packages, all women and children are prescribed juice. The reduction of total juice in the revised food packages results in a total phased-in cost savings of approximately $627 million over the course of FY2018 through FY2022, as compared to the current food packages. In contrast, increasing the value of the CVV for all women and children in the revised food package leads to an estimated total phased-in cost increase of approximately $780 million over the course of FY2018 through FY2022.

Major Cost Differences of Food Package Items Within Each Food Package

To further explore the sources of the cost differences, the committee evaluated the total phased-in cost differences of each food package item within each food package. Table U-6 presents each food package item revision that resulted in a total phased-in cost difference of at least $25 million in cost saving or increases over the course of FY2018 through FY2022, as compared to the total cost of the corresponding item in the current food packages. The major total cost differences summarized in the table not only reflect the specific revisions to the items and the quantity prescribed, but also the distribution of participants across the different food packages. Because food package IV-B comprises the largest participant group (approximately 36 percent of food package recipients), relatively small changes lead to more drastic cost differences. For example, the CVV in the revised food package IV-B would increase by $3 per month compared to the current food package,[8] leading to an estimated $246 million increase in

[8] Participants do not received adjustments in the CVV until the inflated value inflates crosses a $1 increment. The CVV for food package IV is currently $8 per month. By 2018, it is expected to cross the next $1 increment and be adjusted to $9 per month.

TABLE U-5 Phased-in Total Food Cost and Cost Differences (FY2018 Through FY2022) Between the Current and Revised Food Packages by Food Package Item Category, in Descending Order of Additional Costs

Food Package Item[a]	Total Phased-in Food Costs, FY2018 Through FY2022 ($, millions)[b]		Total Phased-in Cost Difference, FY2018 Through FY2022 ($, millions)[c]
	Current Food Packages	Revised Food Packages	
Cash value voucher	1,886.9	2,666.4	+779.5
Canned fish	51.9	165.5	+113.5
Jarred infant vegetables and fruits	578	659.4	+81.4
Eggs	513.5	513.6	+0.2[d]
Infant food meat	52.1	32.6	−19.4
Breakfast cereal	1,321.8	1,300.0	−21.7
Infant formula, postrebate	3,321.2	3,279.8	−41.5[d]
Cheese[e]	45.9	0	−45.9
Infant cereal	142.6	64.4	−78.1
Milk	3,747.7	3,662.2	−85.5
Legumes and peanut butter	410.4	286.9	−123.6
Whole wheat bread	559.5	406.9	−152.6
Juice	1,251.6	625.0	−626.6

NOTES: Phased-in estimates assume full implementation of the proposed revisions in state agencies serving one-third of all WIC participants as of April 1, 2018. All other state agencies are assumed to implement the proposed revisions as of FY2020.

[a] Broadly describes the food package item category. Cost differences include assumptions about substitutions and selection of allowable options within each category.

[b] Calculated by summing the food cost of each specific food package item from FY2018 through FY2022. To account for the phased-in implementation, the food costs for FY2018 and FY2019 are one-third the estimated unadjusted food costs. Phased-in and unadjusted food costs are identical for FY2020 through FY2022. The estimated phased-in total food costs reflect assumptions about redemption, substitutions, prices, and program participation.

[c] Cost differences were calculated by subtracting the estimated phased-in food costs for the current food packages from the estimated food costs for the revised food packages. Negative values (−) indicate that the revised food packages result in cost savings as compared to the current food packages. Positive values (+) indicate that the revised food packages result in cost increases as compared to the current food packages. Row totals may not be exact owing to independent rounding.

[d] This analysis assumes the proposed revisions will incentivize partially (mostly) breastfeeding food packages for mother–infant dyads. Accordingly, the cost estimates for the revised food package anticipates a 5 percent shift of fully formula-fed dyads to the partially (mostly) breastfed participant categories in the year after full implementation of the food package revisions. The participant shift is assumed to take place in FY2021. The shift is expected to be sustained, but to not recur in FY2022. The projected cost difference is attributed solely to this shift, rather than revisions to the food item in the food package.

[e] Describes the total food cost and cost difference of cheese as a separate food package category for food package VII. The costs associated with cheese as a substitution option for fluid milk is incorporated into the estimates for the milk category.

TABLE U-6 Revisions to Food Package Items That Lead to Major Total Phased-in Cost Differences from FY2018 Through FY2022, by Food Package

Food Package	Food Package Revision	Total Phased-In Cost Difference, FY2018 Through FY2022 ($, millions)[a]
I	• No revision leading to a major cost difference[b]	—
II	• Infant vegetable and fruit redemption is projected to increase with the addition of the CVV substitution option	+69
	• Infant cereal is reduced	-71
III	• No revision leading to a major cost difference[c]	—
IV-A	• Cash value voucher is increased	+107
	• Canned fish is added to the food package	+27
	• Milk[d] is reduced	-45
	• Whole wheat bread[e] is reduced	-52
	• Juice is reduced	-116
IV-B	• Cash value voucher is increased	+246
	• Canned fish is added to the food package	+62
	• Legumes and peanut butter are reduced	-47
	• Whole wheat bread[e] is reduced	-119
	• Juice is reduced	-264
V-A	• Cash value voucher is increased	+129
	• Milk[d] is reduced	-29
	• Legumes and peanut butter are reduced	-37
	• Juice is reduced	-84
V-B	• Cash value voucher is increased	+26
VI	• Cash value voucher is increased	+65
	• Juice is reduced	-109
VII	• Cash value voucher is increased	+200
	• Cheese[f] is eliminated as its own food package item	-46

NOTES: The committee defined a major total cost difference as a revision within a specific food package resulting in a total phased-in cost difference of at least $25 million over the course of FY2018 through FY2022. The major total cost differences not only reflect the specific revisions to the items and the quantity prescribed, but also the distribution of participants across the different food packages. Food packages that represent a smaller proportion of WIC participants generally have fewer major cost differences. Not all savings and costs are reflected in the table.

continued

TABLE U-6 Continued

[a] Phased-in estimates assume full implementation of the proposed revisions in state agencies serving one-third of all WIC participants as of April 1, 2018. All other state agencies are assumed to implement the proposed revisions as of FY2020. Cost differences were calculated by subtracting the estimated cost for the current food package item from the estimated costs corresponding to the food item in the revised food package. Negative values (–) indicate that the revised food packages result in cost savings compared to the current food packages. Positive values (+) indicate that the revised food packages result in cost increases compared to the current food packages.

[b] This analysis assumes the incentives in the proposed revisions will result in a 5 percent shift of fully formula-fed mother–infant dyads to the partially (mostly) breastfed participant categories in the year after full implementation of the food package revisions across the entire WIC program under the phased-in assumption. The total amount of formula prescribed in the revised food packages I and II is expected to decrease because of this shift in participants. For food package I, the total cost difference for FY2018 through FY2022 is expected to result in $22.5 million in savings.

[c] Because food package III recipients comprise a small proportion of food package recipients, all food package revisions resulted in total phased-in cost differences of less than $25 million over the course of FY2018 through FY2022.

[d] The estimated cost differences for milk includes assumptions about the proportion of participants purchasing fluid milk (e.g., whole milk, 2%), milk alternatives (e.g., lactose-free milk, soy-based beverage), and substitutions (e.g., cheese, yogurt).

[e] The estimated cost difference for whole wheat bread includes assumptions about the proportion of participants purchasing options available under the current food packages and proposed revisions (e.g., corn tortillas, instant oatmeal).

[f] The proposed revisions remove cheese as a separate food package category prescribed to food package VII participants. Cheese remains as substitution option for milk across all children's and women's food packages.

estimated total phased-in costs, as compared to the current food package. In contrast, the CVV for fully breastfeeding women (food package VII)—who comprise approximately 3 percent of food package recipients—would increase by $24 per month in the revised food packages, and would only lead to an estimated $200 million increase in estimated phased-in costs.

Cost Differences of Food Package Items Over Time

The preceding sections broadly evaluate the cost implications of each food package item, summed across all projected years. As presented in Table U-7, the phased-in costs differences are not static over the course of FY2018 through FY2022 and reflect assumptions of the analysis. Cost differences in FY2018 and FY2019 are markedly lower than in subsequent years, for example, because they reflect the phased-in implementation of the revised food package. The values for these 2 years are one-third of the unadjusted value. The cost differences for FY2018 are further reduced, because the values only encompass a 6-month period.

TABLE U-7 Phased-in Cost Differences Between the Current and Revised Food Packages by Food Package Item Category, by Fiscal Year

	Phased-in Cost Differences of the Revised Food Packages Compared to Current Food Packages ($, millions)[b]				
Food Package Item[a]	FY2018[c,d]	FY2019[d]	FY2020	FY2021	FY2022
Cash value voucher	+36.5	+73.9	+224.1	+229.7	+215.2
Canned fish	+5.0	+10.3	+31.6	+32.9	+33.7
Jarred infant vegetables and fruits	+3.6	+7.5	+22.9	+23.4	+24
Eggs	0	0	0	+0.1	+0.1
Infant food meat	-0.9	-1.8	-5.5	-5.6	-5.7
Breakfast cereal	-1.0	-2.0	-6.2	-6.2	-6.3
Infant formula, postrebate	0	0	0	-20.5	-21.0
Cheese[e]	-2.0	-4.2	-12.9	-13.2	-13.5
Infant cereal	-3.5	-7.2	-22.0	-22.5	-23.0
Milk	-3.9	-8.1	-24.7	-24.1	-24.7
Legumes and peanut butter	-5.5	-11.3	-34.8	-35.6	-36.4
Whole wheat bread	-6.8	-14.1	-43.4	-43.6	-44.6
Juice	-27.9	-57.7	-176.9	-179.9	-184.2

NOTES: Phased-in estimates assume full implementation of the proposed revisions in state agencies serving one-third of all WIC participants as of April 1, 2018. All other state agencies are assumed to implement the proposed revisions as of FY2020.

[a] Broadly describes the food package item category. Cost differences include assumptions about substitutions and selection of allowable options within each category.

[b] Cost differences were calculated by subtracting the estimated phased-in food cost for each item in the current food packages from the estimated food costs of the corresponding item in the revised food packages. Negative values (–) indicate that the revised food packages result in cost savings as compared to the current food packages. Positive values (+) indicate that the revised food packages result in cost increases as compared to the current food packages.

[c] This analysis assumes the earliest date of implementation of the proposed changes would be April 1, 2018. Accordingly all estimates for FY2018 only encompass a 6-month period.

[d] Phased-in cost differences in FY2018 and FY2019 are 33.3 percent of the unadjusted cost differences.

[e] Describes the cost difference of cheese as a separate food package category for food package VII. The costs associated with cheese as a substitution option for fluid milk is incorporated into the estimates for the milk category.

Some of the variations in cost differences over time are solely due to assumptions regarding participation. In FY2021 and FY2022, infant formula is projected to cost less and eggs are projected to cost slightly more in the revised food packages as compared to the current food packages. The analysis does not assume changes in quantities or percent redeemed between the current and revised food packages for either food package item. Instead, the cost differences result from the 5 percent shift in fully formula-fed mother–infant dyads to partially (mostly) breastfeeding food packages that the committee projects to take place in FY2020 for the revised food packages. The slight increase in egg costs in the revised food packages is attributed to the women shifting from being classified as partially (minimally) breastfeeding at more than 6-months postpartum (i.e., receiving food package N/A) to partially (mostly) breastfeeding (i.e., receiving the revised food package V-B).

Most of the projected variations in cost differences over time are the result of a complex interplay among several factors. The CVV serves as a prime example. The proposed revisions add value to the CVV across all food packages for women and children. In FY2020 and FY2022, the CVV for women in the revised food package VII is projected to be adjusted for inflation by \$1, increasing to \$36 and \$37 per month, respectively. Similarly, an inflation adjustment of \$1 is projected for the revised food package V-B (for partially [mostly] breastfeeding women), increasing the CVV to \$26 per month. Also during FY2021, the committee anticipates a 5 percent shift of fully formula-fed dyads to partially (mostly) breastfed food packages, which would shift a portion of postpartum women to the larger CVV in the revised food package V-B (as compared to the revised food package VI CVV). These adjustments and assumptions in the revised food packages do not have a dramatic effect on total cost differences because participants in food packages VII and V-B make up a small proportion of the total WIC population. In FY2022, however, the trajectory of the cost difference for the CVV changes, decreasing from +\$230 million in FY2021 to +\$215 million in FY2022. This is the result of a \$1 inflation adjustment that is projected to affect all food packages for women in the current food packages. Although the revised CVV values result in positive cost differences (i.e., cost increases) as compared to the CVV values in the current food packages for each fiscal year assessed, the difference across the years is not consistent. Assumptions regarding the CVV are detailed in the "Cost Effect Methodology" section that follows. Alternative assumptions and their effects on total cost differences are tested in the "Uncertainty" section later in this appendix.

Cost Estimate Methodology

This analysis projects costs of each food package in the current and revised sets of food packages through FY2022. The committee estimated the monthly costs of a food package by multiplying the projected number of recipients of the package, the average proportion of each food package item projected to be redeemed, and the estimated prices of each item in the food package and then summing these values within the food package. This process was repeated for each food package. Monthly costs were multiplied by 12 to arrive at annual estimates for each fiscal year in the analysis (FY2018[9] through FY2022). The sections that follow detail how the committee projected participation, redemption, and prices.

The presented estimates only encompass the cost of supplemental foods to the state agency. Administrative costs are not included. Although state and local WIC providers will likely incur additional administrative burden associated with the proposed revisions initially, such as updating their Management Information Systems and retraining staff, the committee was not in a position to quantify the costs of such changes.

Participation

The *WIC Participation and Program Characteristics 2014: Food Package Report* (USDA/FNS, 2016a) and average participation by participant category from administrative data posted on FNS's website[10] (USDA/FNS, 2016b) both describe WIC program participation by food package. While each provides a slightly different portrait of participation, neither directly provides the number of individuals who claim each specific food package type (outlined in Table U-1). The committee used both data sources to estimate the average number of participants who are actually issued a food instrument each month.

The 2014 Food Package Report is the only data source that provides insight into the distribution[11] of participants across the 27 specific types of food packages. While the data used for the Food Package Report are the most comprehensive available on the topic of specific food package assignments, there are limitations including, but are not limited to:

- *The dataset captured all individuals certified to receive benefits during the month of April of the assessment year, regardless of whether the food benefits were claimed.* The total number of participants in the Food Package Report's analyses, therefore, is higher than average monthly participation counts derived from other sources

[9] FY2018 in this analysis only encompasses 6 months. As such, monthly estimates were multiplied by 6 rather than 12.

[10] Administrative data includes all state agencies, Indian Tribal Organizations, and territories.

[11] Throughout this appendix, the phrase "food package distributions" or simply "distributions" refers to the proportions of a WIC participant group assigned specific food packages. It does not refer to the physical distribution or claiming of the food benefit.

of administrative data, which generally reflect those that claimed benefits from the WIC agency.

- *The food package type variable in the dataset is still considered to be in the testing phase.* Because of this, the Food Package Report notes: "Findings should be treated as suggestive rather than definitive" (USDA/FNS, 2016a).
- *The dataset only includes WIC participants in Puerto Rico; Washington, DC; and 48 states.*[12] Louisiana and New Mexico did not provide information on specific food package assigned to participants. Furthermore, other territories and Indian Tribal Organizations were not included in the dataset. As such, the distributions of the food packages within the participant categories approximates, but may not necessarily represent, that which exists across all participating agencies.
- *The dataset had variable levels of missing data.* The Food Package Report notes that "the information provided by state agencies on food package types is not entirely complete or reliable" (USDA/FNS, 2016a).
- *In the data received from states, participants were recorded as being part of one of five certification categories: pregnant women, breastfeeding women, postpartum women, infants, and children.* The breastfeeding category encompasses fully breastfeeding women (intended to be food package VII); partially (mostly) breastfeeding women up to 1-year postpartum (intended to be food package V); partially (minimally) breastfeeding women up to 6-months postpartum (intended to be food package VI); and partially (minimally) breastfeeding women, 6- to 12-months postpartum (no food package). In the analyses performed in the Food Package Report, the breastfeeding certification category was separated into fully and partially breastfeeding women by dichotomizing the participants based on prescription of food package VII. Food package VII, however, can also be assigned to women pregnant with or partially (mostly) breastfeeding multiples, so this approach to subgrouping can only closely approximate the number of fully breastfeeding women in the dataset. Furthermore, partially (minimally) breastfeeding women more than 6-months postpartum are eligible for WIC services but do not receive a food package. Agencies differed in their approach to reporting the food package associated with these participants. Some reported a null food package (food package "N/A") while most did not report a food package.

[12] This statement specifically pertains to Table C.1 in the Food Package Report, "Food Packages Assigned by Participant Category (2014)."

- *Some participant categories appeared to be assigned discordant food packages.* A small fraction of participants were reportedly assigned a food package that did not correspond with their participant category (e.g., an infant receiving food package IV-A). Some of the discrepancy is attributed to how age was calculated in the dataset (e.g., an infant aged into the children's food package during the month of April may still be counted as an infant). Another potential source of the discrepancies is that agencies may prescribe an updated food package without recertifying the participant when their status changes. Women, for example, may take up to 6-weeks postpartum to recertify based on breastfeeding status. During this period, such women would continue to receive the prenatal food package V despite being postpartum.

The distributions presented in the 2014 Food Package Report were applied to the average monthly national participation for FY2015, to arrive at participation estimates that reflect individuals issued food benefits in a given month. Because the Food Package Report and administrative data posted on FNS's website assess participation levels differently, the following adjustments and assumptions were made:

- The data used in the 2014 Food Package Report are collected on a biennial basis, and are the most current portrait of specific food package prescription distributions. The committee presumed that the food package distributions would not be substantially different between FY2014 and FY2015.
- Due to rounding, not all food package distributions within each participant category presented in the 2014 Food Package Report summed to 100 percent. To account for this in the RIA, the following was done:
  - Specific food packages assigned "<0.1 percent" were set to zero for pregnant women, partially breastfeeding women, infants, and children, as the distributions within each of the participant categories summed to 100 percent without accounting for such values.
  - The three food package types assigned a "<0.1 percent" for postpartum women were replaced with a value of 0.03 percent, so the distribution for the participant category summed to 100 percent rather than 99.9 percent.
  - All values ≥0.1 percent in the infant participant category were divided by 1.001 to scale the distribution for the participant category to 100 percent rather than 100.1 percent.
- The percent of a participant group assigned a "Missing" food package type in the Food Package Report was assumed to represent

certified WIC participants who did not claim benefits in a given month. This type of participant is represented in the Food Package Report dataset, but not in the administrative totals presented on FNS's website. To arrive at food package distributions representing only participants claiming their food instrument, the percent assigned "Missing" were removed from each participant category, and the remaining food package distributions were scaled to 100 percent within each participant category. Scaled distributions were then applied to the FY2015 administrative participation data, by participant category. This assumption has implications particularly for the partially breastfeeding women participant category. Since not all states used a null food package ("N/A") to report on partially (minimally) breastfeeding women more than 6-months postpartum (i.e., a participant group that does not receive a food instrument), the slightly higher rate of missing food package assignments for the partially breastfeeding woman participant category could be due to this subgroup being inadequately captured in the data. The extent to which this occurred, however, could not be determined or accounted for in this analysis.

- The Food Package Report includes a null food package ("N/A") which is noted to be assigned to minimally breastfeeding women more than 6-months postpartum who do not receive food benefits but still participate in WIC. According to FNS, this type of WIC participant is captured in the administrative dataset. Because the goal of this analysis is to assess costs related to the food benefit, participants assigned the "N/A" food package were not included in the cost profiles for the current food package (see "Cost Estimate Methodology" for additional details). The final participant count used in this RIA is therefore slightly lower than the total average participation derived from the administrative data.
- Discordance between the food package and the participant category were largely disregarded for the purposes of this analysis, since the primary goal was to determine the number of participants prescribed as specific food package. However, assumptions had to be made for food package V. In the Food Package Report, more than 1 percent of women in the postpartum participant category were assigned food package V, which is intended for pregnant and partially (mostly) breastfeeding women. It was presumed that these participants were women who had given birth within the previous 6 weeks and were still receiving the prenatal food package, and would therefore receive food package V-A (pregnant) in the revised food package structure. This assumption had minimal effect on

overall cost, as postpartum women represented less than 1 percent of participants receiving food package V.

The integration of the 2014 Food Package Report and average participation by category from FNS administrative data allowed the committee to estimate the number of participants actively being issued each of the specific food packages in FY2015. This served as the base for both the current and proposed cost estimates.

Estimating participation for FY2018 through FY2022 The forecasted levels of WIC participation through FY2022 are an extrapolation of FY2015 WIC participation levels based on the relationship between WIC participation and the general economy. During and following the economic recession of 2008–2009, WIC participation grew. As that recession waned, WIC participation declined. As the general economy is forecasted to moderately improve and then stabilize, the committee expects that WIC participation levels will decrease initially, then slightly increase and stabilize through FY2022.

To extrapolate WIC participation into the future, the committee quantified the relationship between WIC participation levels and economic conditions, using regression analysis. The number of unemployed persons served as a measure of economic conditions. Regression analysis showed a strong correlation between the number of unemployed persons and WIC participation. This correlation was used to predict WIC participation based on the Federal Reserve's forecast of unemployment rates and the Bureau of Labor Statistics's forecast of the civilian labor force (BLS, 2013). Based on these data and the relationship between WIC participation and unemployment, the committee forecasts WIC participation to decline by 2.2 percent between FY2015 and FY2018. From FY2018 to FY2022, the committee forecasts WIC participation to increase by 1.5 percent. The FY2022 participation levels are forecasted to be 0.7 percent lower than the FY2015 levels. The relative changes in participation used in this RIA are summarized in Table U-8. The committee assumed the relative change would be experienced the same across all participant categories. Projected participation for the current food packages, by food package type, is presented in Table U-9. These values served as the participant multipliers for estimating costs of the current food packages.

Anticipating a Shift in Fully Formula-Fed Mother–Infant Dyads Under the Proposed Revisions

Participation projections are identical between the current and proposed revised food packages, with one exception. The committee anticipates the

TABLE U-8 Forecasted Relative Change in Total Participation

Fiscal Year	Relative Change in Participation[a]
2016[b]	-1.1%
2017[b]	-0.9%
2018	-0.2%
2019	1.2%
2020	0.1%
2021	0.1%
2022	0.1%

NOTES: The base year of this analysis is FY2015. The committee estimated FY2015 participation from the 2014 Food Packages Report and 2015 average annual program participation from data posted on FNS's website (USDA/FNS, 2016a,b).

[a] The relative change describes the percent by which total participation increased or decreased, relative to the total participation in the preceding fiscal year. Total participation in FY2016, for example, was projected to be 1.1 percent lower than total participation in FY2015.

[b] Year not included in the cost estimates presented in this RIA, but it was necessary to arrive at total participation projections for FY2018 through FY2022.

proposed revision to the categorization of partial (mostly) breastfeeding dyads in the first month will result in a shift of 5 percent of formula-fed infants (food packages I-FF-A, I-FF-B, and II-FF), 5 percent of postpartum and partially (minimally) breastfeeding women less than 6-months postpartum (food package VI recipients), and 5 percent of women classified as receiving the N/A food package to their respective partially (mostly) breastfeeding categories. The shift of women assigned the food package N/A to V-B slightly increases the total number of participants issued food benefits under the proposed revisions, as compared to the projections for the current food packages. The 5-percent shift was selected based on data presented in USDA/FNS (2011) that indicated the 2009 food package resulted in an approximately 8 to 11 percent shift of women out of the partially breastfeeding food package. The shifts were largely due to the fully formula-feeding food packages. The 5 percent value used in this analysis was therefore considered a conservative estimate for the number of participants that would shift back to the partially (mostly) breastfeeding category. The committee anticipates that the shift will take place after all the revisions have been implemented in all states and will be sustained but not recur in subsequent years. Accordingly, the shift has been incorporated in FY2021 participation estimates, which corresponds to the year after full implementation under the phased-in assumption. Projected participation under the proposed revisions by specific food package is presented in

Table U-10. These values served as the participant multipliers for estimating food package costs under the proposed revisions.

Redemption

Three sources of data were used to estimate and project redemption for each item in the current and revised food packages: (1) anonymized redemption data provided by FNS (hereafter referenced as the FNS redemption dataset), (2) redemption data provided by six individual WIC agencies, and (3) a 2014 Altarum report detailing redemption in Kentucky, Michigan, and Nevada as they transitioned to EBT (USDA/ERS, 2014).

Redemption data provided by FNS USDA-FNS provided the committee with 12 months (August 2013 through July 2014) of WIC redemption data from a convenience sample of 6 WIC state agencies, representing five of the seven regions of the country (the FNS redemption dataset). The identities of the states were not known to the committee. The states were diverse in terms of size and did not include Indian Tribal Organizations or territories.[13]

For each state, each month's worth of data included the following information: a description of the main food package item category (e.g., "legume"); the subcategory of food (e.g., "canned beans," "dry beans"); size and measure of the container purchased (e.g., 16 ounces); number of containers redeemed; average price for the container; and the total amount paid by WIC for that specific item (see the "Prices" section for use of the cost data). Because states agencies varied in their reporting approach—some providing specific descriptions of the items purchased (e.g., "soft corn tortilla"), while others only provided general descriptions (e.g., "whole grains, all types")—redemption estimates collectively describe the main food package item category, rather than individual food items. To arrive at redemption estimates from the FNS redemption dataset, the following steps were taken for each state:

- The number of units purchased in a given month was standardized by multiplying the container size by the number of containers redeemed, summing the total amount purchased across the various container sizes, and, where applicable, dividing by a food package-appropriate unit size. For example, ounces of fish purchased in the month was determined across all container sizes (3.75 to 20 ounces), summed, and divided by 30 to arrive at number of 30-ounce units purchased.

[13] As characterized by USDA-FNS.

TABLE U-9 Projected Participation by Food Package Type, Current Food Packages

Participant Category	Specific Food Package	Projected Participation				
		FY2018	FY2019	FY2020	FY2021	FY2022
Infants, 0 to less than 6 months						
0 less than 1 month infants						
Partially (mostly) breastfed	I-BF/FF-A	17,659	17,871	17,889	17,906	17,924
0 less than 4 months infants						
Fully breastfed	I-BF-A	64,749	65,526	65,591	65,657	65,723
Fully formula-fed	I-FF-A	333,554	337,557	337,895	338,232	338,571
1 to less than 4 months infants						
Partially (mostly) breastfed	I-BF/FF-B	66,711	67,511	67,579	67,646	67,714
4 to less than 6 months infants						
Fully breastfed	I-BF-B	31,393	31,770	31,802	31,834	31,865
Partially (mostly) breastfed	I-BF/FF-C	47,090	47,655	47,703	47,750	47,798
Fully formula-fed	I-FF-B	204,057	206,505	206,712	206,919	207,126
Subtotal		*765,213*	*774,395*	*775,170*	*775,945*	*776,721*
Infants, 6 to less than 12 months						
Fully breastfed	II-BF	111,839	113,181	113,294	113,407	113,521
Partially (mostly) breastfed	II-BF/FF	105,953	107,224	107,331	107,439	107,546
Fully formula-fed	II-FF	694,815	703,153	703,856	704,560	705,264
Subtotal		*912,606*	*923,558*	*924,481*	*925,406*	*926,331*
Participants with qualifying conditions						
Infants	All[a]	184,436	186,649	186,836	187,023	187,210

Children	All[a]	62,184	62,930	62,993	63,056	63,119
Women	All[a]	1,197	1,211	1,213	1,214	1,215
Subtotal		*247,817*	*250,791*	*251,042*	*251,293*	*251,544*
Children						
1 to less than 2 years	IV-A	1,229,645	1,244,401	1,245,646	1,246,891	1,248,138
2 to less than 5 years	IV-B	2,813,121	2,846,878	2,849,725	2,852,575	2,855,427
Subtotal		*4,042,766*	*4,091,279*	*4,095,371*	*4,099,466*	*4,103,566*
Women						
Pregnant	V	744,902	753,841	754,595	755,350	756,105
Partially (mostly) breastfeeding	V	129,145	130,695	130,826	130,957	131,088
Subtotal		*874,048*	*884,536*	*885,421*	*886,306*	*887,193*
Postpartum and partially (minimally) breastfeeding, <6-months postpartum	VI	685,082	693,303	693,996	694,690	695,385
Fully breastfeeding	VII	256,034	259,106	259,365	259,625	259,884
Partially (minimally) breastfeeding, >6-months postpartum	N/A[b]	64,768	65,545	65,610	65,676	65,742
Total[c]		***7,783,566***	***7,876,969***	***7,884,846***	***7,892,731***	***7,900,623***

NOTES: Participation was regressed on unemployment from the U.S. Bureau of Labor Statistics, and projections were based on projected unemployment from the Federal Reserve.

[a] Food package III recipients are prescribed food packages appropriate for their age and physiological state. There are specific food packages within food package III for women, infants, and children that correspond to specific food packages I, II, IV, V, VI, and VII.

[b] Women who are minimally breastfeeding and with infants more than 6 months of age that receive more formula than is allowed for a partially breastfed infant do not receive a food benefit. These women, however, are eligible to continue to receive other benefits through WIC, such as breastfeeding support, nutrition education, and health and social services referrals (USDA/FNS, 2013a). This group of participants is included in one of the committee's assumption regarding the revised food package cost estimates, and is therefore included in the above table.

[c] Total number of food package recipients does not include women assigned food package N/A.

TABLE U-10 Projected Participation Under the Proposed Revisions, by Food Package Type

Participant Category	Food Package Type	Projected Participation				
		FY2018	FY2019	FY2020	FY2021[a]	FY2022
Infants, 0 to less than 6 months						
0 to less than 1 month infants						
Partially (mostly) breastfed	I-BF/FF-A	17,659	17,871	17,889	21,446	21,468
0 to less than 4 months infants						
Fully breastfed	I-BF-A	64,749	65,526	65,591	65,657	65,723
Fully formula-fed	I-FF-A	333,554	337,557	337,895	321,321	321,642
1 to less than 4 months infants						
Partially (mostly) breastfed	I-BF/FF-B	66,711	67,511	67,579	81,018	81,099
4 to less than 6 months infants						
Fully breastfed	I-BF-B	31,393	31,770	31,802	31,834	31,865
Partially (mostly) breastfed	I-BF/FF-C	47,090	47,655	47,703	58,096	58,154
Fully formula-fed	I-FF-B	204,057	206,505	206,712	196,573	196,769
Subtotal		*765,213*	*774,395*	*775,170*	*775,945*	*776,721*
Infants, 6 to less than 12 months						
Fully breastfed	II-BF	111,839	113,181	113,294	113,407	113,521
Partially (mostly) breastfed	II-BF/FF	105,953	107,224	107,331	142,667	142,809
Fully formula-fed	II-FF	694,815	703,153	703,856	669,332	670,001
Subtotal		*912,606*	*923,558*	*924,481*	*925,406*	*926,331*
Participants with qualifying conditions						
Infants	All[b]	184,436	186,649	186,836	187,023	187,210
Children	All[b]	62,184	62,930	62,993	63,056	63,119
Women	All[b]	1,197	1,211	1,213	1,214	1,215
Subtotal		*247,817*	*250,791*	*251,042*	*251,293*	*251,544*

Children, 1 to up to 5 years						
1 to less than 2 years	IV-A	1,229,645	1,244,401	1,245,646	1,246,891	1,248,138
2 to less than 5 years	IV-B	2,813,121	2,846,878	2,849,725	2,852,575	2,855,427
Subtotal		*4,042,766*	*4,091,279*	*4,095,371*	*4,099,466*	*4,103,566*
Women						
Pregnant	V-A	744,902	753,841	754,595	755,350	756,105
Partially (mostly) breastfeeding	V-B	129,145	130,695	130,826	168,975	169,144
Postpartum and partially (minimally) breastfeeding, <6-months postpartum	VI	685,082	693,303	693,996	659,956	660,616
Fully breastfeeding	VII	256,034	259,106	259,365	259,625	259,884
Partially (minimally) breastfeeding, >6-months postpartum	N/A[c]	64,768	65,545	65,610	62,392	62,455
Total[d]		***7,783,566***	***7,876,969***	***7,884,846***	***7,896,015***	***7,903,911***

NOTES: Participation was regressed on unemployment from the U.S. Bureau of Labor Statistics, and projections were based on projected unemployment from the Federal Reserve.

[a] This analysis assumes the proposed revisions will incentivize partially (mostly) breastfeeding food packages for mother–infant dyads. Accordingly, the participation projections for the revised food package anticipates a 5 percent shift of fully formula-fed dyads to the partially (mostly) breastfed participant categories in the year after full implementation of the food package revisions. The participant shift is assumed to take place in FY2021. The shift is expected to be sustained, but to not recur in FY2022.

[b] Food package III recipients are prescribed food packages appropriate to their age and physiological state. There are specific food packages for women, infants, and children within food package III that correspond to specific food packages I, II, IV, V, VI, and VII.

[c] Women who are minimally breastfeeding and with infants more than 6 months of age that receive more formula than is allowed for a partially breastfed infant do not receive a food benefit. These women, however, are eligible to continue to receive other benefits through WIC, such as breastfeeding support, nutrition education, and health and social services referrals (USDA/FNS, 2013a). The anticipated shift in fully formula-fed dyads to the partially (mostly) breastfeeding categories includes women who are more than 6-months postpartum. Accordingly, 5 percent of women who did not qualify for a food package under the current food packages are anticipated to qualify for food package V-B under the proposed revisions.

[d] Total number of food package recipients does not include women assigned food package N/A.

- The number of standardized units purchased in a given month was then averaged across the 12 months for each food package item category.
- The average number of standardized units purchased in a month was divided by the number of participants expected to receive the food item and accounted for differences in monthly maximum allowances by food package (e.g., the equation used to estimate juice redemption accounted for the different maximum amounts prescribed children and the various food packages for women). To keep the identity of the state agencies anonymous, FNS inputted average monthly participation by participant category for each state into a spreadsheet that contained the redemption equations created by the committee, and returned the overall unweighted average redemption across the state agencies per food package item.[14] Through this process, FNS identified one of the six states as a clear outlier, and removed it from the averages (personal communication, K. Castellanos-Brown, USDA-FNS, June 22, 2016). As such, redemption estimates are calculated from five of the six state agency datasets provided by FNS.

Redemption estimates based on the FNS data have both strengths and limitations for the purposes of estimating and projecting costs associated with the food benefit. One of the strengths is that the data reflect actual purchases made by WIC participants with their food instrument. The data capture the range of container sizes that participants chose to purchase, and also include state-specific options for substitutions. Using redemption data, rather than making assumptions based on average quantity prescribed to participants, has the potential to better reflect the actual food costs. Limitations of the existing data, however, affect generalizability. The data only provide insight into the total number of units purchased in a given month or over the course of the year and were not currently reported in a way that could be used to see how redemption differed across specific food packages when an item was not unique to a single food package (e.g., breakfast cereal redemption may not be the same for children as it is for women). Furthermore, the FNS data could also not be used to arrive at redemption estimates for certain food package items. Redemption of milk and cheese, for example, could not be determined because cheese is offered not only as a separate food item provided in food package VII, but also as a substitution option for milk across children's and women's food packages. The data also predated the authorization of yogurt as a milk substitution option.

[14] The committee was provided with unweighted averages to preserve the anonymity of the states included in the FNS dataset.

Redemption data provided by individual state agencies From the data provided by FNS, the committee was able to estimate redemption for most of the standard items prescribed to children and women. Some redemption of estimates, however, could not be determined. In these instances, publicly available redemption data from individual state agencies were averaged and used in the analysis. The six agencies that provided redemption data included California (February 2015 through February 2016), the Chickasaw Nation (April 2015 through March 2016), Kentucky (November 2014 through May 2015), Massachusetts (March through August 2015), Texas (July and August 2015), and Wyoming (May 2015). Not all of the state agencies provided redemption estimates for all food items. Although the redemption estimates derived from these sources were WIC-specific, they were relatively limited in scope and not necessarily representative of WIC participants nationally.

Calculating Redemption for Current and Revised Food Package Items

The redemption rates derived from the data provided by FNS and the data provided by individual state agencies were applied to the current food packages and served as the base for the redemption projections under the proposed revised food packages. The committee used a 2014 report from Altarum (USDA/ERS, 2014), which provided insight into three types of redemption practices (full-, partial-, and nonredemption) to develop data-based assumptions for the redemption behaviors in the revised food packages (detailed in Appendix R). Redemption estimates that were based only on assumptions about full-, partial-, and nonredemption were considered "implied redemption rates." Implied redemption rates, however, do not account for behavioral changes, such as those that might result from the offering of new substitution options. Accordingly, the committee made slight adjustments to account for such changes. Table U-11 outlines the redemption rates applied to the current and revised food packages.

Applying redemption rates to the food packages The committee applied the calculated and projected redemption rates to the current and proposed monthly maximum allowances) for all food packages. Tables U-12 and U-13 summarize the estimated average amount redeemed for each food item for the current and revised food packages, respectively. The projected average amounts redeemed for each food package item serves as the quantity multipliers used in the estimation of total food costs.

TABLE U-11 Redemption Estimates and Projections for Food Package Items for Current and Revised Food Packages

	Current Food Packages		Revised Food Packages		
Food Package Item	Redemption Rate	Applicable Food Packages Type	Redemption Rate	Applicable Food Packages	Rationale for Revised Redemption Projection
Breakfast cereal	60[a]	IV-A, IV-B, V, VI, VII	54	IV-A, IV-B, V-A, V-B, VI, VII	10% (6 percentage point) decrease because state-level redemption data indicate that whole grain cereals are less preferred in some states and the number of options in the revised packages are reduced.
Cash value voucher	77[a]	IV-A, IV-B, V, VI, VII	75	IV-A, IV-B, V-A, V-B, VI, VII	Slightly decreased because additional voucher value may not be redeemed at the same rate; projected redemption also accounts for time costs of preparation of vegetables and fruits.
Cheese[b]	70[c]	VII	NA	NA	Cheese, as its own food package item, has been removed under the proposed revisions.
Eggs	80[a]	IV-A, IV-B, V, VI, VII	80	IV-A, IV-B, V-A, V-B, VI, VII	No change.
Fish	69[a]	VII	68	IV-A, IV-B, V-A, V-B, VI, VII	Projected value is the implied redemption rate.[d]
	NA	IV-A, IV-B, V, VI			
Formula	94[e]	I-BF/FF-A, I-BF/FF-B, I-BF/FF-C, I-FF-A, I-FF-B, II-BF/FF, II-FF	94	I-BF/FF-A, I-BF/FF-B, I-BF/FF-C, I-FF-A, I-FF-B, II-BF/FF, II-FF	No change.
Infant cereal	47[f]	II-BF, II-BF/FF, II-FF	57[g,h]	II-BF, II-BF/FF, II-FF	Increased because the amount prescribed is reduced and the amount provided in the current food packages exceeded recommended amounts.

Infant food vegetables and fruits	51[f]	II-BF, II-BF/FF, II-FF	65[h,i]	II-BF, II-BF/FF, II-FF	Increased because of the added CVV substitution option.
Infant food meat	31[c]	II-BF	43[g,h]	II-BF	Increased because the amount prescribed is reduced and the substitution option of canned fish is added.
Juice	70[a]	IV-A, IV-B, V, VI, VII	78[g,j]	IV-A, IV-B	Increased because the amount prescribed is reduced and individuals who prefer the CVV substitution will shift to that option (i.e., individuals who prefer juice will be issued and redeem juice).
			79[g,j]	V-A, V-B, VII	
			NA	VI	Juice is removed from food package VI under the proposed revisions.
Legumes and peanut butter	51[a]	IV-A, IV-B, V, VI, VII	53[g,j]	IV-A, IV-B, V-A, V-B, VI, VII	Increased redemption because of the additional options (canned legumes) and reduced amounts.
Milk	75[k]	IV-A	87	IV-A	Used the implied redemption rate;[d] public comments and redemption indicate that whole milk is a preferred food, so do not anticipate full yogurt substitution.
	71[c]	IV-B	80[j]	IV-B	Used the implied redemption rate[d] and increased it by 4 percentage points because of the additional yogurt substitution option.
	56[c]	V, VI, VII	66[j]	V-A, V-B	
			59[j]	VI	Used the implied redemption rate[d] and increased it by 3 percentage points because of the additional yogurt substitution option.
			68[j]	VII	
Whole grains	53[a]	IV-A, IV-B, V, VII	60	IV-A, IV-B, V-A, V-B, VII	Increased because of the increased options and allowable size range; redemption set to redemption of breakfast cereal in the current food packages.

continued

TABLE U-11 Continued

NOTES: The food package items listed in this table describe the broad categorization of the item, and encompass the allowable options and substitutions. NA = not applicable.

[a] The U.S. Department of Agriculture's Food and Nutrition Service (FNS) provided the committee with 12 months (August 2013 through July 2014) of price and redemption data from a convenience sample of six WIC state agencies, representing five of the seven regions of the country. The identity of the agencies was not known to the committee. The states were diverse in terms of size and did not include Indian Tribal Organizations or territories. FNS identified one of the states as an outlier and removed its data from the average redemption estimates. Accordingly, estimates presented in the table are based on data from five of the six states.

[b] Cheese as its own food package item.

[c] Based on redemption data provided by the Chickasaw Nation, Kentucky, Massachusetts, and Texas.

[d] The committee used the redemption rates in the current food packages and the distribution of redemption shares (full, partial, nonredeemers) provided in a 2014 report from Altarum to calculate an implied redemption rate under the proposed revisions. The implied redemption rate accounts for the change in quantity prescribed to participants, primarily driven by the assumed average amount redeemed by partial redeemers. Although these values account for changes in amounts prescribed, they do not account for changes in composition or substitution options. The implied redemption rate does not account for behavioral changes.

[e] The revised redemption rate is approximately the average of the implied redemption rate (Altarum) and the revised redemption rate for the CVV; it is also the actual average redemption rate from Altarum so represents a reasonable redemption rate.

[f] Based on redemption data provided by the Chickasaw Nation, Kentucky, Massachusetts, and Wyoming.

[g] Used the Altarum report average to account for bimodal distribution of redemption. Bimodal distribution refers to cases where the tails of the distribution (none and full redemption) had a relatively large share of the redemptions and the "partial redemptions" were a small share (USDA/ERS, 2014).

[h] Redemption projection is or closely approximates the average redemption from the Altarum report, and therefore represents a reasonable projection.

[i] Based on redemption data provided by the California, Kentucky, and Massachusetts.

[j] Approximately a 5 percent increase from the Altarum implied redemption rate.

[k] Based on redemption data provided by the Chickasaw Nation, Kentucky, and Massachusetts.

SOURCES: Personal communication, K. Castellanos-Brown, USDA-FNS, redemption data provided to the committee, June 30, 2016; USDA/ERS, 2014; redemption data provided to the committee by individual states. Data are available in the public access file for this study (Email: paro@nas.edu).

TABLE U-12 Estimated Average Amount Redeemed for Each Food Package Item Food Package Type, Current Food Packages

Food Package Type	Foods Package Item	Unit	Monthly Maximum Allowance	Estimated Average Amount Redeemed[a]
Food package I: Infants, 0 to less than 6 months				
I-BF-A	Infant formula	Prepared fl oz	0	0
I-BF-B	Infant formula	Prepared fl oz	0	0
I-BF/FF-A	Infant formula	Prepared fl oz	104[b]	98
I-BF/FF-B	Infant formula	Prepared fl oz	424[b]	399
I-BF/FF-C	Infant formula	Prepared fl oz	510[b]	479
I -FF-A	Infant formula	Prepared fl oz	861[b]	809
I -FF-B	Infant formula	Prepared fl oz	948[b]	891
Food package II: Infants, 6 to less than 12 months				
II-BF	Infant cereal	Ounces	24	11
	Jarred infant food vegetables and fruits	Ounces	256	131
	Jarred infant food meat	Ounces	77.5	24
II-BF/FF	Infant formula	Prepared fl oz	371[b]	349
	Infant cereal	Ounces	24	11
	Jarred infant food vegetables and fruits	Ounces	128	66
II-FF	Infant formula	Prepared fl oz	683[b]	642
	Infant cereal	Ounces	24	11
	Jarred infant food vegetables and fruits	Ounces	128	66
Food package III: Participants with qualifying conditions				
III[c]				
Food package IV: Children, 1 to up to 5 years				
IV-A	Cash value voucher	Voucher ($)	8	6
	Juice	Ounces	128	90
	Milk, whole	Quarts	16	12
	Breakfast cereal	Ounces	36	22
	Whole wheat bread	16 oz	2	1
	Legumes or peanut butter[d]	16 oz/18 oz[e]	1	0.5
	Eggs	Dozen	1	0.8

continued

TABLE U-12 Continued

Food Package Type	Foods Package Item	Unit	Monthly Maximum Allowance	Estimated Average Amount Redeemed[a]
IV-B	Cash value voucher	Voucher ($)	8	6
	Juice	Ounces	128	90
	Milk, reduced-fat	Quarts	16	11
	Breakfast cereal	Ounces	36	22
	Whole wheat bread	16 oz	2	1
	Legumes or peanut butter[d]	16 oz/18 oz[e]	1	0.5
	Eggs	Dozen	1	0.8
Food package V: Pregnant and partially (mostly) breastfeeding women, up to 1-year postpartum				
V	Cash value voucher	Voucher ($)	11	9
	Juice	Ounces	144	101
	Milk, reduced-fat	Quarts	22	12
	Breakfast cereal	Ounces	36	22
	Whole wheat bread	16 oz	1	0.5
	Legumes and peanut butter[f]	16 oz/18 oz[e]	2	1
	Eggs	Dozen	1	0.8
Food package VI: Nonbreastfeeding postpartum women and partially (minimally) breastfeeding women, up to 6-months postpartum				
VI	Cash value voucher	Voucher ($)	11	9
	Juice	Ounces	96	67
	Milk, reduced-fat	Quarts	16	9
	Breakfast cereal	Ounces	36	22
	Legumes or peanut butter[d]	16 oz/18 oz[e]	1	0.5
	Eggs	Dozen	1	0.8
Food package VII: Fully breastfeeding women, up to 1-year postpartum				
VII	Cash value voucher	Voucher ($)	11	9
	Juice	Ounces	144	101
	Milk, reduced-fat	Quarts	24	13
	Cheese	16 oz	1	0.7
	Breakfast cereal	Ounces	36	22
	Whole wheat bread	16 oz	1	0.5
	Legumes and peanut butter[f]	16 oz/18 oz[e]	2	1
	Eggs	Dozen	2	2
	Canned fish	Ounces	30	21

TABLE U-12 Continued

NOTES: The food package items listed in this table describe the broad categorizations and encompass the allowable options and substitutions.

[a] Calculated by multiplying the monthly maximum allowance by the redemption rate for the applicable food package and food package item. Value represents the estimated average quantity purchased by participants issued the specific food package.

[b] Weighted average of the monthly maximum allowances of the three different forms of infant formula. Weights were 0.78 for reconstituted powder, 0.12 for reconstituted liquid concentrate, and 0.10 for ready-to-feed, and were derived from the 2014 Food Package Report (USDA/FNS, 2016a).

[c] Food package III recipients were not uniquely identified in the redemption data. Accordingly, the committee assumed the redemption estimates in the current food packages and corresponding redemption projections applied to all participants categorically eligible to be prescribed the food item (i.e., a child prescribed food package III was assumed to be prescribed all of food package IV foods). With the exception of WIC formulas, the committee used both the monthly maximum allowances and the overall redemption rates for the standard food packages to arrive at corresponding food package III estimates. Owing to a lack of data on the reimbursement and costs to the program associated with exempt infant formulas and WIC-eligible nutritionals, estimates for food package III only encompass supplementary foods. The committee did, however, make one exception regarding WIC formula. The 2014 Food Package Report indicated that at least 40 percent of infant formula prescribed to partially (mostly) breastfed and fully formula fed infants is nonexempt (USDA/FNS, 2016a). Some nonexempt specialty formulas, such as thickened formulas, are reportedly covered by rebate contracts (USDA/ERS, 2004). Accordingly, the committee applied the proportion of nonexempt formula prescribed to the monthly maximum allowances for each of the infant food packages in food package III. The 94-percent redemption rate was then applied to those quantities and used in cost estimates. Because the quantity of infant formula did not change in the revised food package, this assumption is not expected to affect the estimated cost difference between the food packages.

[d] Food package IV and VI recipients can select from either peanut butter or legumes each month. They do not receive both in a given month.

[e] The 16 oz corresponds to the size of the dried legumes. States may also authorize four 16 oz cans (64 oz total) in lieu of the dried legumes. The 18 oz corresponds to size of the peanut butter. Although states may authorize smaller containers of canned legumes (15- to 16-oz) and peanut butter (16- to 18-oz), this analysis uses maximum container size for each.

[f] Food package V and VII recipients are prescribed both legumes and peanut butter each month.

Prices

As described in the preceding "Redemption" section, FNS provided the committee with 12 months' worth of anonymized redemption data from six state agencies (August 2013 through July 2014).[15] The data included the

[15] As was previously discussed, one of the states included in the six states dataset produced outlier redemption estimates when average participation was inputted into the redemption equations. The outlier state was omitted from the average redemption estimates. In looking at price per unit across the six states, however, there were no clear outliers. As such, all six states were included in price estimates.

TABLE U-13 Projected Average Amount Redeemed for Each Food Package Item Under the Proposed Revisions, by Food Package Type

Food Package Type	Foods Package Item	Unit	Monthly Maximum Allowance	Projected Average Amount Redeemed[a]
Food package I: Infants, 0 to less than 6 months				
I-BF-A	Infant formula	Prepared fl oz	0	0
I-BF-B	Infant formula	Prepared fl oz	0	0
I-BF/FF-A	Infant formula	Prepared fl oz	104[b,c]	98
I-BF/FF-B	Infant formula	Prepared fl oz	424[b]	399
I-BF/FF-C	Infant formula	Prepared fl oz	510[b]	479
I -FF-A	Infant formula	Prepared fl oz	861[b]	809
I -FF-B	Infant formula	Prepared fl oz	948[b]	891
Food package II: Infants, 6 to less than 12 months				
II-BF	Infant cereal	Ounces	16	9
	Jarred infant food vegetables and fruits	Ounces	128	83
	Jarred infant food meat	Ounces	40	17
II-BF/FF	Infant formula	Prepared fl oz	371[b]	349
	Infant cereal	Ounces	8	5
	Jarred infant food vegetables and fruits	Ounces	128	83
II-FF	Infant formula	Prepared fl oz	683[b]	642
	Infant cereal	Ounces	8	5
	Jarred infant food vegetables and fruits	Ounces	128	83
Food package III: Participants with qualifying conditions				
III[d]				
Food package IV: Children, 1 to up to 5 years				
IV-A	Cash value voucher	Voucher ($)	12	9
	Juice	Ounces	64	50
	Milk, whole	Quarts	12	10
	Breakfast cereal	Ounces	36	20
	Whole wheat bread	24 oz[f]	1	0.6
	Legumes and peanut butter	16 oz/18 oz[e]	0.7[g]	0.4
	Eggs	Dozen	1	0.8
	Canned fish	Ounces	3.3[h]	2.3

TABLE U-13 Continued

Food Package Type	Foods Package Item	Unit	Monthly Maximum Allowance	Projected Average Amount Redeemed[a]
IV-B	Cash value voucher	Voucher ($)	13	9
	Juice	Ounces	64	50
	Milk, reduced-fat	Quarts	14	11
	Breakfast cereal	Ounces	36	20
	Whole wheat bread	24 oz[f]	1	0.6
	Legumes or peanut butter	16 oz/18 oz[e]	0.7[g]	0.4
	Eggs	Dozen	1	0.8
	Canned fish	Ounces	3.3[h]	2.3
Food package V-A: Pregnant women				
V-A	Cash value voucher	Voucher ($)	15	11
	Juice	Ounces	64	51
	Milk, reduced-fat	Quarts	16	11
	Breakfast cereal	Ounces	36	20
	Whole wheat bread	24 oz[f]	1	0.6
	Legumes and peanut butter	16 oz/18 oz[e]	1[i]	0.5
	Eggs	Dozen	1	0.8
	Canned fish	Ounces	3.3[h]	2.3
Food package V-B: Partially (mostly) breastfeeding women, up to 1-year postpartum				
V-B	Cash value voucher	Voucher ($)	25	19
	Juice	Ounces	64	51
	Milk, reduced-fat	Quarts	13	11
	Breakfast cereal	Ounces	36	20
	Whole wheat bread	24 oz[f]	1	0.6
	Legumes and peanut butter	16 oz/18 oz[e]	1[i]	0.5
	Eggs	Dozen	1	0.8
	Canned fish	Ounces	10	7
Food package VI: Nonbreastfeeding postpartum women and partially (minimally) breastfeeding women, up to 6-months postpartum				
VI	Cash value voucher	Voucher ($)	15	11.3
	Milk, reduced-fat	Quarts	16	9.4
	Breakfast cereal	Ounces	36	19.5
	Legumes and peanut butter	16 oz/18 oz[e]	1[i]	0.5

continued

TABLE U-13 Continued

Food Package Type	Foods Package Item	Unit	Monthly Maximum Allowance	Projected Average Amount Redeemed[a]
	Eggs	Dozen	1	0.8
	Canned fish	Ounces	3.3[b]	2.3
Food package VII: Fully breastfeeding women, up to 1-year postpartum				
VII	Cash value voucher	Voucher ($)	35	26.3
	Juice	Ounces	64	50.8
	Milk, reduced-fat	Quarts	16	10.9
	Breakfast cereal	Ounces	36	19.5
	Whole wheat bread	24 oz[f]	1	0.6
	Legumes and peanut butter	16 oz/18 oz[e]	1[i]	0.5
	Eggs	Dozen	2	1.6
	Canned fish	Ounces	20	13.6

NOTES: The food package items listed in this table describe the broad categorizations and encompass the allowable options and substitutions.

[a] Calculated by multiplying the monthly maximum allowance by projected redemption for the applicable food package and food package item. Value represented the projected average quantity purchased participants issued the specific food package.

[b] Weighted average of the monthly maximum allowances of the three different forms of infant formula. Weights were 0.78 for reconstituted powder, 0.12 for reconstituted liquid concentrate, and 0.10 for ready-to-feed and were derived from the 2014 Food Package Report (USDA/FNS, 2016a).

[c] The committee proposes to allow partially (mostly) breastfed infants up to 364 reconstituted fl oz of infant formula in the first 30 days of life after a breastfeeding assessment by a competent professional authority. Because the committee upholds the provision that issuance of formula to a breastfed infant should not be standard practice and the amount is determined on a case-by-case basis, the monthly maximum allowance of 104 reconstituted fl oz was retained for this analysis. The cost effect of changing the monthly maximum allowance to 364 reconstituted fl oz is evaluated in the "Uncertainties" section of this appendix.

[d] Food package III recipients were not uniquely identified in the redemption data. Accordingly, the committee assumed the redemption estimates in the current food packages and corresponding redemption projections applied to all participants categorically eligible to be prescribed the food item (i.e., a child prescribed food package III was assumed to be prescribed all of food package IV foods). With the exception of WIC formulas, the committee used both the monthly maximum allowances and the overall redemption rates for the standard food packages to arrive at corresponding food package III estimates. Owing to a lack of data on the reimbursement and costs to the program associated with exempt infant formulas and WIC-eligible nutritionals, estimates for food package III only encompass supplementary foods. The committee did, however, make one exception regarding WIC formula. The 2014 Food Package Report indicated that at least 40 percent of infant formula prescribed to partially (mostly) breastfed and fully formula fed infants is nonexempt (USDA/FNS, 2016a). Some nonexempt specialty formulas, such as thickened formulas, are reportedly covered by rebate contracts (USDA/ERS, 2004). Accordingly, the committee applied the proportion of nonexempt formula

TABLE U-13 Continued

prescribed to the monthly maximum allowances for each of the infant food packages in food package III. The 94-percent redemption rate was then applied to those quantities and used in cost estimates. Because the quantity of infant formula did not change in the revised food package, this assumption is not expected to affect the estimated cost difference between the food packages.

[e] The 16 oz corresponds to the size of the dried legumes. The proposed revisions will require all state agencies to authorize four 16-oz cans (64 oz total) in lieu of the dried legumes. The 18 oz corresponds to the size of the peanut butter. All women receive 2 lb of legumes and 18 oz of peanut butter in a quarter. Although states may authorize smaller containers of canned legumes (15- to 16-oz) and peanut butter (16- to 18-oz), this analysis uses maximum container size for each.

[f] The proposed revisions to the whole wheat bread category would allow participants to choose from a range of bread sizes, 16 to 24 oz. The maximum amount that a participant could purchase under the proposed revisions (24 oz) is used in this analysis.

[g] This value reflects the average amount prescribed over the course of 3 months and should not be interpreted as an amount provided on a monthly basis. Under the proposed revisions, food packages IV-A and IV-B recipients receive legumes, peanut butter, and canned fish in rotation over a 3 month period. This rotation scheme results in legumes and peanut butter being issued in 2 out of 3 months, averaging to 0.667 allotments (an allotment corresponds to 16 oz of legumes; 18 oz of peanut butter) per month.

[h] This value reflects the average amount prescribed over the course of 3 months and should not be interpreted as an amount provided on a monthly basis. Under the proposed revisions, food packages IV-A, IV-B, V-A, and VI recipients are prescribed 10 oz of fish once every 3 months. This averages to 3.33 oz per month.

[i] Under the proposed revisions, all women receive 2 lb of legumes and 18 oz of peanut butter once each in quarter.

number and sizes of containers purchased, the average price per container for each container size, and the total amount the WIC agency paid for each size of the food item. Given the range of container sizes purchased for each food package item, the number of units purchased was standardized by multiplying the container size by the number of containers redeemed, summing the total amount purchased across the various container sizes, and, where applicable, dividing by a food package-appropriate unit size. The total amount the agency paid for the food item (across all container sizes) was divided by the total number of standardized units purchased to arrive at a price per unit.

The FNS redemption dataset captures WIC shopping behaviors not readily quantifiable from other sources of food prices. For example, the data were presumed to encompass the range of approved vendors where participants choose to use their WIC food instruments. The prices themselves reflect the choices participants actually made while at the vendor. Prices are inclusive of the substitutions and state-authorized allowable options selected by participants. Although the extent to which the FNS redemption dataset was representative of program participants at large could not be determined, the committee prioritized its use owing to its specificity to the WIC population.

The FNS redemption dataset, however, could not be used to estimate prices for select food package items. Infant formula was not included in the FNS redemption dataset. The FNS redemption dataset also predated allowing yogurt as a substitution option for fluid milk. Finally, the FNS redemption dataset did not contain the range of whole wheat bread and allowable options being proposed for the revised food packages. For these items, prices were drawn from the 2014 IRI Consumer Network database.

Composite prices for the food items State agencies that contributed information to the FNS redemption dataset varied in the level of detail about the purchased item. Some provided specific descriptors of the subcategory (e.g., "nonwhole grain breakfast cereal") while other only provided broad descriptions (e.g., "breakfast cereal: all types"). Because of this, the price estimates derived from the FNS redemption dataset collectively describe the main food package item category, which includes corresponding substitution and state-authorized allowable option selections made within that category. This approach, however, could not be used for five food package items: infant formula, infant food meat (revised food package only), milk, peanut butter and legumes, and whole wheat bread (revised food package only). For these items, the committee developed composite prices for each of the food package items, as outlined below:

- Infant formula prices were not included in the FNS redemption dataset. The committee, therefore, drew retail price data for liquid concentrate, powdered, and ready-to-feed infant formulas from the 2014 IRI Consumer Network database. The prices for unprepared infant formula were converted to prices per prepared fluid ounce. The average costs per prepared fluid ounce were weighted to reflect the distribution of infant formula types purchased through WIC. The weights were derived from the 2014 Food Package Report (USDA/FNS, 2016a): 0.78 (powdered), 0.12 (liquid concentrate), and 0.10 (ready-to-feed). Based on the FY2010 WIC Food Cost Report (USDA/FNS, 2013b), postrebate costs of infant formula are approximately 35 percent of prerebate costs. Given the rebate data were from 2010, the committee evaluated the stability of rebates between 2010 and 2015.[16] With the exception of 2011, rebates between 2010 and 2015 were relatively stable. Accordingly, the

[16] Rebates were reported as "rebates billed" before 2013 and "rebates received" after 2013. These were considered equivalent for the purpose of estimating rebate changes over time.

postrebate cost to the agency was estimated to be approximately 35 percent of the weighted average price per prepared fluid ounce.

- Under the proposed revisions, fully breastfed infants ages 6 to less than 12 months are prescribed 40 ounces of infant food meat, with the option of 10 ounces substituted with canned fish. Given the relatively low redemption of infant food meat and feedback from the public regarding infant food meat, the committee assumed food package II-BF recipients would make use of the 10-ounce substitution option. The weights used to calculate the composite were 0.75 for infant food meat and 0.25 for canned fish. The redemption projection presented in Table U-11 was applied to this composite value.
- In both the current and revised food packages, legumes and peanut butter are prescribed to participant under two different schemes. Accordingly, the different food packages and food package versions needed different weights for calculating composite prices. The weights accounted for the two different forms of legumes that can be authorized (dried and canned). The 2015 WIC Food Package Policy Options II Final Report (USDA/FNS, 2015b) reported that 85 percent of WIC participants are served by state agencies that allow canned legumes as an allowable option. Under the proposed revisions, all state agencies would have to authorize canned legumes as an allowable option. Table U-14 summarizes the weighting scheme used to calculate composite prices for the legume and peanut butter category.
- Allowable options and substitutions in the milk category include milk,[17] yogurt, cheese, soy beverage, and tofu. In both the current and revised food packages, children issued food package IV-A are prescribed whole milk, while all other food packages only prescribed the option of reduced-fat milk, low-fat milk, or nonfat milk. In the FNS redemption dataset, the cost of whole milk was slightly more than reduced-fat, low-fat, and nonfat milks, indicating a single price for fluid milk could not be used for this analysis. Milk prices are a weighted composite of the price of fluid milk, soy beverage, and lactose-free milk. Weights were based on redemption data provided by Texas and Wyoming. Tofu was redeemed for less than 1 percent of milk purchases in the available redemption data, and therefore was omitted from the milk composite price.

[17] Allowable forms of milk include fluid, evaporated, and dry milks. Allowable types include whole, reduced-fat (2%), low fat, nonfat, buttermilk, acidophilus, lactose-free, lactose-reduced, ultra-high-temperature (UHT) milk, and kosher milks. Under the current rule, some state agencies also authorize flavored milk.

TABLE U-14 Weighting Schemes Used to Calculate Composite Prices for Legumes and Peanut Butter for Current and Revised Food Packages

Food Package Version	Food Package	Maximum Monthly Allowance	Weights Used to Calculate Composite Legumes and Peanut Butter Price			Assumptions
			Legumes		Peanut Butter	
			Canned	Dried		
Current	IV-A, IV-B, and VI	1 lb legumes (64 oz canned)[a] or 18 oz peanut butter	0.186	0.314	0.500	Assumes half of food package IV and VI recipients choose peanut butter and half choose legumes; canned beans account for 37.2% of legume purchases while dried legumes account for 62.8%[b]
	V and VII	1 lb legumes (64 oz canned)[a] or 18 oz peanut butter	0.186	0.314	0.500	Legumes and peanut butter are both provided, so are equally weighted; canned beans account for 37.2% of legume purchases while dried legumes account for 62.8%[b]
Revised	IV-A and IV-B	1 lb legumes (64 oz canned) and 18 oz peanut butter prescribed over the course of 3 months[c]	0.211	0.289	0.500	Legumes and peanut butter are both provided in a 3-month cycle, so are equally weighted; canned beans were assumed to account for 42.2% of legume purchases while dried legumes account for 57.8%[d]

V-A, V-B, VI, and VII	2 lb legumes (128 oz canned) and 18 oz peanut butter prescribed over the course of 3 months[e]	0.281	0.385	0.333	Legumes are provided twice and peanut butter is provided once in a 3-month cycle, so are weighted in a 2 to 1 ratio; canned beans were assumed to account for 42.2% of legume purchases while dried legumes account for 57.8%[c]

NOTES: The weights summarized in this table were used to calculate composite prices for the legume and bean category in each food package. lb = pound; oz = ounces.

[a] Most, but not all, state agencies, currently authorize canned as an allowable form of legumes.

[b] Ratio was calculated from the FNS redemption dataset. Because the identity of the state agencies was unknown, the committee could not verify that states authorized both dried and canned options for legumes. It was therefore assumed that the ratio reflected the current state of authorized options for legumes.

[c] Under the proposed revisions, legumes, peanut butter, and canned fish are each prescribed once in a 3-month rotation. The weights presented in the table reflect contributions to the unit price used to estimate total costs. The 3-month rotation pattern is accounted for in this analysis through the value used for the monthly maximum allowance (0.66 allotments per month).

[d] To account for the proposed revision that all states authorized canned legumes, the proportion of legume purchases attributable to canned was increased. The committee assumed the proportion of legume purchases attributable to canned legumes would increase by 5 percentage points (from 37.2 to 42.2 percent).

[e] Under the proposed revisions, legumes and peanut butter are prescribed in a 3-month rotation. Legumes (2 lb or 128 oz canned) and peanut butter (18 oz) are each prescribed once. Because this averages to one allotment (either 1 lb of legume or one 18 oz container of peanut butter) each month, the weights reflect the 2 to 1 ratio across the 3-month period.

Furthermore, because the quantity of milk prescribed differs across the food packages, and the maximum allowed substitutions differ for food package VII, a single weighting scheme of milk, yogurt, and cheese could not be applied. For the current food packages, the committee assumed maximum substitution of cheese and yogurt. For the revised food packages, the committee weighted the maximum cheese and yogurt substitution options. Table U-15 summarizes the weighting scheme used to calculate composite prices for the milk food package item category.

- Proposed changes to the specifications and allowable options in the whole wheat bread category necessitated new prices. Prices for 100% whole wheat bread (18- to 24-ounce sizes),[18] corn tortillas (16 to 24 ounces), and oatmeal (16 to 24 ounces) were used in the cost estimates for the proposed revisions. While other allowable options for the whole wheat bread category exist (e.g., brown rice, bulgur, whole wheat pasta), nationally representative data on the distribution of redemption in context of the different options authorized by states were not available to the committee. Weights for the whole wheat bread (0.755), corn tortillas (0.185), and oatmeal (0.060) were estimated from redemption data from the Chickasaw Nation, Texas, and Wyoming.

Inflating unit prices to FY2015 prices The two sources of price data encompassed different timeframes; the FNS redemption dataset values were from August 2013 through July 2014 and the IRI Consumer Network prices were from calendar year 2014. To create a common base year, prices were inflated to FY2015 prices using Bureau of Labor Statistics Consumer Price Index (CPI) adjustments.[19] To accomplish this, the average item-specific CPI for FY2015 was divided by the average CPI for the time frame encompassed by the available unit price. The FY2015 prices were used to create the composite prices described in the preceding section. Table U-16 outlines the item-specific inflation rates and resulting FY2015 unit and composite prices for each food item used in this analysis.

Projecting prices after FY2015 For years after FY2015, prices for items that are prescribed as a fixed quantity (e.g., 16 quarts of milk) were inflated using the Congressional Budget Office's March 2015 Baseline Thrifty Food

[18] The 2014 IRI Consume Network price of the 16-ounce size of 100% whole wheat bread was not included in the price estimate under the proposed revisions because the committee anticipates the expansion of allowable bread sizes will result in the 16-ounce size eventually being removed from the market. The 16-ounce size was initially manufactured and distributed to comply with current WIC specifications for whole wheat bread.

[19] See http://data.bls.gov/cgi-bin/dsrv?cu (accessed March 12, 2017).

TABLE U-15 Weighting Schemes Used to Calculate Composite Prices for Milk for the Current and Revised Food Packages

Food Package Version	Food Package	Maximum Monthly Allowance	Substitution Scheme Used to Develop the Composite Milk Price Weights[a]	Weights Used to Calculate Composite Milk Price		
				Milk	Cheese	Yogurt
Current	IV-A	16 qt	12 qt milk + 1 lb cheese + 1 qt yogurt	0.750[b]	0.063	0.063
	IV-B	16 qt	12 qt milk + 1 lb cheese + 1 qt yogurt	0.750[c]	0.063	0.063
	V	22 qt	18 qt milk + 1 lb cheese + 1 qt yogurt	0.818[c]	0.045	0.045
	VI	16 qt	12 qt milk + 1 lb cheese + 1 qt yogurt	0.750[c]	0.063	0.063
	VII	24 qt	19 qt milk + 1.5 lb cheese + 0.5 qt yogurt	0.792[c]	0.063	0.021
Revised	IV-A	12 qt	8 qt milk + 1 lb cheese + 1 qt yogurt[d]	0.667[b]	0.083	0.083
	IV-B	14 qt	11 qt milk + 0.5 lb cheese + 1.5 qt yogurt	0.786[c]	0.036	0.107
	V-A	16 qt	13 qt milk + 0.5 lb cheese + 1.5 qt yogurt	0.813[c]	0.313	0.094
	V-B	16 qt	13 qt milk + 0.5 lb cheese + 1.5 qt yogurt	0.813[c]	0.313	0.094
	VI	16 qt	13 qt milk + 0.5 lb cheese + 1.5 qt yogurt	0.813[c]	0.313	0.094
	VII	16 qt	12 qt milk + 1 lb cheese + 1 qt yogurt	0.750[c]	0.063	0.063

NOTES: The weights summarized in this table were used to calculate composite prices for the milk category in each food package. The unit price for milk is per quart, cheese is per pound, and yogurt is per quart. The substitution ratio is 1 lb of cheese for 3 qt of milk and 1 qt of yogurt for 1 qt of milk. Because the unit price for cheese is per pound and the substitution ratio is 3:1 cheese to milk, weights do not sum to one. qt = quart(s); lb = pound(s).

[a] Schemes reflect high-price substitution scenarios for each food package. In the current food packages, the maximum number of quarts of milk that can be substituted are 4 (food packages IV–VI) and 6 (food package VII). A maximum of 1 qt of milk can be substituted for yogurt. No more than 1 lb of cheese can be substituted in food packages IV–VI and 2 lb in food package VII. Under the proposed revisions, all women and children can substitute 1 qt of yogurt and 1 lb of cheese for 4 qt of milk, or 2 qt of yogurt for 2 qt of milk. Food package VII recipients can also substitute 2 lb of cheese for 6 qt of milk. Substitution schemes for revised food packages average the substitution options unless otherwise noted.

[b] Milk price that is weighted is a composite of the price of whole milk (weight: 0.983), soy beverage (weight: 0.008), and lactose-free milk (weight: 0.009). Weights were based on redemption data provided by Texas and Wyoming. Tofu was redeemed for <1 percent of milk purchases in the available redemption data and therefore was omitted from the milk composite price.

continued

TABLE U-15 Continued

[c] Milk price that is weighted is a composite of the average price of reduced-fat, low-fat, and nonfat milk (weight: 0.975); soy beverage (weight: 0.011); and lactose-free milk (weight: 0.013). Weights were based on redemption data provided by Texas and Wyoming. Tofu was redeemed for <1 percent of milk purchases in the available redemption data and therefore was omitted from the milk composite price.

[d] Given the high redemption rate and public feedback received about whole milk, the committee made the assumption that substitution of 2 qt of yogurt may not be a likely scenario for food package IV-A. The substitution scheme used in the weighting, therefore, only represents the cheese and yogurt pattern. This is the higher-price substitution scenario, so cost differences for this food package are most likely conservative.

Plan estimates (CBO, 2015) The inflation assumptions are presented in Table U-17.

Inflating the cash value voucher The CVV does not inflate the same way as items prescribed as a fixed quantity. Instead, its inflation depends on an annual average of the CPI for fresh fruits and vegetables (7 C.F.R. § 246.16). Under the current rule, the average CPI for fresh fruits and vegetables from April 2006 through March 2007 is assigned to FY2008 and considered the baseline CPI. Each subsequent year follows the same pattern (e.g., FY2009 value is the average CPI from April 2007 to March 2008). To inflate the CVV, the average CPI for the fiscal year being considered is divided by the baseline CPI value and multiplied by the base values of each CVV ($8 for children, $10 for women). Participants only receive an increase in value when the inflated CVV crosses a $1 increment. Provision of the CVV in dollar increments, rather than prescribing the exact inflated value, is easier from an administrative perspective, as adjustments only have to be made periodically. It also decreases participant burden, as the benefit is provided in a round number and a consistent value month to month. This inflation approach was used for estimating the costs of the current food packages in this analysis.

Under the proposed revisions, all women and children receive a CVV of higher value. Had the committee kept FY2008 as the baseline CPI value under the proposed revisions, in FY2018 the $12, $15, $25, and $35 CVVs would already have been inflated to $13, $17, $28, and $39, respectively, because of the inflation that will have taken place in the decade between FY2008 and FY2018. Accordingly, the CVV under the proposed revision required a new inflation baseline, which was assumed to be the first year of implementation (FY2018).

The CPI values used in the inflation of the CVV encompass the 6 to 18 months prior to the fiscal year they describe. Accordingly, actual CPI

TABLE U-16 FY2015 Price per Unit for Each Food Package Item and Calculated Composite Using Item-Specific Inflation Rates

Food Package Item	Item-Specific Inflation Rate[a]	FY2015 Price	Unit
Individual Food Package Items			
Infant formula, liquid concentrate[b]	0.99996[c]	0.067	Prepared fl oz, postrebate
Infant formula, powder[b]	0.99996[c]	0.064	Prepared fl oz, postrebate
Infant formula, ready-to-feed[b]	0.99996[c]	0.080	Prepared fl oz, postrebate
Infant cereal	1.01097	0.264	Ounce
Infant food, vegetables and fruits	1.01097	0.165	Ounce
Infant food, meat	1.01097	0.403	Ounce
Beans, dried[b]	1.04713	1.503	Pound
Beans, canned[b]	1.00257	4.058	64 oz
Peanut butter[b]	0.98294	2.286	18 oz
Juice	1.00853	0.049	Ounce
Cheese[b,d]	1.03901	5.327	Pound
Milk, reduced fat[b]	0.98261	0.818	Quart
Milk, whole[b]	0.98261	0.858	Quart
Milk, lactose-free[b]	0.98261	1.631	Quart
Soy beverage[b]	1.02499	1.819	Quart
Yogurt[b]	0.99596[c]	3.219	Quart
Breakfast cereal (current)[e]	1.00602	0.214	Ounce
Breakfast cereal (revised)[f]	1.00602	0.233	Ounce
Corn tortillas[b]	1.00369[c]	2.264	24 oz
Oatmeal[b]	1.00369[c]	4.143	24 oz
Whole wheat bread (current)[b]	1.00608	2.354	16 oz
Whole wheat bread (revised)[b,f]	1.00369[c]	2.650	24 oz
Eggs	1.15757	2.169	Dozen
Fish, canned[b,g]	1.01228	0.202	Ounce
Calculated Food Package Composites			
Infant formula[h]		0.066	Prepared fl oz, postrebate
Infant food, meat (revised)[i]		0.353	Ounce
Legumes and peanut butter[j]			
Food packages IV-A, IV-B, V, VI and VII (current)		2.370	Per one allotment[k]
Food packages IV-A and IV-B (revised)		2.434	Per one allotment[k]

continued

TABLE U-16 Continued

Food Package Item	Item-Specific Inflation Rate[a]	FY2015 Price	Unit
Food packages V-A, V-B, VI, and VII (revised)		2.483	Per one allotment[k]
Milk[l]			
Food package IV-A (current)		1.189	Quart
Food package IV-B (current)		1.164	Quart
Food package V (current)		1.076	Quart
Food package VI (current)		1.164	Quart
Food package VII (current)		1.065	Quart
Food package IV-A (revised)		1.294	Quart
Food package IV-B (revised)		1.195	Quart
Food package V-A, V-B, and VI (revised)		1.151	Quart
Food package VII (revised)		1.164	Quart
Whole wheat bread (revised)[m]		2.667	24 oz

[a] Item-specific inflation rates were calculated using the U.S. Bureau of Labor Statistics Consumer Price Index (CPI). The selected CPI was matched to the closest food category for each food package item. The inflation rate was calculated by dividing the average of the item-specific CPI for FY2015 by the average of the item-specific CPI for the time period encompassed by the estimated price. Unless otherwise noted, the time period encompassed by the estimated price being inflated is August 2013 through July 2014. Values greater than 1 indicate FY2015 prices increased; values less than 1 indicate prices decreased.

[b] Item was used to calculate a composite price listed in the lower portion of the table.

[c] Price data were drawn from the IRI Consumer Network database. The inflation rate was calculated by dividing the average of the item-specific CPI for FY2015 by the average of the item-specific CPI from January through December 2014.

[d] In the current food packages, cheese is prescribed to food package VII recipients as a separate item. In both the current and revised food packages, cheese is offered as a substitution option for milk. Cheese, therefore, is used as an individual item and in the calculated composites.

[e] In the current food packages, whole grain must be the primary ingredient in at least one-half of breakfast cereals authorized by the state agency. The price reflects the average price per ounce of all breakfast cereals purchased in the FNS redemption dataset.

[f] In the revised food packages, all breakfast cereals authorized by a state agency must adhere to the "whole grain-rich" criteria as outlined by USDA-FNS for the school lunch program. The price reflects the average price per ounce of all breakfast cereals described as "whole grain breakfast cereal" purchased in the FNS redemption dataset.

[g] Canned fish is prescribed as an individual food package item in the current food packages (food package VII) and the revised food packages (food packages IV–VII). Additionally, canned fish is offered as a substitution option for infant food meat in food package II-BF. Canned fish, therefore, is used as an individual item and in a calculated composite.

[h] Weights were derived from the 2014 Food Package Report (USDA/FNS, 2016a): 0.78 (powdered), 0.12 (liquid concentrate), and 0.10 (ready-to-feed). All prices were based on prepared fl oz of each infant formula type.

TABLE U-16 Continued

[i] Weights used to calculate the composite were 0.75 for infant food meat and 0.25 for canned fish.

[j] Weighting schemes are presented in Table U-12.

[k] An "allotment" corresponds to 1 lb of legumes, 64 oz of canned legumes, or 18 oz of peanut butter.

[l] Weighting schemes are presented in Table U-13.

[m] Weights used to calculate the composite were: 0.76 (whole wheat bread [revised]), 0.19 (corn tortillas), and 0.06 (oatmeal).

values were used through FY2017 of this analysis. The committee could not identify forecasts for the retail price of fresh vegetables and fruits that extended to FY2022. A forecast for 2017 projected a 1 to 2 percent relative change in price from FY2016 (USDA/ERS, 2016). Therefore, a relative change in average CPI of 1.5 percent was used for FY2018 through FY2022. The CPI value assumptions and associated percent increase are summarized in Table U-18. The cost effect of using alternate baseline years for the CPI inflation values for the revised food packages are tested in the "Uncertainties" section of this analysis.

When the assessment year's CPI is divided by the baseline year value, it represents the percent increase relative to baseline. Because this percent is applied to the initial CVV value, larger CVVs will cross the $1 increment sooner than smaller CVVs. These differences become more pronounced

TABLE U-17 Inflation Assumptions for Food Package Items Prescribed as a Fixed Quantity, FY2016–FY2022

Year	Thrifty Food Plan (inflation rate)[a]
FY2016[b]	1.026
FY2017[b]	1.020
FY2018	1.020
FY2019	1.021
FY2020	1.021
FY2021	1.023
FY2022	1.023

NOTES: The base year of this analysis is FY2015.

[a] Rate is relative to the fiscal year preceding it. Prices for FY2016, for example, were projected to be 2.6 percent higher than in FY2015.

[b] Year not included in the cost estimates presented in this RIA, but it was necessary to arrive at price estimates for FY2018 through FY2022.

SOURCE: CBO, 2015.

TABLE U-18 Consumer Price Index for Fresh Vegetables and Fruits: Assumptions for Inflating the CVV for Current and Revised Food Packages

Year	CPI for Fresh Fruits and Vegetables	Change Relative to Baseline CPI Value, Inflation Rate	
		Current[a]	Revised[b]
FY2015[c]	332.5[d]	1.093	NA
FY2016[c]	340.0[d]	1.117	NA
FY2017[c]	341.1[d]	1.121	NA
FY2018	346.2[e]	1.138	0[f]
FY2019	351.4[e]	1.155	1.015
FY2020	356.6[e]	1.172	1.030
FY2021	362.0[e]	1.190	1.046
FY2022	367.4[e]	1.207	1.061

NOTES: CPI = Consumer Price Index; NA = not applicable.

[a] The baseline CPI value is 304.3 and is assigned to FY2008.

[b] The baseline CPI value is 346.2 and is assigned to FY2018.

[c] Year not included in the cost estimates presented in this RIA, but was necessary to arrive at CVV inflation estimates for FY2018 through FY2022.

[d] Actual values based on available CPI values.

[e] Projected CPI values, based on a 1.5 percent relative increase in CPI each fiscal year.

[f] Baseline value under the proposed revisions.

with higher CVV values. Given this, in this analysis, the CVVs that are issued as substitution options (i.e., half of infant food vegetables and fruits for a $10 CVV; all infant food vegetables and fruits for a $20 CVV; all juice for $3 CVV) are not added to the participant's CVV value, but are instead inflated separately. Table U-19 presents the effect of the CPI projections on the CVVs for the current and revised food packages.

UNCERTAINTIES

The estimated costs of the current food packages and proposed revised food packages are sensitive to key assumptions made in the preceding sections. The cost implications of several of these assumptions are tested below. The uncertainty scenarios specifically evaluate changing one or multiple assumptions about the revised food package and evaluating the cost effects. The "*primary analysis*" refers to the assumptions, food costs, and cost differences presented in the preceding sections of this appendix. "*Base assumption*" refers to the specific assumption(s) used in the primary analysis.

TABLE U-19 Projected Incremental Increases in Cash Value Vouchers for the Current and Revised Food Packages

	CVV Values, as Prescribed to WIC Participants								
	Current		Revised						
Year	Initial Value, \$8[a]	Initial Value, \$10[b]	Initial Value, \$3[c]	Initial Value, \$10[d]	Initial Value, \$12[e]	Initial Value, \$15[f]	Initial Value, \$20[g]	Initial Value, \$25[h]	Initial Value, \$35[i]
FY2015[j]	\$8[k]	\$10[k]							
FY2016[j]	\$8[k]	\$11[k]							
FY2017[j]	\$8[k]	\$11[k]							
FY2018	\$9	\$11	\$3	\$10	\$12	\$15	\$20	\$25	\$35
FY2019	\$9	\$11	\$3	\$10	\$12	\$15	\$20	\$25	\$35
FY2020	\$9	\$11	\$3	\$10	\$12	\$15	\$20	\$25	\$36
FY2021	\$9	\$11	\$3	\$10	\$12	\$15	\$20	\$26	\$36
FY2022	\$9	\$12	\$3	\$10	\$12	\$15	\$21	\$26	\$37

NOTES: Under current WIC regulations (7 C.F.R. §246.16), the CVV inflates based on an annual average CPI value, as compared to a baseline CPI value. WIC participants, however, do not receive an increase in CVV until the inflated value exceeds a dollar increment. The CVV values in the table are inflated based on projected changes in average CPI values presented in Table U-16 and establishing FY2018 as the new baseline year under the proposed revisions. No values are presented for FY2015 through FY2017 under the proposed revisions because the changes are not anticipated to be implemented until FY2018. CPI = Consumer Price Index; CVV = cash value voucher.

[a] Initial values of the CVV prescribed to food packages IV-A and IV-B in the current food packages.
[b] Initial values of the CVV prescribed to food packages V, VI, and VII in the current food packages.
[c] Initial values of the CVV prescribed when substituted for juice under the proposed revisions.
[d] Initial values of the CVV prescribed when substituted for half of jarred infant food vegetables and fruits under the proposed revisions.
[e] Initial values of the CVV prescribed to food packages IV-A and IV-B under the proposed revisions.
[f] Initial values of the CVV prescribed to food packages V-A and VI under the proposed revisions.
[g] Initial values of the CVV prescribed when substituted for all jarred infant food vegetables and fruits under the proposed revisions.
[h] Initial values of the CVV prescribed to food packages V-B under the proposed revisions.
[i] Initial values of the CVV prescribed to food packages VII under the proposed revisions.
[j] Year not included in the cost estimates presented in this RIA, but was necessary to arrive at CVV inflation estimates for FY2018 through FY2022.
[k] Inflation is based on actual CPI data.

For each uncertainty scenario tested, the phased-in cost differences are presented. The phased-in cost differences presented for each assumption scenario (i.e., base assumption, each uncertainty scenario) indicate that the cost effect as it relates to the current food packages. Negative values (–) indicate that the specific scenario costs less than the current food packages, while a positive value (+) indicates the specific scenario costs more than the current food packages. The cost differences between the base assumption and each uncertainty scenario are also presented. These describe how much the base assumption costs or saves, as compared to the tested uncertainty scenario. For these differences, a negative value (–) indicates that the base assumption used in the primary analysis costs less than the uncertainty scenario; a positive value (+) indicates that the base assumption costs more than the uncertainty scenario.

The cost differences presented in this section must be considered in context of estimated overall food costs of the current and revised food packages. Over the course of FY2018 through FY2022, the food packages in this analysis are projected to cost approximately $17 billion, averaging to approximately $3.9 billion per year, both under the current and revised food packages.

Assumptions About the CVV

The CVVs are estimated to cost approximately $780 million more in the revised food packages as compared to the CVVs in the current food packages. The proposed revisions allow for a CVV to be a substitution options for juice and jarred infant food vegetables and fruits. Given the CVV's increased prominence in the revised food packages, it is paramount to evaluate different aspects of the assumptions underlying the primary cost analysis.

Different CVV Redemption Projections Under the Proposed Revisions

In the primary analysis, CVV redemption was estimated to be 77.2 percent in the current food packages and 75.0 percent in the revised food packages The cost implications of two alternative redemption scenarios are presented in Table U-20. Scenario 1 shows that increasing the redemption assumption to 85 percent for the revised food packages would result in the estimated $220.4 million savings projected in the primary analysis becoming $135.1 million in additional costs, as compared to the current food packages ($355.5 million in additional costs as compared to the base assumption). Similarly, scenario 2 shows that lower redemption of the revised CVV (65 percent redemption) results in an additional $355.5 million savings from FY2018 through FY2022, as compared to the base

TABLE U-20 Projected Phased-in Cost Difference of WIC Food Package Revisions, Increase or Decrease in Redemption Assumption of Cash Value Voucher

Scenario	CVV Assumption, Percent Redeemed	Phased-in Cost Differences of the Revised Food Packages Compared to Current Food Packages ($, millions)[a]					
		FY2018	FY2019	FY2020	FY2021	FY2022	Total Cost Difference, FY2018 Through FY2022
Base assumption[b]	75	–6.4	–14.8	–47.7	–65.0	–86.6	–220.4
Uncertainty scenario 1[b]	85	+10.2	+18.8	+53.4	+37.0	+15.8	+135.1
Cost difference of base assumption as compared to uncertainty scenario 1[c]		**–16.6**	**–33.6**	**–101.1**	**–101.9**	**–102.3**	**–355.5**
Base assumption[b]	75	–6.4	–14.8	–47.7	–65.0	–86.6	–220.4
Uncertainty scenario 2[b]	65	–23.0	–48.4	–148.8	–166.9	–188.9	–575.9
Cost difference of base assumption as compared to uncertainty scenario 2[c]		**+16.6**	**+33.6**	**+101.1**	**+101.9**	**+102.3**	**+355.5**

NOTES: This table shows the phased-in cost difference between the revised and current food packages, along with the cost differences between different redemption assumptions for the revised CVV (85 and 65 percent redemption) and the current food packages. The primary analysis of the RIA assumes 75 percent redemption of the revised CVVs. All other assumptions in the primary analysis remain constant. Column and row totals may not be exact owing to independent rounding. CVV = cash value voucher.

[a] Phased-in estimates assume full implementation of the proposed revisions in state agencies serving one-third of all WIC participants as of April 1, 2018. All other state agencies are assumed to implement the proposed revisions as of FY2020.

[b] Describes the increases or savings of the base assumption or uncertainty scenario ("assumption scenario") as compared to the current food packages. Negative values (–) indicate that the assumption scenario costs less than the current food packages. Positive values (+) indicate that the assumption scenario costs more than the current food packages.

[c] Describes the increases or savings of the base assumption as compared to the uncertainty scenario. Negative values (–) indicate that the base assumption costs less than the uncertainty assumption. Positive values (+) indicate that the base assumption costs more than the uncertainty scenario.

assumptions in the primary analysis. This lower redemption assumption for the CVVs in the revised food packages results in a total cost savings of approximately $580 million over the course of FY2018 through FY2022, as compared to the current food packages.

Different CPI Inflation Scenarios

The CVV inflation rate depends on the baseline CPI value to which all subsequent years are compared. In the primary analysis, actual inflation rates were available through FY2017; values thereafter are projections. The CPI value assigned to FY2018 has significant implications, as it is expected to serve as the new CVV inflation baseline for the revised food packages. Based on Economic Research Service forecast (USDA/ERS, 2016), the committee estimated a 1.5 percent relative change in average CPI from FY2017 to FY2018 and in each year thereafter.

Table U-21 presents the cost differences of changing these assumptions about relative change in CPI values.[20] In scenario 1, a higher relative change in just FY2018 (relative increase of 5 percent rather than 1.5 percent) leads to an additional $34.1 million in savings from FY2018 through FY2022, resulting in an estimated total cost savings of $255 million, as compared to the current food packages. When the base assumption inflation rate is maintained for FY2018, but increased to 5.0 percent in all subsequent years (scenario 2), the proposed revisions would decrease cost savings by $42.6 million over FY2018 through FY2022. Scenario 3 assumes a 5.0 percent inflation rate across all years, which would cost $19.8 million more than the total phased-in cost estimate of the primary analysis. In contrast, a 5.0 percent deflation from FY2017 to FY2018 followed by inflation of 1.5 percent in each subsequent year (scenario 4) would cost an additional $130 million compared to the base assumptions in the primary analysis, over the course of FY2018 through FY2022. Finally, when the initial deflation assumption is followed by a higher relative inflation rate (5 percent rather than 1.5 percent; scenario 5), the total costs are approximately $229 million more than the total costs of the base assumptions for the revised food packages. This is the only tested CPI inflation scenario that results in the proposed revisions costing more than the current food packages during FY2018 through FY2022.

Another CPI inflation scenario assumption is the baseline year to which all subsequent years are compared in the revised food packages. Table U-22 explores the cost differences associated with different CPI base years for the revised food packages. In scenario 1, changing the base year to inflate the

[20] The CPI values presented in this section are relative to the immediately preceding year. Increasing or decreasing the CPI value in one year effects all subsequent years.

revised CVV FY2015 would cost an additional $128 million over FY2018 through FY2022, as compared to using FY2018 as the base year. Both scenarios 2 and 3 demonstrate that there are relatively small costs effects of selecting either FY2016 or FY2017 as the base year for CVV inflation in the revised food packages.

Different Levels of Substitution for CVV

Under the proposed revisions, food package II recipients can receive a $10 ("partial substitution") or a $20 ("full substitution") CVV in lieu of the 64 ounces and 128 ounces of jarred infant food vegetables and fruits, respectively. To maintain cost neutrality, the committee selected the dollar value of the CVVs based on estimated FY2015 prices of jarred infant food vegetables and fruits. The base assumptions in the primary analysis, however, project slightly higher redemption of CVVs compared to jarred infant food vegetables and fruits. Furthermore, jarred infant food vegetables and fruits inflate differently than the CVV. While jarred infant food vegetables and fruits are projected to progressively inflate between FY2018 and FY2022, the CVV value prescribed to participants does not adjust until FY2022, when the $20 CVV inflates to $21.

The base assumption in the primary analysis is that 0 percent of participants select the CVV substitution option. Table U-23 summarizes the cost effects of different levels of partial and full substitution of jarred infant food vegetables and fruits. Given the redemption and inflation assumptions, substitutions of jarred infant food vegetables and fruits with CVVs initially cost slightly more but eventually lead to additional cost savings beginning in FY2020. The net cost effect of substitution for CVVs in food package II are $5.1 million (scenario 1, 50 percent of infants selecting partial substitution) to $11.4 million (scenario 4, 100 percent selecting full substitution) of additional savings, as compared to the base assumption of no substitution in the revised food packages.

Under the proposed revisions, a $3 CVV can be substituted for the 64 ounces of juice prescribed in children's and women's food packages. The CVV amount was the closest dollar increment to the estimated cost of 64 fluid ounces of juice based on FY2015 prices, which was estimated to be $3.15. In contrast to jarred infant food vegetables and fruits, the redemption rate of juice is projected to be slightly higher than the overall redemption rate of the CVV. The cumulative effect of the slightly lower price and projected redemption means that, under the assumptions of the analysis, substituting a CVV for the juice prescription would lead to increased cost savings (see Table U-24).

TABLE U-21 Projected Phased-in Cost Difference of WIC Food Package Revisions, Assuming Different Consumer Price Index Inflation Rates Used to Inflate the Revised CVV

	Relative Change in CPI Used to Inflate Revised CVV Assumptions, Inflation Rate[a]					Phased-in Cost Differences of the Revised Food Packages Compared to Current Food Packages ($, millions)[b]					
Scenario	FY2018	FY2019	FY2020	FY2021	FY2022	FY2018	FY2019	FY2020	FY2021	FY2022	Total Difference, FY2018 Through FY2022
Base assumption[c]	1.015	1.015	1.015	1.015	1.015	-6.4	-14.8	-47.7	-65.0	-86.6	-220.4
Uncertainty scenario 1[c]	1.050	1.015	1.015	1.015	1.015	-6.4	-14.8	-64.7	-82.0	-86.6	-254.5
Cost difference of base assumption as compared to uncertainty scenario 1[d]						**0.0**	**0.0**	**+17.0**	**+17.1**	**0.0**	**+34.1**
Base assumption[c]	1.015	1.015	1.015	1.015	1.015	-6.4	-14.8	-47.7	-65.0	-86.6	-220.4
Uncertainty scenario 2[c]	1.015	1.050	1.050	1.050	1.050	-6.4	-13.6	-45.8	-62.3	-49.8	-177.9
Cost difference of base assumption as compared to uncertainty scenario 2[d]						**0.0**	**-1.2**	**-1.9**	**-2.7**	**-36.8**	**-42.6**
Base assumption[c]	1.015	1.015	1.015	1.015	1.015	-6.4	-14.8	-47.7	-65.0	-86.6	-220.4
Uncertainty scenario 3[c]	1.050	1.050	1.050	1.050	1.050	-6.4	-19.3	-45.8	-62.3	-66.8	-200.6
Cost difference of base assumption as compared to uncertainty scenario 3[d]						**0.0**	**4.5**	**-1.9**	**-2.7**	**-19.7**	**-19.8**

Base assumption[c]	1.015	1.015	1.015	1.015	1.015	−6.4	−14.8	−47.7	−65.0	−86.6	−220.4
Uncertainty scenario 4[c]	0.950	1.015	1.015	1.015	1.015	−0.1	−2.0	+7.9	−26.4	−69.5	−90.1
Cost difference of base assumption as compared to uncertainty scenario 4[d]						**−6.3**	**−12.8**	**−55.6**	**−38.6**	**−17.1**	**−130.4**
Base assumption[c]	1.015	1.015	1.015	1.015	1.015	−6.4	−14.8	−47.7	−65.0	−86.6	−220.4
Uncertainty scenario 5[c]	0.950	1.050	1.050	1.050	1.050	−0.1	−0.8	+9.8	−6.7	+5.9	+8.2
Cost difference of base assumption as compared to uncertainty scenario 5[d]						**−6.3**	**−14.0**	**−57.5**	**−58.3**	**−92.5**	**−228.6**

NOTES: This table shows the phased-in cost difference between the revised and current food packages, along with the cost differences between different CVV CPI inflation assumptions and the current food packages. The primary analysis of the RIA assumes that the CPI for fresh fruits and vegetables will increase 1.5 percent relative to each preceding year, from FY2018 through FY2022. The uncertainty scenarios test different relative change values and patterns of relative change. All other assumptions in the primary analysis remain constant. Column and row totals may not be exact owing to independent rounding. CPI = Consumer Price Index; CVV = cash value voucher.

[a] Inflation rates describe the relative change in prices compared to the preceding year. Values greater than 1 indicate prices increased; values less than 1 indicate prices decreased.

[b] Phased-in estimates assume full implementation of the proposed revisions in state agencies serving one-third of all WIC participants as of April 1, 2018. All other state agencies are assumed to implement the proposed revisions as of FY2020.

[c] Describes the increases or savings of the base assumption or uncertainty scenario ("assumption scenario") as compared to the current food packages. Negative values (–) indicate that the assumption scenario costs less than the current food packages. Positive values (+) indicate that the assumption scenario costs more than the current food packages.

[d] Describes the increases or savings of the base assumption as compared to the uncertainty scenario. Negative values (–) indicate that the base assumption costs less than the uncertainty assumption. Positive values (+) indicate that the base assumption costs more than the uncertainty scenario.

TABLE U-22 Projected Phased-in Cost Difference of WIC Food Package Revisions, Changing the Base Comparison Year for CVV Inflation

Scenario	Base Year for CVV Inflation in the Revised Food Packages	Phased-in Cost Differences of the Revised Food Packages Compared to Current Food Packages ($, millions)[a]					
		FY2018	FY2019	FY2020	FY2021	FY2022	Total Cost Difference, FY2018 Through FY2022
Base assumption[b]	FY2018	-6.4	-14.8	-47.7	-65.0	-86.6	-220.4
Uncertainty scenario 1[b]	FY2015	-5.8	-13.6	-31.1	-8.6	-32.4	-91.6
Cost difference of base assumption as compared to uncertainty scenario 1[c]		**-0.6**	**-1.2**	**-16.6**	**-56.4**	**-54.1**	**-128.8**
Base assumption[b]	FY2018	-6.4	-14.8	-47.7	-65.0	-86.6	-220.4
Uncertainty scenario 2[b]	FY2016	-6.4	-14.0	-46.5	-62.6	-72.3	-201.8
Cost difference of base assumption as compared to uncertainty scenario 2[c]		**0.0**	**-0.8**	**-1.2**	**-2.3**	**-14.3**	**-18.6**

Base assumption[b]	FY2018	-6.4	-14.8	-47.7	-65.0	-86.6	-220.4
Uncertainty scenario 3[b]	FY2017	-6.4	-14.0	-46.5	-62.6	-73.8	-203.4
Cost difference of base assumption as compared to uncertainty scenario 3[c]		**0.0**	**-0.8**	**-1.2**	**-2.3**	**-12.8**	**-17.1**

NOTES: This table shows the phased-in cost difference between the revised and current food packages, along with the cost differences between different base years for CVV inflation and the current food packages. The primary analysis of the RIA assumes that the base year of the CVV inflation is FY2018. All other assumptions in the primary analysis remain constant. Column and row totals may not be exact owing to independent rounding. CVV = cash value voucher.

[a] Phased-in estimates assume full implementation of the proposed revisions in state agencies serving one-third of all WIC participants as of April 1, 2018. All other state agencies are assumed to implement the proposed revisions as of FY2020.

[b] Describes the increases or savings of the base assumption or uncertainty scenario ("assumption scenario") as compared to the current food packages. Negative values (–) indicate that the assumption scenario costs less than the current food packages. Positive values (+) indicate that the assumption scenario costs more than the current food packages.

[c] Describes the increases or savings of the base assumption as compared to the uncertainty scenario. Negative values (–) indicate that the base assumption costs less than the uncertainty assumption. Positive values (+) indicate that the base assumption costs more than the uncertainty scenario.

TABLE U-23 Projected Phased-in Cost Difference of WIC Food Package Revisions, Changing Assumptions About Substitution of Cash Value Vouchers for Jarred Infant Food Vegetables and Fruits

Scenarios	Jarred Infant Food Vegetables and Fruit, Percent of Participants Substituting for CVV[a]	Phased-in Cost Differences of the Revised Food Packages Compared to Current Food Packages ($, millions)[b]					
		FY2018	FY2019	FY2020	FY2021	FY2022	Total Cost Difference, FY2018 Through FY2022
Base assumption[c]	0	–6.4	–14.8	–47.7	–65.0	–86.6	–220.4
Uncertainty scenario 1[c]	50 (partial)	–6.2	–14.7	–48.4	–66.8	–89.4	–225.6
Cost difference of base assumption as compared to uncertainty scenario 1[d]		**–0.2**	**–0.1**	**+0.7**	**+1.8**	**+2.9**	**+5.1**
Base assumption[c]	0	–6.4	–14.8	–47.7	–65.0	–86.6	–220.4
Uncertainty scenario 2[c]	100 (partial)	–6.0	–14.7	–49.1	–68.6	–92.3	–230.7
Cost difference of base assumption as compared to uncertainty scenario 2[d]		**–0.4**	**–0.1**	**+1.4**	**+3.6**	**+5.8**[e]	**+10.3**[e]
Base assumption[c]	0	–6.4	–14.8	–47.7	–65.0	–86.6	–220.4
Uncertainty scenario 3[c]	50 (full)	–6.0	–14.7	–49.1	–68.6	–87.8	–226.1
Cost difference of base assumption as compared to uncertainty scenario 3[d]		**–0.4**	**–0.1**	**+1.4**	**+3.6**	**+1.2**[e]	**+5.7**[e]
Base assumption[c]	0	–6.4	–14.8	–47.7	–65.0	–86.6	–220.4
Uncertainty scenario 4[c]	100 (full)	–5.7	–14.5	–50.6	–72.1	–89.0	–231.8
Cost difference of base assumption as compared to uncertainty scenario 4[d]		**–0.8**	**–0.3**	**+2.9**	**+7.2**	**+2.4**	**+11.4**

Base assumption[c]	0	−6.4	−14.8	−47.7	−65.0	−86.6	−220.4
Uncertainty scenario 5[c]	25 (partial), 25 (full)	−6.1	−14.7	−48.8	−67.7	−88.6	−225.8
Cost difference of base assumption as compared to uncertainty scenario 5[d]		**−0.3**	**−0.1**	**+1.1**	**+2.7**	**+2.0**	**+5.4**

NOTES: This table shows the phased-in cost difference between the revised and current food packages, along with the cost differences of different assumptions regarding jarred infant food vegetables and fruits substitution for CVV. All other assumptions in the primary analysis remain constant. Column and row totals may not be exact owing to independent rounding. CVV = cash value voucher.

[a] Under the proposed revisions, 64 oz of jarred infant food vegetables and fruits can be substituted for a $10 CVV ("partial") and all 128 oz can be substituted for a $20 CVV ("full"). Values in the column correspond to the percent of food package II recipients that choose to be prescribed a CVV instead of the jarred infant food vegetables and fruits.

[b] Phased-in estimates assume full implementation of the proposed revisions in state agencies serving one-third of all WIC participants as of April 1, 2018. All other state agencies are assumed to implement the proposed revisions as of FY2020.

[c] Describes the increases or savings of the base assumption or uncertainty scenario ("assumption scenario") as compared to the current food packages. Negative values (–) indicate that the assumption scenario costs less than the current food packages. Positive values (+) indicate that the assumption scenario costs more than the current food packages.

[d] Describes the increases or savings of the base assumption as compared to the uncertainty scenario. Negative values (–) indicate that the base assumption costs less than the uncertainty assumption. Positive values (+) indicate that the base assumption costs more than the uncertainty scenario.

[e] Cost differences for 100 percent of food package II recipients opting for partial substitution and cost difference for 50 percent of food package II recipients opting for full substitution are not identical because of CVV inflation assumptions. The $20 CVV prescribed to recipients opting for full substitution is projected to inflate in FY2022 to a level in which the value prescribed would increase to $21. The $10 CVV is not projected to inflate to $11 during this time period.

TABLE U-24 Projected Phased-in Cost Difference of WIC Food Package Revisions, Changing Assumptions About Substitution of Cash Value Vouchers for Juice

Scenario	Juice, Percent of Participants Substituting for CVV[a]	Phased-in Cost Differences of the Revised Food Packages Compared to Current Food Packages ($, millions)[b]					
		FY2018	FY2019	FY2020	FY2021	FY2022	Total Cost Difference, FY2018 Through FY2022
Base assumption[c]	0	-6.4	-14.8	-47.7	-65.0	-86.6	-220.4
Uncertainty scenario 1[c]	50	-8.4	-19.5	-63.6	-83.0	-106.7	-281.2
Cost difference of base assumption as compared to uncertainty scenario 1[d]		**+2.0**	**+4.7**	**+15.9**	**+18.1**	**+20.2**	**+60.8**
Base assumption[c]	0	-6.4	-14.8	-47.7	-65.0	-86.6	-220.4
Uncertainty scenario 2[c]	100	-10.5	-24.2	-79.5	-101.1	-126.9	-342.1
Cost difference of base assumption as compared to uncertainty scenario 2[d]		**+4.1**	**+9.4**	**+31.8**	**+36.1**	**+40.3**	**+121.6**

NOTES: This table shows the phased-in cost difference between the revised and current food packages, along with the cost differences of different assumptions regarding jarred infant food vegetables and fruits substitution for CVV. All other assumptions in the primary analysis remain constant. Column and row totals may not be exact owing to independent rounding. CVV = cash value voucher.

[a] Under the proposed revisions, 64 fl oz of juice prescribed to women and children can be substituted for a $3 CVV. Values in the column correspond to the percent of women and children that choose to be prescribed a CVV instead of the juice.

[b] Phased-in estimates assume full implementation of the proposed revisions in state agencies serving one-third of all WIC participants as of April 1, 2018. All other state agencies are assumed to implement the proposed revisions as of FY2020.

[c] Describes the increases or savings of the base assumption or uncertainty scenario ("assumption scenario") as compared to the current food packages. Negative values (–) indicate that the assumption scenario costs less than the current food packages. Positive values (+) indicate that the assumption scenario costs more than the current food packages.

[d] Describes the increases or savings of the base assumption as compared to the uncertainty scenario. Negative values (–) indicate that the base assumption costs less than the uncertainty assumption. Positive values (+) indicate that the base assumption costs more than the uncertainty scenario.

Assumptions About Use of "Up to" Amounts

The primary analysis assumes that infant formula prescription practices will remain unchanged between the current and revised food packages. Table U-25 projects the cost effects of different formula prescription practices for the revised food packages. In Scenario 1, prescribing all infants in food package I-BF/FF-A the maximum "up to" amount of infant formula would result in approximately $20 million in additional costs in the revised food packages, over the course of FY2018 through FY2022, as compared to the base assumption used in the primary analysis. The revised food packages would still be projected to cost approximately $201 million less than the current food packages, over the course of FY2018 through FY2022. In contrast, if the average amount of infant formula prescribed across all food packages was 95 percent of the maximum "up to" amount for each food package (scenario 2), the total cost savings of the revised food packages would increase by $145 million over the course of the FY2018 through FY2022, as compared to the base assumption used in the primary analysis. This would result in an estimated $366 million in total savings as compared to the current food packages.

Assumptions About Shifts in Fully Formula-Fed Dyads

A key assumption of the primary analysis is that, under the proposed revisions, 5 percent of fully formula-fed mother–infant dyads will shift to corresponding fully (mostly) breastfeeding food packages. The committee considered the 5 percent shift conservative, given evidence that the 2009 food package, which allowed women to either choose between formula-feeding or fully breastfeeding in the infant's first month of life, resulted in an approximately 7 to 11 percent shift of dyads from breastfeeding to formula-feeding (USDA/FNS, 2011).

Table U-26 presents the cost effect of this assumption. The cost differences only affect FY2021 and FY2022, because the base assumption is that the shift would occur 1 year after full implementation in all state agencies under the phased-in implementation scheme. Assuming no shift in participants in the revised food packages (scenario 1) would cost approximately $25 million more over the course of FY2018 through FY2022, as compared to the assumption of a 5 percent shift. A 3 percent shift of participants would decrease estimated total cost savings by $9.9 million (scenario 2), while an 8 percent shift would increase estimated total cost savings by $14.8 million (scenario 3), as compared to the base assumption in the primary analysis. If the shift only occurs for infants less than 6 months old and women less than 6 months postpartum, the estimated total cost savings of

TABLE U-25 Projected Phased-in Cost Difference of WIC Food Package Revisions, Changing the Maximum Amount of Formula in Food Packages I and II

Scenario	Maximum Formula Assumption, Amount Change	Phased-in Cost Differences of the Revised Food Packages Compared to Current Rule ($, millions)[a]					
		FY2018	FY2019	FY2020	FY2021	FY2022	Total Cost Difference, FY2018 Through FY2022
Base assumption[c]	Identical to Current Food Package[b]	-6.4	-14.8	-47.7	-65.0	-86.6	-220.4
Uncertainty scenario 1[c]	All I-BF/FF-A recipients prescribed maximum "up to" amount	-5.6	-13.1	-42.6	-58.8	-80.3	-200.5
Cost difference of base assumption as compared to uncertainty scenario 1[d]		**-0.8**	**-1.6**	**-5.1**	**-6.1**	**-6.3**	**-19.9**
Base assumption[c]	Identical to Current Food Package[b]	-6.4	-14.8	-47.7	-65.0	-86.6	-220.4
Uncertainty scenario 2[c]	95% of maximum "up to" amounts	-13.0	-28.5	-89.6	-105.9	-128.5	-365.5
Cost difference of base assumption as compared to uncertainty scenario 2[d]		**+6.6**	**+13.7**	**+41.9**	**+41.0**	**+41.9**	**+145.1**

NOTES: This table shows the phased-in cost difference between the proposed revisions and the current rule, along with the cost differences of different assumptions regarding the maximum amount of formula in food packages I and II. All other assumptions in the primary analysis remain constant. Column and row totals may not be exact owing to independent rounding.

[a] Phased-in estimates assume full implementation of the proposed revisions in state agencies serving one-third of all WIC participants as of April 1, 2018. All other state agencies are assumed to implement the proposed revisions as of FY2020.

[b] Base assumptions for maximum formula under the proposed revisions are as follows: I-BF/FF-A (104 fl oz), I-BF/FF-B (424 fl oz), I-BF/FF-C (510 fl oz), I-FF-A (861 fl oz), I-FF-B (948 fl oz), II-BF/FF (371 fl oz), II-FF (683 fl oz). The formula amounts are the weighted average of the monthly maximum allowances across the different forms of infant formula. The base assumption is that the quantity of formula prescribed will remain unchanged.

[c] Describes the increases or savings of the base assumption or uncertainty scenario ("assumption scenario") as compared to the current food packages. Negative values (–) indicate that the assumption scenario costs less than the current food packages. Positive values (+) indicate that the assumption scenario costs more than the current food packages.

[d] Describes the increases or savings of the base assumption as compared to the uncertainty scenario. Negative values (–) indicate that the base assumption costs less (provides more savings) than the uncertainty assumption. Positive values (+) indicate that the base assumption costs more than the uncertainty scenario.

TABLE U-26 Projected Phased-in Cost Difference of WIC Food Package Revisions, Changing Assumptions About Percent of Fully Formula-Fed Dyads Shift to Partially (Mostly) Breastfed Food Packages

Scenario	Dyadic Shift Assumption, Percent of Fully Formula-Fed Projected to Shift[a]	Phased-in Cost Differences of the Revised Food Packages Compared to Current Food Packages ($, millions)[b]					
		FY2018	FY2019	FY2020	FY2021	FY2022	Total Cost Difference, FY2018 Through FY2022
Base assumption[c]	5	–6.4	–14.8	–47.7	–65.0	–86.6	–220.4
Uncertainty scenario 1[c]	0	–6.4	–14.8	–47.7	–52.8	–74.0	–195.7
Cost difference of base assumption as compared to uncertainty scenario 1[d]		**0.0**	**0.0**	**0.0**	**–12.1**	**–12.5**	**–24.7**
Base assumption[c]	5	–6.4	–14.8	–47.7	–65.0	–86.6	–220.4
Uncertainty scenario 2[c]	3	–6.4	–14.8	–47.7	–60.1	–81.5	–210.6
Cost difference of base assumption as compared to uncertainty scenario 2[d]		**0.0**	**0.0**	**0.0**	**–4.9**	**–5.0**	**–9.9**
Base assumption[c]	5	–6.4	–14.8	–47.7	–65.0	–86.6	–220.4
Uncertainty scenario 3[c]	8	–6.4	–14.8	–47.7	–72.2	–94.1	–235.2
Cost difference of base assumption as compared to uncertainty scenario 3[d]		**0.0**	**0.0**	**0.0**	**+7.3**	**+7.5**	**+14.8**

Base assumption[c]	5	–6.4	–14.8	–47.7	–65.0	–86.6	–220.4
Uncertainty scenario 4[c]	5 (only dyads <6-months postpartum)[d]	–6.4	–14.8	–47.7	–57.5	–78.9	–205.30
Cost difference of base assumption as compared to uncertainty scenario 4[d]		**0.0**	**0.0**	**0.0**	**–7.5**	**–7.7**	**–15.1**

NOTES: This table shows the phased-in cost difference between the revised and current food packages, along with the cost differences of different assumptions regarding the percent of fully formula-fed mother–infant dyads shifting to partially (mostly) breastfeeding food packages. All other assumptions in the primary analysis remain constant. Column and row totals may not be exact owing to independent rounding.

[a] The shift describes the percent of participants prescribed food package I-FF-A, I-FF-B, II-FF, VI, and N/A shifting to corresponding partially (mostly) breastfeeding food packages. Approximately 21 and 79 percent of participants shifting from food package I-FF-A were assigned to food packages I-BF/FF-A and I-BF/FF-B, respectively. All women shifting from being classified as more than 6-months postpartum (i.e., food package N/A) were assigned to food package V-B. The shift is projected to occur in the year after full implementation of the proposed revisions (FY2021). The effect on participation is expected to be sustained but additional shifts are not projected in subsequent years.

[b] Phased-in estimates assume full implementation of the proposed revisions in state agencies serving one-third of all WIC participants as of April 1, 2018. All other state agencies are assumed to implement the proposed revisions as of FY2020.

[c] Describes the increases or savings of the base assumption or uncertainty scenario ("assumption scenario") as compared to the current food packages. Negative values (–) indicate that the assumption scenario costs less than the current food packages. Positive values (+) indicate that the assumption scenario costs more than the current food packages.

[d] Describes the increases or savings of the base assumption as compared to the uncertainty scenario. Negative values (–) indicate that the base assumption costs less (provides more savings) than the uncertainty assumption. Positive values (+) indicate that the base assumption costs more than the uncertainty scenario.

the revised food packages would decrease by $15.1 million over the course of FY2018 through FY2022, as compared to the base assumption.

Assumption About Milk Redemption

Milk and its associated substitutions and allowable options play a key role in the projected differences between the revised and current food packages. Under the proposed revisions, the projected redemption for milk increased by varying degrees because of different initial redemption estimates, the increase in the amount of yogurt allowed as a substitution, the reduction in the amount prescribed (excluding food package VI), and substitution options that eliminate the dangling quart of milk. Table U-27 evaluates the cost implications of increases and decreases in projected milk redemption. If the projected redemption rates were each underestimated by 5 percentage points (scenario 1), the proposed revisions would cost $21.8 million more than the current food packages over the course of FY2018 through FY2022. In contrast, lower redemptions of milk would lead to greater cost savings under the proposed revisions (scenarios 2 and 3).

ALTERNATIVES

The committee considered several alternatives to current food package items and amounts that were ultimately rejected. Some of these alternatives and the committee's rationale for not including them in the revised food packages are outlined in the sections that follow. As with the uncertainty scenarios, the "*primary analysis*" refers to the set of base assumptions that led to a total phased-in cost savings of $220 million for the revised food packages as compared to the current food packages, over the course of FY2018 through FY2022.

For each alternative tested, the phased-in cost differences are presented. The phased-in cost differences presented for each scenario (i.e., base assumption, each alternative) indicate the cost effect as it relates to the current food packages. Negative values (–) indicate the specific scenario costs less than the current food packages, while a positive value (+) indicates the specific scenario costs more than the current food packages. The cost difference between the base assumption and the alternative are also presented. These describe how much the base assumption costs or saves, as compared to the tested alternative. For these differences, a negative value (–) indicates the base assumption used in the primary analysis costs less than the alternative; a positive value (+) indicates the base assumption costs more than the alternative. This section presents select alternatives tested by the committee.

More Canned Fish

To support the DGA's recommendation to increase seafood intake, the committee proposes adding canned fish to all children's and women's food packages and offering it as a substitution option for jarred infant food meat. To maintain cost neutrality and create incentives for partially (mostly) and fully breastfeeding women, different quantities and rotation patterns were created for canned fish. The amount prescribed in food packages IV-A, IV-B, V-A, and VI are relatively low compared to the DGA recommended intake. Table U-28 shows the cost effects of prescribing additional canned fish to these food packages. Increasing the prescribed amount to 20 ounces every 3 months for these food packages (alternative 1) costs approximately $122 million more than the base assumption. Alternative 1 would be considered cost neutral from FY2018 through FY2022, as the total food package costs would be approximately $99 million less than the projected costs for the current food packages (from FY2018 through FY2022). However, the parameter of cost neutrality the committee was operating under was plus or minus $0.10 per-participant cost per month, based on FY2015 prices. When 20 ounces of canned fish every 3 months is used in this pricing scenario, the revised food packages would cost $0.37 more per-participant per month than the current food packages. Alternative 2 shows that 10 ounces per month in the food packages would cost approximately $23 million more than the current food packages.

Maintain the 16-Ounce Requirement for Whole Wheat Bread

Based on available data to the committee, the 16- to 24-ounce whole wheat bread and allowable options will cost more per ounce than the 16 ounces authorized in the current food packages. Allowing the range of sizes and simultaneously decreasing the total number of ounces prescribed to food package IV recipient helped the committee to arrive at a cost neutral food package. Table U-29 shows the cost implications of maintaining the current whole wheat bread regulations as they exist in the current food packages. This alternative would cost an estimated $154 million more than the base assumptions for the revised food packages. While keeping the 16-ounce requirement would be cost neutral compared to the current food packages (approximately $67 million less than the current food packages over the course of FY2018 through FY2022), the committee considered two factors as benefits that are anticipated to increase redemption: (1) the ease of shopping for participant with the range of authorized bread sizes, and (2) the expansion of stocking options for vendors.

TABLE U-27 Projected Phased-in Cost Difference of WIC Food Package Revisions, Changing Assumptions About Percent of Fully Formula-Fed Dyads Shift to Partially (Mostly) Breastfed Food Packages

Scenario	Milk Redemption Assumption, Percent Point Change[a]	Phased-in Cost Differences of the Revised Food Packages Compared to Current Food Packages ($, millions)[b]					
		FY2018	FY2019	FY2020	FY2021	FY2022	Total Cost Difference, FY2018 Through FY2022
Base assumption[c]	[d]	–6.4	–14.8	–47.7	–65.0	–86.6	–220.4
Uncertainty scenario 1[c]	+5	+4.3	+7.4	+20.4	+4.80	–15.1	+21.8
Cost difference of base assumption as compared to uncertainty scenario 1[e]		**–10.7**	**–22.2**	**–68.1**	**–69.8**	**–71.5**	**–242.2**
Base assumption[c]	[d]	–6.4	–14.8	–47.7	–65.0	–86.6	–220.4
Uncertainty scenario 2[c]	–5	–17.2	–37.0	–115.8	–134.7	–158.0	–462.7
Cost difference of base assumption as compared to uncertainty scenario 2[e]		**+10.7**	**+22.2**	**+68.1**	**+69.8**	**+71.4**	**+242.2**
Base assumption[c]	[d]	–6.4	–14.8	–47.7	–65.0	–86.6	–220.4
Uncertainty scenario 3[c]	–10	–27.9	–59.2	–183.9	–204.5	–229.4	–704.9
Cost difference of base assumption as compared to uncertainty scenario 3[e]		**+21.5**	**+44.4**	**+136.2**	**+139.5**	**+142.9**	**+484.5**

NOTES: This table shows the phased-in cost difference between the revised and current food packages, along with the cost differences of different assumptions regarding the redemption of milk and associated substitutions and allowable options. All other assumptions in the primary analysis remain constant. Column and row totals may not be exact owing to independent rounding.

[a] The term "milk" encompasses substitutions and allowable options, including cheese, yogurt, soy beverage, and tofu. The redemption assumptions are applied to the food package-specific milk composite price.

[b] Phased-in estimates assume full implementation of the proposed revisions in state agencies serving one-third of all WIC participants as of April 1, 2018. All other state agencies are assumed to implement the proposed revisions as of FY2020.

[c] Describes the increases or savings of the base assumption or uncertainty scenario ("assumption scenario") as compared to the current food packages. Negative values (–) indicate that the assumption scenario costs less than the current food packages. Positive values (+) indicate that the assumption scenario costs more than the current food packages.

[d] Base assumptions for the redemption rates of milk under the proposed revisions are as follows: IV-A (87.00 percent), IV-B (79.53 percent), V-A and V-B (65.61 percent), VI (58.54 percent) and VII (67.96 percent). All tested uncertainty scenarios added and subtracted a set value from each of the redemption rates.

[e] Describes the increases or savings of the base assumption as compared to the uncertainty scenario. Negative values (–) indicate that the base assumption costs less (provides more savings) than the uncertainty assumption. Positive values (+) indicate that the base assumption costs more than the uncertainty scenario.

TABLE U-28 Projected Phased-in Cost Difference of WIC Food Package Revisions, Prescribing Additional Fish to Food Packages IV-A, IV-B, V-A, and VI

Scenario	Quantity of Fish Prescribed to Food Packages IV-A, IV-B, V-A, and VI	Phased-in Cost Differences of the Revised Food Packages Compared to Current Food Packages ($, millions)[a]					
		FY2018	FY2019	FY2020	FY2021	FY2022	Total Cost Difference, FY2018 Through FY2022
Base assumption[b]	10 oz once every 3 months	–6.4	–14.8	–47.7	–65.0	–86.6	–220.4
Alternative 1[b]	20 oz once every 3 months	–1.0	–3.6	–13.4	–30.0	–50.8	–98.8
Cost difference of base assumption as compared to alternative 1[c]		**–5.4**	**–11.2**	**–34.3**	**–35.0**	**–35.8**	**–121.6**
Base assumption [b]	10 oz once every 3 months	–6.4	–14.8	–47.7	–65.0	–86.6	–220.4
Alternative 2[b]	10 oz per month	4.4	7.6	20.9	4.9	–15.0	22.8
Cost difference of base assumption as compared to alternative 2[c]		**–10.8**	**–22.4**	**–68.6**	**–69.9**	**–71.6**	**–243.2**

NOTES: This table shows the phased-in cost difference between the revised and current food packages, along with the cost differences of alternative quantities of canned fish prescribed to participants receiving food packages IV-A, IV-B, V-A, and VI. All other assumptions in the primary analysis remain constant. Column and row totals may not be exact owing to independent rounding.

[a] Phased-in estimates assume full implementation of the proposed revisions in state agencies serving one-third of all WIC participants as of April 1, 2018. All other state agencies are assumed to implement the proposed revisions as of FY2020.

[b] Describes the increases or savings of the base assumption or alternative as compared to the current food packages. Negative values (–) indicate that the base assumption or alternative costs less than the current food packages. Positive values (+) indicate that the base assumption or alternative costs more than the current food packages.

[c] Describes the increases or savings of the base assumption as compared to the alternative. Negative values (–) indicate that the base assumption costs less (provides more savings) than the uncertainty assumption. Positive values (+) indicate that the base assumption costs more than the uncertainty scenario.

TABLE U-29 Projected Phased-in Cost Difference of WIC Food Package Revisions, Maintaining the 16-Ounce Whole Wheat Bread Requirement

Scenario	Bread Prescription and Specification for Food Packages IV-A, IV-B, V-A, V-B, and VII	Phased-in Cost Differences of the Revised Food Packages Compared to Current Food Packages ($, millions)[a]					
		FY2018	FY2019	FY2020	FY2021	FY2022	Total Cost Difference, FY2018 Through FY2022
Base assumption[b]	All are prescribed 16–24 oz per month	−6.4	−14.8	−47.7	−65.0	−86.6	−220.4
Alternative[b]	Women are prescribed 16 oz per month; children are prescribed 32 oz (two 16 oz) per month	+0.4	−0.7	−4.3	−20.7	−41.3	−66.5
Cost difference of base assumption as compared to alternative[c]		**−6.8**	**−14.2**	**−43.4**	**−44.3**	**−45.3**	**−153.9**

NOTES: This table shows the phased-in cost difference between the revised and current food packages, along with the cost differences of alternative quantities of whole wheat bread prescribed to participants receiving food packages IV-A, IV-B, V-A, V-B and VII. All other assumptions in the primary analysis remain constant. Column and row totals may not be exact owing to independent rounding.

[a] Phased-in estimates assume full implementation of the proposed revisions in state agencies serving one-third of all WIC participants as of April 1, 2018. All other state agencies are assumed to implement the proposed revisions as of FY2020.

[b] Describes the increases or savings of the base assumption or alternative as compared to the current food packages. Negative values (–) indicate that the base assumption or alternative costs less than the current food packages. Positive values (+) indicate that the base assumption or alternative costs more than the current food packages.

[c] Describes the increases or savings of the base assumption as compared to the alternative. Negative values (–) indicate that the base assumption costs less (provides more savings) than the uncertainty assumption. Positive values (+) indicate that the base assumption costs more than the uncertainty scenario.

Separate Vouchers for Vegetables and Fruits

Analyses presented in the DGA indicate that vegetable consumption across all age groups (ages 2 years and older) and fruit consumption among adolescents and adults do not currently meet the recommended intake ranges. The committee responded to these data by increasing the CVVs across all children's and women's food packages, and providing options for substituting food package items for a CVV. Given the shortfall in vegetable intake, in particular, the committee considered splitting the benefit into a vegetable CVV and a fruit CVV. Such a benefit would require state and local agencies to develop participant materials communicating why and how the benefits differ. Although this would create an opportunity to separately adjust vegetable and fruit prescriptions and encourage recipients to buy both vegetables and fruits, implementation would be challenging. USDA-FNS would need to provide state agencies with clear guidance on what items would qualify as a vegetable and which would qualify as a fruit. Vendors, particularly small vendors, would need clear guidance on how to implement such a classification into their systems. While these challenges are not insurmountable, the committee considered the simplicity of the

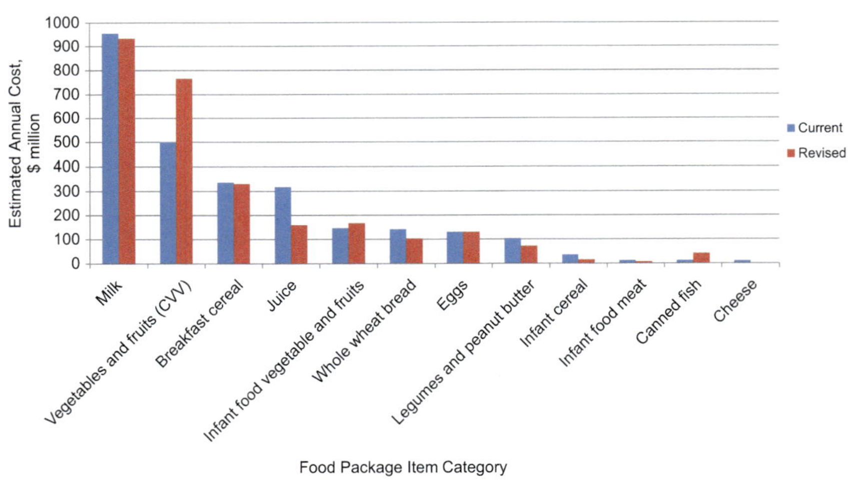

FIGURE U-1 Estimated annual cost of food package item categories, current and revised food packages, FY2015.
NOTES: The food package item categories encompass substitutions and allowable options. Estimates for the revised food packages include the 5 percent participant shift from the fully formula-fed mother–infant dyads to partially (mostly) breastfeeding food packages. Vegetables and fruits (CVV) estimates for the current food packages use $11 for all women's food packages. CVV = cash value voucher.

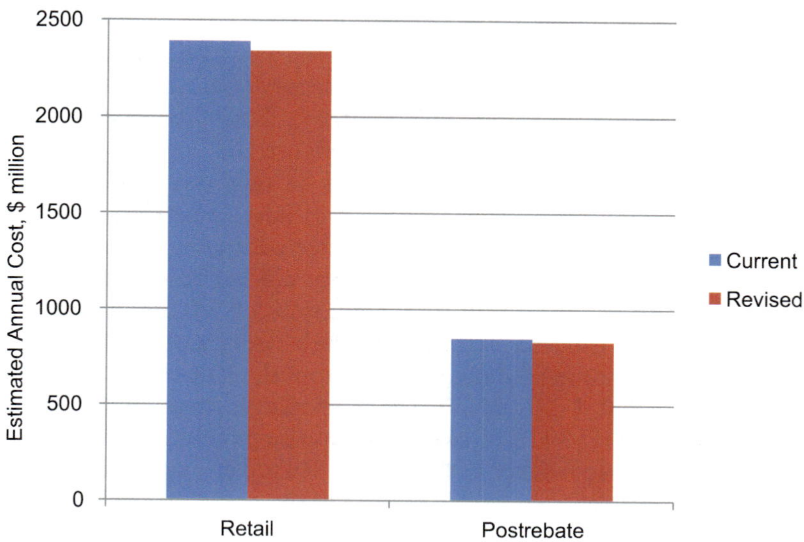

FIGURE U-2 Estimated annual cost of infant formula, current and revised food packages, FY2015.
NOTES: Estimates for the revised food packages include the 5 percent participant shift from the fully formula-fed mother–infant dyads to partially (mostly) breastfeeding food packages.

single CVV more favorable in the proposed revised food packages at this time.

MARKET ANALYSIS

The food package revisions will result in changes in the quantities and types of foods that WIC participants buy with their WIC food benefit. While the market effects of the changes are difficult to accurately quantify, the committee expects them to be minor.

Based on the assumptions in the primary analysis, the committee estimated the total value of WIC sales for each food item using the quantities in the current and revised food packages for FY2015.[21] Figure U-1 shows the estimated sales for each category prescribed in the current food packages

[21] To reflect current regulations, women's CVV in this portion of the analysis is $11 for the current food package. The committee acknowledges that this inflation-based increase in CVV was not effective until FY2016. Using a $10 CVV for women in this portion of the analysis would result in the estimated annual cost of fruits and vegetables to be approximately $483 million for the current food package.

side-by-side with estimates for the revised package. Each food item represents the food item category, which encompasses assumptions about substitutions and allowable options within that category (e.g., yogurt and cheese substitution are included in the milk category). Estimated sales of infant formula using retail prices are presented in Figure U-2.

Changes in total sales are estimated to be relatively small for most food categories, with the possible exception of juice, vegetables and fruits, and milk. However, WIC sales of each of these categories are a small portion of the total retail market. The committee did not have access to data that would enable an estimate of total retail sales of WIC food categories. Instead, the analysis is based on the committee's assessment of likely market effects using aggregate retail data available from the RIA conducted for the Interim Rule (7 C.F.R. § 246, 2007). The estimates presented in that RIA are summarized in Table U-30. WIC sales of juice were estimated to be 2 percent of the total retail juice market in the Interim Rule. WIC sales of vegetables and fruits were estimated to be 2.7 percent of the retail vegetable and fruit market. In the interim rule, sales of milk were estimated to be 4.4 percent of the retail milk market, and cheese sales were estimated to be 2 percent of the retail cheese market. While it is difficult to accurately gauge how sales of any individual product within that composite will be affected, data for the dairy products examined in the Interim Rule suggest that effects of the

TABLE U-30 Estimated Percent of the Market Attributed to WIC Sales, as Presented in the Interim Rule Regulatory Impact Analysis

	Estimated WIC Percent of the Market of the Interim Rule Food Packages Calendar Year 2005	
WIC Food Item	Assuming No Substitutions	Assuming Full Substitution
Formula	65.5	56.3
Beans	8.9	9.5
Peanut butter	4.8	4.8
Milk	4.5	4.4
Adult cereal	4.1	4.1
Juice	2.0	2.0
Vegetables and fruits	2.7	2.7
Eggs	2.3	2.3
Cheese	2.0	2.0
Bread	0.5	0.6
Canned fish	0.6	0.6

SOURCE: 7 C.F.R. § 246, 2007.

proposed revisions will be small. The categories estimated to experience the largest changes in sales under the revised packages represent small shares of their respective total retail markets, and the committee expects minimal market effects as a consequence of the revision to the food package.

REFERENCES

AAP (American Academy of Pediatrics). 2014. *Pediatric nutrition.* 7th ed. Edited by R. E. Kleinman and F. R. Greer. Elk Grove Village, IL: American Academy of Pediatrics.

AHA (American Heart Association). 2015. *Fish and omega-3 fatty acids.* http://www.heart.org/HEARTORG/HealthyLiving/HealthyEating/HealthyDietGoals/Fish-and-Omega-3-Fatty-Acids_UCM_303248_Article.jsp (accessed August 30, 2016).

BLS (U.S. Bureau of Labor Statistics). 2013. *The U.S. economy to 2022: Settling into a new normal.* http://www.bls.gov/opub/mlr/2013/article/the-u-s-economy-to-2022-settling-into-a-new-normal-16.htm (accessed October 3, 2016).

CBO (U.S. Congressional Budget Office). 2015. *Supplemental Nutrition Assistance Program —CBO's March 2015 baseline.* https://www.cbo.gov/sites/default/files/51312-2015-03-SNAP.pdf (accessed October 3, 2016).

CDC (U.S. Centers for Disease Control and Prevention). 2015. *National vital statistics system: Birth data.* http://www.cdc.gov/nchs/births.htm (accessed December 21, 2016).

DHS (U.S. Department of Homeland Security). 2014. *2013 yearbook of immigration statistics.* http://www.dhs.gov/publication/yearbook-2013 (accessed December 21, 2016).

FDA/EPA (U.S. Food and Drug Administration/Environmental Protection Agency). 2014. Fish: What pregnant women and parents should know. Silver Spring, MD: U.S. Food and Drug Administration. http://www.fda.gov/downloads/Food/FoodborneIllnessContaminants/Metals/UCM400358.pdf (accessed December 21, 2016).

HHS (U.S. Department of Health and Human Services). 2015. *Healthy People 2020: Maternal, infant, and child health objectives.* https://www.healthypeople.gov/2020/topics-objectives/topic/maternal-infant-and-child-health/objectives (accessed December 21, 2016).

IOM (Institute of Medicine). 2006. *WIC food packages: Time for a change.* Washington, DC: The National Academies Press.

NWA (National WIC Association). 2013. *The role of WIC in public health.* https://s3.amazonaws.com/aws.upl/nwica.org/WIC_Public_Health_Role.pdf (accessed December 21, 2016).

Oldways Whole Grain Council. 2015. *Whole grain statistics.* http://wholegrainscouncil.org/newsroom/whole-grain-statistics (accessed December 21, 2016).

USDA/ERS (U.S. Department of Agriculture/Economic Research Service). 2004. *WIC and the retail price of infant formula.* http://www.ers.usda.gov/media/330246/fanrr39-1_1_.pdf (accessed October 3, 2016).

USDA/ERS. 2005. *Interstate variation in WIC food package costs: The role of food prices, caseload composition, and cost-containment practices.* https://www.ers.usda.gov/publications/pub-details/?pubid=46844 (accessed March 26, 2017).

USDA/ERS. 2014. *Transition to EBT in WIC: Review of impact and examination of participant redemption patterns: Final report.* http://altarum.org/sites/default/files/uploaded-publication-files/Altarum_Transition%20to%20WIC%20EBT_Final%20Report_071614.pdf (accessed December 21, 2016).

USDA/ERS. 2016. *Food price outlook—Consumer Price Index, changes in food price indexes, 2014 through 2017.* http://www.ers.usda.gov/data-products/food-price-outlook.aspx (October 3, 2016).

USDA/FNS (U.S. Department of Agriculture/Food and Nutrition Service). 2006. *Special Supplemental Nutrition Program for Women, Infants and Children (WIC): Revisions in the WIC food packages*. Proposed Rule, 7 C.F.R. § 246.

USDA/FNS. 2007a. *Special Supplemental Nutrition Program for Women, Infants and Children (WIC): Revisions in the WIC food packages*. Interim Rule, 7 C.F.R. § 246.

USDA/FNS. 2007b. *Special Supplemental Nutrition Program for Women, Infants and Children (WIC): Revisions in the WIC food packages; additional data for RIA*. http://www.fns.usda.gov/sites/default/files/WICfoodpkg-additionaldataforRIA.pdf (accessed October 3, 2016).

USDA/FNS. 2007c. *WIC participant and program characteristics 2006*. http://www.fns.usda.gov/sites/default/files/pc2006.pdf (accessed December 21, 2016).

USDA/FNS. 2011. *Evaluation of the birth month breastfeeding changes to the WIC food packages*. http://www.fns.usda.gov/sites/default/files/BirthMonth.pdf (accessed December 21, 2016).

USDA/FNS. 2012. *Special Supplemental Nutrition Program for Women, Infants, and Children (WIC) Erroneous Payments to Vendors: Annual Estimates for FY 2011*. http://www.fns.usda.gov/sites/default/files/WICErroneousPayment_2011.pdf (accessed October 3, 2016).

USDA/FNS. 2013a. *Breastfeeding promotion in WIC: Current federal requirements*. http://www.fns.usda.gov/wic/breastfeeding-promotion-wic-current-federal-requirements (accessed October 3, 2016).

USDA/FNS. 2013b. *Fiscal year 2010 WIC food cost report*. http://www.fns.usda.gov/sites/default/files/WICFoodCost2010_0.pdf (accessed October 3, 2016).

USDA/FNS. 2014a. *WIC food packages Final Rule - Regulatory impact analysis (RIA)*. https://www.regulations.gov/document?D=FNS-2006-0037-2586 (accessed October 3, 2016).

USDA/FNS. 2014b. *Special Supplemental Nutrition Program for Women, Infants, and Children (WIC): Revisions in the WIC food packages*. Final Rule, 7 C.F.R. § 246.

USDA/FNS. 2014c. *Whole grain resource for the national school lunch and school breakfast programs: A guide to meeting the whole grain-rich criteria*. http://www.fns.usda.gov/sites/default/files/WholeGrainResource.pdf (accessed October 3, 2016).

USDA/FNS. 2015a. *About WIC—WIC at a glance*. http://www.fns.usda.gov/wic/about-wic-wic-glance (accessed December 21, 2016).

USDA/FNS. 2015b. *WIC food packages policy options II, final report*. http://www.fns.usda.gov/wic-food-package-policy-options-ii (accessed December 21, 2016).

USDA/FNS. 2016a. *WIC participant and program characteristics 2014: Food package report*. http://www.fns.usda.gov/wic-participant-and-program-characteristics-2014-food-package-report (accessed August 30, 2016).

USDA/FNS. 2016b. *Monthly data—state-level participation by category and program costs*. http://www.fns.usda.gov/pd/wic-program (accessed October 3, 2016).

USDA/FNS. 2016c. *August 2016 EBT detail status report*. http://www.fns.usda.gov/sites/default/files/wic/August2016EBTDetailStatusReport.pdf (accessed October 3, 2016).

USDA/FNS. 2016d. *Breastfeeding policy and guidance*. http://www.fns.usda.gov/sites/default/files/wic/WIC-Breastfeeding-Policy-and-Guidance.pdf (accessed October 3, 2016).

USDA/HHS (U.S. Department of Agriculture/U.S. Department of Health and Human Services). 2016. *Dietary Guidelines for Americans 2015–2020*. https://health.gov/dietaryguidelines/2015 (accessed August 29, 2016).

Appendix V

Committee Biosketches

Kathleen M. Rasmussen, Sc.D., R.D. (*Chair*), is the Nancy Schlegel Meinig Professor of Maternal and Child Nutrition, Division of Nutritional Sciences, at Cornell University. Dr. Rasmussen is internationally known for her research on maternal and child nutrition, particularly in the areas of pregnancy and lactation. She has served as program director for Cornell's National Institutes of Health (NIH)–sponsored training grant in maternal and child nutrition since 1986 and has also directed a training grant in international maternal and child nutrition. Dr. Rasmussen has taught a nationally recognized course in maternal and child nutrition for graduate students since 1980 and has taught a unique course on public health nutrition for undergraduate students since 1998. As part of her commitment to mentoring future leaders in nutrition, Dr. Rasmussen serves as the principal faculty member at the Dannon Nutrition Leadership Institute, which she helped to develop in 1998. She has received the Excellence in Nutrition Education Award and also the Mentorship Award from the American Society for Nutrition. The American Public Health Association honored her for her research accomplishments with their Agnes Higgins Award in 2012. Dr. Rasmussen has served as president of the American Society of Nutritional Sciences and also as president of the International Society for Research on Human Milk and Lactation. She has been associate dean and secretary of the university faculty and served a 4-year term on Cornell's Board of Trustees as one of its faculty-elected members. Dr. Rasmussen has been a member of several expert committees at the National Academies of Sciences, Engineering, and Medicine, including the Committee on Scientific Evaluation of the Special Supplemental Nutrition Program Women, Infant, and Children

Nutrition Risk Criteria. Recently, she served as the chair of the Committee on Reexamination of Institute of Medicine Pregnancy Weight Guidelines and then as chair of a committee to disseminate these new guidelines. She received her A.B. degree from Brown University in molecular biology and both her Sc.M. and Sc.D, degrees from Harvard University in nutrition.

Shannon E. Whaley, Ph.D. (*Vice Chair*), is the Director of Research and Evaluation for Public Health Foundation Enterprises (PHFE) Women, Infant, and Children Program (WIC), the largest local agency WIC program in the nation. In her 16 years of experience on the front lines of WIC, Dr. Whaley has become an expert in understanding both how the program functions and how it can be maximally effective in achieving positive health outcomes for the families WIC serves. Dr. Whaley's expertise is in the planning, development, and evaluation of programs designed to optimize the healthy development of children and families served by WIC. Her work spans a broad range of topics including childhood nutrition and obesity, prevention of prenatal alcohol use, promotion of early literacy for low-income children, and examination of the impact of the recent WIC food package change on WIC participants. Dr. Whaley's work includes controlled research studies as well as implementation of community-based interventions using evidenced-based practices. In her role at PHFE WIC, Dr. Whaley has been successful in supporting her work with public and private grants that support research endeavors as well as enhance core WIC services. She supervises graduate students from local universities and has mentored a postdoctoral researcher who recently moved on to a full-time academic position. Dr. Whaley also serves as Chair of the Evaluation Committee of the National WIC Association and in this role works closely with other WIC programs to advance the national WIC research agenda. Dr. Whaley received her undergraduate degree in psychology from Pomona College, and her Ph.D. in developmental psychology from University of California, Los Angeles.

Susan S. Baker, M.D., Ph.D., is professor, Department of Pediatrics, professor and co-chief, Digestive Diseases and Nutrition Center, University of Buffalo School of Medicine. She also serves as the laboratory director for the Gastroenterology Laboratory at Women and Children's Hospital of Buffalo. Dr. Baker is the program director for the Pediatric Gastrointestinal Fellowship program. Her research focus is on liver (hepatology), nutrition, pediatric gastroenterology, and pediatrics. Dr. Baker worked in Africa and established two new programs in Gastroenterology and Nutrition at the University of Massachusetts Medical Center and the Medical University of South Carolina before moving to Buffalo. She has published many peer-reviewed articles, chapters, reviews, as well as having edited four medical textbooks and one nonmedical book. Dr. Baker is recognized as a leader in the field, having served as the chairperson of the American Academy of Pediatrics Committee on Nutrition, the chairperson of the American Board of Pediatrics, subboard of Gastroenterology, and numerous other national and international advisory groups including the National Academies of Sciences, Engineering, and Medicine, U.S. Department of Agriculture, and the U.S. Food and Drug Administration representative to the CODEX expert committee on infant formula. Dr. Baker received her M.D. from Temple University School of Medicine and her Ph.D. from Massachusetts Institute of Technology.

Marianne P. Bitler, Ph.D., is professor of economics in the Department of Economics at the University of California, Davis, and a faculty research associate at the National Bureau of Economic Research, in the programs on Children and Health Economics. Dr. Bitler is also a visiting scholar at the San Francisco Federal Reserve Bank; and a research fellow at the Institute for the Study of Labor in Bonn, Germany. Previously, she was a professor of economics at the University of California, Irvine, a postdoctoral fellow and then an economist at the RAND Corporation, a research fellow at the Public Policy Institute of California, and an economist on the Board of Governors of the Federal Reserve in the Division of Research and Statistics (where she worked on the Survey of Small Business Finances). Her research interests include labor economics, health economics, public economics, and applied microeconomics. Her publications include several on participation in and effects of the Special Supplemental Nutrition Program for Women, Infants, and Children (WIC) program, which appeared in the *Journal of Human Resources*, the *Review of Agricultural Economics*, and the *Journal of Policy Analysis and Management*. Dr. Bitler has a B.S. degree in mathematics from The Pennsylvania State University, and a Ph.D. in economics from the Massachusetts Institute of Technology.

Patsy M. Brannon, Ph.D., R.D., is professor, Division of Nutritional Sciences, Cornell University, where she has also served as dean of the College of Human Ecology. Prior to moving to Cornell University, Dr. Brannon was chair, Department of Nutrition and Food Science, University of Maryland. She has also served as visiting professor, Office of Dietary Supplements, National Institutes of Health. Her research focus includes nutritional and metabolic regulation of gene expression, especially as relating to human development, the placenta, and exocrine pancreas. She was a member of the Committee on Dietary Reference Intakes for Vitamin D and Calcium, and she is currently a member of the Food and Nutrition Board. Dr. Brannon is a member of a number of professional and scientific associations and has served on the Executive Board of the American Society for Nutrition.

She has received numerous awards, including the Pew Faculty Scholar in Nutrition award as well as the Centennial Laureate award from Florida State University. Dr. Brannon received her Ph.D. from Cornell University in nutritional biochemistry.

Alicia L. Carriquiry, Ph.D., M.Sc., is a distinguished professor of liberal arts and sciences and professor of statistics at Iowa State University. Dr. Carriquiry research interests include Bayesian statistics and general methods. Her recent work focuses on nutrition and dietary assessment, as well as on problems in genomics, forensic sciences, and traffic safety. Dr. Carriquiry is an elected member of the International Statistical Institute and a fellow of the American Statistical Association and of the Institute of Mathematical Statistics. She has served on the executive committees of the Institute of Mathematical Statistics, the American Statistical Association, and of the International Society for Bayesian Analysis, and she has served on the Council of the International Statistical Institute. She has served on several committees of the National Academies of Sciences, Engineering, and Medicine and was elected a member of the National Academy of Medicine in 2016. Dr. Carriquiry received an M.Sc. in animal science from the University of Illinois, and an M.Sc. in statistics and a Ph.D. in statistics and animal science from Iowa State University.

David E. Davis, Ph.D., is an associate professor in the Department of Economics at South Dakota State University. Dr. Davis studies industrial organization, currently focusing on the effects of food assistance programs on market interactions. Dr. Davis previously held a position with the Economic Research Service of the U.S. Department of Agriculture, where he studied food markets. He has researched the Special Supplemental Nutrition Program for Women, Infants, and Children (WIC) and infant formula markets, and analyzed the effects of WIC cost-containment practices for creating interstate variation in WIC food package costs. He has expertise in empirical microeconometrics: applications of panel data methods to empirical investigations of industrial organization and market power. Dr. Davis received his Ph.D. from the University of Oregon in economics.

Mary Kay Fox, M.Ed., is senior fellow and area leader for nutrition policy research at Mathematica Policy Research. Ms. Fox has more than 25 years of research experience with child nutrition and food assistance programs. She has conducted research on the adequacy and quality of diets consumed by children, from birth through adolescence, and has examined the contributions of school- and child care–based meal programs to children's dietary intakes and obesity risk. She was a co-principal investigator on the 2002 and 2008 Feeding Infants and Toddler Studies, which examined feeding practices and food and nutrient intakes among infants, toddlers, and preschoolers from birth to 48 months of age. Ms. Fox conducted a comprehensive review of research literature on the impacts of the Special Supplemental Nutrition Program for Women, Infants, and Children (WIC) program on health- and nutrition-related outcomes. She is currently directing the Food and Nutrition Service WIC-Medicaid II study, which is updating the landmark WIC-Medicaid study conducted in the early 1990s. Ms. Fox served on the Institute of Medicine Committee to Review Child and Adult Care Food Program Meal Requirements, as well as the Committee on Nutrition Standards for the National School Lunch and Breakfast Programs, and the Committee on the Consequences of Sodium Reduction in Populations. Ms. Fox has an M.Ed. in nutrition from Tufts University.

Tamera J. Hatfield, M.D., Ph.D., is a board-certified obstetrician-gynecologist specializing in maternal–fetal medicine at the University of California, Irvine. She treats high-risk pregnancy patients and has a particular interest in managing maternal conditions that complicate pregnancy. Dr. Hatfield's research interests include using magnetic resonance imaging (MRI) to evaluate brain injury as it relates to perinatal risk factors, weight gain during pregnancy among obese patients, and preeclampsia. She is involved with teaching residents, fellows, and medical students and previously served on the Council on Resident Education in Obstetrics and Gynecology. Dr. Hatfield received her M.D. from the University of California, Irvine, where she also completed a residency in obstetrics and gynecology and a fellowship in maternal–fetal medicine. In addition, she holds a Ph.D. in behavioral neuroscience from the University of North Carolina at Chapel Hill. She is a member of the Society for Maternal Fetal Medicine and the American College of Obstetricians and Gynecologists.

Helen H. Jensen, Ph.D., is professor of economics and leads a research group focused on food and nutrition programs in the Center for Agricultural and Rural Development of Iowa State University, an internationally recognized research center that addresses issues of the food, agricultural, and natural resource sectors. Her research interests include the design of food and nutrition programs and policies, assessment of nutritional enhancement of foods, food demand and markets, linkages between agricultural policies and nutrition, and food-safety regulations. She has led projects that analyze food demand, and that involve dietary, nutritional, and health assessment as well as the design and implementation food consumption surveys in the United States as well as in several developing countries. Dr. Jensen was elected Fellow of the Agricultural and Applied Economics Association (AAEA) in 2012 and completed a term on the AAEA Executive Board of Directors. She has served on several committees of the National Academies of Science, Engineering, and Medicine, including the Institute of Medicine (IOM) Committee on Child and Adult Care Food Program Meal, and the National Research Council (NRC) and IOM Committee on Risk-Characterization for Decision-Making at the U.S. Food and Drug Administration. She chaired the IOM and NRC's True Cost of Food Workshop planning committee and is a member of the Food Forum. Dr. Jensen holds a Ph.D. in agricultural economics from the University of Wisconsin.

Rachel K. Johnson, Ph.D., M.P.H., R.D., is the Robert L. Bickford, Jr., Professor of Nutrition and Professor of Medicine at the University of Vermont. Dr. Johnson served as Dean of the College of Agriculture and Life Sciences at the University of Vermont from 2001 to 2008 and as Associate Provost for Faculty Affairs from 2009 to 2011. Dr. Johnson's research expertise covers pediatric nutrition and obesity, dietary intake methodology, diet and cardiovascular disease, and national nutrition policy. She was appointed to the Year 2000 Dietary Guidelines Advisory Committee. She served on the Panel on Dietary Reference Intakes (DRIs) for the macronutrients for the Institute of Medicine. Dr. Johnson served on the President's Council on Fitness, Sports and Nutrition Science Board from 2011 to 2014 and was Chair of the American Heart Association Nutrition Committee from 2012 to 2014. Dr. Johnson holds a Ph.D. in Nutrition from the Pennsylvania State University, an M.P.H. from the University of Hawaii, and is a registered dietitian.

Angela Odoms-Young, Ph.D., is associate professor in the Department of Kinesiology and Nutrition at the University of Illinois at Chicago (UIC) College of Applied Health Sciences and an Institute of Health Research and Policy Fellow. Dr. Odoms-Young's research is focused on understanding social, cultural, and environmental determinants of dietary behaviors and diet-related diseases in low-income and minority populations. Her current projects include studies to evaluate the impact of the new WIC food package on dietary intake, weight status, and chronic disease risk in 2- to 3-year-old low-income children and vendor participation; identify strategies to improve program participation and retention among WIC-eligible children; evaluate the efficacy of a community-based participatory weight loss intervention in African American women; and examine community engagement approaches to promote food justice. Prior to joining UIC, Dr. Odoms-Young served on the faculty of Northern Illinois University in Public Health and Health Education. She completed a Family Research Consortium Postdoctoral Fellowship examining family processes in diverse populations at the Pennsylvania State University and the University of Illinois at Urbana-Champaign and a Community Health Scholars Fellowship in community-based participatory research at the University of Michigan School of Public Health. She received her M.S. in human nutrition and Ph.D. in community nutrition from Cornell University.

Rafael Pérez-Escamilla, Ph.D., is professor of Epidemiology and Public Health, and director of the Global Health Concentration and the Office of Public Health Practice at the Yale School of Public Health. His public health nutrition and food security research has led to improvements in breastfeeding protection, promotion and support programs and prevention of iron deficiency anemia among infants, as well as improvements in household food insecurity measurement and community nutrition programs worldwide. His health disparities research focuses on the impact of community health workers on improving behavioral and metabolic outcomes among Latinos with type 2 diabetes. He is a member of the National Academies of Sciences, Engineering, and Medicine's Food and Nutrition Board, and he served on the 2010 and 2015 U.S. Dietary Guidelines Advisory Committees. He chaired the Institute of Medicine (IOM) Planning Workshop Committee Updating the USDA National Breastfeeding Campaign and served on the Committee to Reexamine the IOM Pregnancy Weight Guidelines. He is past chair of the American Society for Nutrition's Global Nutrition Council and President of the International Society for Research in Human Milk and Lactation (ISRHML). He has served on the editorial boards of the *Journal of Nutrition*, the *Journal of Human Lactation, Global Food Security,* and the *Journal of Hunger and Environmental Nutrition*. He received a B.S. in chemical engineering from the Universidad Iberoamericana in Mexico City and an M.S. in food science and a Ph.D. in nutrition from the University of California, Davis.

A. Catharine Ross, Ph.D., is professor and occupant of the Dorothy Foehr Huck Chair of Nutrition in the Department of Nutritional Sciences at Pennsylvania State University. As a nutritional biochemist, Dr. Ross has studied cellular factors involved in the biosynthesis and transport of vitamin A molecules. Her focus has been on the cellular basis of vitamin A homeostasis. She also investigates the role of retinoids in immune function, principally antibody production, and in neonatal lung development. She served as editor-in-chief of the *Journal of Nutrition* from 2004 to 2013. Dr. Ross has received numerous awards, including the Mead-Johnson Award and the Osborne and Mendel Award from the American Society for Nutrition. She is active within a range of professional societies, including the American Association of Immunologists, Sigma Xi, and the American Physiological Society, and has served on a number of committees for the American Society for Nutrition and the Federation of the American Societies for Experimental Biology. Dr. Ross is a Fellow of the American Association for the Advancement of Science and a member of the National Academy of Medicine. She chaired the Committee on Dietary Reference Intakes for Vitamin D and Calcium and is a member of the Food and Nutrition Board. Dr. Ross received her Ph.D. from Cornell University in biochemistry and molecular and cell biology.

Charlene Russell-Tucker, M.S.M., R.D., is the chief operating officer (COO) for the Connecticut State Department of Education. As COO, Ms. Russell-Tucker leads priority project management functions to help improve the planning, efficiency, service, and delivery effectiveness of the department's programs and services. In addition to broad agency efforts, she also directly provides leadership and oversight to the department's Office of Student Supports and Organizational Effectiveness. Her prior position was associate commissioner for the Connecticut State Department of Education. In this role Ms. Russell-Tucker was responsible for the administration of the Division of Family and Student Support Services which comprises three bureaus: the Bureau of Choice Programs; the Bureau of Health/Nutrition, Family Services and Adult Education; and the Bureau of Special Education. She provides leadership and support in developing and implementing effective family and student support programs and services to assist schools and other educational partners in improving student performance. Prior to her appointment as Associate Commissioner, Ms. Russell-Tucker was chief of the Bureau of Health and Nutrition Services and Child/Family/School Partnerships at the Connecticut State Department of Education. The bureau was strategically positioned within the department to support the social, emotional, physical, and mental health of students and families in order to achieve success in school and in life. Its initiatives and services include school-family-community partnerships, child nutrition programs, school health promotion/mental health services/school nurses, nutrition education, safe and drug-free schools program, 21st century community learning centers/after-school programs, family resource centers, young parents program, and education of homeless children and youth. Ms. Russell-Tucker is past president of the Connecticut Dietetic Association and the Child and Adult Care Food Program National Professional Association. She is also an adjunct faculty member at a local college where she teaches business management courses in the program for nontraditional students. She received her M.S. in management from Albertus Magnus College in New Haven, Connecticut, and is a registered dietitian.

Index

A

C

F

G

H

J

M

N

O

P

S

T

U

V

W

Y

Z